ENDOCRINE SECRETS

Third Edition

ENDOCRINE SECRETS

Third Edition

MICHAEL T. McDERMOTT, M.D.

Professor of Medicine
Division of Endocrinology, Metabolism & Diabetes
University of Colorado School of Medicine
Denver, Colorado

HANLEY & BELFUS, INC./Philadelphia

Publisher: HANLEY & BELFUS, INC.
Medical Publishers
210 South 13th Street
Philadelphia, PA 19107
(215) 546-7293; 800-962-1892
FAX (215) 790-9330
Web site: http://www.hanleyandbelfus.com

Note to the reader: Although the information in this book has been carefully reviewed for correctness of dosage and indications, neither the authors nor the editor nor the publisher can accept any legal responsibility for any errors or omissions that may be made. Neither the publisher nor the editor makes any warranty, expressed or implied, with respect to the material contained herein. Before prescribing any drug, the reader must review the manufacturer's current product information (package inserts) for accepted indications, absolute dosage recommendations, and other information pertinent to the safe and effective use of the product described.

Library of Congress Cataloging-in-Publication Data

Endocrine secrets / edied by Michael T. McDermott.—3rd ed.
    p. ; cm—(The Secrets Series®)
  Includes index.
  ISBN 1-56053-449-4 (alk. paper)
    1. Endocrinology—Examinations, questions, etc. 2. Endocrine
glands—Diseases—Examinations, questions, etc. I. McDermott, Michael T., 1952-
II. Series.
  [DNLM: 1. Endocrine Diseases—physiopathology—Examination Questions.
WK 18.2 E56 2001]
RC649 .M36 2001
616.4'0076—dc21

                                       2001039197

ENDOCRINE SECRETS, 3rd edition   ISBN 1-56053-449-4

Last digit is the print number: 9 8 7 6 5 4 3 2 1

CONTENTS

VII. MISCELLANEOUS

CONTRIBUTORS

Arnold A. Asp, M.D., F.A.C.P.
Department of Clinical Investigation, Brooke Army Medical Center, Ft. Sam Houston, Texas

Jennifer A. Baquero, M.D.
Endocrinology- Metabolic Service, Walter Reed Army Medical Center, Washington, DC.

Linda A. Barbour, M.D., M.S.P.H.
Associate Professor of Medicine, Division of Endocrinology, Metabolism & Diabetes, Department of Medicine, University of Colorado School of Medicine, Denver, Colorado

Holly A. Batal, M.D.
Assistant Professor of Medicine, Department of Medicine, University of Colorado School of Medicine, Denver, Colorado

Brenda K. Bell, M.D.
Endocrinologist, private practice, Lincoln, Nebraska

Daniel H. Bessesen, M.D.
Associate Professor of Medicine, Division of Endocrinology, Metabolism & Diabetes, University of Colorado School of Medicine, Denver, Colorado

Tamis M. Bright, M.D.
Assistant Professor of Medicine, Assistant Medical Residency Program Director, and Chief, Division of Endocrinology, Department of Medicine, Texas Tech University School of Medicine, El Paso, Texas.

Henry B. Burch, M.D.
Associate Professor of Medicine, Department of Medicine, Uniformed Services University of the Health Sciences, Bethesda, Maryland, and Endocrine-Metabolic Service, Walter Reed Army Medical Center, Washington, DC.

Reed S. Christensen, M.D.
Staff Endocrinologist, Tripler Army Medical Center, Honolulu, Hawaii

Stephen Clement, M.D.
Associate Professor of Medicine, Division of Endocrinology, Georgetown University School of Medicine, and Director, Georgetown Diabetes Center, Washington, DC

William E. Duncan, M.D., Ph.D.
Associate Professor and Director, Division of Endocrinology, Uniformed Services University of the Health Sciences, Bethesda, Maryland, and Chief, Endocrinology, Diabetes and Metabolism Service, Walter Reed Army Medical Center, Washington, DC.

James E. Fitzpatrick, M.D.
Associate Professor, Department of Dermatology, University of Colorado School of Medicine, Denver, Colorado

Robert H. Gates, M.D.
Chief, Department of Medicine, Brooke Army Medical Center, Ft. Sam Houston, Texas

William J. Georgitis, M.D.
Clinical Professor of Medicine, Division of Endocrinology, Metabolism and Diabetes, University of Colorado School of Medicine, Denver, Colorado

Bryan R. Haugen, M.D.
Associate Professor of Medicine, Division of Endocrinology, Metabolism and Diabetes, University of Colorado School of Medicine, Denver, Colorado

James V. Hennessey, M.D.
Associate Professor of Medicine, Division of Endocrinology, Brown University School of Medicine, Providence, Rhode Island

Fred D. Hofeldt, M.D.
Clinical Professor of Medicine, Division of Endocrinology, Metabolism and Diabetes, University of Colorado School of Medicine, Denver, Colorado

Robert E. Jones, M.D.
Associate Professor of Medicine, Division of Endocrinology, Metabolism and Diabetes, Department of Internal Medicine, University of Utah School of Medicine, Salt Lake City, Utah

Wendy M. Kohrt, Ph. D.
Professor of Medicine, Division of Geriatric Medicine, University of Colorado School of Medicine, Denver, Colorado

Homer J. LeMar, Jr., M.D.
Chief, Department of Medicine, William Beaumont Army Medical Center, El Paso, Texas

Elliot G. Levy, M.D.
Clinical Professor of Medicine, University of Miami School of Medicine, and Endocrinologist in private practice, Miami, Florida

Michael T. McDermott, M.D.
Professor of Medicine, Division of Endocrinology, Metabolism & Diabetes, University of Colorado School of Medicine, Denver, Colorado

Robert C. McIntyre, M.D.
Assistant Professor of Surgery, Department of Surgery, University of Colorado School of Medicine, Denver, Colorado

Christopher D. Raeburn M.D.
Department of Surgery, University of Colorado School of Medicine, Denver, Colorado

Robbie J. Rampy, M.D.
Department of Medicine, William Beaumont Army Medical Center, El Paso, Texas

Jane E.-B. Reusch, M.D.
Associate Professor of Medicine, Division of Endocrinology, Metabolism & Diabetes, University of Colorado School of Medicine, and Research Associate, Veterans Affairs Medical Center, Denver, Colorado

Terri Ryan-Turek, R.D., C.D.E.
Diabetes Educator and Dietician, Endocrinology, Metabolism and Diabetes Practice, University of Colorado Hospital, Denver, Colorado

Mary H. Samuels, M.D.
Associate Professor of Medicine, Division of Endocrinology, Diabetes and Clinical Nutrition, Oregon Health Sciences University, Portland, Oregon

Leonard R. Sanders, M.D., F.A.C.P.
Chairman, Division of Nephrology, Staff Endocrinologist, Lovelace Health Systems, Albuquerque, New Mexico

Virginia Sarapura, M.D.
Associate Professor of Medicine, Division of Endocrinology, Metabolism & Diabetes, University of Colorado School of Medicine, Denver, Colorado

Robert S. Schwartz, M. D.
Professor of Medicine, Head, Division of Geriatric Medicine, University of Colorado School of Medicine, Denver, Colorado

Kenneth J. Simcic, M.D.
Associate Professor of Medicine, University of Texas School of Medicine, San Antonio, and Brooke Army Medical Center, Ft. Sam Houston, Texas

Robert H. Slover, M.D.
Assistant Professor of Pediatrics, Pediatric Endocrinology, University of Colorado School of Medicine

Robert C. Smallridge, M.D.
Professor of Medicine, Mayo Medical School, and Chair, Endocrinology Division, Mayo Clinic, Jacksonville, Florida

Rodney J. Sparks, M.D.
Department of Medicine, William Beaumont Army Medical Center, El Paso, Texas

Elizabeth Stephens, M.D.
Assistant Professor of Medicine, Division of Endocrinology, Diabetes and Clinical Nutrition, Oregon Health Sciences University, Portland, Oregon

Derek J. Stocker, M.D.
Endocrine-Metabolic Service, Walter Reed Army Medical Center, Washington, DC.

Sharon Travers, M.D.
Assistant Professor of Pediatrics, Pediatric Endocrinology, University of Colorado School of Medicine

Robert A. Vigersky, M.D.
Associate Professor of Medicine, Department of Medicine, Uniformed Services University of the Health Sciences, Bethesda, Maryland, and Endocrine-Metabolic Service, Walter Reed Army Medical Center, Washington, DC.

Margaret E. Wierman, M.D.
Associate Professor of Medicine, Division of Endocrinology, Metabolism & Diabetes, and Chief, Division of Endocrinology, Veterans Affairs Medical Center, Denver, Colorado

Susan T. Wingo, M.D.
Instructor of Medicine, Department of Medicine, Uniformed Services University of the Health Sciences, Bethesda, Maryland, and William Beaumont Army Medical Center, El Paso, Texas

Philip S. Zeitler, M.D.
Assistant Professor of Pediatrics, Pediatric Endocrinology, University of Colorado School of Medicine

Sharon Zemel, M.D.
Assistant Professor of Pediatrics, Pediatric Endocrinology, University of Colorado School of Medicine

PREFACE TO THE THIRD EDITION

It is a great privilege to be entrusted with the health care of a fellow human being. No less of a privilege is the training of new generations of care providers to continue the important work of health care. I again wish to express my sincere gratitude to the authors who have so generously contributed their time and talents to this book. In doing so, they will help many more patients than they will ever see. And finally, I urge our students to be lifelong learners for, as physicians, this is a fundamental need and a solemn responsibility.

Michael T. McDermott, M.D.

DEDICATION OF THIRD EDITION

I dedicate this book to my mother, Chloe, and my father, Gene, both of whom left this life far too soon, and to my wonderful wife, Libby, and my children, Jenny, Mac, Andi and Megan.

I. Fuel Metabolism

1. DIABETES MELLITUS

Stephen Clement, M.D.

1. What is diabetes mellitus?

A chronic disorder characterized by the abnormal metabolism of fuels, particularly glucose and fat. By tradition, the diagnosis of diabetes rests on the demonstration of an abnormality in glucose tolerance. The array of entities called diabetes mellitus is linked by the common abnormality of glucose intolerance and the potential for developing complications from altered glucose and lipid metabolism.

Types of Diabetes Mellitus and Other Categories of Glucose Intolerance

CLINICAL CLASSES	DISTINGUISHING CHARACTERISTICS
Type 1 diabetes mellitus (formerly called insulin-dependent diabetes)	Beta cell destruction, usually leading to absolute insulin deficiency. Beta cell loss may be immune mediated or idiopathic. Patients may be any age and are usually non-obese. All patients eventually require insulin for glucose control and survival. This requirement may occur rapidly, as in children or young adults, or slowly as in older adults. Patients are prone to ketoacidosis.
Type 2 diabetes mellitus (formerly called non–insulin-dependent diabetes)	Patients have both insulin resistance and relative insulin deficiency. Often associated with obesity or an increase in visceral (truncal) fat. Ketoacidosis seldom occurs spontaneously but may occur with stress. Patients often can be treated without insulin.
Other types of diabetes	Associated with specific conditions and syndromes (see next table).
Impaired glucose homeostasis	Stages of impaired glucose metabolism that are abnormal but do not meet the criteria for diabetes mellitus or impaired fasting glucose.
Gestational diabetes	Any degree of glucose intolerance with onset or first recognition during pregnancy.

Adapted from American Diabetes Association: Report of the Expert Committee on the Diagnosis and Classification of Diabetes Mellitus. Diabetes Care 20:1183–1196, 1997.

Other Types of Diabetes Mellitus and Impaired Glucose Tolerance

Secondary to:	Examples:
Pancreatic disease	Pancreatectomy, hemochromatosis, cystic fibrosis, chronic pancreatitis
Endocrinopathies	Acromegaly, pheochromocytoma, Cushing's syndrome, primary aldosteronism, glucagonoma
Drugs and chemical	Certain antihypertensive drugs, thiazide diuretics, glucocorticoids, estrogen-containing preparations, psychoactive agents, catecholamines, pentamidine, and anti-HIV medications
Associated with:	Examples:
Insulin-receptor abnormalities	Acanthosis nigricans
Genetic syndromes	Hyperlipidemia, muscular dystrophies, Huntington's chorea
Miscellaneous conditions	Malnutrition ("tropical diabetes")

For a more complete list, see American Diabetes Association: Report of the Expert Committee on the Diagnosis and Classification of Diabetes. Diabetes Care 20:1183–1196, 1997.

2. Describe how diabetes is diagnosed.

The criteria for diagnosing diabetes were updated in 1997 to make screening easier. It is important to perform the fasting glucose test in the morning (i.e, before 9 A.M.), since the glucose level drops after this time and may give a false negative reading.

Diagnosis of Diabetes

	TEST		
STAGE	FASTING PLASMA GLUCOSE (FPG)*	CASUAL PLASMA GLUCOSE	ORAL GLUCOSE TOLERANCE TEST (OGTT)
Diabetes	FPG ≥ 126 mg/dL (7.0 mmol/L)†	Casual plasma glucose ≥ 200 mg/dL (11.1 mmol/L) plus symptoms‡	Two-hour plasma glucose (2hPG) ≥ 200 mg/dL§
Impaired glucose homeostasis	Impaired fasting glucose = FPG ≥ 110 and < 126 mg/dL		Impaired glucose tolerance = 2hPG ≥ 140 and < 200 mg/dL
Normal	FPG < 110 mg/dL		2hPG < 140 mg/dL

*The morning FPG is the preferred test for diagnosis, but any one of the three is acceptable. In the absence of unequivocal hyperglycemia with acute metabolic decompensation, one of the three tests should be repeated on a different day to confirm the diagnosis.
†Fasting is defined as no caloric intake for at least 8 hr.
‡ Casual = any time of day without regard to time since last meal; classic symptoms are polyuria, polydipsia, and unexplained weight loss.
§OGTT should be performed using a glucose load containing the equivalent of 75 g anhydrous glucose dissolved in water. The OGTT is not recommended for routine clinical use.

3. What is the prevalence of diabetes?

An estimated 16 million Americans, or 5.9% of the population, have diabetes. Approximately 1 million have type 1 diabetes and 15 million have type 2 diabetes. An estimated 5.4 million Americans have type 2 diabetes and are unaware of it. The prevalence of type 2 diabetes is increasing dramatically in the U.S. and worldwide as populations become more sedentary and obese.

4. Should presumably healthy people be screened for diabetes?

Yes. Undiagnosed type 2 diabetes is common in the United States. Often the early symptoms of increased thirst, fatigue, and increased urination are ignored and do not prompt the person to seek medical attention. For this reason, many people with diabetes have the disease for several years before detection, thus increasing the risk for long-term complications.

Criteria for Testing for Diabetes in Asymptomatic, Undiagnosed People*

Persons without risk factors for diabetes should be tested at age 45 yr and retested at 3-yr intervals
Testing should be considered at a younger age or carried out more frequently in people who
- Are obese (body mass index ≥27 kg/m^2)
- Have a family history of diabetes
- Are members of a high-risk ethnic population (e.g., African-American, Hispanic, Native American)
- Have delivered a baby weighing 9 lb or have been diagnosed with gestational diabetes
- Are sedentary
- Have a history of polycystic ovarian syndrome
- Have hypertension or dyslipidemia
- On previous testing had impaired glucose tolerance or impaired fasting glucose (IFG)

*The OGTT or FPG test may be used to diagnose diabetes; however, in clinical settings the morning FPG test is greatly preferred because of ease of administration, convenience, acceptability to patients, and lower cost.
From American Diabetes Association: Screening for Diabetes. Diabetes Care 24:S21–24, 2001.

5. Describe the effect of genetics on type 1 diabetes.

The interplay between genetics and environment in diabetes is complex and still not well understood. Monozygotic twins have a 20–50% concordance for type 1 diabetes. The cumulative risk for siblings of diabetic patients is 6–10% vs. 0.6% for the general population. Regarding the effect of parental genes, the offspring of women with type 1 diabetes have a lower risk of disease (2.1%) than the offspring of men with type 1 diabetes (6.1%). The reason for this disparity is unknown. The susceptibility for type 1 diabetes is associated with the genetic expression of certain proteins coded by the HLA region of the major histocompatibility complex. These proteins are present on the surface of lymphocytes and macrophages and are considered essential for triggering the autoimmune destruction of the beta cells. Although all of the genetic markers (HLA and others) for type 1 diabetes are not known, future progress in this field will allow population screening for genetic susceptibility.

6. What is the role of genetics in the development of type 2 diabetes?

The familial clustering of type 2 diabetes suggests a strong genetic component to the disease. Monozygotic twins have a 60–90% concordance for type 2 diabetes. The cumulative risk for type 2 diabetes in siblings of diabetic patients is 10–33% vs. 5% for the general population. Offspring of women with type 2 diabetes have a twofold to threefold greater risk for developing diabetes than do offspring of men with the disease. The exact mode of inheritance for type 2 diabetes is not known but is thought to be polygenic. Specific mutations that are associated with risk for type 2 diabetes have been identified, but many of these genes are widely found in the population at large. Because type 2 diabetes is so commonly associated with obesity, many investigators suspect that genes which predispose to obesity are associated with type 2 diabetes as well. There appears to be a strong interplay between genetic and environmental influences for causing type 2 diabetes. One illustration of this is the demonstration of higher fasting insulin levels for every weight category in offspring of two parents with type 2 diabetes compared with controls. High insulin levels are a marker for insulin resistance and are predictive of progression to type 2 diabetes.

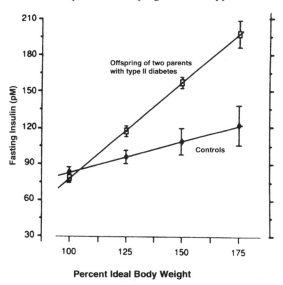

Fasting insulin levels in offspring of two parents with type 2 diabetes according to weight category. (From Warram JH, Martin BC, Krolewski AS, et al: Slow glucose removal rate and hyperinsulinemia precede the development of type 2 diabetes in the offspring of diabetic parents. Ann Intern Med 113:909–915, 1990, with permission.)

7. Discuss the pathogenesis of type 1 diabetes.

For type 1 diabetes, the primary pathogenic step is the activation of host T-lymphocytes against specific antigens present on the patient's own beta cells. These activated T-cells orchestrate a slow destruction of the beta cells via the recruitment of T- and B-lymphocytes, macrophages, and cytokines. Morphologic study of the pancreases of children who died at the onset of diabetes have shown an inflammatory infiltrate of mononuclear cells confined to the islets—called **insulitis.** The final result is total destruction of the beta cells over a span of years. The finding of high-titer islet-cell antibodies (ICAs) in the serum of a child is highly predictive for progression to type 1 diabetes.

Various antigens that are expressed by the beta cell have been implicated as the target for the autoimmune attack. Candidate antigens include insulin itself and a 64-kilodalton protein (now recognized as glutamic acid decarboxylase [GAD]). The triggering event for T-cell activation against these autoantigens is unknown but may involve the exposure to some environmental substance that is antigenically similar to the autoantigen. The T-cells that are activated against this environmental antigen can then cross-react with the antigen on the beta cells—a process called **molecular mimicry**. Suspected environmental triggers for type 1 diabetes are viruses, toxins, and foods. For example, exposure to cow's milk in the first 6 weeks of life has been implicated in the development of type 1 diabetes in genetically susceptible children. Viruses may trigger type 1 diabetes via molecular mimicry or by direct alteration of the beta cell, causing abnormal expression of autoantigens or by direct destruction of the beta cells.

8. What is the pathogenesis of type 2 diabetes?

The pathogenesis of type 2 diabetes is unclear but appears to be multifactorial. The earliest defect that can be detected is insulin resistance, manifested as elevated plasma insulin levels—either fasting or after an oral or intravenous glucose tolerance test. This abnormality can be seen as early as late adolescence and may precede the development of diabetes by one or two decades. In this early stage, insulin resistance is seen even in the absence of obe-

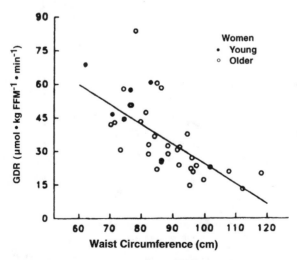

Relationship between insulin resistance measured by the euglycemic clamp technique and waist circumference in women with various degrees of glucose tolerance. A high glucose disposal rate (GDR) = insulin-sensitive. A low GDR = insulin-resistant (r = –0.71, p < 0.01 for women; r = _0.65, p < 0.01 for men [graph not shown]). (From Kohrt WM, Kirwan JP, Staten MA, et al: Insulin resistance in aging is related to abdominal obesity. Diabetes 42:273, 1993, with permission.)

sity. Prospective studies indicate that the inheritance of this insulin resistance trait is necessary but not sufficient for the development of diabetes. The development of diabetes does not occur in genetically susceptible people who maintain close to ideal body weight. Only genetically susceptible people who become obese are affected. Obesity, particularly truncal obesity, is associated with further insulin resistance and is postulated to place an increased demand on the beta cells.

The figure above shows the relationship between waist circumference (measure of truncal obesity) and insulin sensitivity in women with various degrees of glucose tolerance. Women with the smallest waist measurements were the most insulin-sensitive compared with women with the largest waist measurements. An identical relationship was demonstrated for men.

For people genetically susceptible to type 2 diabetes, the beta cells are able to compensate, to a point, for the insulin resistance. Recent studies suggest that imparied insulin secretion and insulin resistance are independent predictors for the development of type 2 diabetes. The point when beta cell failure occurs is often the point when clinical diabetes is diagnosed. Progression from insulin resistance to beta cell failure has been clearly demonstrated in humans. Similarly, animal models for type 2 diabetes progress in a predictable fashion through various stages of insulin resistance and insulin deficiency.

9. Describe what causes beta cell failure in type 2 diabetes.

The cause for the failure of beta cells to "keep up" with the increased demand in type 2 diabetes is unclear. Subtle defects in beta cell function have been described early in the course of the disease. One provocative theory is that glucose itself, once above the normal range, may actually be "toxic" to the beta cells (glucose toxicity). This theory is supported by a number of animal studies that demonstrate that beta cells fail to respond appropriately to glucose when ambient glucose levels are maintained above 120 mg/dL. The studies suggest that glucose itself may contribute to a vicious cycle of increasing blood glucose levels and decreasing beta-cell function. This acquired defect in beta cell function appears to be reversible, once the glucose levels are normalized.

Other causes for beta-cell dysfunction have been implicated in type 2 diabetes, including genetically determined reduction of beta cell mass and the accumulation of amyloid-like

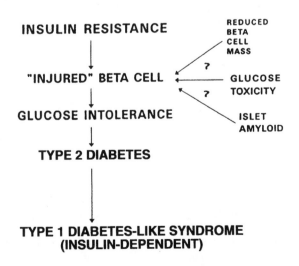

Natural history of type 2 diabetes

fibrils in the beta cells (amylin). Free fatty acids, which are often elevated in uncontrolled type 2 diabetes, have also been implicated as a beta cell toxin, a phenomenon referred to as "lipotoxicity." The relative contribution of these factors is not known. Over the course of the disease, beta-cell function in type 2 diabetes diminishes and can eventually progress to an entity similar to type 1 diabetes, manifested by profound insulin deficiency and a predisposition to ketosis. (See figure below.)

10. How does the liver contribute to sustaining fasting hyperglycemia in type 2 diabetes?
   The fasting glucose level is determined by the balance between glucose utilization by peripheral tissues and hepatic glucose production. In the nondiabetic state, the basal fasting insulin level is sufficient to suppress hepatic glucose production and maintain glucose levels in the normal range. In type 2 diabetes, however, the circulating insulin level is not sufficient to suppress hepatic glucose production, which increases in the late phases of diabetes progression and becomes the major contributor to fasting hyperglycemia. Therefore, in the advanced stages in the development of type 2 diabetes, insulin resistance, insulin deficiency, and increased hepatic glucose production play a role in sustaining hyperglycemia. A comparison of the known pathogenic factors for type 1 and type 2 diabetes is provided below.

Comparison of Known Pathogenic Factors for Types 1 and 2 Diabetes

PATHOGENIC FACTOR	TYPE 1 (INSULIN-DEPENDENT)	TYPE 2 (NON–INSULIN-DEPENDENT)
Genetic	Disease risk associated with specific HLA haplotypes	Strong familial clustering, but a specific gene marker not identified
Environmental	? Viral-triggered autoimmunity ? Ingested antigens (e.g., cow's milk)	Sedentary lifestyle, obesity ? Drugs
Autoimmunity	Yes	No
Other	?	? Reduced beta cell mass ? Amylin ? Glucose "toxicity"

Adapted from a lecture by Michael Bush, M.D., unpublished.

11. Describe the insulin resistant syndrome, or syndrome X of Reaven.
   Reaven coined the term *syndrome X* to describe a constellation of abnormalities often seen together: hyperinsulinemia, impaired glucose tolerance, hypertension, increased plasma triglycerides, and decreased high-density lipoprotein cholesterol concentrations. A sixth feature closely associated with the syndrome is truncal obesity. This clustering of abnormalities often occurs in patients at risk for or with previously diagnosed type 2 diabetes and suggests a single etiologic factor. Although a genetic marker for the syndrome has not been determined, tissue resistance to glucose uptake is universally found. Implications of syndrome X are that patients with even mild glucose intolerance are at increased risk for atherosclerotic disease due to associated lipid and blood pressure abnormalities. Correction of these disorders should be addressed at the etiologic level of the syndrome, namely insulin resistance.

12. What is resistin?
   Claire Steppan and colleagues at the University of Pennsylvania recently discovered a novel peptide secreted by adipocytes that causes insulin resistance in animals and impairs insulin-induced glucose transport in vitro. The investigators named this new protein resistin. Resistin levels are elevated in both genetic and diet-induced obesity. Neutralization by anti-resistin IgG resulted in a drop in blood glucose and an improvement in insulin sensitivity in insulin resistant diabetic mice. Treatment of animals with the antidiabetic drugs called thiazolidinediones causes a decline in expression of resistin messenger RNA. This finding may

explain how this class of drugs improves insulin action. It is hoped that further research on the physiology of this novel protein will result in a better understanting of the molecular basis for insulin resistance in obesity and diabetes and point the direction to more effective medications.

13. What constitutes optimal treatment for type 1 diabetes?

The treatment strategies for type 1 diabetes have changed dramatically over the past decade. Before 1980, standard insulin therapy consisted of a fixed dose of one or two injections of a mixture of regular and neutral protamine Hagedorn (NPH) insulin, a fixed diet and exercise regimen, and urine glucose testing. The availability of self-monitoring blood glucose testing (SMBG), the use of multiple-dose insulin regimens, and the evolution of the diabetes treatment team have allowed a marked improvement of glycemic control in the motivated patient. Improved glycemic control has been shown to reduce the risk for long-term diabetic complications.

14. Describe the Diabetes Control and Complications Trial (DCCT) model for management of type 1 diabetes.

The DCCT showed a 34–76% reduction in clinically meaningful retinopathy in type 1 diabetic patients using intensive diabetes therapy compared with patients randomized to standard diabetes therapy. Marked reductions in albuminuria and neuropathy also were seen. An adverse effect of intensive therapy is a threefold increase in severe hypoglycemia. The implementation of intensive therapy requires that the patient monitor his or her blood glucose 4–8 times per day and use a multiple-dose (three or more injections) insulin regimen or an insulin infusion pump. The patient must count the exact amount of carbohydrate (CHO) ingested or use the diabetic exchange system to make rational decisions on insulin adjustment.

Intensive therapy is best managed by a specialized team consisting of a certified diabetes educator (CDE), nurse, dietitian, behavioral medicine specialist, and physician with special training in intensive therapy (usually an endocrinologist). Patient contact with the team is frequent, consisting of monthly clinic visits and often weekly telephone contacts for review of SMBG results. A computer modem or fax is now frequently used to transmit SMBG results. Frequent adjustments are made in the insulin, food, and exercise regimen.

Based on the DCCT results, the American Diabetes Association recommends that "patients should aim for the best level of glucose control they can achieve without placing themselves at undue risk for hypoglycemia or other hazards associated with tight control." The use of continuous subcutaneous insulin infusion (CSII) via a small insulin pump has become a popular way of providing more precise insulin delivery. The CSII delivers a rapid-acting insulin (regular or lispro insulin) via continuous infusion. The patient gives additional "boluses" of insulin before meals and when needed for hyperglycemia. A typical work sheet for instructing patients in CSII therapy is shown:

INSULIN PUMP SETTINGS FOR

1. BASAL RATE
   1st basal rate: 12 midnight to —————— : —————/hr
   2nd basal rate: ————— to————— : —————/hr
   3rd basal rate: ————— to ————— : —————/hr
2. MEAL PLAN/INSULIN BOLUS   INSULIN BOLUS

Breakfast	—— BR ——	Fruit ——	Milk	(—— g CHO) ——units
Lunch	—— BR ——	Fruit ——	Milk	(—— g CHO) ——units
Dinner	—— BR ——	Fruit ——	Milk	(—— g CHO) ——units
Snack	—— BR ——	Fruit ——	Milk	(—— g CHO) ——units

One unit of insulin will cover *approximately* ————— g CHO.

3. SUPPLEMENTAL INSULIN

    Give one extra unit bolus for every —————— points your BG is above ——.
    Give supplemental insulin only after waiting at least 4 hr since last insulin bolus.

4. TIMING (for lispro insulin)

    If BG is 80–150, give bolus 10 min before meal.
    If BG is >150, give bolus 15 min before meal.
    If BG is <80, give bolus and eat immediately.

5. HYPOGLYCEMIA

    Treat hypoglycemia with —— g fast-acting CHO, then 15 g bread exchange or 1 milk.

6. EXERCISE

Reduce meal bolus by —— units before exercise.

For prolonged exercise, reduce basal rate to ——/hr during and —— hr after exercise.

7. BG GOALS

Fasting ——————, 2 hr after meal ——————————, 3 A.M. >60 mg/dL.

15. Is intensive diabetes therapy cost-effective?

    Analyses of the cost-effectiveness suggest that the potential reduction in cost for treating diabetic complications (laser photocoagulation, dialysis, hospitalization for amputations and rehabilitation) justifies the cost of personnel and supplies to support intensive diabetes therapy. The risk-benefit ratio for intensive therapy may be less favorable for prepubertal children, patients with far advanced complications, and patients with coronary or cerebral vascular disease.

16. Can glycemic control be improved without resorting to intensive therapy?

    The DCCT model for type 1 diabetes management is considered the gold standard. However, various simple alterations in insulin management may yield improvements in glycemic control as well. In our experience, simply splitting the evening insulin dose so that the regular insulin is taken before dinner and the NPH is taken before bed stabilizes nocturnal glycemic control. The rationale is that the NPH insulin taken before bed does not peak until 5–6 A.M. For people with a prominent dawn phenomenon (increased insulin requirements due to counterregulatory hormones), this regimen covers the increased requirement and minimizes the chance of nocturnal hypoglycemia. The evening NPH can then be adjusted more easily to control the fasting glucose level.

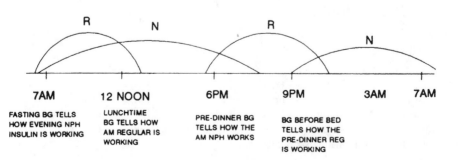

WHEN IS YOUR INSULIN WORKING?

REG: ONSET 45 MIN
PEAK 2 HOURS
DURATION 6 HOURS

NPH: ONSET 3 HRS
PEAK 6-7 HRS
DURATION 13 HRS

R   N   R   N

7AM   12 NOON   6PM   9PM   3AM   7AM

FASTING BG TELLS HOW EVENING NPH INSULIN IS WORKING

LUNCHTIME BG TELLS HOW AM REGULAR IS WORKING

PRE-DINNER BG TELLS HOW THE AM NPH WORKS

BG BEFORE BED TELLS HOW THE PRE-DINNER REG IS WORKING

17. Describe the approach to the patient with a labile blood glucose profile.

A careful history, searching for causes of glucose variability, is essential for optimizing a diabetes regimen. The presence and cause of hypoglycemic reactions are crucial information because hypoglycemia often leads to overtreatment with carbohydrate, causing hyperglycemia. Hypoglycemia also may blunt the patient's ability to respond to subsequent hypoglycemic episodes in the ensuing 24 hours. (See chapter 3.) A common strategy for optimizing a diabetes regimen is as follows:

- Address and abolish causes of hypoglycemia
- Optimize the fasting glucose
- "Fine tune" the regimen to optimize the pre- and postprandial glucose readings
- Address special situations (increased exercise, dining out, travel, infections, intercurrent illnesses)
- Use hemoglobin Alc (glycohemoglobin) levels to follow progress

Troubleshooting an Insulin Regimen

- Check accuracy of SMBG
- Pharmacokinetics
    - Insulin drawing and mixing (be careful with regular/Lente mix)
    - Injection sites (abdomen > arms > thighs)
    - ?Injecting into active limbs
    - Potency of insulin (storage)
    - Timing of regular insulin (?30 min before meals)
- Fasting hyperglycemia: Somogyi vs. dawn phenomenon
- Nutrition
    - Timing of meals
    - ?Food binges
    - ?Consider gastroparesis
- Exercise
    - Acute hypoglycemia
    - Delayed hypoglycemia (especially with prolonged exercise)
- Alcohol: delayed hypoglycemia
- Drugs (e.g., glucocorticoids)
- Stress
- Illness
- Hormonal: e.g., menses (insulin requirements may increase at midcycle and decrease on first day of menses)

18. What is lispro insulin?

Lispro insulin is an insulin analog that was developed to have a faster onset of action than traditional regular insulin. Traditional regular insulin forms hexamers, both in solution and in the subcutaneous tissue. These hexamers delay the diffusion of the insulin from the subcutaneous space into the circulation. For this reason, synthetic insulin analogs that remain as monomers when injected have been developed. Lispro insulin was developed by changing the natural sequence of the human insulin beta chain at the amino acid positions 28 and 29 from the native sequence of proline-lysine to lysine-proline. This simple change in amino acid sequence hinders the ability of insulin to form dimers or hexamers by a factor of 300 compared with regular insulin. The result is an insulin that has an onset of action of approximately 15 minutes and duration of action of approximately 3 hr. Clinical trials have shown lower postprandial blood glucose levels and a lower incidence of hypoglycemia with lispro insulin. Lispro insulin may be useful in patients who prefer to take their insulin immediately before a meal or who have difficulty with frequent hypoglycemic episodes.

19. What is the United Kingdom Prospective Study (UKPDS)?

The UKPDS is the largest and longest prospective study on type 2 diabetes ever conducted. Investigators recruited 5,102 patients with newly diagnosed type 2 diabetes in 23 centers within the U.K. between 1977 and 1991. Patients were followed for an average of 10 years to determine the impact of intensive therapy using pharmocologic agents vs. dietary therapy alone. The study also tested the efficacy of intensive blood pressure control vs. "less tight blood pressure control." The results of the study showed a significant reduction in microvascular complications in patients randomized to the intensive therapy arm. Tight blood pressure was associated with a reduction in both microvascular and macrovascular events. When the entire cohort of patients was studied together, the mean HbA1c level for the duration of the study was a strong positive predictor of all diabetes-related endpoints, including death, amputation, myocardial infarction, and stroke.

20. Based on the UKPDS and other studies, describe the optimal treatment for type 2 diabetes.

Because type 2 diabetes is a heterogeneous disorder and patients may have other comorbid illnesses, treatment must be individualized. The most common mistake in management is to label type 2 diabetes as "borderline" or to neglect treatment completely. Patients with fasting glucose levels ≥126 mg/dL or postprandial glucose levels >200 mg/dL, even though asymptomatic, are at risk for diabetic complications.

The optimal treatment strategy for type 2 diabetes is one that normalizes blood glucose levels by increasing insulin sensitivity, normalizes blood pressure, and normalizes the lipid profile. The lifestyle interventions of diet and exercise can dramatically enhance insulin sensitivity in sufficiently motivated patients. The initial intervention should include providing a specific prescription for an aerobic exercise program. Insulin sensitivity can be enhanced with a program as simple as brisk walking for 20 minutes daily. The exercise program should fit the patient's lifestyle and schedule. An optimal program is one in which the patient can be part of a supervised exercise group. Dietary intervention should include an initial evaluation by a dietitian and personalized follow-up visits or classes. The goal should be modest but steady weight loss (if appropriate). Target levels for key tests are as follows: HbA1c <7%, blood pressure ≤130/80 mm Hg, and low-density lipoprotein cholesterol ≤100 mg/dL.

21. If diet and exercise are not successful in reaching target goals in glucose control, what medications are available?

Several classes of medications are available for optimizing glycemic control in patients with type 2 diabetes. Sulfonylureas (glipizide, glyburide, glimepiride) work by stimulating the pancreas to produce more insulin. Metformin acts to improve insulin sensitivity, predominantly at the site of the liver. Acarbose and Miglitol slow the absorption of ingested carbohydrates by inhibiting the hydrolysis (breakdown) of dietary disaccharides. Thiazolidinediones directly enhance insulin sensitivity at the site of the muscle and fat cell by mechanisms still to be understood. These medications can be used as monotherapy or in various combinations to achieve the desired glucose levels.

Site of Action of Various Drugs for Type 2 Diabetes

DRUG	PANCREAS	LIVER	MUSCLE/FAT	GASTROINTESTINAL TRACT
Sulfonylureas/Repaglinide	X			
Metformin		X		
Acarbose/Miglitol				X
Rosiglitazone/Pioglitazone		X	X	

22. What is BIDS therapy?

The addition of a dose of bedtime NPH insulin to the current regimen of sulfonylurea is called bedtime insulin, daytime sulfonylurea (BIDS) therapy. The rationale is that bedtime insulin is a potent inhibitor of hepatic glucose production—the cause of fasting hyperglycemia (see pathogenesis of type 2 diabetes). By titrating the NPH dose upward, the fasting glucose level can often be safely normalized with only minimal risk of hypoglycemia. With a normal fasting glucose, the daytime sulfonylurea is often then able to control the glucose level during the day.

The technique of BIDS therapy can be learned quickly in the outpatient setting with the help of a diabetes nurse educator. A popular initial treatment dose is 6–10 units NPH before bedtime. The dose can be increased every 3–4 days by two units until the fasting blood glucose is in the 80–120 mg/dl range. Once this level is achieved, efficacy of the program can be monitored by having the patient test his or her blood glucose before breakfast and the evening meal. If the fasting morning blood glucose is normalized but the evening glucose is elevated, then traditional twice-a-day insulin therapy is indicated.

23. Have standards been established for the medical care of patients with diabetes mellitus?

Yes. The American Diabetes Association publishes minimal standards of care. These standards are evidence-based and updated by health care providers from diverse fields of expertise. For example, the standards state that patients should have a complete history and physical examination at the initial visit. Laboratory testing should include a fasting lipid profile and glycosylated hemoglobin (HbA1c) level. Surveillance for complications should include an annual physical examination, ophthalmologic examination, and urinalysis. (See also chapter 4.) Laboratory follow-up should include HbA1c test at least semiannually in all patients and quarterly in insulin-treated patients and patients with poorly controlled type 2 diabetes.

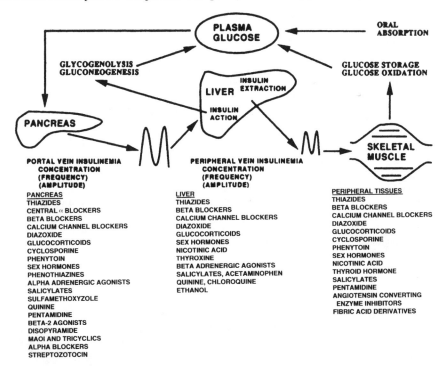

Potential sites of action for drugs influencing glucose metabolism. (From Pandit MK, Burke J, Gustafson AB, et al: Drug-induced disorders of glucose intolerance. Ann Intern Med 118:529, 1993, with permission.)

24. What is the role of diabetes education in the management of diabetic patients?
Few chronic diseases require the patient to participate in his or her own care as much as is required for diabetes. The quality and intensiveness of diabetes education often determine success or failure in diabetes management. Diabetes education is provided by all health care providers. However, active input by a diabetes nurse educator and dietitian is considered essential for optimal care. These professionals not only can enhance adherence to the treatment regimen, but they can address barriers to compliance and resolve obstacles that may not be obvious to the physician. (For review, see reference 10.)

BIBLIOGRAPHY

1. American Diabetes Association: Implications of the Diabetes Control and Complications Trial. Diabetes Care 16:1517–1520, 1993.
2. American Diabetes Association: Implications of the United Kingdom prospective diabetes study. Diabetes Care 21:2180-2184, 1998.
3. American Diabetes Association: Report of the expert committee on the diagnosis and classification of diabetes mellitus. Diabetes Care 20:1183–1196, 1997.
4. American Diabetes Association: Standards for Medical Care for patients with diabetes mellitus. Diabetes Care 24(supp 1):S33–S43, 2001.
5. DeFronzo RA: Pharmacologic therapy for type 2 diabetes mellitus. Ann Intern Med 131:281–303, 1999.
6. Kahn SE.: The importance of the B-cell in the pathogenesis of type 2 diabetes mellitus. Am J Med 108(6A):2S–8S, 2000.
7. Holleman F, Hoekstra JB: Insulin Lispro. N Engl J Med 337:176–183, 1997.
8. Immunology and diabetes. Diabetes Rev 1(entire volume), 1993.
9. Leahy JL, Bonner-Weir GC: B-cell dysfunction induced by chronic hyperglycemia. Diabetes Care 15:442–455, 1992.
10. Muhlhauser I, Berger M: Diabetes education and insulin therapy: When will they ever learn? J Intern Med 233:321–326, 1993.
11. Pandit MK, Burke J, Gustafson AB, et al: Drug-induced disorders of glucose tolerance. Ann Intern Med 118:529–539, 1993.
12. Reaven G: Role of insulin resistance in human disease. Diabetes 37:1595–1607, 1988.
13. Soneru IL, Agrawal L, Murphy JC, et al: Comparison of morning or bedtime insulin with and without glyburide in secondary sulfonylurea failure. Diabetes Care 16:896–901, 1993.
14. Spiegelman BM: PPAR-gamma: Adipogenic regulator and thiazolidinedone receptor. Diabetes 47:507–517, 1998.
15. Steppan CM, Bailey ST, Bhat S, et al: The hormone resistin links obesity to diabetes. Nature 409:307–312, 2001.
16. Statton IM, Adler AI, Neil AW, et al: Association of glycaemia with macrovascular and microvascular complications of thpe 2 diabees (UKPDS 35). BMJ 321:405–412, 2000.
17. Warram JH, Martin BC, Krolewski AS, et al: Slow glucose removal rate and hyperinsulinemia precede the development of type II diabetes in the offspring of diabetic parents. Ann Intern Med 113:909–915, 1990.
18. Weyer C, Bogardus C, Tataranni PA, Pratley RE.: Insulin resistance and insulin secretory dysfunction are independent predictors of worsening of glucose tolerance during each stage of type 2 diabetes development. Diabetes Care 24:89–94,2000.

2. INTENSIVE INSULIN THERAPY

Elizabeth Stephens, M.D., and Terri Ryan-Turek, R.D., C.D.E.

1. What is intensive insulin therapy (IIT)?

Intensive insulin therapy (IIT) involves the utilization of multiple daily injections (MDIs) of insulin (both long- and immediate-acting formulations) or an insulin pump in an effort to mimic normal pancreatic function and consequently obtain the best diabetes control possible. IIT has also been called flexible insulin therapy or basal-bolus insulin therapy. These terms are used in an attempt to describe the components of this treatment as well as emphasize the move away from the standard morning and evening insulin doses. The idea behind IIT is to utilize a regimen that more closely approximates the way a healthy body produces insulin in response to food consumed and activity performed. The basal, or background, insulin is used to control glucose excursions between meals due to the production of glucose by the liver. The immediate-acting insulin is given with meals to compensate for changes in glucose levels that result from the food ingested. In general, IIT is a complex regimen that takes many hours of education and practice for patients to understand and utilize effectively. However it is important to recognize that IIT is just one aspect of overall "intensive therapy." Other critical components include:

- Frequent self-monitored blood glucose (SMBG) and the establishment of targeted or goal blood glucose levels. Only with the information from SMBG can a person observe how his or her insulin regimen is controlling blood glucose levels and follow the response to changes in insulin doses, timing and other factors.
- An understanding of diet composition, specifically carbohydrate content and the impact that certain foods have on SMBG.
- The incorporation of algorithms, using correction factors and carbohydrate/insulin ratios for the adjustment of insulin according to food intake and glucose levels.

As you might predict, the initiation of intensive therapy requires a great deal of training for the patient, since the effort is geared toward making him or her capable of utilizing the information to make decisions about therapy. To provide thorough training, the best approach is to utilize a diabetes management team that includes a certified diabetes educator, a nutritionist and a psychologist or medical social worker in addition to the physician who cares for the patient. In most cases, these teams exist in diabetes centers with experience in intensive diabetes management. With the expertise and experience of the diabetes team, initiation and follow-up of intensive therapy will be much more successful.

2. Describe any studies that support optimal diabetes management to decrease chronic complications from diabetes mellitus.

In the 1990s there were three major studies that documented the importance of intensive glucose management as a means to decrease the risk of complications in patients with diabetes. These studies include the Diabetes Control and Complications Trial (DCCT), the United Kingdom Prospective Diabetes Study (UKPDS) and the Kumamoto Study. Below is a brief summary of these trials describing the questions addressed, the study design and the results obtained.

- The DCCT was a trial started in 1983, designed to compare the effect of intensive and

conventional diabetes therapy in people with type 1 diabetes. These therapies were defined by the following criteria:
- Intensive therapy: designed to achieve near normal blood glucose values, (goal preprandial blood glucose between 70 and120 mg/dL and goal postprandial blood glucose < 180 mg/dL) using three or more insulin injections daily or an insulin pump.
- Conventional therapy: one to two insulin injections per day with absence of symptoms of hyperglycemia or hypoglycemia.

In this study, 1441 patients were stratified according to the absence (primary prevention) or presence (secondary intervention) of retinopathy and were randomized to intensive or conventional treatment. Cases were followed on average for 6.5 years, and the appearance or progression of retinopathy as well as neurologic, cardiovascular and neuropsychological changes were assessed regularly. A brief summary of the results from this study are shown in the table below.

*Comparison of DCCT and Kumamoto Studies**

	DCCT	KUMAMOTO
	Type 1 diabetes	Type 2 diabetes
Retinopathy	63%†	60%‡
Nephropathy§	54%	74%
Neuropathy	60%	—

*Percentages indicate the reduction in risk associated with intensive insulin therapy.
†This value is an average of primary prevention cohort (76%) and secondary intervention cohort (54%).
‡Average of primary prevention (68%) and secondary intervention (52%).
§Defined as albuminuria/urine albumin excretion of ≥ 300 mg/day.

- The Kumamoto Study was an 8-year prospective study done in Japanese patients with type 2 diabetes. The objective was to examine whether intensive glycemic control would decrease the frequency or severity of diabetic microvascular complications. The treatment groups were defined by the following:
  - Intensive treatment: utilized short-acting insulin at each meal and intermediate-acting insulin at bedtime to keep fasting blood glucose at < 140 mg/dL, 2-hour postprandial blood glucose at < 200 mg/dL and hemoglobin A1C levels at < 7.0%
  - Conventional treatment: insulin was administered once or twice daily using intermediate-acting insulin only to keep patients free of symptoms of hyperglycemia or hypoglycemia and to maintain fasting blood glucose levels at close to 140 mg/dL.

In the Kumamoto study, 110 patients were divided into two cohorts: the primary prevention cohort (55 patients without retinopathy) and the secondary intervention cohort (55 patients with simple retinopathy). Participants were then randomly assigned to either conventional or intensive therapy. Changes in microvascular complications were assessed regularly over the 8 years that the trial continued. (See the previous table for results.)

The findings from the DCCT and Kumamoto studies demonstrate that glycemic control significantly reduces the risk for the development or progression of microvascular complications, regardless of whether the individual has type 1 or type 2 diabetes. However, given the small number of patients in the Kumamoto study, there was less confidence in the extrapolation of the results to those with type 2 diabetes. This made the findings from the UKPDS critical.
- The UKPDS is the largest and longest study ever performed in patients with type 2 diabetes. In this study 5102 people with newly diagnosed type 2 diabetes were

recruited between 1977 and 1991, and their cases were followed on average for 10 years. The primary questions addressed in this study included: 1) whether intensive use of medication to lower blood glucose levels would result in a reduction of cardiovascular and microvascular complications; 2) whether the use of specific drugs such as sulfonylureas, biguanides or insulin have specific advantages or disadvantages; and 3) whether "tight" or "less tight" blood pressure control utilizing either an angiotensin-converting enzyme (ACE) inhibitor or beta-blocker offered specific advantages or disadvantages.

The incredible amount of information generated from this study with its large number of participants and long duration is far too extensive to be detailed here. Instead, a brief summary of the results and main conclusions are outlined below:

- The UKPDS findings establish that the microvascular complications associated with type 2 diabetes (such as retinopathy, nephropathy and possibly neuropathy) are reduced by lowering blood glucose levels with intensive therapy (goal fasting plasma glucose < 108 mg/dL) compared with conventional therapy (goal fasting plasma glucose < 270 mg/dL). These improvements were seen despite a small difference in overall hemoglobin A1C between groups of only 0.9% (intensive 7.0%; conventional 7.9%). These results support the evidence that hyperglycemia either causes or contributes to the microvascular complications in type 2 diabetes.

- There was no significant effect of lowering blood glucose on cardiovascular complications, with a 16% reduction in the risk of combined fatal or nonfatal myocardial infarction and sudden death observed (p = .052). However epidemiological analysis did show a continuous association between cardiovascular complications and glycemia, such that there was a 25% reduction in diabetes related death and an 18% reduction in combined fatal and nonfatal myocardial infarction for every percentage point decrease in hemoglobin A1C.

- There were no significant differences with regard to diabetic complications when comparing insulin and sulfonylurea therapy, and neither insulin nor sulfonylureas increased cardiovascular events. Because both medications result in higher plasma insulin levels, this finding provides reassurance that it is not insulin that is responsible for cardiovascular or atherosclerotic events. Furthermore, the findings helped to reassure those who remained concerned about the use of sulfonylureas in type 2 diabetes because of the University Group Diabetes Program (UGPD) study. The UGPD, a study done in 200 subjects with type 2 diabetes in the 1960s, had suggested that the use of sulfonylureas (in this study, tolbutamide) resulted in increased cardiovascular mortality. This result, however, was not confirmed in the UKPDS, a study that involved a much larger number of people and a longer duration of treatment.

- The subgroup of obese patients assigned to intensive therapy with metformin had a 32% reduction in the risk of combined diabetes-related endpoints, diabetes-related deaths, all-cause deaths and myocardial infarction. However, there was no significant decrease in microvascular complications in this group, a surprising finding that raised questions about the number of subjects in this group (n = 342) and the frequency of drug crossovers between treatment groups. This uncertainty was increased by the findings in the 537 patients who failed to maintain glucose levels within the target range on sulfonylureas and who were subsequently randomly assigned to have metformin added to their therapy. In this substudy, there was a 96% increase in diabetes-related deaths and a 60% increase in all-cause death in those randomized to have metformin added compared with those continued on sulfonylurea drugs alone. These findings were reanalyzed and felt to be due to a significant reduction in events in those receiving sulfonylureas alone, which occurred by random chance, rather than an effect of the metformin. This was also supported by a meta-analysis of all patients on sulfonylureas plus metformin in the UKPDS that found significant reductions in myocardial infarctions and all diabetes-related end points.

- "Tight blood pressure control" (mean blood pressure, 144/82 mmHg) reduced the risks of cardiovascular and microvascular outcomes with a risk reduction ranging from 24–56% when compared to "less tight blood pressure control" (mean blood pressure, 154/87 mm/Hg). Comparison between antihypertensive treatment with an ACE inhibitor and with a beta-blocker showed that both drugs were about equally effective in lowering blood pressure and in reducing the risk of diabetes-related deaths, myocardial infarctions and microvascular end points. Overall, the study showed a low incidence of nephropathy, and therefore the lack of a difference between beta-blockers and ACE inhibitors in regard to microalbuminuria and proteinuria is of questionable significance.

3. Which patients are candidates for IIT?

All people with diabetes should be considered as potential candidates for intensive insulin regimens, because it has been definitively established that good glycemic control results in fewer complications. The first decision is whether IIT will be implemented as MDI or with an insulin pump. This choice and the degree of intensification must be individualized, based on each patient's personal situation and abilities.

When considering the degree of intensification to be pursued, it is helpful to think about certain characteristics of the patient and the diabetes team that are associated with greater success in the implementation of IIT. The patient characteristics include:

- Motivation and desire to improve glycemic control
- Willingness to perform frequent SMBG (up to 6–10 times/day) and record results
- Time to spend with the dietitian and educator to learn about carbohydrate counting and correction factors to then be able to respond with adjustments in insulin doses
- The understanding and ability to recognize and treat hypoglycemia appropriately
- The understanding and ability to manage sick days and to check for ketones
- A supportive network of family and/or friends who can work with and help the patient in his or her efforts to improve blood glucose control

In addition, it is important to stress that most patients cannot intensify their insulin regimen alone. It requires a cohesive and organized diabetes team that is available for frequent interaction and discussion about results from monitoring, insulin adjustments, etc. It is equally important that this team respond quickly to the results from patients and the information that they provide. It takes a great deal of effort on the part of patients to collect the dietary and SMBG values and insulin dosage information, and this effort should be respected by the team with a timely response.

4. Describe the benefits and risks of insulin pump therapy.

There are multiple benefits and risks to insulin pump therapy that need to be explained to the patient before proceeding with this treatment option. These include the following:

Benefits:

- Reduction in frequency of hypoglycemia. Insulin delivered continuously through an insulin pump provides a much more predictable absorption profile. In contrast, the absorption of long-acting injected insulins can have significant fluctuations, with only 10–52% being absorbed and acting in the anticipated manner. The predictable absorption of insulin given through the insulin pump results in significantly less risk for unexpected hypoglycemic episodes.

- Compensation for the dawn phenomenon. The dawn phenomenon is characterized by a rise in blood glucose levels in the early morning. This is thought to be due to increases in glucose production at that time due to rising serum levels of cortisol and growth hormone. It is currently thought that approximately 80% of patients with type 1 diabetes experience the dawn phenomenon. It is very difficult to compensate for this early morning rise with longer-acting insulins because the timing of the increase is nearly impossible to consistently match with the peak of the injected insulin. However, with an insulin pump, the basal rate can be increased automatically in the early morning to meet the anticipated rise in blood sugar. This match can be extremely effective in treating the dawn phenomenon.
- Improved flexibility of lifestyle. The ability to adjust the amount of insulin delivered in order to adapt to varying mealtimes and activities is an attractive feature of the insulin pump. With injections of long- and short-acting insulin that have less predictable absorption times, patients usually need to eat in response to insulin peaks rather than to their appetites or mealtimes. This can often lead to weight gain. The pump enables a person to adjust his or her insulin doses to meet specific needs at the appropriate times; this helps to eliminate the rigidity of scheduling that can often be demanded by injected insulin.
- Ability to administer very small amounts of insulin to those with extreme insulin sensitivity. Insulin pumps can accurately deliver as little as 0.1 unit of insulin at a time; this can be very useful for extremely insulin-sensitive individuals.

Risks:

- Weight gain. The weight gain associated with IIT in general is due to the decrease in glycosuria and calorie wasting that accompanies poor metabolic control. Intensive therapy results in more efficient glucose utilization or storage, which can cause weight gain. This occurs whether IIT is done by multiple daily injections or by an insulin pump. Patients often need to decrease their caloric intakes and subsequently their insulin doses to compensate for the decline in their average blood sugars. As this balance is reached, body weight usually stabilizes. It is also worth noting that some patients will actually lose weight when using a pump because they are better able to time their insulin doses with meals and are not eating to keep up with the peaks of the longer-acting insulin injections.
- Increased risk for diabetic ketoacidosis (DKA). This occurs primarily because a rapid-acting insulin, such as lispro, is used with the pump. If there is any interruption of insulin delivery, the blood sugar will rise rapidly because there is no long-acting insulin present to compensate. As a result, DKA can develop very quickly. To counteract this risk, there are many safety features incorporated into the newer insulin pumps to alarm the patient if insulin is not being delivered appropriately (e.g., when there is obstruction in the tubing) or if the pump buttons have not been pushed for a certain period of time. (In the event that a person is not conscious, the pump will eventually stop delivering insulin.) Regardless of the presence of safety features, the risk for DKA still exists and has to be recognized and managed by the patient using an insulin pump.
- Worsening of retinopathy. Several studies have documented worsening of retinopathy with rapid improvements in glycemic control. The mechanism of this finding is not clear but may be related to either 1) retinal ischemia—retinal blood flow is increased with chronic hyperglycemia but may decrease significantly with sudden improvement in glycemic control; or 2) insulin-like growth factor (IGF)-1changes in those with poorly controlled type 1 diabetes. IGF-1 levels are generally decreased but may increase with glucose reduction, leading to vessel proliferation and retinopathy. This connection between rapid improvements in blood glucose control and worsening of

retinopathy has led many experts to recommend gradual improvement in glucose levels with frequent ophthalmologic follow-up.

- Increased frequency of hypoglycemia with intensification of metabolic control. Hypoglycemia is the most frequent complication of intensive glucose control, and its significance should not be overlooked as it is estimated that 4% of deaths in those with type 1 diabetes are due to hypoglycemia. It seems that as average blood sugars decline as a result of intensive therapy, the symptoms associated with hypoglycemia, such as sweating and shaking, occur with lower blood glucose levels. What this means is that a person with poorly controlled diabetes might have symptoms of hypoglycemia initially with blood sugars < 80 mg/dL. However with intensification and more frequent hypoglycemia, these symptoms may only be present with blood glucose values of < 50 mg/dL. This change is secondary to increased frequency of hypoglycemia, leading to a lower threshold for the catecholamine discharges that cause the symptoms. In those with very frequent or nocturnal hypoglycemia, these responses may disappear altogether, resulting in hypoglycemia unawareness, a very frightening situation for the patient and provider. This complication again reinforces the importance of SMBG to follow trends and make adjustments to a regimen to achieve the best control possible with the lowest risk of hypoglycemia. In practice, utilization of an insulin pump may actually decrease the frequency of hypoglycemia, as discussed above, by eliminating the variable absorption rate of injected insulin that can produce unexpected and recurrent hypoglycemia.

5. What is an insulin pump, and what types are currently available?

An insulin pump is a battery-operated device about the size of a pager. It is composed of a pump reservoir (which holds the insulin) that is connected to a tube called an "infusion set." The tube is connected to a cannula, which is inserted into the skin and changed every 2–3 days to prevent infection. Through the infusion set and cannula, insulin is delivered subcutaneously in microliter amounts continuously over 24 hours. The wearer programs basal rates that can be changed to manage situations like the dawn phenomenon and nighttime hypoglycemia. At mealtimes, bolus doses of insulin can be administered to provide sufficient insulin for the expected carbohydrate consumption. It is important to note that none of the functions of the pump are automatic. The basal rates need to be set initially, and the bolus doses need to be adjusted depending on the meal ingested and the results of SMBG.

Currently, there are three insulin pump companies in the United States: MiniMed, Disetronic and Animas. Each pump has special features and functions that are unique and help with the flexibility of pump use. To learn more about each of these companies and the pumps they provide, please call or go to the following web sites:

MiniMed: 1-800-MiniMed; www.minimed.com
Disetronic: 1-800-280-7801; www.disetronic.com
Animas: 1-877-937-7867; www.animascorp.com

6. What are the patient responsibilities before insulin pump therapy can be initiated?

A patient must learn a lot of information to be able to operate and utilize an insulin pump safely. Once learned, these practices need to be demonstrated to the diabetes team to confirm the motivation of the patient as well as his or her comprehension of intensive therapy utilizing an insulin pump. These practices include:

- A commitment on the part of the patient and the diabetes team to devote at least 2–3 months to the completion of the pump initiation program.
- The monitoring and recording of SMBG values at least 6–10 times per day in addition to maintaining dietary records.

- Meeting with a diabetes educator for multiple visits before starting to use the pump, a visit with a certified insulin pump trainer on the day of pump initiation and follow-up visits with the diabetes team.
- Watching the pump training video and practicing pump functions at least 2–3 times before wearing the pump.
- A willingness and ability to test SMBG throughout the night for at least 5–10 days while fine-tuning the overnight basal rates. This process includes testing before meals, 2 hours after eating, at midnight, at 3 a.m. and at 6 a.m.; alternatively, one may use a temporary indwelling glucose sensor to adjust basal insulin delivery rates.
- A willingness and ability to fax or e-mail records (of diet and SMBG values) to the diabetes team for at least 1–2 weeks while fine-tuning the basal rates, carbohydrate-to-insulin ratios and high blood glucose correction factors.

It is very important to review all of these criteria before preparing a patient for insulin pump therapy. Often it takes time for a person to clear his or her schedule and deal with other commitments to make the time to spend on the intensification and pump-training process.

7. Explain the difference between basal and bolus insulin coverage.

Basal insulin coverage is the insulin required to manage blood glucose fluctuations due to hepatic glucose production, which occurs primarily in the fasting state. Basal insulin coverage is usually accomplished with injections of long-acting insulin preparations or with the basal infusion function on the insulin pump. Insulin requirements are set and adjustments are made by monitoring premeal blood glucose values.

Bolus insulin coverage is the insulin required to manage glucose excursions following meals. This is usually accomplished by injections of immediate-acting, or sometimes short-acting, insulin preparations or using the bolus function on the insulin pump. Bolus insulin doses are estimated for each meal based on the anticipated carbohydrate content of the meal (carbohydrate counting), the amount of insulin required to cover a given amount of carbohydrate (carbohydrate to insulin ratio) and a high blood glucose correction factor. These concepts are discussed in detail later.

8. What are the currently available long-acting insulins, and how are they used with an MDI regimen?

Long-acting insulins are subdivided more specifically into intermediate-acting and long-acting preparations:

Intermediate-acting
- Neutral protamine Hagedorn (NPH)
- Lente

Long-acting
- Ultralente
- Glargine (new in 2001)

Lantus, Aventis' insulin glargine, is a recombinant basal insulin analog. Lantus has a glycine substitution on the A-chain and an extension on the B-chain of two arginine amino acids. It is a clear, long-acting preparation that cannot be mixed with other insulins because it has a pH of 4. Lantus is taken once daily, at bedtime and has a 24-hour duration of effect. Lantus was approved by the Food and Drug Administration (FDA) in 2000.

These intermediate-acting and long-acting or basal insulins cover the increase in blood glucose that comes from hepatic glucose production due to the action of the counter-regulatory hormones (glucagon, epinephrine, cortisol and growth hormone). It should cover background insulin needs only, independent of food intake and exercise.

Basal insulin is usually 50–60% of a patient's total daily dose (TDD) of insulin. When initiating an MDI insulin regimen, calculate basal insulin requirements by adding up a patient's current TDD, or simply use 0.5–0.7 units/kg body weight and give 50% of this amount as basal insulin. If using NPH or Lente, give 10% of the TDD in the morning (mixed with breakfast insulin) and the remaining 30–40% at bedtime. Using NPH or Lente at bedtime requires a 4th injection but decreases the risk of nocturnal hypoglycemia and targets the rise in glucose from the dawn phenomenon. Ultralente can be initiated as 25% of TDD in the morning and 25% in the evening (mixed with breakfast and dinner insulin). The initial Lantus dose is 50% of TDD at bedtime, and it cannot be mixed with other insulins.

9. Describe the intermediate-acting and long-acting insulins.

Insulin	Onset	Peak*	Duration*
NPH or Lente	1–4 hours	8–12 hours	12–20 hours
Ultralente	3–5 hours	10–16 hours	18–24 hours
Lantus	1–4 hours	None	24 hours

*The peak and duration of insulin action are variable, depending on the injection site (regular and long acting), duration of diabetes, renal function, smoking status and other factors.

10. What are the currently available short-acting insulins and how are they used with MDI regimens and insulin pump therapy?

The short-acting insulins are subdivided into those that are immediate acting and those that are short acting:

Immediate-acting
  • Humalog (lispro; new in 1996)
  • NovoLog (aspart; new in 2001)

Short-acting
  • Regular insulin
  • Velosulin insulin (buffered regular insulin for pumps)

Humalog, Lilly's insulin lispro, is a recombinant human insulin analog created by reversing the amino acids proline and lysine in the human insulin molecule's B chain at positions 28 and 29. NovoLog, NovoNordisk's insulin aspart, is a recombinant human insulin analog created by the substitution of amino acid proline with aspartic acid at position B28. These alterations prevent the normal insulin hexamer formation seen with regular insulin and results in very rapid insulin absorption from subcutaneous sites. Humalog insulin was FDA approved in 1996. NovoLog insulin was FDA approved in 2000; the release date has not been announced. The European version of insulin aspart, NovoRapid, was European Medicines Evaluation Agency (EMEA) approved in 1999. The FDA labels neither of these immediate-acting insulins for use in insulin pumps. However, Humalog is routinely used in insulin pumps.

The immediate-acting, and less commonly the short-acting, insulins are used as boluses to balance the increases in blood glucose (BG) that come from eating meals or snacks containing carbohydrates (starches or sugars). With MDI therapy, these insulins are injected with each meal on a background of basal insulin provided by once- or twice-daily injections of intermediate-acting or long-acting insulin preparations. Insulin pumps use only immediate-acting or short-acting insulin but have two different insulin delivery methods provided by the bolus (mealtime) and basal (background) functions on the device.

11. Describe the action of the immediate-acting and short-acting insulins.

Insulin	Onset	Peak*	Duration*
Humalog	5–15 min.	1–2 hours	3.5–5 hours
NovoLog	10–20 min.	1–3 hours	3–5 hours
Regular	30–60 min.	2–4 hours	6–8 hours

*The peak and duration of insulin action are variable, depending on the injection site (regular and long acting), the duration of diabetes, renal function, smoking status and other factors.

12. When should the immediate-acting and short-acting insulin preparations be taken in relation to meals?

Immediate-acting insulin (Humalog, NovoLog) should be taken immediately (5–10 min) before meals so that its quick peak may coincide with the postprandial glucose peak. There are exceptions to this rule, however. If the premeal blood glucose is high (greater than the usual target range of 80–120 mg/dL), the insulin should be delivered and the meal eaten 15–30 min later to allow the insulin time to begin working. If the patient has gastroparesis or an intercurrent illness interfering with normal food intake, the insulin should be taken after meals. This allows the individual to alter his or her insulin dose if necessary, as early satiety and vomiting may change the actual carbohydrate absorbed compared with the amount consumed.

Regular insulin and Velosulin insulin should be taken 30–45 min before meals. In practice, this is inconvenient and imprecise and may result in hypoglycemia if a meal is delayed or not fully consumed.

13. Define carbohydrate counting and describe how is it used with IIT.

Carbohydrate counting is a tool used to match the peak of glucose after meals with the peak of administered bolus insulin. It replaces the exchange system for patients using IIT. Nutrition guidelines still recommend a balance of carbohydrate, protein and fat at each meal, but carbohydrates are the primary macronutrients that are used to estimate insulin requirements for blood glucose control because they have the greatest effect on blood glucose levels. Carbohydrates are digested and absorbed in about 1–2 hours, depending on the accompanying fat and fiber content of the meal, and are then essentially 100% metabolized into glucose. Bolus insulin, which also peaks in 1–2 hours, is then given to match the timing and magnitude of the postmeal glucose excursion.

14. List the foods that contain carbohydrates.

- Starches
  - Bread, rice, pasta, cereals, starchy vegetables
- Sugars
  - Lactose (e.g., milk and yogurt)
  - Fructose (e.g., canned, fresh and dried fruit and juice)
  - Sucrose (e.g., table sugar and desserts)
- Fiber
  - Cellulose, hemicellulose, lignin, gums or pectins found in fruits, vegetables, whole grains and beans (Fiber is indigestible but is included in total carbohydrate content on labels; subtract from the total carbohydrate if ≥ 5 g/serving)

15. Define a serving of carbohydrate.

Fifteen grams of carbohydrate is considered one serving. Some examples follow:

- Starches
  - 1 slice of bread = ~15 g carbohydrate
  - 1/3 cup cooked rice = ~15 g carbohydrate
- Sugars
  - 1 medium apple = ~15 g carbohydrate
  - 1 2" × 2" unfrosted piece of cake = ~15 g carbohydrate

16. Explain the carbohydrate-to-insulin (C:I) ratio.

This formula is used to estimate how many grams of carbohydrate each unit of immediate-acting insulin (i.e., Humalog, NovoLog) will cover. It is based on a patient's weight
and TDD of insulin, which usually indicates his or her sensitivity to insulin.

17. How do you determine an initial C:I ratio?

1. Begin by adding up the patient's long- and short-acting insulins on his or her current
   therapy.
   - Take into consideration how well the blood glucose is controlled with the current
     therapy based on the hemoglobin A1c. The American Diabetes Association's goal
     for the HbA1c is < 7%.
   - It is recommended that a MDI regimen of two injections of long-acting insulin and
     pre-meal injections of immediate-acting insulin be previously (or concurrently)
     implemented before establishing a C:I ratio.
   - Also assess the frequency of hypoglycemia. The first goal is to decrease hypo-
     glycemia. A HbA1c < 6.5% may indicate excellent control but may also indicate
     frequent hypoglycemia and a need for decreased insulin overall.
2. Divide the TDD of all insulin into 1650 and multiply it by 0.33.
3. Consider the following example of a regimen:
   - 24 units Ultralente in a.m.
   - 8 units regular in a.m.
   - 8 units regular in p.m.
   - TDD = 40 units
   - HbA1c of 8.5% with 2–3 hypoglycemic episodes per month
   - 1650 divided by 40 = 41.25
   - Multiply by 0.33 = 13.61
   - Begin with a C:I ratio of 14:1.

18. How do you adjust the C:I ratio once the initial ratio has been established?

Fine-tuning of a C:I ratio is based on blood glucose records before meals and 2 hours
after meals. The pre-meal blood-glucose goal range is 80–120 mg/dL for most patients using
IIT. Individualized glucose goals should be set based on the patient's situation (complications, history of severe hypoglycemia, understanding and adherence to hypoglycemia treatment and support systems).

If a C:I ratio is correct (when used for a meal containing low to moderate amounts of
fat or fiber), a blood glucose rise of 30–50 mg/dL over the pre-meal value will be seen at
the 2-hour postprandial reading.

Consider the following example:
- Premeal glucose is 100 mg/dL
- 56 g carbohydrate consumed
- 4 units of Humalog taken 10 min before the meal
- 2-hour postprandial glucose is 140 mg/dL
- Review glucose records on multiple days to confirm trend
- If the pattern is consistent, the C:I ratio of 14:1 appears accurate

If the 2-hour postprandial blood glucose is higher or lower than expected, adjust the ratio accordingly. The patient's blood glucose, food and insulin records should be faxed or e-mailed to the health care team weekly for assistance with adjustments.

19. Define the high blood glucose correction factor and how is it used for IIT.
A high blood glucose correction factor is an estimation of the amount that 1 unit of insulin will decrease the blood glucose under normal circumstances. As with the C:I ratio, a correction factor is based on a person's TDD of insulin and sensitivity to insulin.

Many practitioners use a "1500 rule" when working with regular insulin and an "1800 rule" for Humalog insulin. After fine-tuning and adjustments are made, most patients' high blood glucose correction factor falls in between the 1500 and 1800 "rules." Therefore, beginning with a "1650 rule" decreases the time needed for fine-tuning the initial high blood glucose correction factor.

Example of determining an initial correction factor:
- 7 units Ultralente in a.m.
- 7 units Ultralente in p.m.
- 5 units Humalog before each meal
- TDD = 29 units
- HbA1c of 7.2% with 1–2 hypoglycemic episodes per week
- 1650 divided by 29 = 56.9
- Begin with a correction factor of 60:1

To determine the amount of extra insulin needed if the blood glucose is out of the target range (80–120 mg/dL) before a meal, subtract the goal blood glucose (100) from the actual blood glucose and divide by the correction factor.

Example of correction factor usage:
- Correction factor is 60:1
- Blood glucose preprandially is 220 mg/dL
- 220 mg/dL (actual blood glucose) – 100 mg/dL (target blood glucose) = 120 mg/dL
- 120 mg/dL divided by 60 (correction factor) = two additional units of immediate-acting insulin to return the glucose to the target range

20. When should one use a high blood glucose correction?
It is recommended that high blood glucose corrections be taken only before meals or at least 5 hours after the last bolus. If a patient has a glucose level that is higher than expected at the 2-hour postprandial point, he or she may be tempted to take a high blood glucose correction right away. Nonetheless, he or she should be advised to wait the full 5 hours before taking a correction dose to avoid hypoglycemia resulting from overlapping of insulin doses (several hours of the initial insulin dose activity remain at this time) and to help establish a glycemic pattern on which to make permanent adjustments in the C:I ratio or correction factor.

If an individual has a blood glucose that is dangerously high (i.e., > 300 mg/dL) or insists on making high blood glucose corrections less than 5 hours since the last bolus or during the night, he or she should be instructed how to take a smaller correction safely. This would entail taking a half correction (half of the usual amount of insulin needed to lower the blood glucose to the target level) and using a target level of 150 mg/dL rather than 100 mg/dL in the correction calculation. This is because the insulin taken 2 hours earlier still has nearly 3 hours of activity remaining.

21. Discuss how initial basal rates for insulin pump therapy are determined.
Pump therapy proceeds more smoothly if a patient has already established a C:I ratio and correction factor on MDI before transitioning to pump therapy. To calculate an initial basal

rate, take the total current daily pre-pump dose of insulin on MDI and reduce it by 25%. Use 50% of the reduced dose as the total basal dose to be given over 24 hours and 50% as bolus doses for meals based on carbohydrate counting. Start with one basal rate for 24 hours (divide the total basal dose by 24). If a patient is not already using a C:I and correction factor, see the table below for an estimated starting basal rate, C:I ratio and correction factor

Weight (lbs)	Units/kg	TDD	Initial Basal (units/hr)	Initial Correction Factor	Initial C:I
100	0.5	23	0.2-0.4	70:1	25:1
120	0.5	27	0.3-0.5	60:1	20:1
140	0.5	32	0.5-0.7	50:1	17:1
160	0.6	44	0.5-0.7	40:1	12:1
180	0.6	49	0.6-0.8	35:1	11:1
200	0.7	64	0.9-1.1	25:1	9:1
220	0.7	70	1.0-1.2	25:1	8:1
240	0.7	76	1.1-1.3	20:1	7:1

22. How are nighttime basal rate adjustments made?

- Nighttime basal rates should be established before the daytime basal rates are verified. To do so, the patient must do the following the night before:
- Eat the evening meal before 7 p.m.
- Avoid bedtime snacks, restaurant meals or high-fat meals
- Avoid exercise other than typical daily activity
- Avoid alcohol intake
- The patient must then awaken and check his or her blood glucose at 12 midnight, 3 a.m and 6 a.m. to determine if an additional rate is necessary to cover the dawn phenomenon. Alternatively, one may use a temporary indwelling glucose sensor for this process.
- Adjust (increase or decrease) the initial basal rate by 0.1 unit per hour starting 1 hour before the first change (increase or decrease of > 20–30 mg/dL) in blood glucose is seen.
- Continue to make changes until fasting blood glucose in the morning is within the target range (80–120 mg/dL for most patients).
- It may take several days of reviewing e-mailed or faxed blood glucose records for patterns to emerge. Changing more than one element at a time will increase the amount of time required for patterns to emerge (i.e., only change the basal rate, the C:I ratio or the high blood glucose correction factor at any given time).
- Once nighttime basal rates are set, adjustments are made in the C:I ratios and high blood glucose correction factors. Fine tuning of C:I ratios and high blood glucose correction factors requires that the basal rates be accurately set and tested.
- Daytime basal rates are verified next, usually 1–2 weeks after pump initiation. See the patient handout ("Verifying Daytime Basal Rates") for specific instructions.

23. How are daytime basal rate adjustments made?

The morning basal rate should be set by having the patient skip breakfast and check his or her blood glucose levels every 1–2 hours from 7 a.m. to 12 noon. If the blood glucose levels change by more than 20–30 mg/dL during this time, adjust the basal rate for the next day by 0.1 units/hour, starting 1 hour before the glucose change was seen. Once the morning basal rate is set, the afternoon basal rate can be set by having the patient skip lunch and then follow the same monitoring and adjustment procedures. The evening basal rate should

PATIENT HANDOUT:
VERIFYING DAYTIME BASAL RATES

The morning, afternoon and evening basal rates are each tested separately (on different days). This minimizes the length of time you must fast. In deciding when best to verify your rates:
- Choose a day with normal activity only—no exercise.
- Choose a day when you will be able to avoid eating in restaurants.
- Choose a day when you are not changing your infusion set.
- Choose a day when you have not had to treat a severe low or high blood glucose level.

STOP THE TEST AND TREAT AS INSTRUCTED BY YOUR HEALTH CARE TEAM IF
- Your blood glucose falls below 70 mg/dL
- Your blood glucose is above 300 mg/dL

Morning Rates
- Test your morning fasting blood glucose before 7 a.m.
- If your blood glucose is in the range of 80–180 mg/dL, do not eat breakfast
- Test your blood glucose every 1–2 hours until lunch.
- If these tests show your blood glucose changing by more than 20–30 mg/dL (comparing the first reading with the last reading) adjust the basal rate by 0.1 unit per hour beginning 1 hour before seeing the change in blood glucose.

  Example: Your morning fasting blood glucose at 7 a.m. was 110; at 9 a.m. your blood glucose was 100; at 10:30 a.m. it was 110; and at 12 p.m. it was 140. There was a 30 mg/dL change in your blood glucose from, when you had checked it at 7 a.m. Therefore, adjust your basal rate by 0.1 unit per hour starting at 11 a.m. (1 hour before the change occurred).

Afternoon Rates
- Take your usual bolus and eat breakfast before 7 a.m. (or as early as possible).
- Test your blood glucose before lunch. If your blood glucose is in the range of 80–180 mg/dL, skip lunch and its bolus.
- Test your blood glucose every 1–2 hours until the evening meal.
- If these tests show your blood glucose changing by more than 20–30 mg/dL (comparing the first reading with the last reading), adjust the basal rate by 0.1 unit per hour beginning 1 hour before seeing the change in blood glucose. (See example with morning rates.)

Evening Rates
- Take your usual bolus and eat lunch before noon (or as early as possible).
- Test your blood glucose before the evening meal. If your blood glucose is in the range of 80–180 mg/dL, skip the evening meal and its bolus.
- Test your blood glucose every 1–2 hours until bedtime. You could eat a meal or snack before bed if it is too difficult for you to continue fasting.
- If these tests show your blood glucose changing by more than 20–30 mg/dL (comparing the first reading with the last reading) adjust the basal rate by 0.1 unit per hour beginning 1 hour before seeing the change in blood glucose. (See example with morning rates.)

then be set in a similar manner by having the patient skip dinner. The "Verifying Daytime Basal Rates" handout is a useful guide for patients going through this process.

24. List the recommended guidelines for the treatment of hypoglycemia with MDI and pump therapy.

- Dextrose should be taken for a blood glucose of ≤ 70 mg/dL. Dextrose is available in the following products:
  - Glucose tablets
  - Dextrose-based candy (e.g., SweetTarts, Smarties or Spree candies)
  - Glucose gel in tube
- The use of immediate-acting insulins with a shorter duration of effect requires less dextrose to raise the blood glucose than was previously needed with regular insulin.
- If the last immediate-acting insulin dose was 1–3 hours earlier, 15 g dextrose should be taken.
- If the last immediate-acting insulin dose was ≥ 4 hours earlier, only 5–10 g dextrose should be taken.
- After 15–20 min, the blood glucose should be tested again.
- If the repeat glucose is ≤ 70 mg/dL, another 15 g dextrose should be taken.
- If the repeat glucose is ≥ 70 mg/dL, and there are less than 30 min before the next planned meal or snack, no additional action is needed other than to proceed with the meal or snack and to take the appropriate insulin bolus with the meal.
- If the repeat glucose is ≥ 70 mg/dL, and there are more than 30 min until the next meal, an additional 5–15 g of any carbohydrate should be eaten, based on the timing of the last immediate-acting insulin dose, as above.

Fine-tuning the treatment of hypoglycemia helps to avoid wide variations in blood glucose. Rebound hyperglycemia occurs after hypoglycemia for a number of reasons:

- Overtreatment with an inappropriate amount of carbohydrate (≥ 15–30 g or eating until the symptoms stop) will result in hyperglycemia.
- Delayed treatment, inadequate treatment (not enough carbohydrate) or no treatment (i.e., sleeping through a low glucose episode) may also result in hyperglycemia from counter-regulatory hormone release, resulting in increased hepatic glycogenolysis.
- Treatment with a food that contains fat will delay digestion and absorption, thereby prolonging hypoglycemia and causing a counter-regulatory hormone release with subsequent hepatic glycogenolysis.

In contrast, severe hypoglycemia can occur if the hepatic glycogen stores have been depleted from recent frequent hypoglycemic episodes.

25. Discuss the use of glucagon to treat hypoglycemia.

All patients undergoing MDI or pump therapy should be given a glucagon emergency kit prescription and a third party demonstration. Glucagon is used to raise blood glucose when a person is unable to swallow. This may occur either as a result of a seizure or unconsciousness. Family members should receive the following reassuring instructions:

- Glucagon will not raise the blood glucose unless it is low, so it is difficult to make a judgment error. It is a hormone produced in the pancreas, which causes glycogenolysis.
- Write down the three or four steps for administering glucagon on an index card (in clear handwriting) and attach it with a rubber band to the glucagon emergency kit. It may be more comforting to follow recognizable directions in one's own handwriting during an emergency than reading the package insert.
- Practice mixing and drawing glucagon once a year with prescriptions that have expired.

- Glucagon is meant to be given subcutaneously but will work if administered intramuscularly or intravenously.
- The patient should be turned on his or her side to avoid the risk of aspiration if vomiting occurs.

26. List some of the newest items available and those on the horizon to improve blood glucose control and quality of life and to encourage patient self-management.
- Short, fine syringes: Ultrafine (30 gauge, 5/16")
- Insulin pens: Disposable pens with 31-gauge, 5/16" needles
- Insulin pumps (Animas, Disetronic and MiniMed)
- Interstitial fluid glucose monitoring: Continuos glucose monitoring systems (MiniMed)
- GlucoWatch Biographer (Cygnus; FDA approval pending)
- Alternative-site (forearm) blood glucose monitoring:
  - Freestyle meters (Therasense)
  - At Last meters (Amira)
  - Ultra (One Touch)
  - Inhaled insulin (in development)

INSULIN PUMP CASE STUDIES

27. What problems can occur with pump therapy that the on-call physician will need to resolve?

A. Troubleshooting "high-glucose and sick days" case: A 25-year-old woman who has been on an insulin pump for 3 weeks calls. She is very anxious because she just checked her blood sugar and found it to be 380 mg/dL, which is the highest reading that she has ever had. She sounds panicked on the phone and wants to know what to do. She also reports that she last changed the infusion site 2 days ago and has the catheter in the place that she "always uses." She also reports that 45 minutes ago she bolused with 5 units of insulin but did not notice any change in her blood sugar. What should she do? What should you do to educate the patient so she will be more self-sufficient?

Start with the following: Correct the high blood sugar with an insulin pen or syringe first. Then assist the patient using the "Troubleshooting High Blood Glucose While Using an Insulin Pump" handout. Troubleshooting consists of an assessment of the site, tubing, pump, insulin, concurrent illness, ketones, boluses and appropriate carbohydrate counting. If the patient has a concurrent illness, instruct him or her according to the "Sick Day Guidelines for Insulin Pump Users" handout.

B. Exercise case: A 33-year-old traveling sales representative has used a pump for 2 years. He is fairly sedentary and is interested in exercising but is nervous about hypoglycemia. He wants to start playing tennis and is asking what to do about his pump rates.

Each individual must determine the effect of exercise on blood glucose. There are several adjustments of insulin and carbohydrate that can be made to include exercise in a diabetes self-management routine. A few general exercise guidelines are as follows:
- Reduce insulin bolus amounts for meals eaten prior to exercise.
- Eat additional carbohydrates prior to or during exercise without insulin.
- Use a decreased temporary basal rate.
- Use exercise to decrease high blood glucose (with negative ketones).
- For performance and safety, the blood glucose should be between 80 and 150 mg/dL during exercise.

PATIENT HANDOUT:
TROUBLESHOOTING HIGH BLOOD GLUCOSE WHILE USING
AN INSULIN PUMP

Items to Consider that May Affect Blood Glucose	*Action to Take*
Has your blood glucose been over 250 mg/dL two times in a row and you can't explain it? Have you taken one high blood glucose correction with the pump and your glucose is still over 250?	Take high blood glucose correction by *injection*, using a pen or a syringe. Check for ketones. Call physician if moderate or large ketones. Change infusion set.
Is your catheter site red, irritated, painful or bloody?	If yes, change your infusion set.
When was the infusion set last changed?	If your set was changed more than 3 days ago, change your infusion set.
Are there bubbles in the tubing?	Unhook your infusion set at the quick release and clear the bubbles with a priming bolus.
Is your insulin clear?	If not, change the insulin, syringe and infusion set.
Has your insulin been exposed to extreme temperatures?	If yes, change the insulin, syringe and infusion set.
Have you had a low-battery alarm?	If yes, change your batteries as soon as possible. Always change batteries before going to bed.
Is the pump working?	Check your basal rates for accuracy. Check your 24-hour total use of insulin. Do pump self-check found in the pump manual.
Are you ill, stressed, or menstruating?	Contact your health care team regarding adjustments to make in your insulin.
Are you counting carbohydrates?	If yes, go back to basic skills—read labels, weigh or measure servings. If not, contact your health care team for a review.
Was the last meal bolus taken?	Review bolus history on pump to make sure a bolus wasn't missed.

Never forget to tell a patient that they have the same diabetes as they did before their pump! Therefore, if their blood sugar is high and the first correction bolus made with the pump did not correct it, he or she should always take a shot of insulin with a pen or syringe. Then the patient can trouble-shoot the pump using the trouble-shooting list.

If you have determined that the patient is ill, instruct him or her to follow the pump sick day guidelines on the following patient handout ("Sick Day Guidelines for Insulin Pump Users").

PATIENT HANDOUT:
SICK DAY GUIDELINES FOR INSULIN PUMP USERS

These guidelines are for you to use when you are unable to keep food down (have severe vomiting or diarrhea).

- Test your blood glucose at least every 4 hours. Illness can cause your blood glucose to go up even if you can't eat.
- Always take your insulin even if you are unable to eat normally. This may be only your usual basal rate or an increased temporary basal rate if illness increases your blood glucose.
- Drink eight glasses (8 ounces) of water or Pedialyte to avoid dehydration if you are vomiting or have diarrhea or a fever.
- Keep "sick day" foods (containing carbohydrates) on hand if you are unable to eat regular foods. These include

> Regular pop
> Jell-O
> Diluted juice
> Canned fruit
> Pudding
> Popsicles
> Saltine crackers
> Canned soup

- You will need an insulin bolus to cover the carbohydrate content of the foods you are able to eat or drink. If you have been vomiting, you may want to wait until after you eat to take a bolus to make sure you can keep the food down.
- Check for ketones if your blood glucose is over 250 mg/dL or if you are vomiting (even with a normal or low blood glucose). Call your physician if you have moderate or large ketones.
- Take an injection by pen or syringe and change your infusion set (see "Troubleshooting High Blood Glucose" handout) if you have unexplained blood glucose readings over 250 mg/dL.

- After exercise, blood glucose should not drop below 70 mg/dL.
- The less training one has for an exercise, the more likely the blood glucose is to drop.
- Extra blood glucose testing is needed before, during and after exercise when a new exercise regimen is started.
- Intense or lengthy exercise can decrease blood glucose for 24–36 hours.
- For rapid treatment of hypoglycemia, glucose tablets, SweetTarts, Smarties or Sprees are useful and should always be available.
- Wearing medical identification is advised

C. Erratic blood glucose case: A 59 year old woman has a 49-year history of type 1 diabetes mellitus with multiple complications including nephropathy (status post kidney transplant), retinopathy (for which she has had multiple laser treatments), peripheral neuropathy and gastroparesis. She is referred for management of wide variations in blood glucose that have not improved with the use of an insulin pump for 2 months. Her records show the following:

- Variable blood sugars following a restaurant meal consisting of a cheeseburger and medium french fries

- C:I ratio = 8:1; correction factor = 30:1
- Carbohydrate content of meal
    - Cheeseburger = 33 g (13 g fat)
    - French fries = 47 g (19 g fat)
- Insulin doses and blood sugars
    - 11:30 a.m.—100 mg/dL (ate lunch); gave 10.0 units insulin
    - 1:30 p.m.—45 mg/dL (treated with glucose tabs)
    - 3 p.m.—280 mg/dL
    - 5 p.m.—360 mg/dL (corrects with 8.6 units)

What is causing her erratic blood sugars and what pump options are available to help treat this complication of diabetes?

Delayed digestion may occur as a result of gastroparesis, a high fiber intake or a high-fat meal. Gastroparesis combined with a high-fat meal is likely the cause of this patient's low glucose 2 hours after eating and the high glucose 3–5 hours after eating. Most insulin pumps have features called dual wave or extended bolus, which deliver insulin over a period

---

PATIENT HANDOUT:
ADJUSTING INSULIN FOR FAT, FIBER, AND DELAYED DIGESTION

To control blood glucose after meals, the timing of the immediate-acting insulin peak must match the blood glucose peak that occurs from the digestion of a meal. A typical meal is a combination of carbohydrates, fat and protein.

- Carbohydrates are digested and metabolized to blood glucose in about 1–2 hours.
- The higher the fiber, fat and protein content of the meal, the longer the digestion and absorption time will be. Fat, whether it is body fat or dietary fat, will increase insulin resistance.
- Immediate-acting insulin (Humalog or NovoLog) starts working in 5–15 min, peaks in about 1–2 hours and lasts for 3.5–5 hours.

When eating certain types of meals, it may be necessary to make some changes to try to have the Humalog or NovoLog and blood glucose peak in the bloodstream at the same time. Try splitting your dose of insulin in the following ways:

- For *delayed stomach emptying, gastroparesis, or high fiber meals* (> 5 g fiber per serving): Split your usual Humalog or NovoLog dose. Take half of it with the meal and the other half of the dose 1 hour later. (If using an insulin pump, use the dual wave feature—half normal bolus and half square wave or extended bolus.)
- For meals with a *moderate fat* content (any restaurant meal or a meal containing 15–20 g fat): Increase your Humalog or NovoLog insulin dose by 1–2 units and then split that dose in half. Take half of it with the meal and the other half of the dose 1–1.5 hours later. (If using an insulin pump, use the dual wave feature—half normal bolus and half square wave or extended bolus.)
- For meals with a *high fat* content (e.g., pizza, Mexican or Chinese food from a restaurant, biscuits and gravy or a meal containing > 20 g fat): Increase your Humalog or NovoLog insulin by 1–4 units and then split that dose in half. Take half of it with the meal and the other half of the dose 2–3 hours later. (If using an insulin pump, use the dual wave feature—half normal bolus and half square wave or extended bolus.)

of time to match the peak of the insulin to the peak of delayed carbohydrate digestion. A dual wave or extended bolus allows for a normal bolus to be delivered immediately and the second portion of the bolus to be delivered over a duration of time specified by the patient. See the patient handout "Adjusting Insulin for Fat, Fiber and Delayed Digestion" for the typical dual wave or extended bolus duration for delayed digestion.

BIBLIOGRAPHY

1. American Diabetes Association: Implications of the United Kingdom Prospective Diabetes Study. 23(suppl 1):S27, 2000.
2. The Diabetes Control and Complications Trial Research Group: The effect of intensive treatment of diabetes on the development and progression of long-term complications in insulin-dependent diabetes mellitus. N Engl J Med 329:977, 1993.
3. Hirsch IB: Intensive treatment of type 1 diabetes. Med Clin North Am 82:689, 1998.
4. Shichiri M, Kishikawa H: Long-term results of the Kumamoto Study of Optimal Diabetes Control in Type 2 Diabetic Patients. Diabetes Care 23(suppl 2):B21, 2000.

RECOMMENDED PATIENT READING

1. MiniMed Insulin Pump Therapy Book. (Introduction by Jay Skyler, M.D. Editor: Fredrickson L.) Los Angeles, MiniMed, Inc., 1995.
2. Walsh J, Roberts R: Pumping Insulin. San Diego, Torrey Pines Press, 2000.
3. Walsh J, Roberts R, Jovanovic-Peterson L: Stop the Rollercoaster. San Diego, Torrey Pines Press, 1996.

3. ACUTE COMPLICATIONS OF DIABETES MELLITUS

Stephen Clement, M.D., and Michael T. McDermott, M.D.

1. Describe the most common acute complications of diabetes.

Acute complications of diabetes are a direct result of abnormalities in the plasma glucose level: hyperglycemia or hypoglycemia. Initial symptoms of hyperglycemia are increased thirst (polydipsia), increased urination (polyuria), fatigue and blurry vision. If uncorrected, hyperglycemia eventually may lead to diabetic ketoacidosis (DKA) or hyperglycemic hyperosmolar nonketotic syndrome (HHNS). DKA and HHNS have traditionally been considered to be distinct entities. In actuality, they represent parts of a spectrum of a disease process characterized by varying degrees of insulin deficiency, overproduction of counterregulatory hormones and dehydration. In some situations, features of DKA and HHNS may be present concurrently.

Hypoglycemia, another acute complication of diabetes, results from an imbalance between the medication for diabetes treatment (insulin or oral agent) and the patient's food intake or exercise. Because the brain depends almost entirely on glucose for normal function, a dramatic fall in circulating glucose can lead to confusion, stupor or coma.

2. What is DKA?

DKA is a state of uncontrolled catabolism triggered by a relative or absolute deficiency in circulating insulin. The triad of DKA is metabolic acidosis (pH <7.35), hyperglycemia (blood glucose level usually >250 mg/dL) and positive ketones in the urine or blood. The relative or absolute deficiency of insulin is accompanied by a reciprocal elevation in counterregulatory hormones (glucagon, epinephrine, growth hormone and cortisol), causing increased glucose production by the liver (gluconeogenesis) and catabolism of fat (lipolysis). Lipolysis provides the substrate (free fatty acids) for the uncontrolled production of ketones by the liver. The production of ketones leads to acidosis and elevation of the anion gap, which almost always occur in DKA.

3. Discuss the causes of DKA.

Any disorder that alters the balance between insulin and counterregulatory hormones can precipitate DKA. A minority of cases occur in people (generally older) not previously diagnosed with diabetes. Most cases (up to 80%) of DKA, however, occur in people with previously diagnosed diabetes owing to in*adequate insulin* or *intercurrent illness.*

Many patients with recurrent episodes of DKA are found to have deficient knowledge about their insulin regimen or have not been taught how to test their urine for ketones or how to handle their diabetes during times of illness. These are deficiencies in diabetes education.

The most common intercurrent illnesses that may trigger DKA are infection and myocardial infarction. Even local infections such as urinary tract infections or prostatitis have precipitated DKA. Other triggering events include severe emotional stress, trauma and exogenous medications (i.e., corticosteroids, pentamidine) or hormonal changes (i.e., preovulation) in women. DKA is most often associated with type 1 (insulin-dependent) diabetes. However, it also may occur in the older patient with type 2 (non–insulin-dependent) diabetes, particularly when associated with a major intercurrent illness.

4. How is DKA diagnosed?

Prompt diagnosis is essential, because delays may lead to increased morbidity and mortality. Levels of serum electrolytes and glucose should be determined before initiating intravenous fluids in any patient who appears to be dehydrated. Dehydrated patients should routinely be asked if they have any symptoms suggestive of diabetes.

Signs and symptoms suggestive of DKA are rapid or Kussmaul respirations, an acetone odor on the breath, nausea and vomiting and diffuse abdominal pain (seen in 30% of patients). Other important features of the history are symptoms of infection, ischemic heart disease, other possible precipitating factors and pattern of insulin use.

The diagnosis should be suspected if the patient presents with marked hyperglycemia (glucose >300 mg/dL) and metabolic acidosis. An elevated anion gap (>13 mEq/L) is usually, but not always, present. The finding of elevated ketones in the blood or urine in the above setting confirms the diagnosis.

If blood or urine ketones are negative and DKA is strongly suspected, treatment with fluids and insulin should still be initiated. During the course of treatment, the blood and urine ketone tests will become positive. This "delay" in positivity for measured ketones is due to a limitation of the laboratory test for ketones, which detects only acetoacetate. The predominant ketone in untreated DKA is betahydroxybutyrate. As DKA is treated, acetoacetate becomes the predominant ketone, causing the test for ketones to turn positive.

5. How is DKA treated?
First Hour

1. Obtain baseline electrolytes, blood urea nitrogen (BUN), creatinine, glucose, urinalysis, urine/blood ketone measurements and electrocardiogram (ECG).

2. Obtain an arterial blood gas if the patient appears ill or tachypneic or if the serum bicarbonate is low (<10 mEq/L).

3. Start a flow sheet for recording fluid intake, output and laboratory data (see sample flow sheet below).

4. Fluids: Give normal saline, 15 cc/kg/hr (~1 L/hr for 70 kg).

5. Potassium: Look at the T waves on the ECG. If the T waves are peaked or normal,

DIABETIC KETOACIDOSIS FLOW SHEET

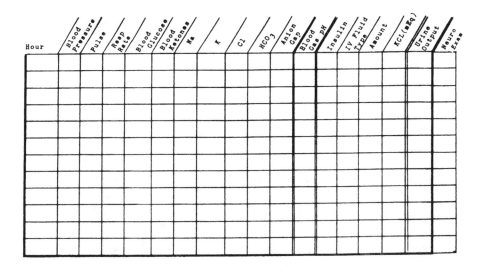

no potassium is necessary initially. If T waves are low or if U waves are present (denoting hypokalemia), add 40 mEq/L of KCl to each liter of intravenous (IV) fluids.

6. Insulin: Give a bolus with 10–20 units IV, followed by a continuous infusion of 5–10 units per hour (0.1 unit/kg/hr). The insulin drip is mixed by adding 500 units of regular insulin to 1 L of normal saline (concentration: 0.5 units/mL). Run the first 50 mL through the IV tubing into the sink before hooking up to the patient. Use *only* regular insulin for IV administration.

7. Look for a precipitating event for DKA (e.g., infection, myocardial infarction).

Second Hour

1. Assess the patient's breathing, vital signs, alertness, level of hydration and urine output.

2. Obtain repeat electrolytes, glucose and urine/blood ketones.

3. Fluids: Continue normal saline at approximately 1 L/hr.

4. Potassium: Adjust KCl supplement in fluids to maintain the serum potassium at 4–5 mEq/L. Anticipate a need for 40 mEq/L replacement per hour as therapy continues.

5. Insulin: Continue the infusion of regular insulin. If the serum glucose drops to <250 mg/dL, change fluids to 5–10% dextrose with saline. The insulin infusion rate may be doubled if the serum glucose does not decline. The optimal rate of glucose decline is 100 mg/dl/hr. The serum glucose level should not be allowed to fall to <250 mg/dL during the first 4–5 hr of treatment.

Third and Subsequent Hours

1. Assess the patient as above.

2. Repeat lab tests as above.

3. Fluids: Adjust infusion rate based on the patient's state of hydration. Consider changing to 0.45% saline if the patient is euvolemic and hypernatremic.

4. Potassium: Adjust supplement in fluids as noted above.

5. Insulin: Continue infusion as long as acidosis is present. Supplement with dextrose as needed. Follow the anion gap. Once the anion gap corrects to normal, the pH is ≥7.3, or the serum bicarbonate is ≥18 mEq/L, the patient can be given a *subcutaneous* dose of regular or lispro insulin to cover a meal. The insulin infusion can be discontinued *30 minutes* after the insulin dose. If the patient is unable to eat, give 5 units of regular or lispro insulin, continue the dextrose solution, and give supplemental regular or lispro insulin every 4 hr based on the blood glucose level (e.g., 5–15 units every 4 hr).

Other Interventions

1. Consider replacing phosphate as potassium phosphate, 10–20 mEq/hr in the IV fluids if the initial serum phosphorus is <1.0 mg/dl.

2. Sodium bicarbonate replacement is not recommended unless other causes of severe acidosis are present (such as sepsis or lactic acidosis) or the arterial pH is very low (pH <6.9). If used, dilute in IV fluids and give over 1 hr.

3. New-onset diabetes and young age are risk factors for cerebral edema. If the patient suddenly develops a headache or becomes confused during therapy, give mannitol, 1 mg/kg, *immediately.*

6. Describe the prognosis for patients with DKA.

If the patient is young and has no intercurrent illnesses and if DKA is adequately managed, the prognosis is excellent. However, when the acidosis is severe, when the patient is elderly or when the intercurrent illness is significant (such as sepsis or myocardial infarction), there is significant mortality. Coma or hypothermia is a particularly poor prognostic sign. Careful monitoring of fluids and electrolytes and treatment of intercurrent illnesses are crucial for optimizing outcome.

7. What is HHNS?

In 1957, Sument and Schwarts described a syndrome of marked diabetic stupor with hyperglycemia and hyperosmolarity in the absence of ketosis. Since their description, the syndrome has been given a number of names, including nonketotic hyperosmolar coma, diabetic hyperosmolar state, hyperosmolar nonacidotic diabetes and hyperglycemic hyperosmolar nonketotic syndrome (HHNS). All of these terms refer to the same entity:

- Marked hyperglycemia (serum glucose ≥600 mg/dl)
- Hyperosmolarity (serum >320 mOsm/L)
- Arterial pH ≥7.3

The syndrome occurs primarily in elderly patients with or without a history of type 2 diabetes and is always associated with severe dehydration. Polyuria and polydipsia often occur days to weeks before presentation of the syndrome. Elderly people are predisposed to the syndrome because they have a higher prevalence of impaired thirst perception. Another compounding problem, impaired renal function (commonly seen in the elderly), prevents clearance of excess glucose in the urine. Both factors contribute to dehydration and marked hyperglycemia. The absence of metabolic acidosis is due to the presence of circulating insulin and/or lower levels of counterregulatory hormones. These two factors prevent lipolysis and ketone production. Hyperglycemia, once triggered, leads to glycosuria, osmotic diuresis, hyperosmolarity, cellular dehydration, hypovolemia, shock, coma and, if untreated, death.

8. List the signs, symptoms and laboratory findings of HHNS.

Altered mental status is the most common reason patients are brought to the hospital. An effective osmolarity of >340 mOsm/L is required for coma to be attributed to the syndrome. To calculate the effective osmolarity, the following equation is used:

$$\text{Effective osmolarity} = 1 \ (Na + K) + \text{glucose}/18$$

The serum sodium (Na) and potassium (K) levels are measured in mEq/L; the serum glucose, in mg/dL. "Effective osmolarity" refers to the true osmolarity seen by the cell. Because urea is freely permeable through membranes, it does not contribute to this condition and is not used in the equation. If the patient's mental status is out of proportion to the effective osmolarity, another etiology for impaired mental state should be sought. For other causes of altered mental state, keep in mine the mnemonic AEIOU TIPSS:

A = Alcohol	T = Trauma
E = Encephalopathy	I = Insulin
I = Infection	P = Psychosis
O = Overdose	S = Syncope
U = Uremia	S = Seizures

Other neurologic signs that may be present include bilateral or unilateral hypo- or hyperreflexia, seizures, hemiparesis, aphasia, positive Babinski sign, hemianopsia, nystagmus, visual hallucinations, acute quadriplegia and dysphagia. Fever is *not* part of the syndrome and if present should suggest an infectious component to the illness. Other physical features are those of profound dehydration. The physical exam and other tests should be performed to search for possible precipitating factors, such as infection, myocardial infarction, cerebrovascular events, pancreatitis, gastrointestinal hemorrhage or exogenous medications.

The hallmark laboratory finding is marked hyperglycemia (often >1000 mg/dL). The serum sodium is often low due to an osmotic shift from hyperglycemia. To correct for this, the following formula is used:

$$\text{Corrected Na} = \text{serum Na} + \frac{1.6 \ (\text{serum glucose} - 100)}{100}$$

Other laboratory abnormalities include elevated BUN and creatinine, hypertriglyceridemia and leukocytosis.

9. Discuss the treatment of HHNS.

After the diagnosis is made, attention should be directed to replacing the patient's fluid deficit. The fluid deficit is usually severe, ranging from 9–12 L. The most critical issue in fluid replacement is having an accurate means of monitoring the patient's level of hydration and response to therapy. In the presence of renal insufficiency or cardiac disease, monitoring may require central venous line access. In the patient with an altered mental state, an indwelling urinary catheter is also usually required. Although there is controversy about whether to use isotonic or hypotonic fluids, the present authors recommend using isotonic (0.9%) saline at a rate of approximately 1–2 L over the first hour until the blood pressure normalizes. After the first hour, the fluids may be changed based on the measured serum sodium level. If the serum sodium is between 145 and 165 mEq/L, a change to half normal saline should be considered to replace the free water deficit. If the serum sodium is lower than 145 mEq/L, then isotonic saline should be continued. Replacement of one half of the calculated fluid deficit over the initial 5–12 hr is recommended, with the balance of the deficit replaced over the subsequent 12 hr. The use of a continuous IV insulin infusion, as described for DKA, has been found to be useful for reducing the glucose levels at a predictable rate. Care must be taken not to induce hypoglycemia. The replacement of other electrolytes, including potassium, is identical to the protocol for DKA.

10. What are the potential complications of HHNS?

Estimates of mortality vary from 20–80%. This high mortality rate has been attributed to the high prevalence of underlying disease or to delay in diagnosis or treatment. Patients with initially normal lung exams and normal chest radiographs have been reported to develop adult respiratory distress syndrome or distinct lung infiltrates during fluid resuscitation. The cause for these findings is unknown but may be an underlying infection that was not initially apparent in the severely dehydrated state. For this reason, repeat physical exam and, when indicated, chest radiographs should be considered as therapy progresses. Other reported complications are coagulopathy, pancreatitis and venous or arterial thrombosis.

11. List the causes of hypoglycemia in diabetes mellitus.

For diabetic patients on sulfonylureas or insulin, hypoglycemia is an "occupational hazard" of the therapy. Particularly in type 1 diabetes, it is impossible to mimic the peaks and troughs of a normal insulin secretory pattern with intermittent subcutaneous insulin injections. Even a perfectly designed insulin regimen can lead to hypoglycemia when the patient even slightly decreases food intake, delays a meal or exercises slightly more than usual. Menstruating women can experience hypoglycemia at the time of menses due to a rapid fall in estrogen and progesterone. Elderly patients given a sulfonylurea for the first time may respond with severe hypoglycemia. In addition to "misadventures" in therapy, patients with diabetes may develop hypoglycemia as a result of a number of other contributing disorders, which are summarized below.

Causes of Postabsorptive (Fasting) Hypoglycemia

1. Drugs: especially insulin, sulfonylureas or alcohol
2. Critical organ failure: renal, hepatic or cardiac failure; sepsis; inanition
3. Hormonal deficiencies: cortisol, growth hormone or both; glucagon + epinephrine
4. Non-β-cell tumor
5. Endogenous hyperinsulinism: β-cell tumor (insulinoma); functional β-cell hypersecretion; autoimmune hypoglycemia; ? ectopic insulin secretion
6. Hypoglycemias of infancy and childhood

From Cryer PE, Gerich JE: Hypoglycemia in insulin-dependent diabetes mellitus: Insulin excess and defective glucose counterregulation. In Rifkin H, Porte E (eds): Ellenberg and Rifkin's Diabetes Mellitus: Theory and Practice, 4th ed. New York, Elsevier, 1990, pp 526–546, with permission.

12. Are some diabetic patients more susceptible to hypoglycemia than others?

Yes. It has been established that some type 1 diabetic patients have a defect in glucose counterregulation. When the blood glucose is lowered experimentally, counterregulatory hormones (glucagon and epinephrine, among others) normally are released. These hormones stimulate glycogenolysis and gluconeogenesis by the liver, resulting in a reversal of hypoglycemia. In some patients with type 1 diabetes, this hormone release is blunted, leading to severe hypoglycemia or delayed recovery from hypoglycemia. This defective counterregulation is often associated with "hypoglycemia unawareness," in which the patient reports having none of the typical neurogenic warning symptoms of hypoglycemia (see table below). In contrast, the predominant signs and symptoms are due to decreased delivery of glucose to the brain—so-called neuroglycopenic symptoms. The cognitive impairment associated with neuroglycopenia may prevent the patient from responding appropriately to self-treat the hypoglycemia. The result may be a traumatic automobile accident, seizure, coma or death.

Clinical Manifestations of Hypoglycemia

NEUROGENIC	NEUROGLYCOPENIC
Diaphoresis	Cognitive impairment
Palpitations	Fatigue
Tremor	Dizziness/faintness
Arousal/anxiety	Visual changes
Pallor	Paresthesias
Hypertension	Hunger
	Inappropriate behavior
	Focal neurologic deficits
	Seizures
	Loss of consciousness
	Death

From Cryer PE, Gerich JE: Hypoglycemia in insulin-dependent diabetes mellitus: Insulin excess and defective glucose counterregulation. In Rifkin H, Porte D (eds): Ellenberg and Rifkin's Diabetes Mellitus: Theory and Practice, 4th ed. New York, Elsevier, 1990, pp 526–546, with permission.

It was previously thought that the development of hypoglycemic unawareness or defective counterregulation was an unpreventable manifestation of autonomic neuropathy from the diabetes. However, recent studies suggest that this disorder may be the body's maladaptation to previous episodes of hypoglycemia. A single episode of hypoglycemia has been shown to reduce autonomic and symptomatic responses to hypoglycemia the following day in normal subjects and in patients with type 1 diabetes. In contrast, meticulous prevention of hypoglycemia has been shown to reverse the defective counterregulation and reestablish the neurogenic symptoms after 3 months. Thus, initial studies suggest that meticulous attention to *prevent* hypoglycemia in patients without established autonomic neuropathy may be beneficial in reversing hypoglycemic unawareness.

13. How is hypoglycemia treated?

Once detected, hypoglycemia is easily self-treated by the patient. For mild hypoglycemia (blood glucose = 50–60 mg/dL), 15 g of simple carbohydrate, such as 4 oz of unsweetened fruit juice or nondietetic soft drink, is sufficient. For more profound symptoms of hypoglycemia, 15–20 g of simple carbohydrate should be ingested quickly and followed by 15–20 g of a complex carbohydrate, such as crackers or bread. Patients who are unconscious should not be given liquids. In this situation, more viscous sources of sugar (honey, glucose gels or cake icing in a tube) can be carefully placed inside the cheek or under the tongue. Alternatively, 1 mg of glucagon may be injected intramuscularly. Glucagon indirectly causes the blood glucose level to increase via its effect on the liver. In the hospital setting, IV dextrose (D-50) is probably more accessible than glucagon and results in a prompt return of consciousness.

Instruction in the use of glucose gels and glucagon should be an essential part of training for people living with insulin-treated diabetic patients. Patients and family members should be instructed not to overtreat hypoglycemia, particularly if it is mild. Overtreatment leads to subsequent hyperglycemia. Patients should also be instructed to test their blood glucose level when symptoms occur to confirm hypoglycemia whenever feasible. If testing is not possible, it is best to treat first. Patients on medication should be instructed to test their blood glucose level before driving a vehicle. If the glucose level is lower than a preset level (e.g., <125 mg/dL), the patient should be instructed to ingest a small source of carbohydrate before driving.

14. Is hypoglycemia a risk of intensive diabetes management?

Yes. Patients in the intensive therapy arm of the Diabetes Control and Complications Trial experienced a threefold increased incidence of severe hypoglycemic episodes compared with the standard therapy group. The potential risk of hypoglycemia must be weighed against the proven benefit of intensive therapy in reducing the risk of microvascular complications. The risk for hypoglycemia can be reduced by frequent blood glucose monitoring, self-adjustment of insulin dosing and self-adjustment of food and exercise. This requires intensive training in diabetes self-management. The risk for hypoglycemia associated with intensive diabetes therapy may outweigh the potential benefit in patients with established autonomic neuropathy, elderly patients or patients unable to perform frequent blood glucose monitoring.

BIBLIOGRAPHY

 1. American Diabetes Association: Hyperglycemic crises in patients with diabetes mellitus. Diabetes care 24(suppl 1):S83–S90, 2001.
 2. Amiel SA, Tamborlane WV, Simonson DC, Sherwin RS: Defective glucose counterregulation after strict glycemic control of insulin-dependent diabetes mellitus. N Engl J Med 316:1376–1383, 1987.
 3. Cryer PE: Hypoglycemia begets hypoglycemia in IDDM. Diabetes 42:1691–1693, 1993.
 4. Cryer PE: Hypoglycemia unawareness in IDDM. Diabetes Care 16(suppl 3):40–47, 1993.
 5. Cryer PE, Gerich JE: Hypoglycemia in insulin-dependent diabetes mellitus: Insulin excess and defective glucose counterregulation. In Rifkin H, Porte D (eds.): Ellenberg and Rifkin's Diabetes Mellitus: Theory and Practice, 4th ed. New York, Elsevier, 1990, pp 526–546.
 6. Delaney MF, Zisman A, Kettyle WM: Diabetic ketoacidosis and hyperglycemic hyperosmolar nonketotic syndrome. Endocrinol Metab Clin North Am 29(4):683–705, 2000.
 7. Fanelli CG, Epifano L, Rambotti AM, et al: Meticulous prevention of hypoglycemia normalizes the glycemic thresholds and magnitude of most neuroendocrine responses to, symptoms of and cognitive function during hypoglycemia in intensively treated patients with short-term IDDM. Diabetes 42:1683–1689, 1993.
 8. Jones TW, Borg WP, Borg MA, et al: Resistance to neuroglycopenia: An adaptive response during intensive insulin treatment of diabetes. J Clin Endocrinol Metab 82:1713–1718, 1997.
 9. Kitabchi AE, Wall BM: Management of diabetic ketoacidosis. Am Fam Physician 60(2):455–464, 1999.
10. Magee MF, Bhatt BA: Management of decompensated diabetes. Diabetic ketoacidosis and hyperglycemic hyperosmolar syndrome. Crit Care Clin 17(1):75–106, 2001.
11. Matz R: Management of the hyperosmolar hyperglycemic syndrome. Am Fam Physician 60(5):1468–1476, 1999.
12. Stagnaro-Green A: Diabetic ketoacidosis: In search of zero mortality. Mt Sinai J Med 57:3–8, 1990.
13. Umpierez GE, Khajavi M, Kitabchi AE: Review: Diabetic ketoacidosis and hyperglycemic hyperosmolar nonketotic syndrome. Am J Med Sci 311(5):225–233, 1996.

4. CHRONIC COMPLICATIONS OF DIABETES MELLITUS

Stephen Clement, M.D., and Michael T. McDermott, M.D.

1. Discuss the common long-term complications of diabetes mellitus.

Although patients with diabetes are susceptible to an extensive array of medical complications, most of these problems can be attributed to particular susceptibility to damage to the eye (retinopathy), the kidney (nephropathy), the peripheral nerves (neuropathy) and the blood vessels (atherosclerosis). The first three categories of complications are relatively specific for diabetes and are characterized by pathologic endothelial changes, such as basement membrane thickening and increased vascular permeability. For this reason retinopathy, nephropathy and neuropathy have been categorized as *microvascular complications* of diabetes. The increased susceptibility to atherosclerosis and its ensuing complications are categorized as *macrovascular complications*.

2. What mechanisms underlie the development of long-term diabetic complications?

The pathophysiology of diabetic complications is far from clear. Chronically elevated glucose levels appear to be a necessary component for the development of complications. The results of the Diabetes Control and Complications Trial (DCCT) (see Chapter 1), as well as extensive animal data, have proved that fact. However, the mechanisms of how increased glucose levels predispose to such varied pathologic findings are only recently being unraveled. Cerami, Vlassara, Brownlee and others have demonstrated that glucose

The chemical structure is known for glucose-protein Schiff bases and Amadori products. Workers have yet to learn the structure of most AGEs and AGE-derived cross-links, but one link has been identified: 2-furanyl-4(5)-(2-furanyl)-1*H*-imidazole, or FFI. (From Cerami A, Vlassara H, Brownlee M: Glucose and aging. Sci Am 256:90–96, 1987, with permission.)

nonenzymatically attaches to proteins. The initial reaction forms an intermediate compound called an Amadori product.

The Amadori product remains in equilibrium with the native protein and glucose. After weeks to years, the Amadori product undergoes a slow and irreversible conversion and cross-linkage to form complex compounds known as advanced glycosylation end-products

(AGEs). These products have been found in the connective tissue of blood vessels, the matrix of the renal glomerulus, the phospholipid component of low-density lipoproteins (LDLs) and as a component of thickened basement membranes. These structural alterations are associated with altered function, such as increased vascular permeability, loss of vascular elasticity, altered enzyme function and reduced clearance of lipoprotein particles. AGEs in the circulation appear to be efficiently cleared by the normal kidney. In diabetic nephropathy, however, the level of circulating AGEs is dramatically elevated. Because these particles may be atherogenic, the buildup of AGEs in the circulation may be a primary contributor to the accelerated atherosclerosis and death seen with diabetic nephropathy. A postulated mechanism for diabetic neuropathy is the accumulation of sorbitol and depletion of myoinositol in the supporting Schwann cells of the nerves. These abnormalities are associated with altered nerve function, demyelinization and axonal damage. Similar alterations have been described in the capillaries of the retina.

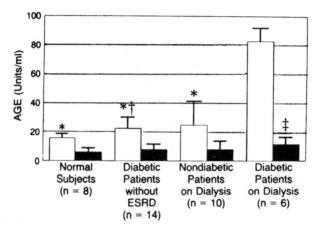

Mean serum levels of AGEs. (From Makita Z, Radoff S, Rayfield EJ, et al: Advanced glycosylation end products in patients with diabetic nephropathy. N Engl J Med 325:836–842, 1991, with permission.

3. What is the cost burden for treating diabetic complications?

The cost burden for the treatment of diabetic complications is significant. Approximately one in seven U.S. health care dollars is spent on a person with diabetes. Age-adjusted direct health care costs for diabetic patients are 2.47-fold higher than the costs for nondiabetic patients. The majority of this increased cost is currently for the treatment of diabetic complications, namely for surgery, diagnostic and therapeutic procedures and inpatient care.

4. Name the most common type of diabetic neuropathy.

The clinical manifestations of diabetic neuropathy are extremely diverse. The most common entity, distal symmetric polyneuropathy, is usually discovered on routine physical exam by the finding of loss of vibration sense in the toes and loss of ankle reflexes. Light touch and pinprick sensation are subsequently lost. Common associated symptoms are numbness and paresthesias of the feet, especially at night. The paresthesias may evolve to severe knife-like or burning pain, which can be quite disabling. Pathologically, the nerves show axonal degeneration. Sensory loss or pain in the hands may also occur but more commonly is a manifestation of entrapment neuropathy, such as carpal tunnel syndrome. Entrapment neuropathies are common in patients with diabetes and may result from increased susceptibility of these nerves to external pressure. Loss of nerve fibers for proprioception can result in an abnormal gait, leading to "pressure spots" on the foot that are signaled by the presence of a thick callus. If untreated, the callus may ulcerate and become infected. Neuropathy, vascular disease and predisposition to infection are the primary pathogenic components for the increased incidence of foot injury and amputation in patients with diabetes.

5. What other peripheral neuropathies are common in diabetics?

A number of other distinct neuropathic syndromes are associated with diabetes. Mononeuropathies may affect the third, fourth, sixth and seventh cranial nerves. Most mononeuropathies are of sudden onset and resolve spontaneously over weeks to months. Third nerve palsy may be preceded by a pricking dysesthesia on the upper lid or retroorbital pain. Third nerve palsy is usually complete, with lateral deviation of the affected eye and ptosis. Pupillary function is usually spared, which may be the only distinguishing feature between diabetic third nerve palsy and a leaking cerebral aneurysm. The pathogenesis of diabetic mononeuropathies is unknown, but the sudden nature of the complication suggests infarction of the nerve fibers.

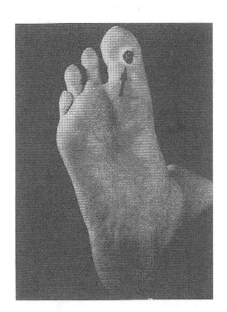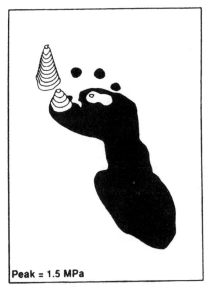

Peak = 1.5 MPa

Left, Photograph from a patient with loss of protective sensation and a neuropathic ulcer under the great toe. *Right*, Computer-generated diagram depicting the peak plantar pressures during the late support phase of gait for the same patient when stepping on a pressure-sensitive plate. Each contour interval depicts an increase above basal pressure. (From Sims DS, Cavanagh PR, Ulbrecht JS: Risk factors in the diabetic foot: Recognition and management. Phys Ther 68:1887, 1988, with permission.)

Neuropathy of the T4–T12 nerves, often referred to as intercostal radiculopathy or truncal neuropathy, may be manifested as pain in the chest or abdomen. The pain may follow a specific dermatome or may cover several dermatomes and be confused with pain from a gastrointestinal or cardiac source. Characteristics of pain suggestive of neuropathy include constant, unrelenting nature, worsening at night and a normal abdominal and chest exam. The diagnosis can be confirmed by nerve conduction studies.

6. Describe the autonomic neuropathies associated with diabetes.

Diabetes is associated with an autonomic neuropathy that is manifested by the impairment of both sympathetic and parasympathetic nerves. Classic signs are resting tachycardia and postural hypotension. A lack of R-R variation on the electrocardiogram during deep breathing, Valsalva maneuver or squatting is used to confirm the diagnosis. A common symptom of cardiovascular autonomic neuropathy is postural dizziness. Gastrointestinal symptoms from autonomic neuropathies are secondary to a lack of peristalsis in the stomach (gastroparesis) or intestine. Symptoms include early satiety, bloating, nausea, belching, abdominal distention, constipation or diarrhea. Urinary bladder dysfunction causing incontinence or urinary retention may be seen. Impotence is a common manifestation of autonomic neuropathy in men with diabetes.

7. What systemic manifestations may be associated with diabetic neuropathies?

Diabetic neuropathic cachexia and *diabetic amyotrophy* are terms that refer to a poorly understood syndrome of painful neuropathy associated with profound weight loss and often depression and anorexia. Physical signs invariably include a distal symmetric sensory polyneuropathy and may reveal wasting of the quadriceps muscle. The pathogenesis of the syndrome is unclear, and most patients undergo an extensive work-up to rule out a possible malignancy. With supportive care, the symptoms slowly resolve and most patients begin to regain weight after 6–12 months.

8. Describe the characteristics of diabetic retinopathy.

The progression of significant diabetic retinopathy may occur without symptoms. The initial visible lesions are microaneurysms that form on the terminal capillaries of the retina. Increased permeability of the capillaries is manifested by the leaking of proteinaceous fluid, causing hard exudates. Dot and blot hemorrhages occur from the leaking of red blood cells. These findings by themselves do not lead to visual loss and are categorized as nonproliferative retinopathy (see table below). Proliferative retinopathy, by contrast, develops when the retinal vessels are further damaged, causing retinal ischemia. The ischemia triggers new, fragile vessels to develop, a process termed neovascularization. These vessels may grow into the vitreous cavity and may bleed into preretinal areas or vitreous, causing significant vision loss. Loss of vision also may result from retinal detachment secondary to the contraction of fibrous tissue, which often accompanies neovascularization. Diabetic macular edema occurs when fluid from abnormal vessels leaks into the macula. It is detected with indirect fundoscopy by the finding of a thickened retina near the macula and is commonly associated with the presence of hard exudates.

Clinical Manifestations of Eye Disease

Nonproliferative diabetic retinopathy
Nonproliferative diabetic retinopathy
• Retinal microaneurysms
• Occasional blot hemorrhages
• Hard exudates
• One or two soft exudates
Preproliferative diabetic retinopathy
• Presence of venous beading
• Significant areas of large retinal blot hemorrhages
• Multiple cotton-wool spots (nerve fiber infarcts)
• Multiple intraretinal microvascular abnormalities
Proliferative diabetic retinopathy
• New vessels on the disc (NVD)
• New vessels elsewhere on the retina (NVE)
• Preretinal or vitreous hemorrhage
• Fibrous tissue proliferation

High-risk proliferative diabetic retinopathy
- NVD with or without preretinal or vitreous hemorrhage
- NVE with preretinal or vitreous hemorrhage

Diabetic macular edema
- Any thickening of retina < 2 disc diameters from center of macula
- Any hard exudate < 2 disc diameters from center of macula with associated thickening of the retina
- Any nonperfused retina inside the temporal vessel arcades
- Any combination of the above

From Centers for Disease Control: The Prevention and Treatment of Complications of Diabetes Mellitus. Department of Health and Human Services, Division of Diabetes Translation, Atlanta, 1991, with permission.

Over a lifetime, up to 70% of patients with type 1 diabetes may develop proliferative retinopathy. In type 2 diabetes, 2% of patients may have significant nonproliferative and even proliferative retinopathy or macular edema at the time of diagnosis of diabetes. This may be due to the long asymptomatic (and undiagnosed) period of hyperglycemia that often occurs in people with type 2 diabetes. Risk factors for the development of retinopathy are duration of diabetes, level of glycemic control and hypertension. Diabetic nephropathy is strongly associated with proliferative retinopathy in type 1 and insulin-treated type 2 diabetes. Other ophthalmologic complications of diabetes are cataracts and open-angle glaucoma.

9. Discuss the characteristics of diabetic nephropathy.

Diabetic nephropathy is currently the leading cause of end-stage renal disease in the United States. The onset and progression of disease follow a relatively predictable pattern. Stage 1 is characterized by renal hypertrophy and an increase in glomerular filtration rate (GFR). Patients with a sustained GFR ≥ 125 cc/min are at particularly high risk for progression of disease. Stage 2 nephropathy is defined by demonstration of histologic changes in the glomerulus, which are distinctive for diabetes. Stage 3 is marked by mildly elevated urinary albumin excretion (microalbuminuria) on a 24-hr or timed urine collection. Normal urinary albumin is less than 30 mg/day. Microalbuminuria is defined as the excretion of 30–300 mg/day. Patients with microalbuminuria are at markedly increased risk for progression to clinical nephropathy. Hypertension is commonly present at this stage, particularly in patients with type 2 diabetes. Stage 4 is defined by Dipstix-positive proteinuria, as measured by routine urinalysis. The urinary albumin excretion in this stage is > 300 mg/day or total protein > 500 mg/day. Hypertension is invariably present. During this stage proteinuria increases and GFR declines slowly but steadily. Stage 5 nephropathy is end-stage renal disease.

10. What is the risk that a diabetic person will develop nephropathy?

Patients with type 1 diabetes are at highest risk for nephropathy, which affects approximately 30%. The risk of nephropathy is about 10 times less for type 2 patients, but because of the overwhelming prevalence of type 2 diabetes, this group currently outnumbers type 1 patients with end-stage renal disease. In addition to glycemic control, genetics plays a key role in determining the risk for diabetic nephropathy. Genes that code for essential hypertension appear to increase the risk. Known risk factors for diabetic nephropathy are listed below along with their risk ratio (RR):
1. A family history of hypertension (RR=3.7)
2. Sibling with diabetic nephropathy (RR>4.0)
3. Black race (RR= 2.6 vs. white race)
4. History of smoking (RR= 2.0)
5. History of poor glycemic control (RR=1.3–2.0)

11. Describe the most common cause of death in persons with diabetic nephropathy.

Diabetic nephropathy places the patient at a markedly increased risk for cardiovascular disease. For example, the cardiovascular and overall mortality for type 2 diabetic Pima Indians with proteinuria is 3.5 times greater than for the same group without proteinuria. Although the cause for this association is not clear, the nephropathy augments any genetic tendency for hypertension and lipid abnormalities. As stated earlier, nephropathy prevents clearance of AGEs, which may be directly atherogenic. Other mechanisms are clearly involved but require further research.

12. What are the characteristics of macrovascular disease in diabetes?

Patients with diabetes are at twofold to fourfold increased risk for both cardiovascular disease (CVD) and peripheral vascular disease compared with the nondiabetic population. Women with diabetes have as high a risk for CVD as men. The commonly identified risk factors for CVD—smoking, hypercholesterolemia and hypertension—adversely affect CVD risk in diabetic persons (see figure below).

The increased risk for CVD from diabetes is due to factors that may be specific for diabetes. For example, the blood in diabetic patients has been found to have increased platelet aggregation, decreased red cell deformability and reduced fibrinolytic activity. The glycation of lipoproteins may lead to decreased clearance by the liver and increased atherosclerosis. The

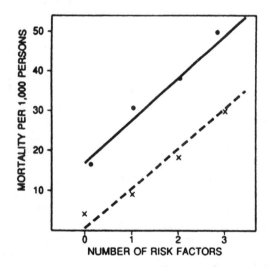

Effect of three major risk factors (hypercholesterolemia, smoking, and diastolic hypertension) on age-standardized cardiovascular disease mortality in 5245 diabetic subjects (solid line) and 350,977 nondiabetic subjects (broken line) between ages 35 and 57 years and free of myocardial infarction at baseline. Follow-up was in 6 years. Abscissa, number of risk factors present. (From Diabetes Care 16(Suppl 2):73, 1993, with permission.)

blood vessels themselves have distinct abnormalities. Long-standing diabetes predisposes the arteries to calcification. In the lower extremity, diabetes is associated with atherosclerotic disease below the knee, but often sparing the foot. This unusual anatomy is often used by the vascular surgeon. Revascularization of the foot using distally placed in situ saphenous bypass grafts often results in healing of limb-threatening foot infections or gangrene.

13. Discuss the clinical manifestations of ischemic heart disease in diabetic patients.

The symptoms of ischemic heart disease in diabetic patients may be more subtle than in nondiabetic patients. Diabetic patients have an increased incidence of "silent" ischemia. Often the patient may experience only some of the autonomic symptoms of ischemia—nausea or sweating—without pain. Diabetic patients may have a higher incidence of congestive heart failure and mortality after myocardial infarction than the nondiabetic population.

14. How important is glycemic control in preventing the chronic complications of diabetes mellitus?

As discussed in the previous chapters, the DCCT, the Kumamoto study and the United Kingdom Prospective Diabetes Study (UKPDS) all established that improving glycemic control effectively reduces the risk of developing microvascular complications (retinopathy, neuropathy and nephropathy) in patients with type 1 and type 2 diabetes mellitus. The UKPDS also demonstrated that glycemic control with metformin reduced the risk of macrovascular disease (coronary artery and cerebrovascular disease) and that control with either sulfonylureas or insulin produced a similar, though not statistically significant, trend for coronary artery disease. Based on these data, the American Diabetes Association recommends that glycemic control be sufficient to maintain the fasting blood glucose level below 120 mg/dL and the hemoglobin A1c below 7%.

15. What treatments are effective for diabetic neuropathy?

There is no known treatment for sensory loss from diabetic neuropathy. Educational programs addressing proper foot care and prevention of foot injury have been shown to reduce the incidence of serious foot lesions. Routine foot examination and early referral to a podiatrist or vascular surgeon for patients with foot lesions are considered essential to prevent limb loss.

Various medications have been tried with mixed success for treatment of painful neuropathy. These medications include nonsteroidal anti-inflammatory drugs, tricyclic antidepressants, anticonvulsant medications, mexiletine, and topical capsaicin. The most effective drug currently available is gabapentin (Neurontin); the starting dose is 300 mg two or three times a day with titration up to a dose of 600 mg three times a day, as needed.

Postural hypotension from autonomic neuropathy is improved by the use of supportive stockings to prevent venous pooling in the legs. Fludrocortisone is effective but must be used cautiously to prevent worsening of hypertension or edema. Other drugs that have demonstrated benefit include clonidine, octreotide, and midodrine. The symptoms of diabetic gastroparesis can be improved by reducing fiber and fat in the diet, by decreasing meal size and by increasing exercise. Metoclopramide has been shown to increase gastrointestinal motility and reduce symptoms in patients with diabetic gastroparesis.

16. Describe the treatment for diabetic retinopathy.

Early detection is essential for successful treatment of diabetic complications. For retinopathy, this requires annual examination (including dilation of the fundus) by a trained specialist, usually an ophthalmologist. If preproliferative or proliferative retinopathy or significant macular edema is detected, laser therapy may be indicated and can prevent significant vision loss. Vitrectomy or retinal surgery may be required for restoration of vision loss due to vitreous hemorrhage or retinal detachment.

17. How is diabetic nephropathy managed?

The progression of diabetic nephropathy can be slowed by aggressive treatment of hypertension. Angiotensin converting enzyme (ACE) inhibitors are the agents of choice for treating hypertension in diabetic patients, as these medications have been shown to have beneficial effects that are independent of blood pressure control. Other antihypertensive agents are also beneficial, but their effects appear to be more closely related to the degree of blood pressure control achieved. The recommended blood pressure goal is 130/80 mmHg. ACE inhibitors have also been shown to attenuate the decline in renal function in normotensive, normoalbuminemic patients with type 2 diabetes. Based on this type of information, one study concluded that treating all type 2 diabetic patients would be a cost-effective strategy; further study of this important question is warranted. Some, but not all, studies have shown that a low-protein diet (<0.6 g/kg/day) can also reduce progression of renal disease in diabetic patients.

18. How can macrovascular disease be prevented in the diabetic population?
    Cardiovascular risk factor reduction should be initiated at the first visit and should be pursued as aggressively in diabetic patients as in patients with known coronary artery disease. Aggressive blood pressure control is strongly supported by recent randomized controlled trials; the currently recommended blood pressure goal is 130/80 mmHg. ACE inhibitors have been reported to be more effective than other antihypertensive agents in preventing CVD events and thus are currently the antihypertensive agents of choice. Control of hyperlipidemia should be pursued just as aggressively; the recommended goal for LDL cholesterol is 100 mg/dL. Improving glycemia often causes a dramatic reduction in the triglyceride level and a modest reduction in LDL cholesterol. If goals for lipids are not achieved through glycemic control, diet and exercise, then antihyperlipidemic drug therapy should be considered. Smoking should be strongly discouraged, while exercise and weight loss (if overweight) should be encouraged. Low-dose aspirin therapy is also recommended; additionally, specific anti-platelet therapy may be considered.

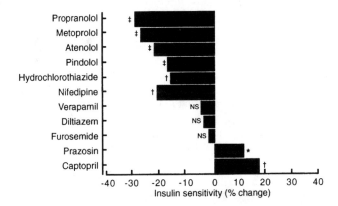

Effect of various antihypertensive drugs on insulin sensitivity. (From Berne C, Pollare T, Lithell H: Effect of antihypertensive treatment on insulin sensitivity with special reference to ACE inhibitors. Diabetes Care 14(Suppl 4):39, 1991, with permission.)

19. Does aggressive lipid-lowering therapy improve cardiac outcomes in diabetic patients?
    Yes. The Scandinavian Simvastatin Survival Study compared the outcome of 4,242 patients with a previous myocardial infarction or angina pectoris and elevated total cholesterol. Patients were randomized to aggressive lipid-lowering therapy with simvastatin or placebo. A post-hoc subgroup analysis of the 202 diabetic participants showed a 55% reduction in major coronary events, including myocardial infarction, in the simvastatin-treated group. At 5.4 yr, total mortality was also reduced by 43%. Statistically significant beneficial results were also reported with pravastatin in the CARE and LIPID studies. Based on these reports, aggressive lipid-lowering therapy should be advocated in all diabetic patients, particularly those with known coronary artery disease.

20. Which therapy—coronary bypass or angioplasty—is the procedure of choice for diabetic patients with multi-vessel coronary artery disease?

Diabetic patients often present with multi-vessel coronary artery disease (CAD). If they do not respond to medical therapy, surgical revascularization or coronary angioplasty is often recommended. Until recently the optimal therapy for diabetic patients with CAD was not known. However, three studies have now demonstrated a significant survival advantage of bypass surgery compared with coronary angioplasty in diabetic patients with multi-vessel CAD. Based on these studies, diabetic patients with multi-vessel CAD should be considered for bypass surgery as the revascularization procedure of choice. Further advances in angioplasty, including the use of stents, may improve the patency rates and outcomes in diabetic patients, but further data are needed before this therapy can be endorsed for multi-vessel disease in diabetic patients.

BIBLIOGRAPHY

1. American Diabetes Association: Aspirin therapy in diabetes. Diabetes Care 24(supp. 1):S62–S63, 2001.
2. American Diabetes Association: Diabetic nephropathy. Diabetes Care 24(supp. 1):S69–S72, 2001.
3. American Diabetes Association: Diabetic retinopathy. Diabetes Care 24(suppl 1):S73–S76, 2001.
4. American Diabetes Association: Implications of the Diabetes Control and Complications Trial. Diabetes Care 24(suppl 1):S25–S27, 2001.
5. American Diabetes Association: Implications of the United Kingdom Prospective Diabetes Study. Diabetes Care 24(suppl 1):S28–S32, 2001.
6. American Diabetes Association: Management of dyslipidemia in adults with diabetes. Diabetes Care 24(suppl 1):S58–S61, 2001.
7. American Diabetes Association: Preventive foot care in people with diabetes. Diabetes Care 24(suppl 1):S56–S57, 2001.
8. American Diabetes Association: Standards of medical care for patients with diabetes mellitus. Diabetes Care 24(suppl 1):S33–S43, 2001.
9. Backonja M, Beydoun A, Edwards KR, et al: Gabapentin for the symptomatic treatment of painful neuropathy in patients with diabetes mellitus: A randomized controlled trial. JAMA 280:1831–1836, 1998.
10. Bypass Angioplasty Revascularization Investigation (BARI) investigators: Comparison of coronary bypass surgery with angioplasty in patients with multi vessel disease. N Engl J Med 335:217–225, 1996.
11. Detre KM, Lombardero MS, Brooks MM, et al: The effect of previous coronary artery bypass surgery on the prognosis of patients with diabetes who have acute myocardial infarction. N Engl J Med 342:989–997, 2000.
12. The Diabetes Control and Complications Trial/Epidemiology of Diabetes Interventions and Complications Research Group: Retinopathy and nephropathy in patients with type 1 diabetes four years after a trial of intensive therapy. N Engl J Med 342:381–389, 2000.
13. Estacio RO, Jeffers BW, Hiatt WR, et al: The effect of nisoldipine as compared with enalapril on cardiovascular outcomes in patients with non-insulin-dependent diabetes and hypertension. N Engl J Med 338:645–652, 1998.
14. Ferris FL, Davis MD, Aiello LM: Treatment of diabetic retinopathy. N Engl J Med 341:667–678, 1999.
15. Garber AJ, Vinik AJ, Crespin SR: Detection and management of lipid disorders in diabetic patients. Diabetes Care 15:1068–1073, 1992.
16. Golan L, Birkmeyer JD, Welch HG: The cost-effectiveness of treating all patients with type 2 diabetes with angiotensin-converting enzyme inhibitors. Ann Intern Med 131:660–667, 1999.
17. Haffner SM, Lehto S, Ronnemaa T, et al: Mortality from coronary heart disease in subjects with type 2 diabetes and in nondiabetic subjects with and without prior myocardial infarction. N Engl J Med 339:229–234, 1998.
18. Kasiske BL, Kalil RSN, Ma JZ, et al: Effect of antihypertensive therapy on the kidney in patients with diabetes: A meta-regression analysis. Ann Intern Med 118:129–138, 1993.

19. Krolewski AS, Canessa M, Warram JH, et al: Predisposition to hypertension and susceptibility to renal disease in insulin-dependent diabetes mellitus. N Engl J Med 318:140–145, 1988.
20. Lewis EJ, Hunsicker LG, Bain RP, et al: The effect of angiotensin-converting enzyme inhibition on diabetic nephropathy. N Engl J Med 329:1456–1462, 1993.
21. Makita Z, Radoff S, Rayfield E, et al: Advanced glycosylation end products in patients with diabetic nephropathy. N Engl J Med 325:836–842, 1991.
22. Meigs JB, Singer DE, Sullivan LM, et al: Metabolic control and prevalent cardiovascular disease in non–insulin-dependent diabetes mellitus (NIDDM): The NIDDM Patient Outcomes Research Team. Am J Med 102:38–47, 1997.
23. Nathan DM: Long-term complications of diabetes mellitus. N Engl J Med 328:1676–1685, 1993.
24. Nelson RG, Pettit DJ, Carraher MJ, et al: Effect of proteinuria on mortality in NIDDM. Diabetes 37:1499–1504, 1988.
25. O'Keefe JH, Miles JM, Harris WH, et al: Improving the adverse cardiovascular prognosis in type 2 diabetes. Mayo Clin Proc 74:171–180, 1999.
26. Pedrini MT, Levey AS, Lau J, et al: The effect of dietary protein restriction on the progression of diabetic and nondiabetic renal diseases: a meta-analysis. Ann Intern Med 124:627–632, 1996.
27. Pyörälä K, Pederson TR, Kjekshus J, et al: Cholesterol lowering with simvastatin improves prognosis of diabetic patients with coronary heart disease: A subgroup analysis of the Scandinavian Simvastatin Survival Study (4S). Diabetes Care 20:614–620, 1997.
28. Ravid M, Brosh D, Levi Z, et al: Use of enalapril to attenuate decline in renal function in normotensive, normoalbuminuric patients with type 2 diabetes mellitus: A randomized, controlled trial.
29. Ritz E, Orth SR: Nephropathy in patients with type 2 diabetes mellitus. N Engl J Med 341: 1127–1133, 1999.
30. Vinik AI, Holland MT, Le Beau JM, et al: Diabetic neuropathies. Diabetes Care 15:1926–1975.

5. DIABETES IN PREGNANCY

Linda A. Barbour, M.D., M.S.P.H., and Jane E.-B. Reusch, M.D.

1. What are the changes in fuel metabolism during normal pregnancy, and what causes glucose intolerance?

Pregnancy is a complex metabolic state that involves dramatic alterations in the hormonal milieu (increases in estrogen, progesterone, prolactin, cortisol, human chorionic gonadotropin, placental growth hormone, and human placental lactogen) as well as an increasing burden of fuel utilization by the conceptus. Metabolically, the first trimester is characterized by increased insulin sensitivity and accelerated starvation with an increased turnover of maternal metabolic fuels and an earlier transition from carbohydrate to fat utilization in the fasting state. The second and third trimesters, in contrast, are characterized by insulin resistance with a nearly 50% decrease in insulin-mediated glucose disposal (assessed by the hyperinsulinemic-euglycemic clamp technique) and a 200–300% increase in the insulin response to glucose in late pregnancy. This serves to meet the metabolic demands of the fetus, which requires 80% of its energy as glucose, while maintaining euglycemia in the mother. Glucose transport to the fetus is augmented by a 5-fold increase in a placental glucose transporter (GLUT-1), which increases transplacental glucose flux even in the absence of maternal hyperglycemia. At the same time, it has been demonstrated that in normal pregnancy there is decreased expression of the GLUT-4 glucose transporter protein in maternal adipose tissue and impaired insulin receptor autophosphorylation in skeletal muscle, both of which contribute to the insulin resistance of pregnancy. Women usually have lower fasting levels of plasma glucose and modestly elevated postprandial glucose excursions associated with maternal hyperinsulinemia. Glucose is not the only fuel altered in normal pregnancy. Amino acids, triglycerides, cholesterol, and free fatty acids are all increased; the latter may serve to further accentuate the insulin resistance of pregnancy.

2. How do fuel changes in pregnancy affect the management of diabetes in the first, second, and third trimesters?

Diabetes should optimally be under tight control before conception. During the first trimester, nausea, accelerated starvation, and increased insulin sensitivity (perhaps owing to estradiol increasing adipocyte insulin binding) may place the mother at risk for hypoglycemia. This is especially true at night when prolonged fasting and continuous fetal glucose utilization place the woman at even a higher risk for hypoglycemia. Women with type 1 diabetes mellitus must have a bedtime snack and usually need to have their evening dose of NPH insulin lowered and moved from suppertime to bedtime to avoid early morning hypoglycemia. Severe hypoglycemia occurs in 30–40% of pregnant women with type 1 diabetes in the first 20 weeks of pregnancy, most often between midnight and 8:00 a.m. Diabetic women who have gastroparesis or hyperemesis gravidarum are at the greatest risk for daytime hypoglycemia. During the first trimester, glycemic control just above the normal range (hemoglobin A1C < 7.0%) may thus be safer than "normal" and may decrease the risk of fetal hypoglycemia. After 20 weeks, peripheral insulin resistance increases insulin requirements, so that it is not unusual for a pregnant woman to require twice as much insulin as she did prior to pregnancy. It has been demonstrated that postprandial hyperglycemia is the strongest risk factor for macrosomia. Therefore, tight glucose control in women with type 1 diabetes often requires insulin administration with each meal. Frequent monitoring allows appropriate insulin dosage adjustments. The mainte-

nance of normal glucose control is the key to prevention of complications such as fetal malformations in the first trimester, macrosomia in the second and third trimesters, and neonatal metabolic abnormalities.

3. What are the essential components of preconception counseling in women with diabetes?

Most important is the message of optimal glucose control prior to conception. In a retrospective study, < 40% of women attempted to achieve optimal glycemic control before
becoming pregnant. Hyperglycemia is a known teratogen. The incidence of congenital
abnormalities in offspring of diabetic mothers in the early era of insulin use was 33%. In the
1970s, 6.5% of offspring had birth defects. Over the past decade, with the advent of home
blood glucose monitoring and more rigid objectives, this percentage has fallen further.
However, four times as many fetal and neonatal deaths and congenital abnormalities
occurred in a group of women who did not receive prenatal counseling in comparison with
those who did. Epidemiologic and prospective studies have shown that the level of HgbA1C
in the 6 months before conception and during the first trimester correlates with the incidence
of major malformations such as neural tube and cardiac defects. The neural tube is completely formed by 4 weeks and the heart by 6 weeks after conception; many women do not
even know they are pregnant at these times. It has been demonstrated that women with a
normal HgbA1C at conception and during the first trimester have no increased risk while
women with a HgbA1C of > 12% have about a 40% risk of major malformations.

Oral hypoglycemic agents such as sulfonylureas and metformin do not appear to be teratogenic, although there is concern about the risks of fetal and neonatal hypoglycemia or
lactic acidosis if pregnant women take these medications. Glyburide has been shown not to
cross the placenta, or to significantly affect fetal insulin levels; however, glyburide was not
given until after 24 weeks gestation in this trial and therefore the effect on embryogenesis
could not be evaluated. There are also no data available on thiazolidinedione exposure
during the first trimester. Accordingly, it is recommended that oral hypoglycemic agents be
avoided during pregnancy with the possible exception of glyburide, which should be limited
to the second and third trimesters, if used at all. However, if a woman conceives while
taking these agents, they should simply be replaced by insulin. Women who are actively
trying to become pregnant should be switched to insulin during the preconception period
because it may take some time to determine the ideal insulin dose prior to the critical time
of embryogenesis.

Women who are taking ACE inhibitors should be counseled that these agents are contraindicated in the second and third trimesters of pregnancy because of the risk of fetal
anuria. Although first trimester exposure alone has not been shown to cause problems,
women who are actively trying to conceive and who have no history of infertility should
probably be switched to a safer agent before pregnancy (calcium channel blocker, methyldopa, hydralazine). A woman who is being treated with an ACE inhibitor for significant diabetic nephropathy and who is not actively trying to conceive should be told to stop her ACE-
inhibitor as soon as she misses a period and to obtain a pregnancy test. At that time she can
be switched safely to an alternative agent. Women with diabetes also have an increased risk
of preeclampsia, particularly if they have hypertension or renal disease. Although mild renal
disease does not seem to be accelerated by pregnancy, women with more severe renal disease are at a very high risk of pregnancy complications and progression of their renal disease. Therefore, women with diabetic nephropathy should be counseled to have their children when their diabetes is optimally controlled and preferably early in the course of their
nephropathy. Proliferative retinopathy may also progress during pregnancy; it is imperative,
therefore, that this condition be optimally treated with laser therapy prior to pregnancy.

Because of the high morbidity and mortality of coronary artery disease in pregnancy, women with multiple cardiac risk factors such as hyperlipidemia, hypertension, smoking, advanced maternal age (>35), or a strong family history should have their cardiac status assessed with functional testing prior to conception. Lipid lowering agents should be discontinued before conception, since there are inadequate data about their safety during pregnancy. However, if a woman has severe hypertriglyceridemia, which places her at high risk for pancreatitis, it may be necessary to continue fibrate therapy if a low fat diet, fish oils, or niacin therapy are not effective or tolerated. All women should also be taking folic acid supplements (1 mg per day) before conception.

Smoking continues to be the leading cause of low birth weight infants in patients with and without diabetes and places the infant at increased risk for respiratory infections, reactive airway disease, and sudden infant death syndrome. Smoking cessation efforts need to be intensified before conception, since agents such as the nicotine patch and Wellbutrin are not approved for use during pregnancy.

4. What is the White Classification of diabetes in pregnancy, and why is it used by obstetricians?

Priscilla White observed that a patient's age at onset of diabetes, the duration of diabetes, and the severity of complications, including vascular disease, nephropathy, and retinopathy, significantly influenced maternal and perinatal outcomes (see table below). She developed a classification scheme in 1949 that has undergone widespread application in the obstetric community because of its predictive value in identifying patients who are at greatest risk for obstetric complications during pregnancy. The updated classification scheme allows physicians to focus and intensify management and fetal surveillance on those patients who have the highest risk of poor maternal and obstetric outcome during pregnancy. Pregestational diabetic women are designated by the letters B,C,D,F,R,T, and H according to their duration of diabetes and complications. There is not a separate classification scheme for type 1 and type 2 diabetes, but the initial scheme was developed for women with type 1 diabetes.

Modified White Classification of Pregnant Diabetic Women

Class	Diabetes onset age (yr)		Duration (yr)	Type of Vascular Disease	Insulin Need
Gestational Diabetes					
A1	Any		Pregnancy	None	None
A2	Any		Pregnancy	None	Yes
Pregestational Diabetes					
B	≥20		<10	None	Yes
C	10-19	OR	10-19	None	Yes
D	<10	OR	≥20	Benign retinopathy	Yes
F	Any		Any	Nephropathy	Yes
R	Any		Any	Proliferative retinopathy	Yes
T	Any		Any	Renal transplant	Yes
H	Any		Any	Coronary artery disease	Yes

5. What are the goals of glucose control for pregnant women with diabetes?

The goals of blood glucose control during pregnancy are rigorous. Optimally, the premeal whole blood glucose should be less than <95 mg/dl, the 1 hour postprandial glucose <140 mg/dl, and the 2 hour glucose <120 mg/dl. Since macrosomia is more strongly related to the postprandial glucose excursions, pregnant diabetic women need to monitor their premeal and postprandial glucose values regularly. Type 1 diabetic patients usually require 3–4 injections per day or an insulin pump to achieve adequate control during pregnancy. Lispro (Humalog) insulin may be especially helpful in women with hyperemesis or gastroparesis because it can be dosed after a successful meal and still be effective. Women with gestational or type 2 diabetes may be able to achieve optimal glycemic control with twice daily injections. However, if postprandial lunch excursions are too high, 3 injections a day of a rapid acting insulin (Lispro) may be necessary. Occasional monitoring in the middle of the night is recommended in women with type I diabetes because of the increased risk of nocturnal hypoglycemia, especially if they have hypoglycemia unawareness. The physician must have a low threshold for bringing the expectant mother into the hospital to optimize education and glycemic control.

Failure to achieve optimal control in early pregnancy may have teratogenic effects or lead to early fetal loss. Poor control later in pregnancy increases the risk of intrauterine fetal demise, macrosomia, and metabolic complications in the newborn. An early dating ultrasound is necessary to accurately determine the gestational age of the fetus, and a formal anatomy scan at 18–20 weeks should be performed to evaluate for fetal anomalies. A fetal echocardiogram should be offered at 20–22 weeks, especially if the HgA1C was elevated during the first trimester.

6. What is the risk of diabetic ketoacidosis (DKA) in pregnancy?

Pregnancy predisposes to accelerated starvation, which can result in ketonuria after an overnight fast. DKA may thus occur at lower glucose levels and may develop more rapidly than it does in nonpregnant individuals. Two studies (involving 7 patients in Great Britain and 20 patients in the United States) reported a risk of fetal loss ranging from 22–35%. Fetal loss frequently occurred before presentation to the hospital. Once the patient was hospitalized and treated, the risk of fetal loss declined dramatically. Risk factors for fetal loss included third trimester glucose > 800 mg/dl; BUN > 21 mg/dl; osmolality > 300 mmol/L; high insulin requirements; and longer duration until resolution of DKA. The fetal heart rate must therefore be monitored continuously until the acidosis has resolved. Neither series reported increased mortality in the mothers. Causes of DKA were similar to those among the general diabetic population, with infection at initial presentation (6 of 20) and poor compliance being the most common. Pyelonephritis is a frequent complication of urinary tract infections in pregnancy and should be immediately evaluated as a possible cause. Tocolytics and corticosteroids may also precipitate DKA. Prenatal care attuned to the signs and symptoms of new-onset diabetes and good metabolic control should allow prevention in most cases.

7. What happens to retinopathy during the diabetic pregnancy?

Progression of retinopathy during pregnancy is well documented. This phenomenon is most prevalent in women with high-risk diabetic eye disease such as severe preproliferative or proliferative retinopathy. Recent data suggest that rapid institution of tight control may be associated with subsequent progression of retinopathy. However it is unclear whether the tight control often achieved during pregnancy or the changes of pregnancy per se, including increased cardiac output, the production of growth factors, and the hypercoagulable state of pregnancy, account for this deterioration. Given this uncertainty, it is best to intensify glycemic control and to stabilize retinopathy before conception. However, laser surgery is as effective in preventing blindness during pregnancy, as it is outside of pregnancy and can be performed safely. Women with low-risk eye disease should be followed by an ophthalmologist during pregnancy, but significant vision-threatening progression of retinopathy is rare in these individuals.

8. Does diabetic nephropathy progress during pregnancy?

Women with pre-existing proteinuria often have a significant progressive increase in protein excretion, frequently into the nephrotic range, in part owing to the 30–50% increase in glomerular filtration rate (GFR) that occurs during pregnancy. In most cases, the proteinuria returns to the pre-pregnancy baseline after delivery. In some patients, however, the protein-uria can become massive and result in significant edema, hypoalbuminemia, and a hyperco-agulable state. While women with mild renal insufficiency are not at an appreciable risk for irreversible progression of their nephropathy, those with more severe renal insufficiency (cre-atinine >2.5 mg/dl) have a 30–50% risk of a permanent pregnancy-related decline in GFR. They are also at extremely high risk of having preeclampsia, a preterm delivery, and a low birth weight infant. Women who have had a successful renal transplant and who are at least 1-2 years out from their transplant with good renal function, good blood pressure control, and a low requirement for anti-rejection medications have a much more favorable outcome than women with severe renal disease who have not received a transplant.

9. What is gestational diabetes? How is it diagnosed?

Gestational diabetes mellitus (GDM) is a glucose-intolerant state with onset or first recog-nition during pregnancy. The incidence of GDM ranges from 2 to 8% of pregnancies through-out the world and is highest in ethnic groups that have a higher incidence of type 2 diabetes (Hispanic Americans, African Americans, Native Americans, and Pacific Islanders). The cri-teria for diagnosis in the United States have recently changed and the Carpenter and Coustan criteria have been adopted by the ADA and the Fourth International Workshop-Conference on Gestational Diabetes. Screening recommendations have been stratified according to low risk status, average risk status, and high risk status of GDM. Most obstetricians employ universal screening of all women at 24–28 weeks which is a reasonable approach, especially in a popu-lation that contains ethnic groups with a higher prevalence of GDM.

SCREENING FOR GESTATIONAL DIABETES

Low Risk Status: Low risk status requires no glucose testing, but this category is limited to those women meeting all of the following criteria:
- Age <25 years
- Weight normal before pregnancy
- Member of an ethnic group with a low prevalence of GDM
- No known diabetes in first-degree relatives
- No history of abnormal glucose tolerance
- No history of poor obstetric outcome or macrosomic infant

High Risk Status: High risk status requires glucose testing as soon as pregnancy is diagnosed and again at 24–28 weeks if the early testing is normal. Women meeting any of these criteria should be tested early:
- Obesity
- Personal history of GDM or previous macrosomic infant
- Glycosuria
- Strong family history of diabetes

Women with a fasting blood glucose >125 mg/dl or a random or postprandial glucose of > 200 mg/dl meet the criteria for GDM and this precludes the need for any glucose challenge. All other high risk status women should be given a 50 gm glucose challenge (Glucola test) or proceed directly to a 100 gm oral glucose tolerance test as soon as they establish prenatal care. If initial testing is normal, repeat testing should be done at 24-28 weeks gestation.

Average Risk Status: These are women who do not fall in the low risk or high risk status. They should receive a 50 g glucose challenge at 24-28 weeks and if positive, undergo diagnostic testing with a 100 g 3 hour oral glucose tolerance test (3 hr OGTT).

---

50 Gram Glucola: The 50 g glucose challenge is the accepted screen for the presence of GDM but, if positive, must be followed by a diagnostic 100 g 3 hour oral glucose tolerance test (3 hr OGTT). A pos-itive screen is in the range of 130–140 mg/dl. The sensitivity and specificity of the test will depend on what threshold value is chosen, and the cutoff may be selected according to the prevalence of GDM in the population being screened. The test does not have to be performed fasting, but a serum sample must be drawn exactly 1 hour after administering the oral glucose.

Criteria for a Positive 50 Gram Glucola Challenge

Glucose > 140 mg/dl (7.8 mmol/l): Identifies ~80% of women with GDM at the cost of performing a 3 hr OGTT in ~15% of patients.

Glucose > 130 mg/dl (7.2 mmol/l): Identifies ~90% of women with GDM at the cost of performing a 3 hr OGTT in ~25% of patients.

100 Gram 3 hour OGTT: The 100 gm 3 hour test must be performed after 3 days of an unrestricted carbohydrate diet and while the patient is fasting. A positive test requires that two values be met or exceeded. One abnormal value should be followed with a repeated 3 hour test 1 month later because a single elevated value increases the risk of macrosomia and one third of patients will ultimately meet the diagnostic criteria for GDM.

Criteria for a Positive 100 gm OGTT	
Fasting glucose:	95 mg/dl
1 hour glucose:	180 mg/dl
2 hour glucose:	155 mg/dl
3 hour glucose:	140 mg/dl

10. What are the risks to the mother with GDM, and what are her risks of subsequently developing type 2 diabetes mellitus?

The immediate risks to the mother with GDM are an increased incidence of cesarean section (~30%), preeclampsia (~20-30%), and polyhydramnios (~20%), which can result in preterm labor. The long-term risks to the mother are related to recurrent GDM pregnancies and the substantial risk of developing type 2 diabetes mellitus. Women with GDM represent a group of patients with an extremely high risk (~50%) of developing type 2 diabetes in the subsequent 5–10 years. Women with fasting hyperglycemia, GDM diagnosed prior to 24 weeks (preexisting glucose intolerance) or obesity, those belonging to an ethnic group with a high prevalence of type 2 diabetes, or who demonstrate impaired glucose tolerance at 6 weeks postpartum have the highest risk. Women with GDM in multiple pregnancies also have a higher risk of developing type 2 diabetes. Counseling with regard to diet, weight loss, and exercise is essential and is likely to improve insulin sensitivity. Such dietary modifications should be adopted by the family, since the infant is also at increased risk of developing impaired glucose tolerance. Whether or not medications that may improve insulin sensitivity (metformin and thiazolidinediones) could be used in this high risk group of patients to prevent the development of type 2 diabetes is under current investigation.

11. What are the risks to the infant of a mother with GDM?

Even with the advent of screening and aggressive management of GDM, the incidence of neonatal complications ranges from 12 to 28%. The most common complication is macrosomia, which places the mother at increased risk of requiring a cesarean section and the infant at risk for shoulder dystocia. Shoulder dystocia can result in Erb's palsy, clavicular fractures, fetal distress, low APGAR scores, and even birth asphyxia when unrecognized. Shoulder dystocia occurs nearly 50% of the time when a 4500 g infant is delivered vaginally. If mothers have poor glycemic control, respiratory distress syndrome may occur in up to 31% of infants while cardiac septal hypertrophy may be seen in 35-40%. With extremely poor glucose control, there is also an increased risk of fetal mortality as a result of fetal acidemia and hypoxia. Common metabolic abnormalities in the infant of a GDM mother include neonatal hypoglycemia, hypocalcemia, hyperbilirubinemia, and polycythemia.

Women with GDM who require insulin or those who are not taking insulin but have suboptimal glycemic control should undergo fetal surveillance at ~32 weeks' gestation, and an earlier delivery should be considered after fetal lung maturity is confirmed by amniocentesis. Ultrasonography can often predict the risk of fetal macrosomia by measuring the abdominal circumference of the fetus at 29–33 weeks. An estimated fetal weight of > 4500 g carries such a high risk of shoulder dystocia that an elective cesarean section is usually recommended.

The long-term sequelae of GDM for offspring are much more controversial. Reports of an increased risk of adolescent obesity and of type 2 diabetes are compelling. Elevated amniotic fluid insulin levels (owing to fetal hyperinsulinemia as a result of maternal hyperglycemia) predicted teenage obesity in one study, independent of fetal weight, and one third of these offspring had impaired glucose tolerance by 17 years of age.

12. What causes women to get gestational diabetes mellitus?

GDM is caused by abnormalities in at least 3 aspects of fuel metabolism: insulin resistance, increased hepatic glucose production, and impaired insulin secretion. Insulin resistance is thought to be due primarily to the effects of increased production of human placental lactogen and placental growth hormone. There is also evidence of a decrease in the number of glucose transporters (GLUT-4) in adipocytes and an abnormal distribution of these transporters that results in reduced ability of insulin to recruit them to the cell surface. Reduced phosphorylation of the insulin receptor makes yet another contribution to insulin resistance in this state. Increased hepatic glucose production results mainly from excessive hepatic gluconeogenesis. Finally, impaired insulin secretion renders the individual unable to meet the requirement for greater insulin production necessitated by the insulin resistance and increased hepatic glucose production. These same pathophysiologic disorders, which are in large part genetically determined, make the GDM patient more likely to develop type 2 diabetes mellitus later in life, when weight gain and aging often contribute further to insulin resistance and impaired insulin secretion.

13. What is the best therapy for women with GDM? Specify the role of insulin and oral diabetes medications.

Women with GDM should be taught home glucose monitoring to ensure that their glycemic goals are being met throughout the duration of pregnancy. At a minimum, weekly fasting blood glucose and postprandial glucose determinations should be obtained. The best therapy for GDM depends entirely on the extent of the glucose intolerance and on the mother's response. In at least half of the cases, diet alone will maintain the fasting and postprandial blood glucose values within the target range. Since postprandial glucose levels have been most strongly associated with the risk of macrosomia, modest carbohydrate restriction to 35–40% of total calories may be helpful to blunt the postprandial glucose excursions. Women who weigh more than 130% of ideal body weight should be restricted to a caloric intake of ~24 kcal/kg and advised to limit their weight gain to no more than 15 lb. None of the oral diabetes medications (sulfonylureas, metformin, acarbose, or the thiazolidinediones) are currently approved for use in pregnancy. However, in a multicenter trial, 400 women with GDM were randomized to receive either insulin or glyburide after 24 weeks' gestation and maternal glycemic control, macrosomia, neonatal hypoglycemia, and neonatal outcome were no different between the groups. Most importantly, the cord serum insulin concentrations were similar in the two groups and glyburide was not detected in the cord serum of any infant.

Women who have fasting blood glucose levels > 95 mg/dl, 1 hour postprandial glucose levels >140 mg/dl or 2 hour postprandial glucose levels > 120 mg/dl should be started on insulin therapy. Those with large for gestational fetuses by ultrasound are also candidates for insulin. GDM can usually be treated with twice daily injections of NPH and Regular insulin, but occasionally postprandial glycemic excursions are so excessive that three times daily mealtime injections of Lispro (Humalog) are necessary. Alternative treatment with glyburide remains to be defined, since it has not yet been approved for use in pregnancy. Hypoglycemia tends to be an infrequent occurrence in these patients because of their underlying insulin resistance.

14. What is the role of exercise in patients with GDM?
It has been demonstrated that moderate exercise is well tolerated in pregnancy. Fetal safety has been established if the maternal heart rate is maintained < 150 beats per minute at durations of less than 1 hour and if the mother is well hydrated and does not get overheated. Two out of three trials in pregnancy have shown that exercise 3 times per week can achieve glycemic control and infant birth weights that are similar to those seen in women who are treated with insulin. Establishing a regular routine of modest exercise during pregnancy may also have long lasting benefits for the GDM patient who clearly has an appreciable risk of developing type 2 diabetes in the future. Home glucose monitoring must be continued throughout pregnancy to determine whether or not insulin therapy will be necessary. Women at risk for preterm labor or conditions predisposing to growth restriction are not candidates for a controlled exercise program.

15. How do diabetes and GDM affect fetal size?
Many theories have been generated over the years to explain the macrosomia associated with diabetes in pregnancy. Overall, the theory of excessive flux of maternal fuel to the conceptus holds the most credence and has the most supportive data. The figure below outlines the hypothesis of Freinkel, recently expanded upon by many authors. Diabetes in pregnancy is associated with increased delivery of glucose and amino acids to the fetus via the maternal circulation. There are also data to suggest that in GDM, glucose transport is facilitated across the placenta by increased expression of a placental glucose transporter. These fuels stimulate increased production of fetal insulin, which promotes somatic growth. Other

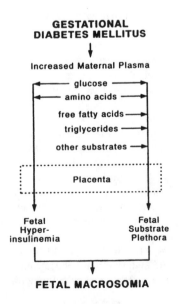

maternal substrates (e.g., free fatty acids, triglycerides) add to the burgeoning supply of fetal substrate and further support excessive growth. It is, therefore, the goal of management of pregnancies complicated by diabetes to normalize the above parameters with good metabolic control. Maternal obesity appears to be an independent risk factor, since some mothers who appear to have optimal metabolic control still give birth to macrosomic infants. Furthermore, macrosomia is not limited to the diabetic population; in fact, approximately 25% of macrosomic infants are born to mothers without GDM. In contrast, some women with type 1 diabetes, particularly those with extensive microvascular disease, may give birth to growth-restricted infants as a result of uteroplacental insufficiency.

16. Explain newborn hypoglycemia. Why does it happen? How should hypoglycemic newborns be followed and treated if necessary?

Approximately 25–50% of infants of diabetic mothers experience neonatal hypoglycemia during the first 4–6 hours of life (glucose < 40 mg/dl). These infants have hyperplastic or hyperfunctioning pancreatic islets because of the preceding intrauterine exposure to chronic glucose and amino acid excess and, as a result, have hyperinsulinemia. Affected infants should be monitored hourly for hypoglycemia until the first full feeding. Glucose reagent strips are not accurate in the low glucose ranges, and therefore all abnormal values need to be confirmed by the laboratory. Asymptomatic hypoglycemia can be treated with oral feedings. Symptomatic hypoglycemia should instead be treated with 300 μg/kg glucagon IV or IM followed by a glucose infusion with a 10% dextrose solution. Higher dextrose concentrations may actually increase insulin secretion and may thus exacerbate the problem.

17. What are the important postpartum management issues that should be addressed in women with pregestational or gestational diabetes?

A number of critical issues including maintenance of glycemic control, diet, exercise, weight loss, blood pressure management, breast feeding, contraception, and postpartum thyroiditis need to be addressed in the postpartum period. It has been demonstrated that the majority of women, even those who have been extremely compliant and who have had optimal glycemic control during pregnancy, have a dramatic worsening of their glucose control after the birth of their infants. Furthermore, many quit seeking medical care for their diabetes. The postpartum period is relatively neglected, therefore, as both the new mother and her physician relax their vigilance. However, this period offers a unique opportunity to institute health habits that could have highly beneficial effects on the quality of life of both the mother and her infant. A weight loss program consisting of diet and exercise should be instituted for women with GDM in order to improve their insulin sensitivity and, it is hoped, to prevent the development of type 2 diabetes. Home glucose monitoring should be continued in the postpartum period because insulin requirements drop almost immediately and often dramatically at this time, increasing the risk of hypoglycemia. Also, women who are candidates for an ACE inhibitor can be started on one of these agents at this time and enalapril has not been shown to appear in breast milk.

Women with a history of GDM should have their glycemic status reassessed at 6 weeks postpartum. Hyperglycemia generally resolves in the majority of patients during this interval but may persist in up to 10%. At the minimum, a fasting blood glucose should be performed to determine if the woman has persistent diabetes (glucose >125 mg/dl) or impaired fasting glucose tolerance (glucose of at least 110 mg/dl). A 75 g 2 hour glucose tolerance test is recommended by many, since a 2 hour value of at least 200 mg/dl establishes a diagnosis of diabetes and a 2 hour value of at least 140 mg/dl but less than 200 mg/dl makes the diagnosis of impaired glucose tolerance. The importance of diagnosing impaired glucose intolerance lies in its value in predicting the future development of type 2 diabetes. In one series, a diagnosis of impaired glucose tolerance was the most potent predictor of the development of type 2 diabetes in women with a history of GDM; 80% of such women developed diabetes in the subsequent 5–7 years. Intensified efforts promoting diet, exercise and weight loss should be instituted in these patients. Nondiabetic women with a history of GDM should then have annual measurements of their fasting glucose levels and lipid profiles.

Women should be encouraged to breast feed unless difficulties in glycemic control arise. None of the oral agents are approved for use while breast feeding, as it appears that the sulfonylureas and metformin cross into breast milk. It is recommended that insulin be continued in diabetic mothers who choose to breast feed. These women require an additional 300– 400 kcal per day to maintain their weight with breast feeding and need to make sure that their calcium intake is at least 1500 mg per day.

Finally, women with type 1 diabetes have been reported to have a 30% incidence of postpartum thyroiditis. Hyperthyroidism can occur in the 2–4 month postpartum period and hypothyroidism may present in the 4–8 month period. Given the significance of this disorder, a TSH measurement should be offered at 6 months postpartum and before this time if a patient has symptoms.

18. What are the contraceptive agents of choice for women with diabetes or who previously had gestational diabetes?

It should be documented at every visit that women are using or have been offered an effective birth control method. The vast majority of contraceptive methods are relatively safe in women with diabetes who do not have poorly controlled hypertension or hypertriglyceridemia and who are not at increased risk for thromboembolic disease. Triglycerides should be measured after the initiation of oral contraceptives in all women with diabetes or a history of GDM because of the significant incidence of hypertriglyceridemia and the associated risk of pancreatitis with oral estrogen use in these women. Low dose combined oral contraceptives have been shown to be effective and to have minimal metabolic effects in women with diabetes. In a retrospective cohort of 904 women with GDM, combined oral contraceptives did not influence the development of type 2 diabetes. Progestational agents such as Norplant, Depo-Provera, and norethindrone are also alternatives, although Depo-Provera and norethindrone may slightly affect carbohydrate tolerance. There is no increase in pelvic inflammatory disease with the use of intrauterine devices in women with well-controlled type 1 or type 2 diabetes after the post-insertion period. Therefore, this may be an attractive choice in older women who do not desire future pregnancies.

BIBLIOGRAPHY

1. American Diabetes Association: Gestational diabetes mellitus. Diabetes Care 23:S77–79, 2000.
2. American Diabetes Association: Preconception care of women with diabetes, Diabetes Care 23:S65–68, 2000.
3. De Viciana M, Major CA, Morgan MA, et al: Postprandial versus preprandial blood glucose monitoring in women with gestational diabetes mellitus requiring insulin therapy. N Engl J Med 333:1237–1241, 1995.
4. Garner P: Type I diabetes and pregnancy. Lancet 346:157–161, 1995.
5. Jones DC, Hayslett JP: Outcome of pregnancy in women with moderate or severe renal insufficiency. N Engl J Med 335:226–232, 1996.
6. Kenshole A, Ray J, Keely E. Type 1 and type 2 diabetes. In Lee RV, Rosene-Montella K, Barbour LA, et al (eds): Medical Care of the Pregnant Patient. Philadelphia, American College of Physicians, 2000, pp 253–272.
7. Kjos SL: Postpartum care of the woman with diabetes. Clinical Obstet Gynecol 43:75–90, 2000.
8. Kjos SL: Peters RJ, Xiang A, et al: Predicting future diabetes in Latino women with gestational diabetes. Diabetes 44:586–591, 1995.
9. Kuhl C: Etiology and pathogenesis of gestational diabetes. Diabetes Care 21:B19–26, 1998.

10. Langer O: Management of gestational diabetes. Clinical Obstet Gynecol 43:106–115, 2000.
11. Langer O, Conway DL, Berkus MD, et al: A comparison of glyburide and insulin in women with gestational diabetes. N Engl J Med 343:1134–8, 2000.
12. Metzger BE, Coustan DR, The Organizing Committee: Summary and recommendations of the Fourth International Workshop-Conference on gestational diabetes mellitus. Diabetes Care 21:B-161–167, 1998.
13. Naylor CD, Sermer M, Chen E , Farine D for the Toronto Trihospital Gestational Diabetes Project Investigators: Selective screening for gestational diabetes. N Engl J Med 337:1591–1596, 1997.
14. Silverman BL, Metzger BE: Impaired glucose tolerance in adolescent offspring of diabetic mothers. Diabetes Care 18:611–617, 1995.
15. Yamashita H, Shao J, Friedman JE: Physiologic and molecular alterations in carbohydrate metabolism during pregnancy and gestational diabetes. Clinical Obstet Gynecol 43:87–98, 2000.

6. INFECTIONS IN DIABETIC PERSONS

Robert H. Gates, M.D.

1. Are diabetic persons more likely to have an infection?

The short answer is yes. While an association with infection is still debated, the medical literature is replete with possible associations between diabetes and particular organisms or specific infectious disease syndromes. Examples include urinary tract infections, periodontitis, and rhinocerebral mucormycosis. Infection is not simply due to elevated serum glucose or the presence of serum ketoacidosis. Infections are more likely related to the effects of diabetes on target end-organs, as exemplified by decreased white cell function and a propensity to vaginal candidiasis. Other associations include peripheral neuropathy and foot ulcerations, incomplete cell basement membranes and bacterial myositis, decreased intestinal motility and salmonella infections, atherosclerosis and pulmonary aspiration. When infections do occur in diabetes, they may take longer to respond to therapy as exemplified by pneumococcal, *Legionella*, and influenza pneumonias.

2. Why do diabetic persons have more infections?

The propensity of diabetic persons to have more infections has been attributed to two broad pathophysiologic categories. The first involves abnormal host defenses. Evidence clearly supports the presence of abnormal white cell function, as shown by diminished ability of polymorphonuclear white cells to perform chemotaxis and phagocytosis, a reduced ability to release degranulation products, decreased production of free oxygen radicals, and impaired intracellular killing of organisms such as *Candida* sp. Defects in cell-mediated immunity, though less well defined, also contribute to the propensity for cryptococcal infection. In addition, poor control of diabetes may lead to malnutrition, which further impairs the function of the cell-mediated immune system.

The second category is end-organ dysfunction secondary to diabetes. This is best exemplified by the presence of neuropathy and vasculopathy, which are discussed more fully later. Other organ systems also have been found to have diabetes-related defects. For example, the propensity of diabetic patients to have staphylococcal and streptococcal infections of the muscles may be due to incomplete cell membrane linings, allowing easy ingress for bacteria.

3. Which infecting organisms are more common or prevalent in diabetes?

Although diabetic patients will usually have the same organisms causing infections as other patients, particular attention should be given to organisms seen more often in diabetic patients related to specific clinical circumstances. For example, in bacteremia associated with soft tissue infection, staphylococci and streptococci are predominant. In urinary tract infections, *Klebsiella* sp. is often found. Vaginitis is usually associated with *Candida* sp. Myositis is usually due to group B streptococci and staphylococci. A mixed aerobic and anaerobic infection is often found in necrotizing soft-tissue infections such as cellulitis or fasciitis.

4. Name the organisms and related infections associated with diabetes mellitus.

Infections and Organisms Associated with Diabetes

ORGANISMS	INFECTIONS
Group B streptococci	Pyomyositis, cellulitis

Staphylococci	Arthritis, pyomyositis, sternal wound infections after coronary artery bypass grafting, tunnel catheter infection in continuous ambulatory peritoneal dialysis
Mucormycoses	Rhinocerebral mucormycosis
Salmonella enteritidis	Gastrotenteritis
Clostridium septicum, mixed gram-negative aerobes and anaerobes	Necrotizing cellulitis and necrotizing fasciitis
Klebsiella sp.	Postoperative urinary tract infections
Candida sp.	Vaginitis, thrush, urinary tract infections
Cryptococcus sp.	Meningitis
Facultative gas-producing	Emphysematous cystitis and pyelonephritis aerobes and anaerobes
Pseudomonas aeruginosa	Invasive external otitis (formerly "malignant" external otitis)

5. Name the postoperative infections that diabetic persons are most prone to develop.

The most common is urinary tract infection. Review of prosthetic hip replacement series revealed a slightly increased risk of urinary tract infections after this procedure but not an increased risk of infection of the prosthetic device itself. However, the best studied postoperative infections in diabetic persons are sternal wound infections after coronary artery bypass grafting with internal mammary artery grafts. Data from these reports are conflicting, but it appears that bilateral internal mammary artery grafts are associated with an increase in sternal infections. Several reports have documented the increased risk of infection of the tunnel of catheters placed for chronic ambulatory peritoneal dialysis.

6. What should diabetic persons be told about the risk of blood-borne pathogens?

Education to prevent the transmission of blood-borne infection is necessary for all persons with diabetes. The risk of transmission of hepatitis B or human immunodeficiency virus (HIV) from a lancet needle, insulin syringe, or finger guard is not well studied but certainly exists. Syringes, platforms, and lancets should be considered medical waste and disposed of properly. Sharps disposal containers should be readily available in the homes of all HIV-infected diabetic patients who require invasive glucose monitoring or insulin therapy. More detailed recommendations are available in the guidelines from the American Association of Dental Examiners.

7. Vascular insufficiency is the most common cause of diabetic foot infection. True or false?

False. Neuropathy is by far the most common underlying reason for foot ulcerations leading to infection. The proposed pathogenesis goes as follows: uneven distribution of pressure on the plantar surface of the foot, perhaps aggravated somewhat by decreased fat within the foot, leads to microtrauma to the tissues, which serves as a portal of entry for bacteria that initially colonize the breaks. Superficial fungal infections likewise may serve as a portal of entry. The patient has no pain response to the initial trauma because of the underlying neuropathy; thus the trauma continues with associated tissue necrosis. Eventually, the motion of the structures within the foot promotes deeper bacterial colonization and spread, with secondary infection leading to increased local inflammation, release of inflammatory mediators, and further compromise in the ability to contain the initial infection. These events result in deep soft tissue and/or bone infection with associated necrosis that ultimately may lead to loss of the lower extremity, with or without associated bacteremia and sepsis.

8. What is the best way to culture a diabetic foot ulcer?

Despite controversy in the medical literature, it is fair to say that the organisms that cause disease in early infection are relatively few in number and often single, with staphylococci predominating. As infection progresses and further tissue necrosis occurs, the likelihood increases dramatically of multiple aerobic organisms and concurrent infection by anaerobic organisms. Swabs of ulcers on diabetic feet are basically worthless. Aspiration by needle through uninvolved tissue has been in vogue from time to time in recent years. The gold standard, of course, is deep biopsy of the involved tissue, with particular emphasis on obtaining bone for culture. A more recent proposal is initial debridement with gauze. Immediately after debridement of the overlying tissue, curettage of the base of the ulcer is performed and the material promptly submitted for culture. Curettage has shown the best correlation with deep biopsy. As a guide to interpretation of the culture, the specimen also should be submitted for Gram stain.

9. Which infection in diabetes causes the most morbidity?

In case you have not guessed by now, the answer is foot infection. Infections of the feet and their sequelae are most likely to lead to hospitalization. Approximately 1 of 5 diabetic patients admitted to the hospital has a foot infection. The estimated annual cost for such hospitalizations is greater than 200 million dollars. Approximately one fourth of the 16 million Americans with diabetes will have foot problems during the course of their disease. Roughly 1 in 15 of such patients will require a limb amputation for ultimate control. The annual rate of amputation is approximately 59.7 per 10,000 diabetics. Indeed, diabetes accounts for approximately one half of the 120,000 amputations performed in the United States each year.

10. Which tests or techniques are the most useful in defining the extent of disease in diabetic foot infections?

The successful management of diabetic foot infections depends on early detection and prompt attention to overt and occult sources of infection that may need to be drained or debrided, such as necrotic tissue, soft tissue abscesses, and particularly bony involvement. Attention also should be directed at the exclusion of macrovascular disease, which may be amenable to immediate corrective therapy with various techniques, such as percutaneous angioplasty, atherectomy, laser-guided atherectomy, and bypass surgery.

Defining the extent of disease plays a key role in duration of therapy and in surgical intervention. Plain radiographs may show abnormalities suggesting involvement of bone with infection; these changes, however, are often difficult to distinguish from those secondary to diabetic osteonecrosis. Bone scans are extremely sensitive for detecting the presence of infection; however, they are highly nonspecific in the setting of possible trauma and diabetic bony involvement. The specificity of bone scans is improved by coupling them with either a gallium scan or an indium-111 white blood cell scan. However, the spatial resolution of the scans is not good enough to allow precise definition of the involved structures. CT scan has proved to be useful for better resolution of the anatomy and associated soft tissue infection but not optimal for the delineation of the extent of bony involvement with infection. In the past several years, MRI has emerged as a key tool for defining the extent of disease. The MRI scan is as sensitive as the bone scan for detecting the presence of disease and at least as specific as the combination of bone scan and gallium or white blood cell scanning. MRI has the added advantage of not exposing the patient to the additional radiation required by a CT scan. The literature is full of reports of previously unsuspected bony or soft tissue involvement, the surgical correction of which led to enhanced resolution of the underlying infection.

11. How can diabetic persons decrease their risk of developing an infection?

The National Diabetes Advisory Board has suggested that more than 50% of lower extremity amputations can be avoided if careful attention is given to general principles. Patients should maintain good glucose control to maximize the function of the body's immune system and to help to prevent end-organ complications that contribute to infection. They also must practice good preventive foot care on a daily basis, be particularly wary of foreign bodies in their shoes, and be especially careful when breaking in a new pair of shoes. Diabetics need to pay close attention to health maintenance, with particular emphasis on available vaccinations to prevent pneumococcal and influenza pneumonia. A multidisciplinary approach to prevention and to management of problems when they occur is the key to success.

12. Does the presence of diabetes change the management of infection?

The presence of diabetes should raise the suspicion of comorbid conditions, such as underlying neuropathy, which may mask the signs and symptoms of disease; accelerated atherosclerotic changes, which may lead to vascular problems; and diminished renal function, which may require monitoring and change in antibiotic therapy. The presence of diabetes also should enhance awareness of the possibility of specific disease presentations, as exemplified by rhinocerebral mucormycosis in diabetic ketoacidosis. Gastroparesis may make the oral route of administration of antibiotics problematic. Cystopathy (poor bladder contractility) and a high rate of involvement of the upper tract in clinical cystitis will contraindicate short course antibiotic therapy. Bacteruria and urinary tract infection are more common in diabetic women than in non-diabetics or in diabetic men. The drugs used in the treatment of diabetes may have adverse interactions with antibiotics, e.g., sulfas like trimethoprim/sulfamethoxazole and macrolides such as clarithromycin may increase the blood levels of oral hypoglycemic agents leading to hypoglycemia. Component drugs in highly active antiretroviral therapy (HAART) can lead to pancreatic injury with worsening hyperglycemia.

13. Does the presence of infection change diabetes?

In addition to the propensity of infections to increase serum glucose levels, there may be persistent and resistant serum ketoacidosis, even in the presence of adequate glucose control. Control of the ketoacidosis usually requires adequate treatment of the underlying infection; in addition to appropriate antibiotics, management may require debridement of involved tissues and/or associated soft tissue abscesses. Infection that causes ketoacidosis is a leading cause of death in diabetes.

14. How can rational decisions be made regarding antibiotic therapy?

The general principles of selection of antibiotic therapy still hold. The setting always should be considered, even though it may be nonproductive. A history of an animal bite may alert the practitioner to the presence of organisms such as *Pasteurella* sp. A history of water exposure may suggest infection with *Aeromonas* sp. A puncture wound through a tennis shoe may lead to early consideration of anti-*Pseudomonas* therapy. The timing of presentation is also important. Early infection is more likely to have a solitary bacterial cause, whereas late disease with extensive necrosis suggests the presence of multiple organisms. The patient's allergies must be considered, along with route of administration of the drug. There is nothing magical about how the drug is delivered, whether it be intravenously or orally, as long as adequate serum levels are achieved with subsequently adequate tissue levels. Renal function should be assessed, because it may require dose modification or antibiotic change. Specific organisms should be considered; for example, with gram-positive organisms, staphylococcal and streptococcal coverage in the diabetic patient with soft tissue–associated bacteremia leads to the use of an antistaphylococcal agent. Urinary tract infection in the diabetic raises the prospect of multiple gram-negative organisms, particularly *Klebsiella* sp. Anaerobes should be covered when tissue necrosis is present.

In addition, the "zebras" listed in question 4 should be considered. Rhinocerebral mucormycosis should be considered in patients with ketoacidosis who present with an eschar in the nose. The patient with relatively subtle signs of meningitis and a negative routine culture may have infection with cryptococci. Emphysematous cystitis or pyelonephritis may be a clue to the presence of anaerobic organisms, such as *Clostridia* sp. or facultative gas-forming, gram-negative aerobes. Multiple antibiotics are available with adequate coverage if appropriate empiric therapy is based on the clinical setting.

15. What are the potential complications of urinary tract infection in the diabetic patient?

The patient with diabetes may have the same complications that any other patient may have, with the additional concern of ketoacidosis. Underlying diabetes-associated bladder neuropathy with poor emptying and functional obstruction in urine flow has been suggested as a unifying pathogenesis that may lead to some complications that occur more frequently:

- **Bacteremia**
- **Renal papillary necrosis** must be considered in patients with severe pyelonephritis, flank pain, hematuria, and slow or no response to therapy. Imaging studies may show obstruction, and histologic examination of urine sediment may reveal papillary fragments.
- **Obstructing fungus ball with candiduria** should be considered in patients with failure to clear candiduria or early relapse after an apparent response to therapy. The presence of a urinary catheter has been noted as a risk factor.
- **Emphysematous cystitis and pyelonephritis** are characterized by the appearance of gas in the bladder or kidney, respectively, with signs and symptoms of severe infection and a high mortality. Gas-forming organisms of the enterobacteriaceae are the usual culprits, although *Clostridia* sp. also may cause infection in the bladder. Surgery to include nephrectomy reduces mortality.
- **Emphysematous pyelitis** is distinct from cystitis and pyelonephritis and denotes gas in the renal collecting system. Although rare and not usually quite as deadly as emphysematous pyelonephritis, the presence of urinary obstruction should make one consider this complication.
- •**Renal and perirenal abscess** should be suspected in the clinical setting that is the same as renal papillary necrosis. Diagnostic imaging studies (i.e., CT scan) help to make the diagnosis.

16. Does diabetes itself have an infectious case?

This fascinating question has been asked and debated for the last 40 years or so in the medical literature. The answer is not completely known. At least for early onset or juvenile diabetes, there appears to be an autoimmune component with a strong individual genetic propensity for the autoimmune destruction of the pancreas over time. Enteroviruses, particularly coxsackie B, have been proposed as the antecedent infection that may trigger the destructive autoimmune response.

BIBLIOGRAPHY

1. Bessman AN, Sapico FL: Infections in the diabetic patient: The role of immune dysfunction and pathogen virulence factors. J Diabetic Complications 6:258–262, 1992.
2. Deresinki S: Infections in the diabetic patient: Strategies for the clinician. Infect Dis Reports 6:1–12, 1995.
3. Joshi N, Caputo GM, Weitekamp MR, Karchmer AW: Infections in patients with diabetes mellitus. N Engl J Med 16: 1906–1912, 1999.

4. Lipsky BA, Pecorano RE, Wheat LJ:The diabetic foot: Soft tissue and bone infection. Infect Dis Clin North Am 4:409–429, 1990.
5. Nelson KE, Vlahov D, Cohn S, et al: Human immunodeficiency virus infection and diabetes intravenous drug users. JAMA 266:2259–2261, 1991.
6. Patterson JE, Andriole VT: Bacterial urinary tract infections in diabetes. Infect Dis Clin North Am 11: 735–750, 1997.
7. Schwartz B, Schuchat A, Oxtoby MJ, et al: Invasive Group B streptococcal disease in adults. JAMA 266:1112–1114, 1991.
8. Shea KW: Antimicrobial therapy for diabetic foot infections. Postgrad Med 106: 85–94, 1999.
9. Wachtel TJ, Tetu-Mouradjian LM, Goldman DL, et al: Hyperosmolality and acidosis in diabetes mellitus. J Gen Intern Med 6:495–502, 1991.
10. Weinstein D, Wang A, Chambers R, et al: Evaluation of magnetic resonance imaging in the diagnosis of osteomyelitis in diabetic foot infections. Foot Ankle 14:18–22, 1993.

7. HYPOGLYCEMIA

Fred D. Hofeldt, M.D., and Holly A. Batal, M.D.

1. What is the definition of hypoglycemia?

Hypoglycemia was defined by the Third International Symposium on Hypoglycemia as a blood glucose value of less than 50 mg/dl (2.8 mmol/L). Clinically, hypoglycemia is defined using Whipple's triad: a low plasma glucose level, symptoms consistent with hypoglycemia, and resolution of these symptoms with correction of the low glucose level.

2. In diagnosing hypoglycemia, what are the important clinical features?

The symptoms of hypoglycemia can be divided into two categories. **Adrenergic symptoms** are catecholamine mediated and include diaphoresis, palpitations, apprehension, anxiety, headaches, and weakness. **Neuroglycopenic symptoms** include reduced intellectual capacity, confusion, irritability, abnormal behavior, convulsions, and coma. The occurrence of symptoms in either the fasting or postprandial state is used to categorize the etiology of the hypoglycemia. The **fasting hypoglycemic disorders** generally result from organic conditions and frequently present with symptoms of neuroglycopenia. **Postprandial hypoglycemia** (reactive hypoglycemia) is thought to arise from a functional disturbance and is usually associated with adrenergic symptoms. Although this separation is important for clinical classification, it is artificial and patients may have mixed-component symptoms.

3. What are the causes of fasting hypoglycemia?

Pancreatic disorders
  Islet beta-cell hyperfunction (adenoma, carcinoma, hyperplasia, nesidioblastosis)
  Islet alpha-cell hypofunction or deficiency
Hepatic disorders
  Severe liver disease (cirrhosis, hepatitis, carcinomatosis, circulatory failure, ascending cholangitis)
  Enzyme defects (glycogen storage disease, galactosemia, hereditary fructose intolerance, familial galactose and fructose intolerance, fructose-1,6-diphosphatase deficiency)
Pituitary-adrenal disorders
  Hypopituitarism, Addison's disease, congenital adrenal hyperplasia
Central nervous system disease (hypothalamus or brainstem)
Muscle (hypoalaninemia?)
Nonpancreatic neoplasms
  Mesodermal tumors (spindle cell fibrosarcoma, leiomyosarcoma, mesothelioma, rhabdomyosarcoma, liposarcoma, neurofibroma, reticulum cell sarcoma)
  Adenocarcinoma (hepatoma, cholangiocarcinoma, gastric carcinoma, adrenocortical carcinoma, cecal carcinoma)
Unclassified
  Excessive loss or utilization of glucose and/or deficient substrate (prolonged or strenuous exercise, fever, lactation, pregnancy, renal glycosuria, diarrheal states, chronic starvation)
  Ketotic hypoglycemia of childhood (idiopathic hypoglycemia of childhood)
Exogenous causes
  Iatrogenic (related to treatment with insulin or oral hypoglycemic agents)
  Factitious (seen especially in paramedical personnel)

Pharmacologic (Akee nut, salicylates, antihistamines, monoamine oxidase inhibitors, propranolol, phenylbutazone, pentamidine, phentolamine, alcohol, angiotensin-converting enzyme inhibitors)

4. What are the causes of postprandial or reactive hypoglycemia?
Reactive to refined carbohydrate (glucose, sucrose)

Reactive hypoglycemia
Alimentary hypoglycemia (previous gastrointestinal surgery, peptic ulcer disease, disordered gastrointestinal motility syndromes, and functional gastrointestinal disease)
Early type 2 diabetes mellitus
Hormonal (hyperthyroidism; hypothyroidism; deficiency of cortisol, epinephrine, glucagon, or growth hormone)
Idiopathic
Other conditions
Deficiency of early hepatic gluconeogenesis (fructose-1,6-diphosphatase deficiency)
Drugs (alcohol, lithium)
Insulinoma
Insulin or insulin-receptor autoantibodies
Reactive to other substrate (fructose, leucine, galactose)

5. What are the artifactual causes of hypoglycemia?
Pseudohypoglycemia occurs in certain chronic leukemias when the leukocyte counts are markedly elevated. This artifactual hypoglycemia reflects utilization of glucose by leukocytes after the blood sample has been drawn. Such a hypoglycemic condition, therefore, is not associated with symptoms. Pseudohypoglycemia also may occur in patients with hemolytic anemia or polycythemia through similar mechanisms. Other artifactual hypoglycemias may be seen with improper sample collection or storage, errors in analytic methodology, or confusion between whole blood and plasma glucose values. The plasma glucose is about 15% higher than corresponding whole blood glucose values.

6. When hypoglycemia occurs, what counterregulatory events occur to spare glucose for brain metabolism?
Glucagon and epinephrine are the dominant counterregulatory hormones. Other hormones that respond to hypoglycemic stress are norepinephrine, cortisol, and growth hormone, but their effects are delayed. The metabolic effects of glucagon and epinephrine are immediate: stimulation of hepatic glycogenolysis and later gluconeogenesis result in increased hepatic production of glucose. Glucagon appears to be the most important counterregulatory hormone during acute hypoglycemia. When glucagon secretion is intact, recovery from hypoglycemia occurs promptly. If glucagon secretion is decreased or absent, catecholamines serve as the principal counterregulatory hormones.

7. Which laboratory tests assist in evaluation of fasting hypoglycemia?
Simultaneous measurement of fasting blood glucose and insulin levels during the occurrence of symptoms is the most important laboratory test. Other potentially important tests include measurement of C-peptide, sulfonylurea levels, renal function, liver function, insulin antibody levels, and plasma cortisol. Hypoglycemia with inappropriate hyperinsulinemia suggests conditions of autonomous insulin secretion, such as those seen in the spectrum of insulinoma (adenoma, carcinoma, hyperplasia and nesidioblastosis) or in the factitious use of insulin or hypoglycemic agents. When the hypoglycemia occurs with correspondingly suppressed insulin values, the noninsulin-mediated causes of fasting hypoglycemia need to be evaluated.

8. Which laboratory tests assist in evaluating patients suspected of having an insulinoma?

In patients with pancreatic insulinomas, inappropriate insulin secretion results in excessive insulin despite the presence of hypoglycemia. During symptomatic hypoglycemia, patients have high insulin values and an increased ratio of insulin to glucose (I/G ratio > 0.33). A similar hormone profile may be seen in patients who have ingested an oral sulfonylurea; a drug screen separates the two entities. Usually proinsulin is less than 10–20% of total fasting insulin immunoreactivity; this proportion is increased in patients with insulinomas (80%) but not in patients with an overdosage of an oral sulfonylurea.

9. Which tests distinguish factitious insulin administration from insulinoma?

The measurement of C-peptide levels during a hypoglycemic episode helps to distinguish these two conditions. Patients with insulinomas have evidence of excessive endogenous insulin secretion as characterized by high values of insulin, proinsulin, and C-peptide during hypoglycemia. Patients who self-administer insulin, in contrast, have suppressed function of beta islet cells; C-peptide levels are low (< 0.5 mg/ml) during hypoglycemia, whereas insulin values are elevated. The presence of insulin antibodies is also strong evidence of exogenous insulin administration. Of note, patients who inadvertently or factitiously take oral sulfonylureas have laboratory results similar to those of the patient with an insulinoma, including an elevated C-peptide value; their proinsulin level, however, is normal, and their sulfonylurea level is elevated.

10. When suspicion of an insulinoma is high but the work-up is inconclusive, what additional studies may be performed?

A supervised 48-hour fast with measurements of glucose and insulin every 6 hours, and any time the patient becomes symptomatic, will unmask the hypoglycemia in most patients with insulinomas. Hypoglycemia is usually evident within 24 hours of fasting. Exercise will often evoke hypoglycemia in the insulinoma patient who remains asymptomatic after 48 hours of fasting.

11. Which conditions cause beta-cell hyperinsulinemia?

In 75–85% of cases the cause of the insulinoma syndrome is a pancreatic islet-cell adenoma. Multiple adenomas (adenomatosis) are present in about 10% of cases. Carcinomas cause 5–6% of cases and an additional 5–10% have islet-cell hyperplasia.

12. If other family members have pancreatic tumors, what condition is suggested?

Multiple endocrine neoplasia type 1 (MEN-1) occurs as an autosomal dominant condition characterized by functioning and nonfunctioning pituitary tumors, parathyroid hyperplasia, and islet-cell tumors, most commonly insulinomas and gastrinomas (Zollinger-Ellison syndrome). Such pancreatic tumors may secrete other polypeptides, including glucagon, pancreatic polypeptide, somatostatin, adrenocorticotropic hormone (ACTH), melanocyte-stimulating hormone (MSH), serotonin, and growth hormone–releasing factor. When this condition is suspected, family members should be screened for the components of MEN-1. However, only about 5–10% of insulinomas are associated with MEN-1.

13. After a diagnosis of pancreatic islet-cell hyperinsulinemia is established, what procedures are helpful to localize the tumor?

Procedures such as ultrasound, celiac angiography, aortography, and abdominal CT scan are frequently insensitive and localize only about 60% of insulinomas. Some insulinomas are extremely small (less than a few millimeters) and easily escape detection. Endoscopic ultrasonography may be useful in these cases. Transhepatic portal venous sampling may localize occult tumors and help to distinguish between an isolated insulinoma and diffuse disease (adenomatosis, hyperplasia, or nesidioblastosis). Intraoperative ultrasound is also useful for localizing pancreatic tumors.

14. If surgical resection is not possible or the patient has metastatic or inoperable carcinoma, adenomatosis, hyperplasia, or nesidioblastosis, what medications may control the hypoglycemia?

Diet (frequent feeding and snacks) is the cornerstone of medical management. The most commonly used medication is diazoxide, which inhibits insulin release. Phenytoin, propranolol, verapamil, and octreotide have also been used. Various chemotherapeutic agents can be used for islet-cell carcinoma.

15. What are the causes of childhood hypoglycemia?

Hyperinsulinemic hypoglycemia in children can be result from the same diseases that cause this condition in adults, although nesidioblastosis is seen more commonly in children. Nesidioblastosis is a type of islet-cell hyperplasia in which primordial pancreatic ductal cells remain undifferentiated islet cells capable of polyhormonal secretion (insulin, gastrin, pancreatic polypeptide, and glucagon). It is the leading cause of hyperinsulinemic hypoglycemia in newborns and infants but may also cause hypoglycemia in adolescents and adults.

Hypoinsulinemic hypoglycemia in infants and young children suggests an inherited disorder of intermediary metabolism, such as the glycogen storage diseases, gluconeogenic disorders (deficiencies of fructose-1,6-diphosphatase, pyruvate carboxylase, and phosphoenolpyruvate carboxykinase), galactosemia, hereditary fructose intolerance, maple syrup urine disease, carnitine deficiency, and ketotic hypoglycemia. Hormonal deficiencies (glucagon, growth hormone, thyroid and adrenal hormones) also may cause hypoglycemia. Furthermore, children are highly susceptible to accidental drug overdose, especially with salicylates and alcohol.

16. What are the most common drugs that cause hypoglycemia in adults?

In adults, drugs are the most common cause of hypoglycemia. Responsible drugs include insulin, the diabetic oral agents, ACE inhibitors, ethanol, propranolol, and pentamidine. An extensive list of drugs associated with hypoglycemia in 1418 cases is included in the reference by Seltzer.

17. How does alcohol cause hypoglycemia?

Ethanol may produce hypoglycemia 6–36 hours after ingestion of even modest amounts (100 g). Alcohol acutely inhibits hepatic gluconeogenesis through alterations of the cytosol $NADH_2/NAD$ ratio. Hypoglycemia from alcohol ingestion generally occurs only in patients who also have impaired glycogenolysis as a result of depletion of hepatic glycogen stores from fasting or chronic malnutrition. It is therefore the combination of acutely impaired gluconeogenesis and ineffective glycogenolysis that results in alcohol-induced hypoglycemia.

18. On occasion, hypoglycemia is caused by non-islet-cell tumors. Which tumors are implicated? What is the mechanism of the hypoglycemia?

Various mesenchymal tumors (mesothelioma, fibrosarcoma, rhabdomyosarcoma, leiomyosarcoma, liposarcoma, and hemangiopericytoma) and organ-specific adenocarcinomas (hepatic, adrenocortical, genitourinary, and mammary) may be associated with hypoglycemia. Hypoglycemia also may occur with pheochromocytomas, carcinoid tumors, and hematologic malignancies (leukemia, lymphomas, and myeloma). The mechanism varies according to the type of tumor, but in many cases hypoglycemia is associated with tumor-related malnutrition and weight loss owing to fat, muscle, and tissue wasting that impairs both hepatic gluconeogenesis and glycogenolysis. In some cases, utilization of glucose by exceptionally large tumors may cause hypoglycemia. Tumors also may secrete hypo-glycemic factors, such as insulin-like growth factor–1 (IGF-1) and, more notably, IGF-2. By binding to hepatic insulin receptors, IGF-2 inhibits hepatic glucose production and thereby promotes hypoglycemia. Also suspect are tumor cytokines, particularly tumor necrosis factor (cachectin). Rarely does a tumor secrete extrapancreatic insulin.

19. What autoimmune syndromes are associated with hypoglycemia?

Autoantibodies directed against insulin receptors or insulin itself may provoke hypo-glycemia. Insulinomimetic anti-receptor antibodies bind to the insulin receptor and mimic insulin action by increasing tissue uptake of glucose. Autoantibodies that bind circulating insulin may undergo dissociation from insulin at inappropriate times, often during the early postprandial fasting period; this acutely raises serum free insulin levels, causing hypoglycemia. Such an autoimmune insulin syndrome has been observed most often in Japanese patients and frequently occurs in the presence of other autoimmune diseases, such as Graves' disease, rheumatoid arthritis, systemic lupus erythematosus, and type 1 diabetes mellitus.

20. What other endocrine disorders are associated with hypoglycemia?

Hypoglycemia may be seen in patients with anterior pituitary insufficiency due to deficient secretion of growth hormone, ACTH, and TSH. In addition, primary adrenal insufficiency and primary hypothyroidism may be associated with either fasting or reactive hypoglycemia.

21. When is hypoglycemia attributed to underlying medical illness?

Frequently, medically ill patients have multiple reasons for developing hypoglycemia, including renal failure, hepatic dysfunction, medications, and poor dietary intake. Hepatic failure leads to hypoglycemia because of the liver's role in gluconeogenesis and glycogenolysis. The hypoglycemia of congestive heart failure, sepsis, and lactic acidosis is also likely owing to hepatic dysfunction. Starvation states, such as anorexia nervosa and protein calorie malnutrition, also cause hypoglycemia.

22. What conditions cause reactive hypoglycemia?

The vast majority of patients with reactive hypoglycemia have idiopathic reactive hypo-glycemia since they have not been found to have any underlying disease of the gastroin-testinal tract (alimentary reactive hypoglycemia), hormone deficiency, or diabetic reactive hypoglycemia. Most patients with idiopathic reactive hypoglycemia have a delayed dis-charge of insulin (dysinsulinism) that occurs inappropriately in conjunction with postpran-dial glucose levels that have peaked and are already beginning to fall. Occasionally, the patient with an insulinoma or pheochromocytoma may present with hypoglycemia that appears to be reactive because it occurs after a meal. Patients with insulin autoantibodies may have a sudden dissociation of insulin from antibody binding in the postprandial state. Reactive hypoglycemia also has been noted in some patients who take prescribed lithium and in those who consume gin-and-tonic cocktails. In the gin and tonic reactive hypo-glycemia, the alcohol impairs epinephrine and growth hormone counter-hormonal respon-siveness to the hypoglycemic stress.

23. What are the characteristics of the hypoglycemia that may occur in patients with malignant pheochromocytomas?

Both reactive and fasting hypoglycemia can occur in these patients. Noteworthy is the observation that severe reactive hypoglycemia may occur following surgical removal of these malignant tumors. Although the mechanism for the hypoglycemia in pheochromocytoma patients remains unknown, most likely the excessive secretion of catecholamines is responsible through stimulation of insulin secretion or through a post-receptor mechanism.

24. What conditions should be considered in the patient self-diagnosed with reactive hypoglycemia?

This type of hypoglycemia may be more correctly termed idiopathic postprandial syndrome. Usually Whipple's triad is not fulfilled, in that chemical hypoglycemia cannot be demonstrated during symptoms. Frequently, underlying neuropsychiatric disease, anxiety, or situational stress reactions are the real culprits of the episodic symptoms, which the patient characterizes or self-diagnoses as reactive hypoglycemia. Although hypoglycemic disorders are uncommon, symptoms suggestive of hypoglycemia are quite common.

25. How is reactive hypoglycemia diagnosed?

Reactive hypoglycemia occurs within 5 hours of food intake (usually between 2 and 4 hours). The diagnosis is made by eliminating other causes of the symptoms and documenting hypoglycemia during the occurrence of symptoms. The supervised 48-hour fast can exclude an insulinoma. The oral glucose tolerance test probably no longer plays a role in the diagnosis.

BIBLIOGRAPHY

1. Arem R: Hypoglycemia associated with renal failure. Endocrinol Metab Clin North Am 18:103–121, 1989.
2. Arky RA: Hypoglycemia associated with liver disease and ethanol. Endocrinol Metab Clin North Am 18:75–90, 1989.
3. Fajans SS, Vinik AI: Insulin-producing islet cell tumors. Endocrinol Metab Clin North Am 18:45–74, 1989.
4. Field JB: Hypoglycemia: Definitions, clinical presentation, classification, and laboratory tests. Endocrinol Metab Clin North Am 18:27–44, 1989.
5. Flanagan D, Wood P, Sherwin R, et al: Gin and tonic and reactive hypoglycemia. J Clin. Endocrinol Metab 83:796-800, 1998.
6. Gorman B, Charboneau JW, James EM, et al: Benign pancreatic insulinoma: Preoperative and intraoperative sonographic localization. AJR 147:929–934, 1986.
7. Hirshberg B, Livi A, Bartlett DL, et al: Forty-eight hour fast: The diagnostic test for insulinoma. J Clin Endocrinol Metab 85: 3222-3226, 2000.
8. Hofeldt FD: Reactive hypoglycemia. Endocrinol Metab Clin North Am 18:185–201, 1989.
9. Haymond MW:Hypoglycemia in infants and children. Endocrinol Metab Clin North Am 18: 211–252, 1989.
10. Lefebve PJ, Andreani D, Marks V, et al: Statement on "postprandial" reactive hypoglycemia. In Hypoglycemia, Serono Symposium. New York, Raven Press, 1987, p 79.
11. Marks V, Teale JD: Tumours producing hypoglycaemia. Endocrine-Related Cancer 5:11-129, 1998.
12. Palardy J, Haurarkova J, Lepage R, et al: Blood glucose measurements during symptomatic episodes in patients with suspected postprandial hypoglycemia. N Engl J Med 321:1421–1425, 1989.
13. Rosch T, Lightdale CJ, Botet JF, et al: Localization of pancreatic endocrine tumor by endoscopic ultrasonography. N Engl J Med 326:1726–1736, 1992.
14. Seltzer HS: Drug-induced hypoglycemia. Endocrinol Metab Clin North Am 18:163–183, 1989.
15. Service FJ: Hypoglycemic disorders. N Engl J Med 332:1144–1152, 1995.
16. Service FJ: Hypoglycemia. In DeGroot LJ (ed): Endocrinology. Philadelphia, W.B. Saunders, 1995, pp 1605–1623.
17. Service FJ, McMahon MM, O'Brien PC, et al: Functioning insulinoma—incidence, recurrence and long term survival of patients. Mayo Clin Proc 66:711–719, 1991.
18. Shapiro ET, Bell GI, Polonsky KS, et al: Tumor hypoglycemia: Relationship to high molecular weight insulin-like growth factor II. J Clin Invest 85:1672–1679, 1990.
19. Skogseid BJ, Eriksson B, Lundquist G, et al: Multiple endocrine neoplasia type I. J Clin Endocrinol 73:281–287, 1991.
20. Whipple AO: The surgical therapy of hyperinsulinism. J Int Chir 3:237–276, 1938.

8. LIPID DISORDERS

Michael T. McDermott, M.D.

1. What are the major lipids in the bloodstream?

Cholesterol and triglycerides are the major circulating lipids. Cholesterol is utilized by cells throughout the body for the synthesis and repair of membranes and intracellular organelles. The adrenal glands and gonads also use cholesterol as a substrate to synthesize adrenal steroid and gonadal steroid hormones. Triglycerides are an energy source that can be stored as fat in adipose tissue or burned as fuel by muscle and other tissues.

2. What are lipoproteins?

Cholesterol and triglycerides are not water-soluble and therefore cannot be transported through the bloodstream as individual molecules. Lipoproteins are large spherical particles that package these lipids into a core surrounded by a shell of water-soluble proteins and phospholipids. Lipoproteins serve as vehicles that transport cholesterol and triglycerides from one part of the body to another.

3. What are the major lipoproteins in the bloodstream?

Chylomicrons, very-low-density lipoproteins (VLDLs), low-density lipoproteins (LDLs), and high-density lipoproteins (HDLs) are the major circulating lipoproteins. Their functions are shown below.

Lipoprotein	Function
Chylomicrons	Transport dietary triglycerides from the gut to adipose tissue and muscle
VLDLs	Transport endogenous triglycerides from the liver to adipose tissue and muscle
LDLs	Transport cholesterol from the liver to peripheral tissues
HDLs	Transport cholesterol from peripheral tissues to the liver

4. What are the apoproteins?

Apoproteins are located on the surface of the lipoproteins. They function as ligands for binding to lipoprotein receptors and as cofactors for metabolic enzymes. Their function are listed below.

Apoprotein	Function
Apoprotein A	Ligand for peripheral HDL receptors
Apoprotein B	Ligand for peripheral and hepatic LDL receptors
Apoprotein E	Ligand for hepatic receptors for remnant particles
Apoprotein C-II	Cofactor for lipoprotein lipase (removes triglycerides from chylomicrons and VLDL, leaving remnant particles)

5. Name some of the other enzymes and transport proteins that are important in lipoprotein metabolism.

Enzyme/Protein	Function
HMG CoA reductase	The rate limiting enzyme in hepatic cholesterol synthesis
Lipoprotein lipase (LPL)	Removes triglycerides from chylomicron and VLDL particles in adipose tissue, leaving remnant particles

Hepatic lipase	Removes remaining triglycerides from remnant particles in the liver, converting them into LDL particles
Lecithin cholesterol acyl transferase (LCAT)	Esterifies cholesterol molecules on the surface of HDL particles, drawing them into the HDL core
Cholesterol ester transfer protein (CETP)	Shuttles esterified cholesterol back and forth between HDL and LDL particles

6. Give a brief summary of overall lipoprotein metabolism.

Triglycerides enter the circulation through the diet (exogenous) or by hepatic synthesis (endogenous). Chylomicrons transport dietary triglycerides and VLDLs transport endogenous triglycerides to adipose tissue and muscle, where lipoprotein lipase (LPL), acting with its co-factor apoprotein C-II, breaks down triglyceride molecules into fatty acids and monoglycerides. Fatty acids then exit the lipoproteins and enter adipose cells, where they are resynthesized into triglycerides and stored as fat or enter muscle cells, where they are burned as fuel. The remnant particles then return to the liver, where hepatic lipase converts the VLDL remnants into LDL particles filled with cholesterol synthesized in the liver. LDL particles transport this cholesterol to peripheral tissues which have LDL receptors that recognize the apoprotein B molecule on the LDL surface. LDL is next internalized and degraded by lysozymes to make cholesterol molecules available for synthesis and repair of membranes and intracellular organelles. Excess LDL particles that are not cleared by LDL receptors remain in the circulation and are later cleared by the scavenger system. Nascent HDL particles, from the liver and intestines, also circulate and dock on peripheral tissues that have receptors for apoprotein A that resides on the HDL particle. Cholesterol molecules attach to the HDL surface and are subsequently esterified and drawn into the HDL core by the enzyme lecithin cholesterol acyl transferase (LCAT). Another protein, cholesterol ester transfer protein (CETP), functions to shuttle cholesterol back and forth between HDL particles bound for the liver and outgoing LDL particles to ensure the proper distribution of cholesterol destined for peripheral utilization or hepatic disposal.

7. Describe the pathogenesis of the atherosclerotic plaque.

LDL particles may be modified by oxidation. Oxidized LDL is preferentially cleared by scavenger macrophages located throughout the body; some lie within or beneath the intima of the arteries. As macrophages engulf LDL particles, they become lipid-laden foam cells, which secrete growth factors that stimulate smooth muscle cell and fibroblast proliferation. The conglomeration of foam cells, smooth muscle cells, and fibroblasts forms the atherosclerotic plaque. These plaques also attract inflammatory cells, which secrete proteolytic enzymes that may weaken the fibromuscular plaque cap and make it prone to rupture. Once rupture occurs, platelets aggregate and release chemicals that promote vasoconstriction and initiate thrombus formation, which may ultimately occlude the artery.

8. Are elevated serum triglyceride levels harmful?

Serum triglyceride levels that exceed 250 mg/dl appear to be associated with atherosclerosis. Triglyceride elevations are often accompanied by low levels of HDL cholesterol and by small, dense LDL particles that are more easily oxidized and that may therefore be more atherogenic. Thus it is unclear whether atherosclerosis results from elevated triglycerides or from the associated changes in HDL and LDL particles that usually accompany hypertriglyceridemia. Triglyceride levels greater than 1000 mg/dl significantly increase the patient's risk of developing acute pancreatitis.

9. What is lipoprotein(a)?

Apoprotein(a) has approximately 85% amino acid sequence homology with plasminogen. When an apoprotein(a) molecule binds to an apoprotein B on the surface of an LDL particle, the new particle is referred to as lipoprotein(a). Excessive lipoprotein(a) promotes atherosclerosis, possibly because it is easily oxidized and engulfed by macrophages and/or because it inhibits thrombolysis.

10. What are the primary dyslipidemias?

Primary dyslipidemias are inherited disorders of lipoprotein metabolism. The major primary dyslipidemias are listed below.

Primary Dyslipidemia	Phenotype
Familial hypercholesterolemia	↑↑Cholesterol
Familial combined hyperlipidemia	↑Cholesterol and ↑triglycerides
Familial dysbetalipoproteinemia	↑Cholesterol and ↑triglycerides
Polygenic hypercholesterolemia	↑Cholesterol
Familial hypertriglyceridemia	↑Triglycerides

11. What is familial hypercholesterolemia?

Familial hypercholesterolemia is an inherited disease characterized by extreme elevations of serum cholesterol but normal serum triglyceride levels. The disorder is usually caused by a genetic mutation resulting in absent or deficient LDL receptors in peripheral tissues; some cases, however, result from a genetic mutation producing a defective apoprotein B that cannot be recognized by LDL receptors. Homozygous patients frequently have serum cholesterol levels of 800–1200 mg/dl and die of coronary artery disease (CAD) before age 20 years. Heterozygotes have cholesterol levels of 300–600 mg/dl and often manifest CAD before age 50 years. Tendon xanthomas are characteristic of this disorder.

12. What is familial combined hyperlipidemia?

Familial combined hyperlipidemia is an inherited disorder characterized by variable elevations of both serum cholesterol and triglycerides. The condition results from excessive hepatic synthesis of apoprotein B and, therefore, excessive production of apoprotein B–rich VLDL and LDL particles. Affected patients typically have elevations of both cholesterol and triglycerides, although the levels of each may vary greatly over time. These patients are prone to develop premature CAD.

13. What is familial dysbetalipoproteinemia?

Familial dysbetalipoproteinemia is an inherited condition characterized by significant and relatively balanced elevations of both serum cholesterol and triglycerides. It is sometimes referred to as type III hyperlipidemia. This disorder results from an abnormal apoprotein E phenotype (E2/E2), which binds poorly to hepatic receptors and thus impairs the clearance of circulating VLDL remnants by the liver. Affected patients often develop premature CAD. Planar xanthomas in the creases of the palms and soles of the feet are a characteristic finding in patients with this disorder.

14. What is polygenic hypercholesterolemia?

Polygenic hypercholesterolemia, which is characterized by mild to moderate elevations of serum cholesterol alone, is the most common type of inherited hypercholesterolemia. This condition generally occurs when two or more mild defects of cholesterol metabolism combine to elevate the serum cholesterol level. Affected patients have an increased risk of developing CAD.

15. What is familial hypertriglyceridemia?

Familial hypertriglyceridemia is an inherited condition characterized by moderate to severe elevations of serum triglycerides with normal serum cholesterol levels. The disorder results from excessive hepatic triglyceride synthesis, producing triglyceride-enriched VLDL particles. It is not known to be associated with a high risk of CAD. However, if serum triglyceride levels are sufficiently elevated, affected individuals are at an increased risk for the development of acute pancreatitis.

16. How do you distinguish among familial combined hyperlipidemia (FCH), familial dysbetalipoproteinemia (FDL) and familial hypertriglyceridemia (FHT)?

Because FCH and FDL are characterized by combined elevations of both cholesterol and triglycerides, additional tests may be necessary to make the distinction. Patients with FCH have increased serum apoprotein B levels, whereas patients with FDL have an E2/E2 apoprotein E phenotype and a broad beta band on lipoprotein electrophoresis. Since FCH and FHT may both present with isolated hypertriglyceridemia, an apoprotein B measurement, which will be elevated only in FCH, can help to distinguish these two disorders.

17. Name the secondary dyslipidemias.

The secondary dyslipidemias are serum lipid elevations that result from systemic diseases such as diabetes mellitus, hypothyroidism, nephrotic syndrome, renal disease, obstructive liver disease, and dysproteinemias. Lipids also may be increased by medications such as beta blockers, diuretics, estrogens, progestins, androgens, retinoids, corticosteroids, cyclosporine, phenothiazines, anticonvulsants, and certain antiviral agents used in the treatment of HIV infection. These dyslipidemias usually improve when the primary disorder is treated or the offending drugs are discontinued.

18. What is the cause of severe elevations of serum triglycerides?

Triglyceride levels above 1000 mg/dl are considered to be severely elevated and pose a very high risk for the development of acute pancreatitis. Most patients with such severe triglyceride elevations have a combination of a primary triglyceride disorder, such as familial hypertriglyceridemia or familial combined hyperlipidemia, and a secondary disorder, most commonly poorly controlled diabetes mellitus, alcohol abuse, or the use of HIV medications.

19. When should lipid disorders be treated?

The National Cholesterol Education Program (NCEP) guidelines are based on CAD risk factors and the serum LDL cholesterol level. Individual patients are considered to have a risk factor for each of the following criteria they meet: male sex with age over 45 years, female sex with age over 55 years, family history of premature CAD (before age 45 in a male relative and age 55 in a female relative), smoking, hypertension, diabetes mellitus, and a serum HDL level less than 35 mg/dl. An HDL level greater than 60 mg/dl warrants subtraction of one risk factor. Risk factors are totaled and patients are placed into one of three categories for treatment decisions based on their LDL levels.

Patient Risk	Goal	Diet, if	Drugs, if
No CAD, <2 risk factors	LDL < 160	LDL > 160	LDL > 190
No CAD, 2 or more risk factors	LDL < 130	LDL > 130	LDL > 160
Known CAD	LDL < 100	LDL > 100	LDL > 130

The American Diabetes Association recommends treating to a goal LDL cholesterol level of 100 mg/dl in all diabetic patients. Triglyceride levels above 200 mg/dl should be treated with diet. Drugs should be added if the triglycerides exceed 500 mg/dl after dietary intervention.

20. What dietary alterations lower serum cholesterol and triglycerides?
Serum cholesterol generally can be lowered approximately 5–10% by decreasing dietary intake of cholesterol and saturated fats. The American Heart Association step 1 or step 2 diet is recommended. Serum triglycerides often respond to the same measures coupled with reductions in the intake of refined carbohydrates, starches, and alcohol. Increasing dietary fiber also appears to be beneficial.

21. What medications most effectively lower serum LDL cholesterol?

Medication	LDL reduction (%)
Statins	20–60
Bile acid resins	15–25
Niacin	15–25
Fibrates	10–15

22. Do the statins differ in LDL-lowering potencies?
Yes. The currently available statins and their approximate LDL-lowering capabilities are as follows:

Medication	LDL reduction (%)
Fluvastatin	15–25
Lovastatin	25–35
Pravastatin	25–35
Cerivastatin	25-35
Simvastatin	30–40
Atorvastatin	40–60

23. What medications significantly lower triglycerides?

Medication	Triglyceride reduction (%)
Fibrates	30–50
Niacin	20–30
Statins	10–20
Fish oils	Variable

24. What medications most effectively raise serum HDL cholesterol levels?

Medication	HDL increase (%)
Niacin	10–25
Fibrates	10–20
Statins	5–10

25. Is aggressive reduction of serum LDL cholesterol with medication an effective strategy for primary prevention of CAD?
There have been two large prospective primary prevention trials, the West of Scotland Study (WOSCOPS) and the Air Force/Texas Coronary Atherosclerosis Prevention Study (AFCAPS/TexCAPS) examining this question. In both studies, LDL cholesterol reduction with statin medications (pravastatin in WOSCOPS; lovastatin in AFCAPS/TexCAPS) significantly reduced the risk of developing a first myocardial infarction and the need for coronary revascularization procedures.

26. Is aggressive reduction of serum LDL cholesterol with medication an effective strategy for secondary prevention in patients with established CAD?
This question has been addressed by three large prospective secondary prevention trials, the Scandinavian Simvastatin Survival Study (4S), the Cholesterol and Recurrent Events

Trial (CARE), and the Long-Term Intervention with Pravistatin in Ischemic Disease Study (LIPID). These studies clearly demonstrated that aggressive LDL cholesterol lowering with statins (simvastatin in 4S, pravastatin in CARE and LIPID) significantly reduces the risk of recurrent myocardial infarctions, cardiovascular death, strokes, and the need for revascularization procedures. The Atorvastatin Versus Revascularization Treatment Study (AVERT) also found that aggressive LDL cholesterol reduction with atorvastatin was more effective in reducing ischemic events than was coronary angioplasty.

27. Can established CAD lesions be reduced by lipid lowering therapy?
Angiographic studies have demonstrated that aggressive lipid-lowering programs can halt progression or induce regression of coronary lesions in patients with known CAD (FATS Study) or previous bypass surgery (Post CABG Study).

28. Do interventions that raise serum HDL cholesterol or lower triglycerides have a significant effect on coronary events?
The Helsinki Heart Study (HHS) and the Veterans Affairs High Density Lipoprotein Cholesterol Intervention Study (VA-HIT) examined the effects of gemfibrozil in dyslipidemic patients without (HHS) and with (VA-HIT) known CAD. In both studies, a 6-8% increase in HDL cholesterol associated with a 30-40% reduction in serum triglycerides significantly lowered the incidence of subsequent major CAD events.

29. Is antioxidant therapy effective in preventing CAD?
Because LDL is oxidized before it is taken up by scavenger macrophages, antioxidant therapy with vitamin E, vitamin C, and beta carotene has come under investigation. Evidence suggests that higher vitamin E intakes are associated with a lower risk of developing CAD in both men and women. Although there is no definitive prospective proof of efficacy, vitamin E supplements have been recommended as adjunctive therapy by many experts.

30. What role does inflammation play in the atherosclerotic process?
Inflammation within the atherosclerotic plaque may make the plaque less stable and more likely to rupture, thereby precipitating an acute ischemic event. Highly sensitive measurements of C-reactive protein (hsCRP), a nonspecific marker of inflammation, have been developed and studied as possible markers to identify patients at increased risk for the development of coronary events. Such a marker might aid providers in making decisions about which patients to treat more aggressively. However, the role of this marker in the evaluation of CAD at this point remains to be determined.

31. Outline an approach to the treatment of a patient with hypercholesterolemia.
The patient with hypercholesterolemia should first be instructed on an American Heart Association (AHA) diet, which is low in cholesterol and saturated fats, and should be advised to exercise, doing at least 30 minutes of aerobic work daily. Any secondary causes of hypercholesterolemia, such as hypothyroidism, should also be treated. If the serum LDL cholesterol level is more than 30 mg/dl above the risk-stratified NCEP goal levels, it is appropriate to prescribe a statin medication. The patient should be reevaluated in 3 months, at which time he/she should be queried about compliance and side effects, particularly muscle aches and/or weakness. Blood samples should be obtained for a lipid profile, AST or ALT, and creatine kinase (CK).

When the LDL goal is not met, an increase in the statin dosage should be considered. In general, approximately a 6% further LDL reduction can be expected for each dosage increment above the initial statin dose. Once a statin is half the maximal dose or above, one may also consider adding either a bile acid resin or niacin. Bile acid resins should be avoided in patients with concomitant triglyceride elevations and niacin should be avoided, or used cautiously, in patients with diabetes mellitus, gout, or peptic ulcer disease. A high risk patient, particularly someone with familial hypercholesterolemia, who continues to have substantial LDL elevations despite the above measures, may benefit from more aggressive and costly measures such as plasmapheresis or specific LDL pheresis.

32. How should you manage the patient with hypertriglyceridemia?

The patient with hypertriglyceridemia should be counseled on an AHA diet with additional emphasis on reducing the intake of refined carbohydrates, starches and alcohol. A daily aerobic exercise regimen is also recommended. Secondary causes of hypertriglyceridemia, such as uncontrolled diabetes mellitus, alcohol abuse, and the use of HIV medications, should be addressed and corrected, if possible.

Drug therapy should be considered if triglyceride levels remain above 250 mg/dl and should definitely be initiated for triglyceride levels above 500 mg/dl. Fibrates (gemfibrozil, fenofibrate) are the most potent agents for treatment of this condition, although niacin is also effective. Niacin may be used as monotherapy or may be added to fibrates for patients who remain hypertriglyceridemic. Niacin should be avoided, or used with caution, in patients with diabetes mellitus, gout and peptic ulcer disease. Fish oils containing omega-3 fatty acids (eicosapentaenoic acid—EPA; docosahexaneoic acid—DHA) may also be added for nonresponders. The desired intake of combined EPA and DHA is 3000–6000 mg/day. Statins also have modest triglyceride lowering effects.

Serum triglyceride levels above 1000 mg/dl must be lowered quickly because of the high risk of precipitating acute pancreatitis. Medications alone are not effective when triglyceride levels are this high. Patients must immediately be placed on a very low fat (less than 5% fat) diet until the triglyceride level is less than 1000 mg/dl. Such a diet lowers serum triglycerides approximately 20% each day. Contributing factors that can be altered, such as poorly controlled diabetes mellitus and alcohol abuse, must simultaneously be addressed. Once serum triglyceride levels are less than 1000 mg/dl, the most effective medications to further reduce serum triglycerides are the fibrates. If these medications do not lower serum triglycerides sufficiently, niacin, fish oils, or a statin may be added to the regimen.

33. How does one treat the patient with mixed hyperlipidemia?

For the patient with an elevated LDL cholesterol level and serum triglycerides between 200 and 400 mg/dl, attention should first be focused on LDL reduction with diet, exercise, treatment of secondary hyperlipidemias, and statin therapy. If serum triglyceride levels remain above 250 mg/dl once LDL levels are below the goal, one may consider the addition of a fibrate (gemfibrozil, fenofibrate) or niacin. In doing so, one must be fully aware of the increased risk of provoking a myopathy (elevated CK, and even rhabdomyolysis) with combination therapy. Muscle symptoms and serum CK levels must therefore be carefully monitored in such patients.

When the patient with mixed hyperlipidemia has a triglyceride level of 400–1000 mg/dl, triglyceride management should be addressed first. Treatment consists of diet, exercise, correction of secondary hyperlipidemias, and drug therapy with either a fibrate or niacin. Once triglyceride levels are below 400 mg/dl, persistently elevated LDL levels should be treated either with a statin or niacin, again with vigilant monitoring for the development of myopathy.

If the serum triglyceride level is greater than 1000 mg/dl, the patient should be treated, as discussed in question 32, with a very low fat (less than 5% fat) diet until the triglyceride level is less than 1000 mg/dl and then with triglyceride lowering medications.

BIBLIOGRAPHY

1. Brown G, Albers JJ, Fisher LD, et al: Regression of coronary artery disease as a result of lipid-lowering therapy in men with high levels of apolipoprotein B. N Engl J Med 323:1289–1296, 1990. (FATS Study.)
2. Criqui MG, Heiss G, Cohn R, et al: Plasma triglyceride level and mortality from coronary artery disease. N Engl J Med 328:1220–1225, 1993.
3. Diaz MN, Frei B, Vita JA, Keaney JF: Antioxidants and atherosclerotic heart disease. N Engl J Med 337:408–416, 1997.
4. Downs JR, Clearfield M, Weis S, et al: Primary prevention of acute coronary events with lovastatin in men and women with average cholesterol levels: Results of AFCAPS/TexCAPS. Air Force/Texas Coronary Atherosclerosis Prevention Study. JAMA 279:1615–1622, 1998. (AFCAPS/TexCAPS Study.)
5. Expert Panel on Detection, Evaluation, and Treatment of High Blood Cholesterol in Adults: Summary of the second report of the National Cholesterol Education Program (NCEP) Expert Panel on Detection, Evaluation, and Treatment of High Blood Cholesterol in Adults (Adult Treatment Panel II). JAMA 269:3015–3023, 1993.
6. Gordon DJ, Rifkind BM: High density lipoprotein—the clinical implications of recent studies. N Engl J Med 321:1311–1316, 1989.
7. Henkin Y, Como JA, Oberman A: Secondary dyslipidemia. Inadvertent effects of drugs in clinical practice. JAMA 267:961–968, 1992.
8. Jha P, Flather M, Lonn E, et al: The antioxidant vitamins and cardiovascular disease. Ann Intern Med 123:860–872, 1995.
9. Knopp RH: Drug treatment of lipid disorders. N Engl J Med 341:498-511, 1999.
10. Kroon AA, van Asten WNJC, Stalenhoef AFH: Effect of apheresis of low-density lipoprotein on peripheral vascular disease in hypercholesterolemic patients with coronary artery disease. Ann Intern Med 125:945–954, 1996.
11. Levine GN, Keaney JF, Vita JA: Cholesterol reduction in cardiovascular disease. Clinical benefits and possible mechanisms. N Engl J Med 332:512–521, 1995.
12. The Lipid Study Group: Prevention of cardiovascular events and death with pravastatin in patients with coronary heart disease and a broad range of initial cholesterol levels. N Engl J Med 339:1349–1357, 1998. (LIPID Study.)
13. Manninen V, Elo MO, Frick MH, et al. Lipid alteration and decline in the incidence of coronary heart disease in the Helsinki Heart Study. JAMA 260:641–651, 1988. (Helsinki Heart Study.)
14. Pitt B, Waters D, Brown WV, et al: Aggressive lipid-lowering therapy compared with angioplasty in stable coronary artery disease. N Engl J Med 341:70–76, 1999. (AVERT Study)
15. The Post Coronary Artery Bypass Graft Trial Investigators: The effect of aggressive lowering of low-density lipoprotein cholesterol levels and low-dose anticoagulation on obstructive changes in saphenous-vein coronary-artery bypass grafts. N Engl J Med 336:153–162, 1997. (Post CABG Study.)
16. Prosser LA, Stinnett AA, Goldman PA, et al: Cost-effectiveness of cholesterol-lowering therapies according to selected patient characteristics. Ann Intern Med 132:769–779, 2000.
17. Rich-Edwards JW, Manson JE, Hennekens CH, et al: The primary prevention of coronary heart disease in women. N Engl J Med 332:1758–1766, 1995.
18. Ridker PM, Hennekens CH, Buring JE, Rifai N: C-reactive protein and other markers of inflammation in the prediction of cardiovascular disease in women. N Engl J Med 342:836–843, 2000.
19. Rosenson RS: Low levels of high density lipoprotein cholesterol (hypoalphalipoproteinemia). An approach to management. Arch Intern Med 153:1528–1538, 1993.
20. Rubins HB, Robins SJ, Collins D, et al: Gemfibrozil for the secondary prevention of coronary heart disease in men with low levels of high-density lipoprotein cholesterol. N Engl J Med 341:410–418, 1999. (VA-HIT Study.)
21. Sacks FM, Pfeffer MA, Moye LA, et al: The effect of pravastatin on coronary events after myocardial infarction in patients with average cholesterol levels. N Engl J Med 335:1001–1009, 1996. (CARE Study.)
22. Scandinavian Simvastatin Survival Study Group: Randomised trial of cholesterol lowering in 4444 patients with coronary heart disease: The Scandinavian Simvastatin Survival Study (4S). Lancet 344: 1383–1389, 1994. (4S Study.)

23. Scanu AM (moderator): Lipoprotein(a) and atherosclerosis. Ann Intern Med 115:209–218, 1991.
24. Schectman G, Hiatt J. Dose-response characteristics of cholesterol-lowering drug therapies: Implications for treatment. Ann Intern Med 125:990–1000, 1996.
25. Shepherd J, Cobbe SM, Ford I, et al: Prevention of coronary heart disease with pravastatin in men with hypercholesterolemia. N Engl J Med 333:1301–1307, 1995. (WOSCOPS Study.)
26. Walden CC, Hegele RA: Apolipoprotein E in hyperlipidemia. Ann Intern Med 120:1026–1036, 1994.

9. OBESITY

Daniel H. Bessesen, M.D.

1. What is obesity?

Obesity is a degree of overweight that is associated with increases in morbidity and mortality. The concept of "ideal body weight" originated with the Build and Blood Pressure Study published in 1959 and followed up in 1979. That study provided the data that were the basis of the Metropolitan Life Insurance tables used by most primary care physicians over the plast 30 years. That data demonstrated a j-shaped relationship between body weight and mortality. People who weighed less than or more than a certain amount experienced excessive mortality rates. The concept of an ideal body weight has subsequently been questioned. More recent studies suggest that the increase in mortality observed in underweight individuals was related to smoking (smokers weigh less than nonsmokers) and preexisting cancer, which were not controlled for in earlier studies. Newer data demonstrate that the relationship between body weight and mortality is more linear when corrected for preexisting illness and smoking. This relationship has been shown for women in the large Nurses Health Study cohort and men in the Harvard Alumni Study, for example, and it holds as people age as well, as demonstrated by the recent American Cancer Society study.

2. Describe how obesity is diagnosed.

With a decreasing interest in the use of ideal body weight tables, most experts advocate the use of the body mass index (BMI) to diagnose obesity. The BMI is calculated by dividing weight in kilograms by height in meters squared. A BMI of 25 or less is normal; 25–29.9, overweight; 30–34.9, mild obesity; 35–39.9, moderately obese; and >40, severe or morbid obesity.

It is not only the BMI that determines the health risks of obesity, but also the distribution of fat. A growing number of studies have demonstrated that excessive adipose tissue in a central or upper-body distribution (android or male pattern) is associated with a greater risk of adverse health consequences than lower-body obesity (gynoid or female pattern). Previously, the ratio of the waist circumference to the maximum circumference of the hips was used to describe central fat distribution. However, more recently it has been appreciated that it is the absolute amount of central fat that confers adverse health risks. For this reason, the waist circumference is now the favored measure to risk stratify patients based on fat distribution. High risk is conferred in men by a waist circumference greater than 40 inches (>102 cm) and in women by a waist circumference greater than 35 inches (>88 cm). Waist circumference is most useful in risk stratifying individuals whose BMI is between 25 and 30. In this intermediate risk area, those with an increased waist circumference deserve greater efforts directed at preventing further weight gain, while those with a smaller waist circumference can be reassured that their weight does not pose major health hazards.

3. Discuss the health consequences of obesity.

Obesity is clearly associated with some of the most common illnesses affecting contemporary society, including diabetes; hypertension; hyperlipidemia; coronary artery disease; degenerative arthritis; gallbladder disease; and cancer of the endometrium, breast, prostate, and colon. The incidence of these conditions rises steadily as body weight increases. (See figures below.) It is surprising how risks increase with even modest gains in weight. Health risks are magnified with advancing age and a positive family history of these diseases.

Body Weights in Pounds According to Height and Body Mass Index*

Body Weight (pounds)

Height (inches)																	
58	91	96	100	105	110	115	119	124	129	134	138	143	148	153	158	162	167
59	94	99	104	109	114	119	124	128	133	138	143	148	153	158	163	168	173
60	97	102	107	112	118	123	128	133	138	143	148	153	158	163	168	174	179
61	100	106	111	116	122	127	132	137	143	148	153	158	164	169	174	180	185
62	104	109	115	120	126	131	136	142	147	153	158	164	169	175	180	186	191
63	107	113	118	124	130	135	141	146	152	158	163	169	175	180	186	191	197
64	110	116	122	128	134	140	145	151	157	163	169	174	180	186	192	197	204
65	114	120	126	132	138	144	150	156	162	168	174	180	186	192	198	204	210
66	118	124	130	136	142	148	155	161	167	173	179	186	192	198	204	210	216
67	121	127	134	140	146	153	159	166	172	178	185	191	198	204	211	217	223
68	125	131	138	144	151	158	164	170	177	184	190	197	203	210	216	223	230
69	128	135	142	149	155	162	169	176	182	189	196	203	209	216	223	230	236
70	132	139	146	153	160	167	174	181	188	195	202	209	216	222	229	236	243
71	136	143	150	157	165	172	179	186	193	200	208	215	222	229	236	243	250
72	140	147	154	162	169	177	184	191	199	206	213	221	228	235	242	250	258
73	144	151	159	166	174	182	189	197	204	212	219	227	235	242	250	257	265
74	148	155	163	171	179	186	194	202	210	218	225	233	241	249	256	264	272
75	152	160	168	176	184	192	200	208	216	224	232	240	248	256	264	272	279
76	156	164	172	180	189	197	205	213	221	230	238	246	254	263	271	279	287
77	160	168	177	185	193	202	210	219	227	235	244	252	261	269	278	286	294
78	164	173	181	190	198	207	216	224	233	242	250	259	268	276	285	293	302
BMI =	**19**	**20**	**21**	**22**	**23**	**24**	**25**	**26**	**27**	**28**	**29**	**30**	**31**	**32**	**33**	**34**	**35**

Body Weights in Pounds According to Height and Body Mass Index* (continued)

Body Weight (pounds)

Height (inches)	36	37	38	39	40	41	42	43	44	45	46	47	48	49	50	51	52
58	172	177	181	186	191	196	201	205	210	215	220	224	229	234	239	244	248
59	178	183	188	193	198	203	208	212	217	222	227	232	237	242	247	252	257
60	184	189	194	199	204	209	215	220	225	230	235	240	245	250	255	261	266
61	190	195	201	206	211	217	222	227	232	238	243	248	254	259	264	269	275
62	196	202	207	213	218	224	229	235	240	246	251	256	262	267	273	278	284
63	203	208	214	220	225	231	237	242	248	254	259	265	270	278	282	287	293
64	209	215	221	227	232	238	244	250	256	262	267	273	279	285	291	296	302
65	216	222	228	234	240	246	252	258	264	270	276	282	288	294	300	306	312
66	223	229	235	241	247	253	260	266	272	278	284	291	297	303	309	315	322
67	230	236	242	249	255	261	268	274	280	287	293	299	306	312	319	325	331
68	236	243	249	256	262	269	276	282	289	295	302	308	315	322	328	335	341
69	243	250	257	263	270	277	284	291	297	304	311	318	324	331	338	345	351
70	250	257	264	271	278	285	292	299	306	313	320	327	334	341	348	355	362
71	257	265	272	279	286	293	301	308	315	322	329	338	343	351	358	365	372
72	265	272	279	287	294	302	309	316	324	331	338	346	353	361	368	375	383
73	272	280	288	295	302	310	318	325	333	340	348	355	363	371	378	386	393
74	280	287	295	303	311	319	326	334	342	350	358	365	373	381	389	396	404
75	287	295	303	311	319	327	335	343	351	359	367	375	383	391	399	407	415
76	295	304	312	320	328	336	344	353	361	369	377	385	394	402	410	418	426
77	303	311	320	328	337	345	354	362	370	379	387	396	404	413	421	429	438
78	311	320	328	337	346	354	363	372	380	389	397	406	415	423	432	441	449
BMI =	**36**	**37**	**38**	**39**	**40**	**41**	**42**	**43**	**44**	**45**	**46**	**47**	**48**	**49**	**50**	**51**	**52**

*Each entry gives the body weight in pounds for a person of a given height and bBMI. Pounds have been rounded off. To use the table, find the appropriate height in the left-hand column. Move across the row to a given weight. The number at the top of the column is the BMI for the height and weight.

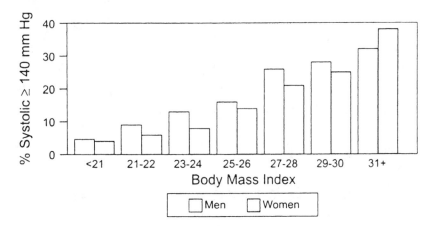

Body mass index and the risk of hypertension. (Canadian Guidelines for Healthy Weights. Cat. no. H39-134 1989e; 1988:69.)

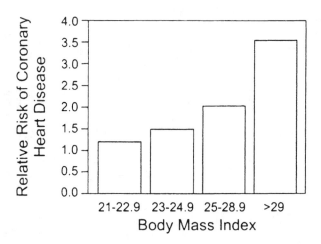

Body mass index and the risk of coronary disease.

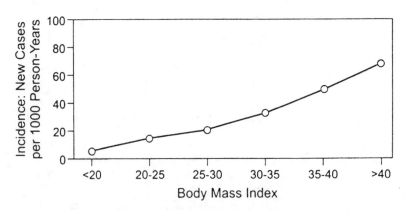

Body mass index and the risk of diabetes. (From Knowler WC, et al: Am J Epidemiol 113:144–156, 1981, with permission.)

4. What are the economic consequences of obesity?

In a study done in 1995, the overall cost of obesity, defined as BMI greater than 30 kg/m^2, totaled $70 billion in 1995 dollars, 7.2% of national health care costs for that year. Included were $16.2 billion for cardiovascular disease, $36.6 billion for diabetes, $7.6 billion for hypertension, and $1.5 billion for breast and colon cancer. This estimate does not include cost of musculoskeletal disorders, which may almost double the total figure. In addition, the loss in wages and productivity attributed to obesity likely exceeds $30 billion per year.

5. Describe the psychological complications of obesity.

Situational depression and anxiety related to obesity are common. The obese person may suffer from discrimination that contributes further to difficulty with poor self-image and social isolation. In one study, obese adolescents were compared with adolescents who had other chronic health problems. Both groups were followed for 7 years. At the end of this period, obese women were 20% less likely to be married, made $6,700/yr less in income, and experienced poverty at a 10% higher rate than controls. This effect was independent of baseline aptitude test scores and socioeconomic status. The concern shown by patients over how their weight affects their lives is profound. It may be difficult or impossible for a care provider who has never experienced discrimination based on obesity to understand the scope of these effects.

6. How common is obesity?

Obesity has reached epidemic proportions in the United States. The National Health and Nutrition Examination Survey [NHANES III]) conducted by the federal government in 1990 demonstrated that one third of all adult Americans were overweight (defined as 20% above ideal body weight) at that time. A more recent study from the Centers for Disease Control found that the prevalence of obesity (defined as a BMI >30 kg/m^2) increased from 12.0% of the adult population in 1991 to 17.9% in 1998. This increase was observed in all states, in both sexes, across age and race groups, and occurred regardless of educational level. The greatest increase in prevalence has been seen in young people ages 18-29 yr.

7. Describe the causes of obesity.

The regulation of body weight is complex with multiple interrelated systems controlling caloric intake, macronutrient content of the diet, energy expenditure, and fuel metabolism. Models of obesity in mice have provided new and fundamental insights into the mechanisms involved in body weight regulation and have helped to foster a change in the way that people think about obesity. Professionals are increasingly viewing obesity as a chronic metabolic disease much like diabetes or hypertension. This model requires a conceptual shift from the previous widely held belief that obesity is simply a cosmetic or behavioral problem. Although the identification of a number of novel gene products involved in the regulation of body weight is exciting, it is important not to forget the complexity of the processes regulating weight. There is a tendency to want a single-gene answer to a this common metabolic problem.

Development of obesity requires a period of positive energy balance; that is, energy intake must exceed energy expenditure. In addition, there must be a dietary source of carbons that ultimately are excessively accumulated as triglycerides within adipose tissue. For this process to occur, the system regulating body weight and composition must be altered, ultimately achieving a new steady state. Maintaining energy balance is one of the most important jobs of any organism. Between ages 20 and 60 yr, the average human eats over 32 tons of food. A sustained negative imbalance between energy intake and expenditure is potentially life-threatening within a relatively short time. To maintain energy balance the organism must assess energy stores within the body; assess the nutrient content of the diet;

determine if the body is in negative energy or nutrient balance; and adjust hormone levels, energy expenditure, nutrient movement, and consumptive behavior in response to these assessments. These tremendously complex events involve thousands of gene products.

8. Do abnormal genes cause obesity?

Obesity is clearly more common in people who have family members who are also obese. A number of studies have shown that the tendency to gain weight in a modern environment, or following a period of overeating, is partly genetically determined. However, the prevalence of obesity has dramatically increased in the past 60 years at a time when there has been almost no change in the human gene pool. The problem of human obesity is a classic interaction between genes and environment. The genes that we possess to regulate body weight evolved somewhere between 200,000 and 1 million years ago. The environmental factors controlling nutrient acquisition and habitual physical activity were dramatically different then. Efforts directed at identifying genes that predispose to obesity not only hold the promise of identifying important pathophysiologic mechanisms, but also may reveal novel targets for therapies.

9. What is leptin? Does abnormal leptin secretion cause obesity?

Leptin is a hormone that is secreted by adipose tissue; it was discovered in 1994. Its name comes from the Greek word *leptos* meaning thin. Leptin was cloned from the ob/ob mouse model of obesity that was first described in 1950. The obese phenotype of this mouse model is transmitted in an autosomal recessive manner. Parabiotic experiments suggested that a normal mouse made obese by tube feeding, monosodium glutamate (MSG) feeding, or ventromedial hypothalamic nucleus lesioning produced a humoral signal that decreased feeding in its parabiotic partner. An ob mouse parabiosed to a normal mouse, however, reduced its intake of food and its body weight. This experiment suggested that the ob mouse had a genetic disorder resulting in ineffective production of the humoral factor that decreased feeding in response to obesity. In ob mice, the administration of leptin produces sustained weight loss through both decreases in food intake and increases in energy expenditure. The weight loss occurs largely from fat mass with little loss in lean body mass.

Leptin is also produced in humans. However, there have been only three cases in which leptin deficiency was identified as a cause of human obesity out of thousands of individuals studied. Many studies have shown that leptin levels are actually increased in obese compared with lean humans. Leptin is secreted by adipose tissue in proportion to its mass. It appears to be a reliable marker of total body adiposity and is highly correlated with other markers of body fat. Much of the leptin in the plasma compartment circulates in a protein-bound form. A number of studies have demonstrated that leptin levels are higher in women than in men and fall with aging. Obese humans have increased levels of free leptin. Most human obesity then is associated with leptin resistance rather than leptin deficiency. Leptin levels fall with prolonged fasting but are unaffected by dietary macronutrient composition. Resistance to exogenous leptin along with obesity can be induced in rats by high-fat feeding. Recent studies in which recombinant human leptin was administered to obese humans found that this hormone did not substantially reduce weight. This disappointing result suggests that the regulation of body weight is controlled by more than just the circulating level of leptin.

Another physiologic role for leptin has recently received attention: regulation of the reproductive axis. It has been known for a long time that marked reductions in the mass of adipose tissue in the body interfere with normal reproductive function. Some investigators hypothesized that leptin evolved less as a satiety hormone and more as a signal to the reproductive axis of adequate fuel stores. In this context it is interesting to note that the ob mouse is infertile and that fertility is restored with leptin administration. Support for this idea has come from recent observations that leptin levels increase just before the onset of sexual maturation in mice and that the time of sexual maturation can be accelerated by the administration of exogenous leptin.

10. Is leptin resistance due to an abnormal leptin receptor?

The family of leptin receptors was cloned from another autosomal recessive animal model of obesity: the db/db mouse. These mice become obese and diabetic. In parabiotic experiments with db mice conjoined to normal mice, no weight reduction was seen in db/db mice. On the contrary, the normal partner quit eating and lost weight. These experiments were interpreted as indicating that the db mouse produced the circulating satiety factor but had a defect in its receptor. In 1995, a group of alternately spliced leptin receptor forms were identified. These proteins can be grouped into short and long forms. The long form contains a single membrane-spanning domain and is related to the class I cytokine receptor family. The short form has a small intracellular domain, is made by the choroid plexus, and may serve as a carrier or transport protein facilitating leptin transport across the blood-brain barrier. A number of studies have suggested that the leptin resistance of obesity may be caused by a reduction in the transport of leptin into the brain. Evidence in support of this hypothesis has come from the demonstration that rats made obese on a high-fat diet are sensitive to leptin injected into the lateral ventricles but resistant to peripherally administered leptin. In addition, a decrease in the ratio of leptin concentration in cerebrospinal fluid and serum has been observed in obese humans. Since then it has become clear that leptin is normally taken up by the central nervous system, probably through the short leptin receptors, where it interacts with the long form of leptin receptors within the hypothalamus. This interaction results in down regulation of neuropeptide Y expression, which is presumed to produce the observed decrease in food intake. Perhaps the most widely studied rodent model of obesity is the Zucker fatty rat (fa). This single-gene autosomal recessive form of obesity has also been attributed to a mutation in the leptin receptor. Recently, a few obese humans have been identified with mutations in the leptin receptor. However, this genetic abnormality is extremely rare and not a common cause of human obesity.

11. Discuss how the melanocortin system is involved in weight regulation.

An unexpected, but potentially very important role of the melanocortin system in body weight regulation was uncovered from studies of the mouse model of obesity known as the agouti mouse. The agouti mouse is so named because of the yellow coat that is one of its distinguishing features. The phenotype of these mice was first detailed in 1927. In addition to the yellow coat, agouti mice are obese and hyperinsulinemic. The gene defect in this mouse model has been identified and involves a peptide (agouti) that competes with alpha melanocortin (MSH) for binding to MSH receptors. The normal protein product of this gene is expressed only in the coat and prevents the binding of MSH to its receptor, thereby changing coat pigmentation from black to yellow. When agouti is ubiquitously expressed, however, obesity develops. The identification of this pathway has highlighted the role of MSH receptors, particularly the MC4R subtype, in the regulation of body weight. Recent molecular experiments have demonstrated that the overexpression of the agouti protein by transgenic means produces a yellow mouse with obesity. This finding definitively demonstrates the pathogenic role of the agouti protein in the obesity of the model. In addition, the inactivation of the MSH-4 receptor (MC4-R) by gene targeting produces mice that develop obesity at maturity, hyperinsulinemia, and hyperglycemia much like the agouti model of obesity. This finding strongly implicates the MC4-R in body weight regulation and in the obesity mediated by the agouti protein. Several drug companies now have drugs that interact with the MC4-R as antagonists. These drugs decrease food intake in rats and reduce body weight. There is hope that these drugs may be useful in treating human obesity.

12. Does a decrease in energy expenditure play a role in the development of obesity?

Development of obesity requires an imbalance between caloric intake and caloric expenditure. For fat mass to increase, there must be an imbalance between the amount of fat deposited compared with the amount of fat oxidized. One possibility is that people become obese because of a reduction in their energy expenditure. There are three components to energy expenditure:

1. **Basal metabolic rate (BMR):** the amount of energy that is needed to keep sodium and potassium where they belong, to keep the body warm, to pump blood, to breathe, and to perform other basic functions.
2. **Energy expended in activity (EA):** the most variable component. It can account for as little as 10–20% of total energy expenditure in people who are bedridden to 60–80% of total energy expenditure in training athletes. This can occur with planned physical activity or with activities of daily living such as stair climbing or even fidgeting. The unconscious component of physical activity has been termed non-exercise activity thermogenesis or NEAT and may be a regulated parameter.
3. **Thermic effect of food (TEF):** a relatively small component of energy expenditure. It represents the increase in energy expenditure that follows the consumption of a meal. Part of the TEF is the energy cost of digesting and storing the food (obligatory). Another small component of the TEF cannot be explained by these processes (facultative).

Total energy expenditure is important because it equals total daily caloric intake when an individual is in energy balance. Total energy expenditure is, in general, linearly related to lean body mass. Studies using indirect calorimetry have shown that obese individuals clearly consume more calories than lean individuals. The obese individual who says that all he or she eats is a small salad may be telling the truth in the short term, but over longer periods, high caloric intakes are required to maintain the obese state. However, the role of alterations in energy expenditure in the development of obesity and the response to dieting is less clear. Increasing evidence suggests that obesity is associated with a relative reduction in energy expended with physical activity. Evidence in favor of this hypothesis comes from the Pima Indians as well as Caucasian obese and reduced obese individuals. The role that reductions in BMR play in weight gain is more controversial. Suffice it to say that regardless of the absolute level of expenditure, obesity results from failure to couple energy intake to energy expenditure accurately. In addition, it now appears that when obese individuals consume a hypocaloric diet, they become more energy efficient, reducing the energy expended per kilogram of lean body mass relative to lean individuals. This compensatory response to dieting would tend to put this individual back into positive energy balance and favor weight regain.

13. Discuss the approaches to treating the obese patient.

Diet, exercise, drugs, surgery, and combinations of these modalities. The specific modality selected should be based on the individual's BMI and associated health problems. A more aggressive treatment approach is warranted in those whose BMI is higher and those with adverse health consequences. Behavioral approaches can be advocated for all overweight and obese patients. Pharmacological treatment should be considered in those whose BMI is greater than 27 kg/m^2 in the presence of medical complications or greater than 30 kg/m^2 in the absence of medical complications. Surgical treatment should be reserved for those with a BMI greater than 40 kg/m^2.

14. What is the goal of a weight loss program?

Before discussing the treatment options with a patient, it is important to decide the goal of the treatment program. What is an appropriate goal for a weight loss program for a given patient? This is a very important question that is not a simple one to answer. There is increasing evidence that many obese individuals have unrealistic expectations about the amount of weight that they might lose through a weight loss program. Most obese individuals would like to reduce down to ideal body weight. They would accept a 20–30% weight loss as adequate but would be disappointed if they only lost 5–10% of their initial weight. These desires stand in stark contrast to the magnitude of weight loss that has been seen with all treatment modalities short of gastric bypass surgery. The most effective diet, exercise, or drug treatment programs available will give roughly a 10% weight loss in most individuals. This degree of weight reduction has been associated with improvements in health associated measures such as lower blood pressure, reductions in low-density lipoprotein (LDL) cholesterol levels, improved functional capacity, and improved insulin sensitivity. However, this degree of weight reduction will be disappointing to most patients unless the goal of the weight reduction program is clearly discussed prior to embarking on any plan. It is important to help the individual adopt more realistic goals for a diet and exercise program. Most experts in this area now feel that a sustained 5–10% weight loss (this would be a 11–22 lb weight loss for someone who initially weighed 220 lb) is a realistic goal with probable medical benefits. The patient's goal may be to lose a lot of weight in a short period of time: "40 lb in 40 days." A more realistic goal may be a gradual, sustained mild weight reduction. Alternatively, prevention of further weight gain may be a reasonable and attainable goal, or the health care provider could encourage the individual to focus on eating and activity habits and not focus on a weight goal at all. With this approach, the patient can succeed in the short term independent of any weight loss. What's more, if he or she goes off the behavioral program, the patient will have relapsed, regardless of what the scale says.

15. Discuss the role of diet in the treatment of the obese patient.

The mainstays of dietary modification in weight loss therapy have been a diet low in fat and reduced in calories. Whatever intervention the clinician makes must be lifelong to be beneficial; therefore, it must be tolerable to the patient. The clinician should assess the current diet with a good nutritional history. This could involve a verbal 24- or 72-hour diet recall. Alternatively, the patient could keep a written 7-day food diary. Assessing meal pattern is important, as many people skip breakfast and eat lunch erratically. Attention should be paid to how often the individual eats out, especially fast food. Then the clinician needs to make suggestions for slow, gradual change.

Simple dietary suggestions include eating three meals per day, eating only at meal times, and eating only one serving. These suggestions help patients to focus on what they are eating, emphasizing making good food choices and controlling portion size. Most people know what they should eat. The problem is that they either do not pay attention to what they eat or do not find a "good diet" palatable. Many of the settings in which care is provided do not allow sophisticated behavioral modification techniques to be taught. The use of commercial programs like Weight Watchers can provide reasonable nutritional counseling along with social support. Many patients are surprised at the cost of these programs, which may be a deterrent to their continued use. However, this kind of program has no risk and may be cheaper in the long term than pharmacological treatment. Unfortunately, many patients have already tried and failed with these approaches before they seek medical attention. The scientific literature supports the notion that for many people, dietary approaches alone are not associated with a high level of success at achieving long-term weight loss.

16. How can a patient's readiness to change his or her diet or physical activity be assessed?

Stages of change theory can help the clinician focus counseling activities within the context of a brief office visit. Prochazka has hypothesized that there are predictable stages that a person goes through before he or she is able to change long-standing behaviors such as diet, physical activity patterns, or smoking. These stages are:

1. *Precontemplative*: Individuals are not even thinking about changing their behavior. The issue is generally lack of perceived benefits to behavior change. For these individuals, perhaps a simple statement about the association between obesity and adverse health consequences may be appropriate, similar to what would be said about smoking cessation.
2. *Contemplative*: Individuals in this stageacknowledge the potential benefits of behavior change but have not yet decided what they are going to do. They are "thinking about it." The important issues to discuss during this stage this are perceived barriers to behavior change. Lack of time, lack of money, or a lack of a sense of control may be preventing progress. Counseling time needs to focus on these barriers as opposed to giving specific behavioral recommendations.
3. *Planning*: Individuals in this stagehave decided that they are going to change their behavior and are developing strategies to do it. They are "reading the book". These individuals need support and encouragement. They may request and benefit from specific suggestions to guide behavior change.
4. *Action*: Individuals in this stage have finished "reading the book," and have embarked on a behavior change program. They are usually excited, maybe even zealous. Sometimes these individuals are seen at an initial visit and may be looking for your support of their current diet or exercise program. Here again, these individuals benefit from encouragement, support, and the provision of objective evidence of the effects, either positive or negative, of their current approach.
5. *Maintenance*: Individuals in this phaseare on an established program that has become second nature. They may need to work on relapse prevention. The counseling time should be spent on looking for situations in which the individual may slip back to older habits and planning strategies to avoid these pitfalls.
6. *Relapse*: Individuals in this phasehave reverted back to a previous pattern of behavior. They may feel like they will always fail. They may say, "I've tried diets. They never work for me." These individuals feel frustrated and they make the care provider feel frustrated. Counseling time with these individuals should acknowledge and reward previous successes. The discussion should also explore what happened in the previous efforts. Can these individuals learn from their past efforts? Why did they fail? Were expectations too high? Were the changes too great? Where did they succeed? What would be reasonable new goals?

Identifying the stage that the patient is in and targeting counseling efforts to that stage may improve the effectiveness of the counseling activities.

17. What is the Atkins' diet?

There are several published diet programs that recently have become popular. These books have been written by individuals who have a particular angle on what constitutes a healthy diet. Each program grows out of a particular bias and is designed to accomplish a particular primary goal. One of these is the Atkins diet. Dr Atkins is a physician who developed his diet to help patients lose weight. His target audience is obese individuals who don't tolerate the usual diet prescription (low calories, low fat). His idea is that hyperinsulinemia is harmful because it promotes fat storage and hunger. He reasons that because insulin goes up as dietary carbohydrate increases, carbohydrate should be restricted. He also feels that carbohydrate in the diet is bad for certain individuals because it promotes wide fluctuations in blood glucose that creates symptoms of fatigue and hunger. His diet is a severely carbohydrate-restricted diet (<20 g/day during the induction phase). This produces what Atkins calls "benign dietary ketosis," which he argues suppresses appetite. He makes very few other dietary restrictions. The diet as practiced is a high-fat, high-protein diet. Atkins does-n't even particularly restrict saturated fat intake. There have been several recent studies that support the idea that some individuals lose a moderate amount of weight on this diet. Atkins is correct in his assertion that some individuals develop increased levels of triglyceride on high-carbohydrate diets. In addition, it is probably true that ketosis is associated with lower levels of subjective hunger. However, many nutrition experts are concerned about the catabolic effects of the hormone profile produced by this diet: very low insulin levels and high levels of counter-regulatory hormones. In addition some individuals might have increases in LDL cholesterol on this diet.

18. Describe the Zone diet.

The Zone diet was developed by Dr. Barry Sears, a PhD who was very interested in the effects of diet on eicosanoids. The goal of his diet is not weight loss per se, but rather "optimizing" health. The target audience, then, is everyone—not just those individuals interested in losing weight. Sears' thesis is that foods are like drugs, in that they have dose response curves. Therefore, one could optimize metabolism (in particular, optimize eicosanoid levels) by eating a diet that has optimal ratios of fat, carbohydrate, and protein. Too much carbohydrate is bad because of hyperinsulinemia; diets containing too little carbohydrate (ketogenic diets) are bad because they promote muscle breakdown and increase counter-regulatory hormones and as a result increase the production of "bad eicosanoids." Specifically he advocates a diet containing 30% protein, 30% fat, and 40% carbohydrate. Like Atkins, he feels that the excessive emphasis on low-fat, high-carbohydrate diets is partly responsible for the increased prevalence of obesity seen recently. He believes that this so-called optimal ratio of macronutrients promotes satiety, and as a result some weight loss will occur without prescribing caloric restriction. Exercise is part of the program, but the program can be adjusted to varying levels of physical activity from fairly sedentary to elite athletes. These concepts are reasonably well grounded in the biology of eicosanoids, but Sears has taken these ideas a bit farther than existing experimental evidence would support. In his book, he cites his own experience using this diet with subjects in a scientific way, but his "experiments" are not published in peer-reviewed journals. There are almost no objective scientific data supporting this diet program.

19. Discuss the Ornish diet.

Dr. Dean Ornish is an exceptionally well-trained medical doctor who was looking for an alternative to bypass surgery for patients with coronary artery disease that was based on nutrition and lifestyle change. His target audience is not obese individuals but rather those with known coronary artery disease. The Ornish diet is not a weight loss diet. It is a "lifestyle change program" incorporating diet—specifically, a very low-fat (10% fat, 10% protein) vegetarian diet with group interactions designed to increase physical activity and decrease "type A" behaviors. Group psychological support, smoking cessation, yoga-based physical activities, and meditation are part of this program. The diet recommendations are an outgrowth of the Pritikin diet of the '70s, also a very low-fat diet. Pritikin-type diets grew out of the belief that since obesity and hyperlipidemia were more common on a modern "high fat" diet, a low-fat diet must be superior. The dietary ideas per se are not based on any particular metabolic theory, and Ornish does not specifically address concerns over how high-carbohydrate diets might cause hyperinsulinemia and increase hunger. In addition, Ornish sees coronary artery disease as part of the whole modern lifestyle of low physical activity, high life stress, and a high-fat diet. His program therefore addresses each of these areas directly. As currently practiced, it is a very labor-intensive program for the care provider and the participants. Ornish has made it a priority to study his ideas with the tools of modern clinical science. He and his collaborators have used the latest techniques in assessing the degree of coronary artery disease and have published their results in excellent peer-reviewed medical journals. In a recent publication, they report on the 5-year follow up of a cohort of 20 patients who were on the program, compared with 15 controls. The subjects experienced a dramatic reduction in anginal events and angiographic evidence of regression of their coronary artery disease. These individuals lost a moderate amount of weight and had reductions in LDL cholesterol but also had reductions in high-density lipoprotein (HDL), or "good," cholesterol and increased levels of triglyceride.

20. What is the blood type diet?

This diet program was developed by a naturopathic physician, Dr. Peter D'Amno. His central idea is that different diets are best for different people. He thinks that blood type is a marker of an individual's genetic background. Specifically, he argues that different blood types arose at different points in our evolution when we were faced with particular nutritional challenges (hunter-gatherers vs. farmers, for example). In addition, Amno argues that blood type antigens interact with certain lectins on foods to directly produce particular health problems. He feels that specific diets should be advised for people of specific blood types. There is no peer-reviewed scientific evidence favoring this overall view. The scientific support for the ideas about the origin of blood types is not strong. The data concerning blood types and lectin binding do not directly relate to the overall diets that Amno advocates. However, the idea that different people with different genetic backgrounds have different responses to different diets seems reasonable and fits with the clinical experience of many health care providers. In fact, this idea may be a very important nutritional principle.

21. What should a clinician do when a patient wants to go on a "fad diet"?

There are several approaches that could be used. The clinician could pick and promote one of these popular diet programs. However, no one is really sure what the right program is, so this may not be the best approach. Probably no single program is right for all patients. A second approach would be to dissuade people from participating in any of these programs. This is certainly the easiest and most common approach. In fact these diets are not currently promoted or even accepted by reputable groups such as the American Heart Association, the American Diabetes Association, or the National Institutes of Health. However it is also hard to completely ignore the often heard testimonials to the effectiveness of these diets, and it seems inappropriate to say these diets don't work when in reality they have not been well studied. A third, and perhaps most acceptable, approach is to try to understand the principles of these diets and provide information and encouragement to patients in their efforts to improve their health. Patients should be encouraged to avoid programs that might hurt them and should be reminded of the need for long-term changes in behavior. The discussion should also focus on realistic goals. Patients can be provided with objective data on which to evaluate their program (e.g., fasting lipid and glucose levels, blood pressure, weight, waist circumference, percent body fat). Try to keep the mood positive yet realistic.

22. What drugs are available to treat obesity?

Phentermine: This medication is chemically related to amphetamine and works predominantly on the neurotransmitter norepinephrine to reduce appetite. The addictive effects of amphetamine are thought to be due to its actions on the neurotransmitter dopamine. Phentermine has substantially less dopaminergic effects than amphetamine and as a result has minimal potential for addiction. It is, however, a central stimulant and can cause nervousness, headache, difficulty sleeping, and tremor in some people. This medication also goes by the trade names: Adipex-P, Fastin, and Ionamin. It effects some weight loss compared with placebo in 50–60% of those who take it, with the average weight loss being in the 5–10% range. Many patients experience mild side effects when using this as a single agent. The average cost is about $30/month. Although fenfluramine, which was used primarily in combination with phentermine (fen/phen), was found to cause cardiac valvulopathy and primary pulmonary hypertension, there is no evidence that phentermine used alone is associated with cardiac valvular and pulmonary vascular toxicity. Phentermine is still on the market but is only Food and Drug Administration (FDA) approved for 3-month use. However, this restriction on long-term use may relate more to ideas about weigh loss medications that were prevalent in the '60s when the FDA reviewed the drug. There are no long-term studies of its safety and efficacy. However it has been on the market and in widespread clinical use longer than any other weight loss agent, and there has been no evidence of serious side effects.

Orlistat: This medication, which goes by the trade name Xenical, is a pancreatic lipase inhibitor. It reduces the absorption of fat by roughly 30% by inhibiting the enzyme responsible for fat digestion. It is given as 120 mg three times a day with meals. Since it is not absorbed into the bloodstream, it is not associated with primary pulmonary hypertension, cardiac valvular disease, or other systemic side effects. Some patients like the fact that it is not an appetite suppressant. The main side effects are due to the malabsorption of fat. Patients who eat a high-fat meal will experience greasy stools and may even have problems with incontinence of stool. In some ways this medications simply enforces a low fat diet. Conversely, if the patient chooses to skip the medication, he or she can eat a high-fat meal without side effects and without the benefit that the medication would otherwise provide. Orlistat became available in May of 1999 and has been widely prescribed since then. The average wholesale price for this drug is $120/month. The average weight loss seen is about 7–8%. The FDA has approved orlistat for long-term use, and there is no specific mention in the package insert of when it should be stopped. This medication may be preferred in those individuals currently using a serotonin-specific reuptake inhibitor (SSRI).

Sibutramine: This medication is a combination norepinephrine and serotonin reuptake blocker. Unlike fenfluramine and dexfenfluramine, it has no serotonin releasing action and therefore is pharmacologically more like the SSRIs that are widely prescribed for the treatment of depression. It is taken at doses ranging from 10–20 mg per day. It produces weight losses in the range of 8–10% at a dose of 20 mg/day. In humans, the drug works primarily by reducing appetite with minimal effects on energy expenditure. Sibutramine has been associated with an increase in blood pressure in some individuals, particularly at the higher doses. It should therefore not be used in people with poorly controlled hypertension. All patients should have their blood pressure monitored closely during the period following initiation of this medicine. The most common side effects are dry mouth, headache, nervousness, and difficulty falling asleep. However, these side effects are generally well tolerated (similar in magnitude to those seen with fen/phen). Sibutramine has now been widely used, and there is no evidence that its use is associated with any serious side effects such as valvular heart disease or pulmonary hypertension. Sibutramine goes by the trade name Meridia and is currently available for roughly $100/month (10 mg/day). The FDA has approved it for the treatment of individuals for 1 year with longer use to be decided by the physician and the patient. Two-year safety and efficacy data are now published, and the FDA may soon approve the use of sibutramine for 2 years. This compound may be preferred in those who desire an appetite suppressant but should not be used in those currently taking an SSRI.

Bupropion: Very preliminary information suggests that bupropion (Wellbutrin) may produce gradual weight loss over as long as 1 year in some individuals. Currently, there is no weight loss indication for this drug, but the manufacturer is pursuing one. While this drug should not currently be prescribed for weight reduction, if a patient is taking a different antidepressant already and he or she does not want to use Xenical, it may be reasonable to have the individual discuss switching to Wellbutrin with their psychiatrist. More data will be available on this drug as relates to weight loss in the next few years.

Herbal Preparations: A number of herbal medications have been purported to have the same mechanism of action as fen/phen but without the side effects. Many of these combinations include the herbal ingredient ephedra, commonly known as ma huang, and the herb *Hypericum perforatum*, also known as St. John's wort. The FDA does not approve of the use of these substances in obese individuals. There have been a number of cases of atrial arrhythmias associated with the use of ephedra, and the chromium contained in some of these products has been found to cause cancer in rats.

Combinations: The combination of phentermine and fluoxetine (Prozac) has been used by some practitioners as an alternative to phentermine and fenfluramine (which was removed from the market). However, there is very limited information on either the long-term safety or efficacy of this combination. Widespread use of this combination, therefore, cannot be advocated at this time. Other options include phentermine and orlistat, sibutramine plus orlistat, and bupropion plus orlistat. Similarly, none of these combinations has been studied in enough detail to recommend their use.

23. How long will a medication need to be taken?

In the past, the FDA would only allow short-term use of weight-loss medicines. However, experts in the field now feel that obesity is a chronic illness just like diabetes or high blood pressure, and that if a medicine is used to help an individual lose weight, it will only work as long as it is taken. This means that if a patient takes a weight loss medicine and loses weight then stops the medicine, he or she is likely to regain the lost weight. This is what happens when someone goes on a diet for a period of time then stops the diet. This so-called yo-yo effect is probably not good for health. Unfortunately, we do not have good data on the safety or effectiveness of these medicines when used for 10–20 yr, the time that they might be used if a person chooses to take them chronically. In general, if a primary care provider and a patient decide to try a weight loss medication, it should be taken for a minimum of 3 months to determine if that individual will lose at least 5–10% of his or her weight. Then consideration should be given to some form of chronic use, given the available information about the risks and potential benefits of the medications. Some patients find that they can restrict their use of the medication to periods when they predict that they are going to have more difficulty adhering to their usual behavioral program.

24. Will the weight reduction afforded by pharmacologic agents improve health outcomes?

The answer to this question is not definitively known at this time. It is clear that the weight reduction afforded by these medications can improve surrogate markers such as blood pressure, cholesterol, and glucose levels in those whose levels were previously elevated. Some individuals find that these medicines reduce the occurrence of obsessive thoughts about eating; this may be their most important therapeutic effect. While it makes intuitive sense that losing weight would enhance your health, it is not yet clear that losing weight *with medications* will improve health. One reasonable approach would be to wait until more research is done to clearly answer this important question. There have been other medicines developed for other conditions, such as ventricular arrhythmias, that everyone thought would improve health, but when studies were done, it actually turned out that the drugs hurt people more than help them. On the other hand, it is clear that increased weight is associated with adverse health risks if nothing is done. The decision on whether the health benefits outweigh the risks and costs of these medicines needs to be made on a case-by-case basis between the primary care provider and the patient based on the best data available to them at that time.

25. What should be done for patients who were exposed to the combination of fenfluramine and phentermine (fen/phen)?

Cardiac valvulopathy was an unexpected complication of this therapy. Cardiac valvulopathy was initially reported in a case series of 24 patients who developed abnormally thickened heart valves, associated with valvular insufficiency by echocardiogram, following treatment with fenfluramine or dexfenfluramine. By September 1997, a total of 144 individuals with valvulopathy associated with these medications had been reported to the FDA; 24% of these individuals required valve replacement surgery, and three died. Fenfluramine and dexfenfluramine were subsequently removed from the market.

It has been demonstrated in several independent series that individuals who received fenfluramine or dexfenfluramine as part of a weight reduction program had a 10–30% risk of developing cardiac valvulopathy by echocardiogram. The most common lesion seen was new aortic regurgitation. In addition, most of those individuals found to have abnormal heart valves on echocardiograms were asymptomatic and did not have audible murmurs by cardiac auscultation. It now appears that valvulopathy was more common in those who took fen/phen for more than 6 months, that it did not appear to progress after stopping these medications, and that it may have even regressed in some individuals. The American Heart Association has recommended that if an individual previously treated with fenfluramine or dexfenfluramine is found to have an abnormal heart valve by echocardiography and is going to have dental work that would warrant antibiotic prophylaxis for other forms of valvular heart disease, the individual should receive antibiotic prophylaxis.

While it would be reasonable to perform echocardiograms on all individuals treated with these anorectic agents, there is currently no consensus that this practice is mandatory. Furthermore, it is not clear at this time how patients identified as having anorectic agent–induced cardiac valvulopathy should be followed or treated. A reasonable course would be to repeat echocardiograms every 6 months in those who are identified as having valvulopathy to ensure that they do not develop progressive cardiac dysfunction. It may be reasonable in an asymptomatic individual to offer echocardiography, to make them aware that they have a 10–30% risk of having an abnormal valve and that they need to know the status of their valves if they are going to have dental work, and then to follow them closely for the development of a murmur or any cardiopulmonary symptoms. If the patient chooses not to have an echocardiogram, that is also acceptable until the natural history of this condition is more clearly defined. The medico-legal implications of either performing or not performing an echocardiogram are not clear at this time.

26. What is the role of exercise in a weight loss program?

The discussion should begin with a physical activity history. Ask about the frequency of engaging in planned physical activity. (Data from the Centers for Disease Control suggest that 30% of Americans engage in no planned physical activity.) Then ask about hours per day of television viewing, computer time, and other sedentary activities. Finally, discuss activities of daily living, including work-related activities. Assess the individual's readiness to change physical activity. Exercise does not provide much weight loss in the short term. This observation is frustrating for many patients. The explanation is that the absolute caloric deficit provided by a moderate exercise program is not sufficient to cause much weight loss over a period of days to weeks. Another problem is that the patient may preserve or even increase lean body mass at a time when fat mass is decreasing. This process may reduce the absolute amount of weight lost. However, the long-term success of a weight loss program is substantially greater if exercise is included.

The American College of Sports Medicine recommends that "all Americans should accumulate at least 30 minutes of moderate physical activity on most days of the week." There are three important points here:

1. *Accumulate*: Three 10-minute bouts of exercise in a day are as good as one 30-minute bout.

2. *Moderate physical activity*: Monitoring and achieving a target heart rate is not necessary. Most people are able to make a subjective assessment of what constitutes moderate physical activity.
3. *On most days of the week*: Frequent activity appears to be important. The goal is to make physical activity part of everyday life.

There now exists a growing body of evidence that fitness conveys health benefits independent of weight loss. In addition increasing physical activity is the number one priority of the Healthy People 2010 national goals. The National Weight Control Registry is a group of 3000 individuals who have been identified because they have successfully lost 30 lb and kept it off for at least 1 year. They self-report 2000 calories per week of physical activity. This suggests that increasing physical activity may be a key component to long-term success in weight reduction.

27. Should liposuction be advocated for obese patients?

In the only controlled trial, weight lost by liposuction was regained. Sometimes the adipose tissue reaccumulated at the same site; other times it reaccumulated elsewhere. Liposuction cannot be advocated as a weight-loss strategy for patients with medically significant obesity.

28. What mechanical methods are available for the treatment of morbidly obese patients?

Morbid obesity has been variably defined as weight that is 100% or 100 lb above ideal. Another definition is a BMI greater than 40. Such people are at high risk for adverse health consequences. Surgical therapy may offer the best long-term chance for reducing body weight. The success rate for gastroplasty or gastric bypass is on the order of 60–70%, and the average weight loss is 30%. When done by an experienced surgeon, the weight loss is maintained long term, as reported in published series out to 15 years of follow up. Many patients experience resolution of diabetes, hypertension, and hyperlipidemia as well as improved rates of employment postoperatively. The complication rate, however, is not trivial, with roughly 20% of patients experiencing some form of postoperative morbidity, including persistent vomiting, wound infections, dehiscence, depression, and pulmonary

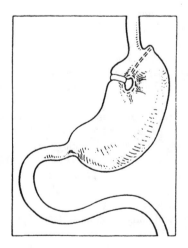 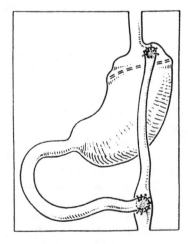

Operations for obesity. Gastroplasty (left) and gastric bypass (right) have been used for the operative treatment of morbid obesity.

complications to name a few. Recently laparoscopy has been used to perform a procedure similar to the banded gastroplasty. Initial results seem to indicate that this form of surgery is less effective than the standard surgical approach.

29. What is a very low-calorie diet (VLCD)? When should its use be considered?

A VLCD is a nutritionally complete diet of 800 kcal/day that produces rapid weight loss. Experienced teams in supervised settings should administer VLCDs. When these diets are used in this manner, complications are rare. The long-term results with VLCDs are no better than with other dietary programs. For this reason, their usefulness is limited. They may be helpful for the patient who needs a short-term loss of weight to reduce the risk of a diagnostic or surgical procedure.

BIBLIOGRAPHY

1. Balsiger BM, Murr MM, Poggio JL, Sarr MG: Bariatric surgery. Surgery for weight control in patients with morbid obesity. Med Clin North Am 84:477–489, 2000.
2. Bray, GA: Obesity. Endocrinol Metab Clin North Am 25:781–1048, 1996.
3. Bray GA, Greenway FL: Current and potential drugs for treatment of obesity. Endocrine Rev 20:805–875, 1999.
4. Brownell KD: The LEARN Program for Weight Control, 7th ed. Dallas, American Health Pub Co, 1997.
5. Colditz GA: Economic costs of obesity and inactivity. Med Sci Sports Exerc 31:S663–S667, 1999
6. Collazo-Clavell ML: Safe and effective management of the obese patient. Mayo Clin Proc 74:1255–1259, 1999.
7. Connolly HM, Crary JL, McGoon MD, et al: Valvular heart disease associated with fenfluramine-phentermine. N Engl J Med 337:581–588, 1997.
8. National Heart Lung and Blood Institute: Clinical Guidelines on the Identification, Evaluation, and Treatment of Overweight and Obesity in Adults. Available at: www.nhlbi.nih.gov/guidelines/obesity/ob_home.htm.
9. National Institutes of Health: The practical guide to the identification, evaluation and treatment of overweight and obesity in adults. Obesity Res 6(suppl 2), 1998.
10. Obesity Issue. JAMA 282:1493–1596, 1999.
11. Rosenbaum M, Leibel RL, Hirsch J: Obesity. N Engl J Med 337:396–407, 1997.
12 Stevens J, Cai J, Pamuk ER, et al: The effect of age on the association between body mass index and mortality. N Engl J Med 338:1–7, 1998.
13 Wolf AM, Colditz GA: Current estimates of the economic cost of obesity in the United States. Obesity Res 6:97–106, 1998.

II. Bone and Mineral Disorders

10. OSTEOPOROSIS

Michael T. McDermott, M.D.

1. What is osteoporosis?

Osteoporosis is defined as a systemic skeletal disease characterized by low bone mass and microarchitectural deterioration of bone tissue with a consequent increase in bone fragility and susceptibility to fracture.

2. What fractures are most commonly associated with osteoporosis?

Fractures of the vertebrae, hips, and distal radius (Colles' fracture) are characteristic, but any fracture may occur.

3. What are the complications of osteoporotic fractures?

Pain and temporary disability result from fractures of any type. Vertebral fractures also cause loss of height and anterior kyphosis, known as "dowager's hump." Hip fractures are associated with permanent disability in approximately 50% of patients and with a significantly increased mortality rate.

4. What two factors contribute most to the risk of developing an osteoporotic fracture?
1. Low bone mass
2. An increased tendency to fall from the standing position

5. How does bone mass change during a person's lifetime?

In women, bone mass normally increases from birth until age 18–20, remains relatively stable until menopause, decreases rapidly in the first 5–10 years after menopause, and then decreases at a slower rate throughout the remaining years of life. Men differ in that they achieve a greater peak bone mass than women and do not normally have a period of rapid bone loss. Low bone mass may result from failure to achieve an adequate peak bone mass during the growing years, from excessive bone loss later in life, or from living to a very old age.

6. What are the major risk factors for developing low bone mass?

Non-modifiable	Modifiable
Age	Low calcium intake
Race (Caucasian, Asian)	Low vitamin D intake
Female gender	Estrogen deficiency
Early menopause	Sedentary lifestyle
Slender build	Cigarette smoking
Positive family history	Alcohol excess (> 2 drinks/day)
	Caffeine excess (> 2 servings/day)
	Medications (glucocorticoids, excess thyroxine)

7. What are the currently accepted indications for bone mass measurement?

The National Osteoporosis Foundation has issued the following recommendations for screening:

Women age 65 and older

Postmenopausal women under age 65, with other risk factors

Postmenopausal women with fractures

Women considering therapy for osteoporosis

Women on hormone replacement therapy for prolonged periods

Medicare considers the following to be indications for bone densitometry utilization:

Estrogen deficiency plus one risk factor for osteoporosis

Vertebral deformity, fracture or osteopenia by x-ray

Primary hyperparathyroidism

Glucocorticoid therapy, $\geq$ 7.5 mg/day of prednisone for $\geq$ 3 months

Monitoring the response to an FDA-approved osteoporosis medication

8. How is bone mass currently measured?

Standard radiographs are inadequate for accurate bone mass assessment. The most accurate and widely used methods in current practice are dual energy x-ray absorptiometry (DEXA), computed tomography (CT), and ultrasound (US). In my opinion, DEXA offers the best accuracy and precision with the least radiation exposure in most patients.

Central densitometry measurements (spine and hip) are the best predictors of fracture risk and have the best precision for longitudinal monitoring. Peripheral densitometry measurements (heel, radius, hands), however, are more widely available and less expensive.

9. Should bone densitometry screening be done at central or peripheral sites?

Because of its availability and low cost, peripheral densitometry has gained great popularity as a screening tool. In many patients, screening with peripheral densitometry is adequate, but the technique is somewhat less sensitive in diagnosing osteoporosis than is central densitometry. Furthermore, densitometry values can vary greatly in the same individual at different skeletal sites. Therefore, even when peripheral bone densitometry values are normal, follow-up central densitometry must still be considered in the following circumstances:

History of fragility fractures

Two or more risk factors for bone loss

Medical conditions associated with bone loss

Medications that cause bone loss

Postmenopausal women not on estrogens, who would consider treatment if bone density is low

Since peripheral densitometry must be followed by central densitometry in some situations and because of the greater accuracy and precision during longitudinal follow-up, I prefer central measurements for all patients who meet the criteria listed in question #7 above.

10. How do you read a bone densitometry report?

The most useful values on the bone densitometry report are the T-score, the Z-score, and the absolute bone mineral density (BMD).

T-score: a comparison of a patient's bone mass to that of young normal subjects. The T-score is the number of standard deviations (SDs) the patient's value is below or above the mean value for young normal subjects (peak bone mass). Thus, a T-score of –2.0 indicates that the patient is 2 SDs below normal peak bone mass. The T-score indicates whether or not the patient has osteoporosis.

Z-score: a comparison of a patient's bone mass to that of age-matched subjects. The Z-score is the number of SDs the patient's value is below or above the mean value for age-matched normal subjects. The Z-score indicates whether or not the patient's bone mass is appropriate for age or whether other factors are likely to account for excessively low bone mass.

Absolute BMD: the actual bone density value expressed in g/cm^2. This is the best parameter to use for calculation of percent changes in bone density during longitudinal follow-up.

11. How is the diagnosis of osteoporosis made?

The diagnosis of osteoporosis is made when a patient has a characteristic osteoporotic fracture or when the T-score on bone densitometry is sufficiently low. The World Health Organization (WHO) criteria for T-score interpretation are as follows:

T-score > –1	Normal
T-score between –1 and –2.5	Osteopenia
T-score < –2.5	Osteoporosis

Thus, a T-score of less than –2.5 makes a diagnosis of osteoporosis even in the absence of a fracture. Before concluding that reduced bone mass or a fracture is due to osteoporosis, one must first rule out other causes of low bone mass.

12. What are the limitations of bone densitometry measurements?

- The WHO diagnostic criteria apply only to postmenopausal white women.
- Disparities exist among bone density values at different sites and with different methods.
- Low bone mass does not necessarily indicate on-going bone loss.
- Low bone mass is not always osteoporosis.
- Bone densitometry cannot distinguish among the causes of low bone mass.

13. What other conditions must be considered as causes of low bone mass?

Osteomalacia	Multiple myeloma
Osteogenesis imperfecta	Rheumatoid arthritis
Hyperparathyroidism	Renal failure
Hyperthyroidism	Idiopathic hypercalciuria
Hypogonadism	Celiac disease
Cushing's syndrome	Mastocytosis

14. Outline a cost-effective evaluation to rule out these possibilities.

A complete history and physical examination should always be performed. Afterward the following tests should be adequate in most patients:

Complete blood count with erythrocyte sedimentation rate
Serum calcium, phosphate, alkaline phosphatase and creatinine
Serum TSH
Serum testosterone (men)
24-hour urine calcium and creatinine

15. What are the most significant risk factors for sustaining a fall from the upright position?

Use of sedatives
Visual impairment
Cognitive impairment
Lower extremity disability
Obstacles to ambulation in the home

16. What nonpharmacologic measures are useful for preventing and treating osteoporosis?

1. Adequate calcium intake:
   1000 mg/day, premenopausal women and men
   1500 mg/day, postmenopausal women and men ≥ age 65 years of age
2. Adequate vitamin D intake: 400–800 units/day
3. Adequate exercise: aerobic and resistance
4. Smoking cessation
5. Limitation of alcohol consumption to 2 drinks/day or less
6. Limitation of caffeine consumption to 2 servings/day or less
7. Fall prevention

17. How do you clinically assess a patient's dietary calcium intake?

Although calcium is present in a variety of foods, the major bioavailable sources are dairy products and calcium-fortified drinks. Ask patients how much milk, cheese, yogurt, and calcium-fortified fruit juice they consume daily, and assign the following approximate calcium contents for their responses:

• Milk	300 mg/cup (8 oz)
• Cheese	300 mg/oz
• Yogurt	300 mg/cup (8 oz)
• Fruit juice with calcium	300 mg/cup (8 oz)

Total these amounts plus 300 mg for the general non-dairy diet, and you have a reasonable estimate of that person's daily dietary calcium intake.

18. How do you ensure an adequate intake of calcium and vitamin D?

Encourage the consumption of low-fat dairy products; this is the safest way to increase calcium intake without increasing the risk of kidney stones. Advise patients according to the estimated calcium content table in question 17. Any shortfalls in dietary calcium intake should be supplemented with calcium tablets or elixirs. Multivitamins contain 400 units of vitamin D per tablet; one or two tablets per day is sufficient for most patients.

19. An understanding of bone remodeling is necessary in order to devise strategies for pharmacological management of osteoporosis. Describe bone remodeling.

Bone remodeling is the process by which old bone is removed and new bone is formed. Osteoclasts are multinucleated giant cells that attach to bone surfaces where they secrete acid and proteolytic enzymes that dissolve underlying bone, leaving a resorption pit. Osteoblasts then move in and secrete osteoid, which is subsequently mineralized with calcium and phosphate crystals (hydroxyapatite), refilling the resorption pit with new bone. Bone remodeling occurs throughout the skeleton as an adaptation to changing mechanical stresses on bone.

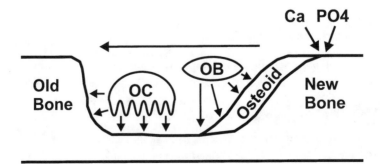

20. What markers are available to assess bone remodeling?

Bone formation	Bone resorption
Serum alkaline phosphatase	Urine N-telopeptides
Serum osteocalcin	Serum N-telopeptides
	Urine pyridinoline crosslinks

21. What pharmacologic agents are available for the prevention and treatment of osteoporosis?

Medications for the prevention and treatment of osteoporosis fall into two main categories: those that inhibit bone resorption and those that stimulate bone formation.

Inhibit bone resorption	Stimulate bone formation
Estrogens	Sodium fluoride
Bisphosphonates	Androgens
Calcitonin	Parathyroid hormone
Raloxifene	Growth hormone / growth factors

22. How effective are the antiresorptive agents in the treatment of osteoporosis?

Medication efficacy is best assessed by the effects on bone mass and on fracture reduction.

Bone mass increments observed over a 2-3 year period:

Medication	Spine	Hip
Alendronate	7–8%	5–6%
Risedronate	4–5%	2–3%
Estrogens	5–6%	3–4%
Raloxifene	2–3%	2–3%
Calcitonin	0–1%	0%

Observed reductions in fracture incidence:

Medication	Spine	Hip
Alendronate	47–50%	51–56%
Risedronate	33–46%	8–58%
Estrogens	42%	No data
Raloxifene	31–49%	0
Calcitonin	33%	0

23. Explain why bone mass increases when patients are treated with medications that inhibit bone resorption.

These medications significantly reduce bone resorption, whereas bone formation initially remains unaffected. As a result, formation temporarily exceeds resorption and bone mass increases. The increase tends to be greater in patients with high turnover osteoporosis because their basal bone formation rate is normal or mildly elevated. Over 6–18 months, however, bone formation gradually declines to the level of resorption and bone mass stabilizes. This phenomenon is referred to as the bone-remodeling transient.

24. Explain how bisphosphonates are used in the treatment of osteoporosis.

The following bisphosphonates are clinically available, although only two (alendronate, risedronate) are FDA-approved for the treatment of osteoporosis because they are the only agents with proven anti-fracture efficacy at both the spine and the hip.

Medication	Dose
Alendronate (Fosamax)	10 mg p.o. q day, 70 mg p.o. q week
Risedronate (Actonel)	5 mg p.o. q day
Etidronate (Didronel)	200 p.o. BID 14 days every 3 months
Pamidronate (Aredia)	30 mg IV every 3 months

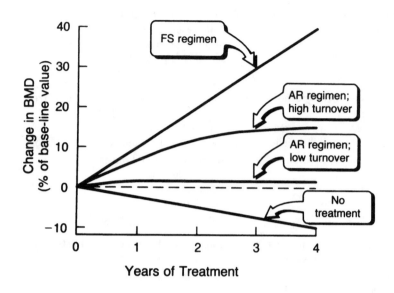

Years of Treatment

The oral bisphosphonates have very poor intestinal absorption that is significantly inhibited by the presence of food or medications in the gastrointestinal tract. Their major side effect is esophageal/gastrointestinal pain. In order to maximize intestinal absorption and to minimize gastrointestinal toxicity, they should be taken first thing each morning on an empty stomach with a full glass of water. The patient should then remain upright and take nothing by mouth for at least 30 minutes after medication ingestion. Alendronate has recently become available in a once-a-week preparation that may provide a more convenient dosing regimen with efficacy, toxicity, and cost that are similar to the daily dose regimen. Risedronate should soon be marketed in a once-a-week preparation as well. Etidronate or pamidronate may be considered in patients who are unable to take one of the FDA approved agents.

25. **Discuss the use of hormone replacement therapy in the management of osteoporosis.**
    The following hormone preparations are commonly used for hormone replacement therapy.

Medication	Dose Regimen
Conjugated estrogens	
Premarin	.625–1.25 mg q day or days 1–25
Estratabs	.625–1.25 mg q day or days 1–25
Estradiol	
Estrace	.5–1.0 mg q day or days 1-25
Estradiol patch	
Estraderm	.05–0.1 mg patch twice a week
Vivelle	.05–0.1 mg patch twice a week
Climara	.05–0.1 mg patch once a week
Combination pills	
Prempro	.625/2.5 mg or .625/5.0 mg (Premarin/Provera) q day
Premphase	.625 mg (Premarin) days 1–14, then
	.625/5.0 mg (Premarin/Provera) days 15–25
OrthoPrefest	1 mg (estradiol) q day for 3 days, then
	1 mg/.09 mg (estradiol/norgestimate) q day for 3 days in repeat cycles

Combination patch
   Combipatch   .05/.14 mg or .05/.25 mg patch (estradiol/norethindrone) twice a week

Medroxyprogesterone
   Provera   2.5 mg qd or 5-10 mg days 15-25

Unopposed estrogens significantly increase the risk of developing endometrial carcinoma. For this reason, women with an intact uterus must take estrogen in combination with progesterone, either cyclically (example: Premarin .625 mg days 1-25, Provera 5-10 mg days 15-25) or daily (example: Premarin .625 mg q day, Provera 2.5 mg q day).

Hormone replacement therapy also appears to moderately increase the risk of developing breast cancer and thromboembolic disease. Counseling about and monitoring for these conditions are therefore indicated in patients on hormone replacement therapy.

26. Discuss the use of selective estrogen receptor modulators (SERMS) in the management of osteoporosis.

Selective estrogen receptor modulators (SERMS) are agents that function as estrogen agonists in some tissues and estrogen antagonists in other tissues. Raloxifene (Evista) is a SERM that has been shown to improve bone mass and to reduce spine fractures; it is FDA-approved for the treatment of postmenopausal osteoporosis. Raloxifene has also been shown to reduce the risk of developing breast cancer. The dose is 60 mg q day. Side effects include hot flashes, leg cramps, and an increased risk of thromboembolic disease similar to that seen with hormone replacement therapy.

27. How is calcitonin used in the management of osteoporosis?

Calcitonin is available as both intranasal (200 units q day) and injectable (100 units q day) preparations. This FDA-approved medication has been shown to modestly improve spinal bone mass and to reduce the incidence of spinal fractures. Potential side effects include nausea, nasal irritation (nasal spray), and skin irritation (injections).

28. Can the antiresorptive agents be used in combination with one another?

Combinations of bisphosphonates and estrogens produce increments in bone mass that are greater than those observed when the drugs are used alone. Similar results have been reported when bisphosphonates are used with raloxifene. There have been no studies to date having sufficient power or duration to adequately demonstrate greater fracture reduction efficacy with combination therapy. Nonetheless, because bone histomorphometry is normal in patients treated with these regimens, it is predicted that they will likely reduce fractures to a greater degree than is seen with single drug therapy.

29. How does PTH therapy stimulate bone formation, and what effects does it have on bone mass?

The most promising bone formation–stimulating agent on the horizon is parathyroid hormone (PTH). PTH is known to stimulate both bone formation and bone resorption in humans. Persistently elevated serum PTH levels, as seen in hyperparathyroidism, stimulate bone resorption more than formation and thereby cause bone loss. However, when PTH is given as single daily injections, the transient PTH bursts disproportionately enhance bone formation. Patients treated with PTH have been reported to have bone mass increments of nearly 15% in the lumbar spine and approximately 5% in the hip over 1–2 year study periods. Furthermore, vertebral fracture risk has been reported to decrease by as much as 65% in treated patients. There are no current studies that have been sufficiently powered to assess hip fractures, but based on bone densitometry changes and normal histomorphometry reports, it is likely that hip fracture risk will also be reduced. It is anticipated that PTH will soon be approved by the FDA and available for the treatment of patients with osteoporosis.

30. How effective are other bone formation stimulating agents?

Sodium fluoride, which appears to directly stimulate osteoblasts, has been reported to increase bone mass by 16–20% over a 4-year period. However, because of lack of convincing anti-fracture efficacy and long-term safety data, this medication is not approved by the FDA for osteoporosis treatment.

Androgens are anabolic agents that also stimulate osteoblastic bone formation. Methyltestosterone (2.5 mg/day) given in combination with estrogens to postmenopausal women has been shown to increase bone mass significantly more than do estrogens alone. Hirsutism, acne, and temporal balding are potential side effects with androgen treatment but are dose-related and therefore may be mild or absent with lower doses. Growth hormone and growth factors also increase bone mass by stimulating bone formation, but these agents remain under investigation and are not yet ready for clinical use, except in patients with documented growth hormone deficiency.

31. What is coherence therapy?

Coherence therapy is a program in which an anti-resorptive medication is used in combination with or alternating with a bone formation–stimulating agent. Recently, combinations of alendronate with PTH and estrogens with PTH have been shown to increase bone mass significantly more than does any single agent alone. Although anti-fracture efficacy has not yet been demonstrated, these findings are very promising, particularly as a treatment approach for patients with very low bone mass.

32. When should medical therapy be initiated for the prevention and treatment of osteoporosis?

The nonpharmacologic measures discussed in question 16 are appropriate for all individuals who want to reduce their risk of developing osteoporosis. The National Osteoporosis Foundation further recommends that pharmacologic therapy be initiated in any patient who has a T-score of –2.0 or less and in patients with a T-score of –1.5 or less in the presence of other osteoporotic risk factors.

33. How common is osteoporosis in men?

Although it occurs more commonly in women, osteoporosis is not a rare disease in men. A 60-year-old man has a 25% lifetime risk of developing an osteoporotic fracture and approximately 30% of all hip fractures worldwide occur in men.

34. How is the diagnosis of osteoporosis made in men?

Currently, there are no adequate data available to determine what level of bone loss significantly increases a man's risk of developing fragility fractures. Although the issue remains controversial, many investigators use the same criteria to diagnose osteoporosis in men as are used in women. According to these criteria, men with T-scores of –2.5 or less have osteoporosis, even in the absence of a preceding fragility fracture. Additional studies are clearly needed in this area.

35. How do you treat osteoporosis in men?

The same nonpharmacologic measures used to treat osteoporosis in women are also appropriate for the treatment of men with this condition. Therefore, men should have 1000–1500 mg/day of calcium, 400 units/day of vitamin D, and adequate exercise. They should be encouraged to discontinue smoking, to limit alcohol consumption, and to limit caffeine consumption. Men also respond well to bisphosphonates, and therefore these agents are appropriate for the treatment of osteoporotic men. Hypogonadal males with osteoporosis should be treated with androgen replacement therapy.

36. How does glucocorticoid therapy cause osteoporosis?

Glucocorticoids in supraphysiologic doses (prednisone dose > 7 mg/day) have several detrimental effects on bone. First, they directly inhibit osteoblastic bone formation. Second, they impair intestinal calcium absorption and promote renal calcium excretion, thereby lowering serum calcium levels sufficiently to increase the secretion of PTH, which then stimulates bone resorption. Finally, they impair secretion of gonadal steroids, which further increases bone resorption. Because they both inhibit bone formation and stimulate bone resorption, glucocorticoids can cause significant bone loss and fractures within 6 months of therapy initiation.

37. When should osteoporosis prevention and treatment measures be instituted in patients taking glucocorticoid therapy?

Nonpharmacologic measures, as discussed above, are indicated in all patients taking glucocorticoids. Pharmacologic intervention should be considered for patients who will be on 7.5 mg/day of prednisone (or an equivalent dose of another glucocorticoid) for at least 3 months, particularly in postmenopausal women and in any individuals who have T-scores of −1.0 or less or who have had fragility fractures.

38. What is the treatment for glucocorticoid-induced osteoporosis?

Patients on glucocorticoid therapy should take calcium (1500 mg/day) and vitamin D (800 units/day). If urinary calcium excretion exceeds 300 mg/day, a thiazide diuretic may be added. Alendronate, risedronate, and etidronate all significantly increase bone mass in patients with glucocorticoid-induced osteoporosis and are the agents of choice for the prevention and treatment of this condition. Calcitonin may also be used in these patients, although its effects are less than those seen with bisphosphonates. Patients with hypogonadism should also receive gonadal steroid replacement.

39. How can falls be prevented?

1. Sedatives should be minimized or discontinued.
2. Visual impairment should be corrected.
3. Ambulatory aids should be used when appropriate.
4. Make the home "fall-proof": adequate lighting, carpeting, handrails, nonslip surfaces in bathrooms, removal of clutter and other obstacles to walking.

BIBLIOGRAPHY

1. Black DM, Cummings SR, Karpf DB, et al: Randomized trial of effect of alendronate on risk of fracture in women with existing vertebral fractures. Lancet 348:1535–1541, 1996.
2. Blake GM, Patel R, Fogelman I: Peripheral or axial bone density measurements? J Clin Densitometry 1:55–63, 1998.
3. Chesnut CH, Silverman S, Andriano K, et al: A randomized trial of nasal spray salmon calcitonin in postmenopausal women with established osteoporosis: The Prevent Recurrence of Osteoporotic Fractures Study. Am J Med 109:267–276, 2000.
4. Cummings SR, Black DM, Cummings SR, et al: Effect of alendronate on risk of fracture in women with low bone density but without vertebral fractures. JAMA 280:2077–2082, 1998.
5. Dawson-Hughes B, Harris SS, Krall EA, Dallal GE: Effect of calcium and vitamin D supplementation on bone density in men and women 65 years of age or older. N Engl J Med 337:670–676, 1997.
6. Delmas P, Bjarnason NH, Mitlak BH, et al: Effects of raloxifene on bone mineral density, serum cholesterol concentrations, and uterine endometrium in postmenopausal women. N Engl J Med 337:1641–1647, 1997.
7. Eastell R: Treatment of postmenopausal osteoporosis. N Engl J Med 338: 736–746, 1998.
8. Ettinger B, Black DM, Mitlak BH, et al: Reduction of vertebral fracture risk in postmenopausal women with osteoporosis treated with raloxifene. JAMA 282:637–645, 1999.

9. Faulkner KG, von Stetten E, Miller P: Discordance in patient classification using T-scores. J Clin Densitometry 2:343–350, 1999.
10. Genant HK, Engelke K, Fuerst T, et al: Noninvasive assessment of bone mineral structure: State of the art. J Bone Min Res 11:707–730, 1996.
11. Gluer C-C: Quantitative ultrasound techniques for the assessment of osteoporosis: Expert agreement on current status. J Bone Miner Res 12:1280–1288, 1997.
12. Grisso JA, Kelsey JL, Strom BL, et al: Risk factors for falls as a cause of hip fracture in women. N Engl J Med 324:1326–1331, 1991.
13. Harper KD, Weber TJ: Secondary osteoporosis: Diagnostic considerations. Endocrinol Metab Clin North Am 27 (2):325–348, 1998.
14. Harris ST, Watts NB, Genant HK, et al: Effects of risedronate treatment on vertebral and nonvertebral fractures in women with postmenopausal osteoporosis. A randomized controlled trial. JAMA 282:1344–1352, 1999.
15. Holloway L, Kohlmeier L, Kent K, Marcus R: Skeletal effects of cyclic recombinant human growth hormone and salmon calcitonin in osteopenic postmenopausal women. J Clin Endocrinol Metab 82:1111–1117, 1997.
16. Hosking D, Chilvers CED, Christiansen, C, et al: Prevention of bone loss with alendronate in postmenopausal women. N Engl J Med 338:485–492, 1998.
17. Kelepouris N, Harper KD, Gannon F, et al: Severe osteoporosis in men. Ann Intern Med 123:452–460, 1995.
18. Khovidhunkit W, Shoback DM: Clinical effects of raloxifene hydrochloride in women. Ann Intern Med 130:431-439, 1999.
19. Klotzbuecher CM, Ross PD, Landsman PB, et al: Patients with prior fractures have an increased risk of future fractures: A summary of the literature and statistical synthesis. J Bone Miner Res 15:721–739, 2000.
20. Liberman UA, Weiss SR, Broll J, et al: Effect of oral alendronate on bone mineral density and the incidence of fractures in postmenopausal osteoporosis. N Engl J Med 333:1437–1443, 1995.
21. Lindsay R, Cosman F, Lobo RA, et al: Addition of alendronate to ongoing hormone replacement therapy in the treatment of osteoporosis: A randomized, controlled clinical trial. J Clin Endocrinol Metab 84:3076–3081, 1999.
22. Lufkin EG, Wahner HW, O'Fallon WM, et al: Treatment of postmenopausal osteoporosis with transdermal estrogen. Ann Intern Med 117:1–9, 1992.
23. Lukert BP, Raisz LG: Glucocorticoid-induced osteoporosis: Pathogenesis and management. Ann Intern Med 112:352–364, 1990.
24. Manolagas SC, Jilka RL: Bone marrow, cytokines and bone remodeling. Emerging insights into the pathophysiology of osteoporosis. N Engl J Med 332:305–311, 1995.
25. Miller PD, Bonnick SL, Rosen CJ: Consensus of an international panel on the clinical utility of bone mass measurements in the detection of low bone mass in the adult population. Calcif Tissue Int 58:207–214, 1996.
26. Miller PD, Zapalowski C, Kulak CAM, Bilezikian JP: Bone densitometry: The best way to detect osteoporosis and to monitor therapy. J Clin Endocrinol Metab 84:1867–1871, 1999.
27. Miller PD, Baran DT, Bilezikian JP, et al: Practical clinical application of biochemical markers of bone turnover. J Clin Densitometry 2:323–342, 1999.
28. Miller PD, Bonnick SL, Johnston CC Jr, et al: The challenges of peripheral bone density testing. Which patients need additional central density skeletal measurements? J Clin Densitometry 1:211–217, 1998.
29. Orlic ZC, Raisz LG. Causes of secondary osteoporosis. J Clin Densitometry 2:79–92, 1998.
30. Orwoll E, Ettinger M, Weiss S, et al: Alendronate for the treatment of osteoporosis in men. N Engl J Med 343: 604–610, 2000.
31. Overgaard K, Hansen MA, Jensen SB, Christiansen C: Effect of calcitonin given intranasally on bone mass and fracture rates in established osteoporosis: A dose-response study. BMJ 305:556–561, 1992.
32. Pak CYC, Sakhaee K, Adams-Huet B, et al: Treatment of postmenopausal osteoporosis with slow release sodium fluoride. Final report of a randomized controlled trial. Ann Intern Med 123:401–408, 1995.

33. Raisz LG: The osteoporosis revolution. Ann Intern Med 126:458–462, 1997.
34. Reginster J-Y, Minn HW, Sorensen OH, et al: Randomized trial of the effects of risedronate on vertebral fractures in women with established postmenopausal osteoporosis. Osteoporos Int 11:83–91, 2000.
35. Reid IR, Ames RW, Evans MC, et al: Effect of calcium supplementation on bone loss in postmenopausal women. N Engl J Med 328:460–464, 1993.
36. Riggs BL, Hodgson SF, O'Fallon WM, et al: Effect of fluoride treatment on the fracture rate in postmenopausal women. N Engl J Med 322:802–809, 1990.
37. Riggs BL, Melton LJ III: The prevention and treatment of osteoporosis. N Engl J Med 327:620–627, 1992.
38. Riggs BL, Khosla S, Melton LJ III: A unitary model for involutional osteoporosis: Estrogen deficiency causes both Type I and Type II osteoporosis in postmenopausal women and contributes to bone loss in aging men. J Bone Miner Res 13:763–773, 1998.
39. Rittmaster RS, Bolognese M, Ettinger MP, et al: Enhancement of bone mass in osteoporotic women with parathyroid hormone followed by alendronate. J Clin Endocrinol Metab 85:2129–2134, 2000.
40. The writing group for the PEPI trial: Effects of hormone therapy on bone mineral density. Results for the postmenopausal estrogen/progestin interventions (PEPI) trial. JAMA 276:1389–1396, 1996.

11. MEASUREMENT OF BONE MASS

William E. Duncan, M.D., Ph.D.

1. Why measure bone mass?

Measurement of bone mass is a very powerful diagnostic, prognostic, and disease management tool. Bone mineral densitometry is used to measure bone mass, to establish the diagnosis of osteoporosis, and to determine the severity of the bone loss. No clinical features, laboratory tests, or other radiographic examinations can reliably identify individuals with osteoporosis. Standard roentgenograms are not sensitive indicators of bone loss, as they do not reliably show osteoporosis until 30–40% of the bone mineral is lost. In addition, an overpenetrated film can produce the appearance of osteoporosis in an individual with a normal bone mass. Thus, bone densitometry is essential for making the diagnosis of osteoporosis. However, while bone densitometry can determine if there is low bone mass, it cannot determine the cause. Thus, bone densitometry must be used along with a complete clinical evaluation, laboratory testing, and other diagnostic studies to determine the cause of and the most appropriate treatment for osteoporosis.

Bone mineral densitometry is also used to predict the risk of subsequent fractures and to monitor changes in bone mass during therapy for osteoporosis. A decreased bone mass is diagnostic for osteoporosis and is the primary determinant of whether a bone will fracture, although bone architecture (connectivity and remodeling) and bone geometry are also important determinants of bone strength. The relationship between bone mass and fracture risk is more powerful than the relationship between serum cholesterol concentration and coronary artery disease. A decrease in bone mass of 1 standard deviation (approximately a 10–12% difference, depending on the bone site) doubles the risk of fracture. A decrease of 2 standard deviations indicates a fourfold increase in risk of fracture, a 3 standard deviation decrease, an eightfold increase in risk, and so on. In comparison, a decrease in the cholesterol concentration of 1 standard deviation increases the risk of coronary artery disease by 20–30%.

2. How does bone densitometry measure bone mass?

All bone densitometry techniques measure the amount of calcium present in bone utilizing an ionizing radiation source, either from a radionuclide or from X-rays, and a radiation detector. Bone densitometry is based on the principle that when a beam of radiation is passed through a bone, the amount of radiation reaching the detector is inversely proportional to the mineral content of the measured bone. The attenuation of the radiation through bone is compared with the attenuation caused by known standards. Thus, the bone mineral content can be determined. The bone mineral content of the bone (or a region of interest within a bone) is then divided by the measured area. The result is the bone mineral density in grams per unit area (g/cm^2). This bone mineral density is not a true volumetric density (g/cm^3) but rather an areal density. In this chapter, bone mass and bone density are used interchangeably and synonymously.

3. What techniques are available to measure bone mass?

The techniques available to measure bone mass include single-photon absorptiometry, single-energy X-ray absorptiometry, dual-photon absorptiometry, dual-energy X-ray absorptiometry, quantitative computed tomography, radiographic absorptiometry and quantitative ultrasound.

When a beam of radiation is passed through a bone, both the bone mineral and the surrounding soft tissue in the region of interest will absorb radiation, although the soft tissue does this to a much lesser extent than does the bone mineral. If the amount of soft tissue surrounding the bone in the region of interest is minimal (as with peripheral sites such as the distal forearm or the heel), a radiation source with single energy is sufficient to measure bone mineral content. The use of a single radioactive energy source (usually iodine 125) is termed single-photon absorptiometry (SPA) or if a X-ray tube is used as the source of radiation, single-energy X-ray absorptiometry (SXA). Thus, SPA and SXA techniques are suitable for measuring bone mass at peripheral sites where there is little interfering soft tissue. SPA was the first technology used to assess bone mass and has been used since the 1960s. This technique is now being replaced by SXA, a method that offers improvements in precision and accuracy, lower cost and less radiation exposure. Peripheral dual-energy X-ray absorptiometry (pDEXA) recently has become available to measure bone density at either the wrist or heel.

If the amount of soft tissue surrounding the bone is significant (as with more central sites such as the spine or hip), a radiation source that has two energy levels must be employed to determine both the amount of soft tissue and bone mineral that is present. If the two energy sources originate from a single isotope (such as Gadolinium 153), the technique is termed dual-photon absorptiometry (DPA). If the dual energy source is an X-ray tube, the technique is termed dual energy x-ray absorptiometry (DEXA). DEXA is the preferred method for measuring bone mass in the United States. In 1997, 89% of bone density tests were performed using DEXA. DEXA can measure the bone mass of the spine, hip or wrist—the most common sites for osteoporotic fractures.

Radiographic absorptiometry (RA), also known as photodensitometry, uses a hand radiograph taken with a special aluminum calibration wedge that is placed on the film. Bone density is calculated relative to the density of the aluminum wedge. This method correlates weakly but significantly with other bone density methods. RA is similar in accuracy and precision to SXA.

Quantitative computed tomography (QCT) can selectively measure the trabecular center of a vertebral body. The measurement of trabecular bone mass has the advantage that this type of bone is more metabolically active and thus reflects bone loss earlier than cortical bone. Bones that contain significant amounts of trabecular bone respond rapidly to osteoporotic therapy for the same reason. Peripheral quantitative computed tomography (pQCT) measures the bone density of the forearm.

Quantitative ultrasound (QUS), while not a true densitometric method, is the most recently approved method for assessing bone in the heel, tibia, or patella. QUS transmits ultrasound waves through the bone and measures the speed of sound (SOS) and the broadband ultrasound attenuation (BUA). Measurement of BUA is based on the principle that the more complex the structure, the greater the attenuation of the ultrasound wave. Thus, BUA determines both density and structure of the bone. The SOS is influenced by the connectivity of the trabeculae. The greater the connectivity, the faster the sound wave will be transmitted through the bone of interest. Therefore, SOS evaluates both bone density and elasticity. It had been hoped that the QUS parameters would provide additional information about bone quality that is not assessed by bone densitometry. However, while the QUS results correlate with bone density by other methods, recent studies have not demonstrated QUS to be superior to bone densitometry for predicting fractures. Therefore, the additional clinical value of the information obtained from QUS technology has yet to be determined.

The following table compares several of the techniques for measuring bone mass.

Comparison of Bone Mass Measurement Techniques

TECHNIQUE	SITES MEASURED	PRECISION ERROR *	ACCURACY ERROR **	RADIATION DOSE (μSV)
SPA	Forearm	1–2%	2–5%	<1
	Calcaneous			
DEXA	Spine	1%	5–8%	1
	Lateral spine	2–3%	5–10%	5
	Proximal femur	1–2%	5–8%	1
	Total body	1%	1–2%	3
QCT	Single-energy (spine)	2–4%	5–10%	60
	Dual-energy (spine)	4–6%	3–6%	90
	Peripheral (radius)	0.5–1.0%	0.5%	<2
QUS	Calcaneous	0.3–3.8%	—	0
	Patella	<2%	—	0

*The error around repeated measurements (reproducibility or coefficient of variation).
**A measure of the agreement between the test result and the true value (accuracy).

4. Discuss the advantages and disadvantages of each bone mass measurement technique.

SPA has the advantages of good accuracy and precision and a very low delivered radiation dose. SPA is limited by its ability to measure bone mass only in the peripheral skeleton, relatively long scan times (10–15 minutes), and short isotope half-life, thus requiring regular replacement of the radioactive source. These disadvantages are overcome by SXA and pDEXA. However, measurement of bone mass at peripheral sites by any technique has serious drawbacks. Discrepancies between bone mass results at peripheral sites, and those of more centrally located sites (hip and spine) may result in underdiagnosis of osteoporosis if peripheral bone sites are the only ones used for bone mass measurement. Methodologies that measure peripheral bone mass may be more useful in the elderly because bone loss at peripheral sites in older individuals approaches that of the spine and hip.

DEXA has the best correlation with fracture risk, requires relatively short scanning times (<5 minutes) and has the ability to measure bone mass in all areas of the skeleton with high accuracy and reproducibility (precision) and with low radiation exposure. This method does not require replacement of the radioactive source. Several drawbacks of DEXA include the initial cost of the machine (more than $100,000) and measurement inaccuracies caused by aortic calcifications, spine implants, compression fractures, and osteoarthritis in the lumbar spine.

QCT is the only technique that is able to measure trabecular bone mass in the spine. This method removes the cortical envelope from the measurement area of the spine. As a result, osteophytes and aortic calcifications do not influence the bone mass values. Also, QCT is the only method that provides a true volumetric bone density. Drawbacks of this technique include higher cost and increased radiation exposure per test, lower accuracy and precision, and measurement of only a single bone site (the spine).

QUS has the advantages of no radiation exposure, being easily transportable, and costing less than other bone measurement technologies. The measurements made by this technique are limited to the peripheral skeleton. Their reproducibility is variable, with the coefficient of variation ranging up to 4%. The poor reproducibility is due to the QUS measurements being very sensitive to positioning of the bone of interest.

5. What are the indications for the measurement of bone mass?

Because of the cost, widespread bone density screening for osteoporosis is not recommended at this time. However, individuals at high risk for osteoporosis should be considered for bone mineral density testing. Measurement of bone mass is indicated whenever a clinical decision will be directly influenced by the outcome of the test. The National Osteoporosis Foundation has recently issued recommendations for appropriate bone mineral density testing. These guidelines are given in the following table. Other indications for measurement of bone mass include X-ray findings suggestive of osteoporosis or vertebral deformity, glucocorticoid therapy for more than 3 months, primary hyperparathyroidism, and treatment for osteoporosis (to monitor therapeutic response).

National Osteoporosis Foundation Guidelines for Bone Mineral Densitometry Testing

- Women ≥65 years of age (regardless of risk factors)
- Postmenopausal women <65 yr of age who have at least one risk factor for osteoporosis other than menopause
- Postmenopausal women who present with fractures
- Women who are considering therapy for osteoporosis and for whom bone mineral densitometry test results would influence this decision
- Women who have been receiving hormone replacement therapy for a prolonged period

6. What do bone densitometry results mean?

The bone densitometry report gives the absolute bone mass measurements (in g/cm^2) which do not provide clinically useful information unless these values are compared with those of reference populations. To do this, the bone mineral density report usually provides two scores: a T-score and a Z-score (see an example of a DEXA report below). The T- and Z-scores are the number of standard deviations above or below the mean bone mass of the comparison population. The T-score compares the patient's bone mass with that of a normal young adult gender- and ethnicity-matched population. This population represents the optimal or peak bone mass for the patient. A patient whose bone mass is 1 standard deviation below that of the young reference population has a T-score of −1.0. At the spine, 1 standard deviation is about 10%, so someone with a T-score of −1.0 has lost about 10% of his or her bone mass. Because the T-score is a measure of bone loss, this value is used to diagnose osteoporosis.

The Z-score compares the patient's bone mass with that of an age-, gender-, and ethnicity-matched reference population. The Z-score is used to determine if the measured bone mass is appropriate for the patient's age. Thus, a Z-score less than expected for a given individual (e.g. less than −2.0) should prompt a search for associated medical or lifestyle conditions (either current or in the past) that may have accelerated bone loss or prevented the patient from reaching peak bone mass in early adulthood. On the other hand, a normal Z-score indicates that the bone loss is age and gender appropriate, and a search for secondary causes of osteoporosis will likely be less successful.

7. How are bone densitometry results interpreted clinically?

In 1994, the World Health Organization (WHO) developed criteria for the diagnosis of osteoporosis and osteopenia in postmenopausal white women using T-scores from any skeletal site. A T-score greater than −1.0 is defined as normal bone mass, a T-score between −1.0 and −2.5 is defined as low bone mass (or osteopenia), and a T-score less than −2.5 is defined as osteoporosis. Established (or severe) osteoporosis was defined as a T-score less than −2.5 with one or more osteoporotic fractures.

There are several caveats about using the WHO classification criteria. These criteria were derived from data pertaining to white postmenopausal women. Thus, applying these definitions to other ethnic groups or to men should be done with caution. The WHO criteria were also not intended to apply to premenopausal women of any ethnicity. The technique used to measure the T-scores is also important. The WHO criteria were developed from stud-

WALTER REED ARMY MEDICAL CENTER

k = 1.229   d0 = 109.2(1.000H)

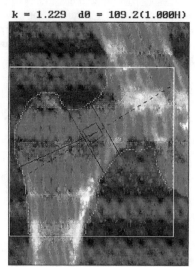

·Jun 1 14:41 2000   [110 x 112]
Hologic QDR-2000 (S/N 2419)
Right Hip V4.76

H06010017   Thu Jun 1 14:32 2000
Name:
Comment:
I.D.:   Sex:
S.S.#:   Ethnic:
ZIP Code: Height:
Scan Code: Weight:
BirthDate: Age:
Physician: DUNCAN
Image not for diagnostic use

   TOTAL BMD CV 1.0%
   C.F.   1.007   1.083   1.000

Region	Area (cm²)	BMC (grams)	BMD (gms/cm²)
Neck	6.51	4.81	0.738
Troch	15.41	9.70	0.629
Inter	23.85	26.58	1.114
TOTAL	45.78	41.09	0.898
Ward's	1.14	0.64	0.559

Midline (116,136)-(18, 76)

Neck	58 x 16 at [-27, 6]
Troch	-8 x 56 at [0, 0]
Ward's	11 x 11 at [-6, 3]

HOLOGIC

WALTER REED ARMY MEDICAL CENTER

Right Hip
Reference Database •

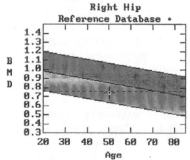

BMD(Neck[R]) = 0.738 g/cm²

H06010017   Thu Jun 1 14:32 2000
Name:
Comment:
I.D.:   Sex:
S.S.#:   Ethnic:
ZIP Code: Height:
Scan Code: Weight:
BirthDate: Age:
Physician: DUNCAN

Region	BMD	T	Z
Neck	0.738	-2.19 75%	-1.01 87%
		(20.0)	
Troch	0.629	-1.52 79%	-1.03 85%
		(20.0)	
Inter	1.114	-0.86 90%	-0.23 97%
		(20.0)	
TOTAL	0.898	-1.34 84%	-0.67 91%
		(20.0)	
Ward's	0.559	-2.28 67%	-0.68 87%
		(20.0)	

• Age and sex matched
T = peak bone mass
Z = age matched   TK   10/25/91

HOLOGIC

Figure 1. Printout of a DEXA Scan of the Hip (personal data deleted)

ies using bone density measurements. Therefore, applying the WHO criteria to bone mass measurements obtained with other technologies (such as QUS) may also be misleading. Finally, these definitions were developed as general guidelines for diagnosis and were not intended to require or restrict therapy for individual patients.

8. Discuss how bone mass measurements are used to determine the need for treatment of osteoporosis.

The physician should use information from bone mass testing in conjunction with knowledge of the patient's specific medical and personal history to determine the best treatment. The bone mineral density results should not be used as the sole determinant for treatment decisions.

The National Osteoporosis Foundation has proposed that women with T-scores less than –2.0 in the absence of risk factors for osteoporosis or women with T-scores less than –1.5 with risk factors should be treated for osteoporosis. Women older than 70 yr having multiple risk factors may be treated without bone mass testing.

9. What bone should be selected for measurement of bone mass?

Bone density of the spine (anteroposterior or lateral views), the hip, the radius, and the whole body can be measured by SXA or DEXA (see examples below). Measurement of bone mass at any skeletal site has value in predicting fracture risk. However, the bone density of the hip is the best predictor of hip fractures. Hip bone mass also predicts fractures at other sites as well as do bone mass measurements at those sites. For these reasons, the hip is the preferred site for measurement of bone mass. While there is significant concordance (r values from 0.6–0.7) between skeletal sites in predicting bone mass from one site to another, there is still enough discordance in bone mass at various sites to not rely on single bone mass measurements to diagnose osteoporosis. This discordance among the various sites is more marked in the early postmenopausal population than in individuals 65 and older. To reduce the likelihood of missing the diagnosis of osteoporosis or osteopenia, bone mass should be measured, if possible, at both the hip and the spine. Measurement of bone mass in the spine may not be possible in the elderly, as the bone mass of the anteroposterior view of the spine might be falsely elevated because of marked aortic calcifications or degenerative joint disease, osteophytes, severe scoliosis, or facet sclerosis of the posterior elements. Likewise, the bone mass of the femur of patients who have hip abnormalities or hip replacement surgery cannot be measured.

Measurement of peripheral bone mass (e.g., the forearm) generally adds little to the evaluation of an individual with postmenopausal osteoporosis, although the forearm appears to be the best site to assess the effects on bone of excess parathyroid hormone activity seen with primary hyperparathyroidism. Furthermore, peripheral bone mass measurements have not yet been shown to be useful for monitoring the effects of therapy for osteoporosis. The best way to follow patients treated for osteoporosis is to monitor central sites (spine and hip), where remodeling occurs at a more substantial pace than in the peripheral sites. Pharmacologic therapy for osteoporosis usually has the greatest effect on the spine, a lesser effect on the hip, and little or no effect on the forearm.

Some bone densitometers have the ability to measure bone mass of the spine using a lateral view. The lateral spine measurement evaluates primarily the vertebral bodies and avoids interference by the posterior elements, such as the pedicles and the articulating and spinous processes. Lateral scanning also can provide morphometric information about the lumbar spine because vertebral deformities (as surrogate measures of vertebral fractures) can be identified. This feature is not commonly used but may be utilized more widely in the future. Densitometry measurements of the lateral spine are less precise, however, making monitoring of serial bone density changes more difficult.

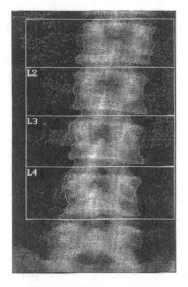

A. AP Spine

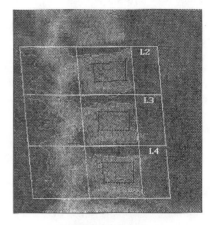

B. Lateral Spine

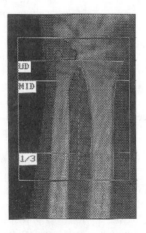

C. Forearm

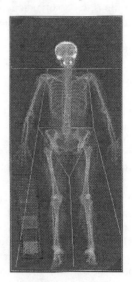

D. Whole Body

Figure 2. Images of Several Skeletal Sites Scanned by a DEXA Bone Densitometer

10. How often should bone mass measurements be repeated?

Patients may undergo one or more follow-up scans. The frequency of bone density measurements is determined in part by the coefficient of variation (CV) of the measurement, which gives an indication of the precision error (or reproducibility) of the technique. The CV is operator and machine dependent and is different for each bone site. The CV is used to calculate the minimum change necessary for two serial bone mass measurements to be considered statistically different. Studies of long-term precision (CV) give values of approximately 1.0% for spine and 1–2% for femoral neck bone mass measurements by DEXA. This means that the smallest difference between two bone mass measurements that is significant is a change of 2.83% at the spine and 5.66% at the femoral neck. In contrast, the average amount of early postmenopausal bone loss from the spine is 1–2 % per year. This annual bone loss is slightly higher than the coefficient of variation of many available bone densitometers. Therefore, to obtain statistically meaningful results, postmenopausal women should not undergo measurements of spine bone mass by DEXA more often than once every 1.4 years. Measurement of bone mass every 6 months is recommended for patients in whom glucocorticoid therapy is being initiated because a rapid rate of bone loss may occur. Patients treated with glucocorticoids may lose as much as 17% of their skeleton in the first 6–12 months of therapy. The federal Bone Mass Measurement Act, passed in 1998, mandates payment for bone densitometry every 2 yr for all at-risk Medicare recipients undergoing therapy for osteoporosis.

Because of differences in calibration between different manufacturers' equipment (and even between machines of the same make and model), the results of serial bone mass determinations should be compared only when the patient has been tested on the same machine and preferably by the same technologist.

11. What conditions limit the accuracy of bone mass measurements?

There are several factors that may limit the accuracy of anteroposterior spine mass measurements if they go unrecognized. Degenerative changes, oral contrast taken for other radiographic studies, and osteophytes will artificially elevate the measured bone density. Anatomic distortions that affect the accuracy of these measurements may also occur from lumbar disc disease, compression fractures, scoliosis, prior surgical intervention, or vascular calcifications in the overlying aorta, which are common in the elderly. Likewise, previous surgery on the hip may alter bone mass. The following figure illustrates some of these anomalies.

12. Interpret the bone mineral density results from the following four patients.

Each patient is a white postmenopausal woman. The bone mass was measured at any skeletal site.

  1. Patient 1:
          T-score = –0.9   Z-score = +0.2
  2. Patient 2:
          T-score = –2.0   Z-score = –0.9
  3. Patient 3:
          T-score = –3.0   Z-score = –1.4
  4 Patient 4:
          T-score = –3.0   Z-score = –2.5

Interpretation:

Patient 1: This woman has a normal bone mass.
Patient 2: This woman has a low bone mass (osteopenia) which is appropriate for her age (the Z-score is greater than -2.0).
Patient 3: This woman has osteoporosis that is appropriate for her age.
Patient 4: This woman has osteoporosis with bone loss that is greater than expected for her age. This bone density finding should prompt a thorough evaluation to rule out secondary causes of osteoporosis (such as hyperthyroidism, malabsorption, Cushing's syndrome, hypogonadism, vitamin D deficiency, excessive alcohol consumption, use of certain drugs, etc.).

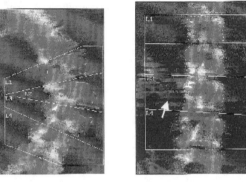 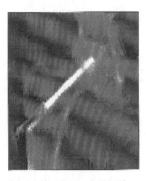

A. Severe Scoliosis   B. Oral Contrast   C. Medullary Rod and Side Plate

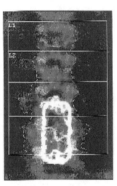 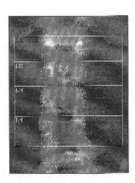 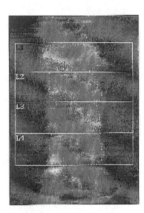

D. Fusion Hardware   E. Laminectomy   F. Compression Fracture (L1)

Figure 3. Distortions that Interfere with Measurement of Bone Mass

BIBLIOGRAPHY

1. Blake GM, Fogelman I: Applications of bone densitometry for osteoporosis. Endocrinol Metab Clin North Am 27:267, 1998.
2. Compston JE, Cooper C, Kanis JA: Bone densitometry in clinical practice. BMJ 310:1507, 1995.
3. Genant HK, Engelke K, Fuerst T, et al.: Noninvasive assessment of bone mineral and structure: State of the art. J Bone Miner Res 11:707, 1996.
4. Gluer CC, Genant HK, Hans D, et al.: Quantitative ultrasound techniques for the assessment of osteoporosis: Expert agreement on current status. J Bone Miner Res 12:1280, 1997.
5. Levis S, Altman R: Bone densitometry: Clinical considerations. Arthritis & Rheumatism 41:577, 1998.
6. Miller PD, Bonnick SL. Clinical application of bone densitometry. In Favus MJ (ed): Primer on the Metabolic Bone Diseases and Disorders of Mineral Metabolism, 4th ed. New York, Raven Press, 1999, p 152.
7. Miller PD, Zapalowski C, Kulak CA, Bilezikian JP: Bone densitometry: The best way to detect osteoporosis and to monitor therapy. J Clin Endocrinol Metab 84:1867,1999.
8. National Osteoporosis Foundation web site: www.nof.org.
9. Pejovic T, Olive DL: Contemporary Use of Bone Densitometry. Clinical Obstet Gynecol 42:876, 1999.
10. The WHO Study Group: Assessment of Fracture Risk and Its Application to Screening for Postmenopausal Osteoporosis. WHO Tech Rep Ser 843. Geneva, World Health Organization, 1994.

12. OSTEOMALACIA AND RICKETS

William E. Duncan, M.D., Ph.D.

1. What are osteomalacia and rickets?

Osteomalacia and *rickets* are terms that describe the clinical, histologic, and radiologic abnormalities of bone that are associated with more than 50 different diseases and conditions. Osteomalacia is a disorder of mature bone, while rickets occurs in growing bone. Mineralization of newly formed osteoid (the bone protein matrix) is inadequate or delayed in both conditions. Thus, in individuals with rickets, defective mineralization occurs both in bones and in cartilage of the epiphyseal growth plates and is associated with growth retardation and skeletal deformities not typically seen in adults with osteomalacia. Although rickets and osteomalacia were initially viewed as distinct clinical entities, the same pathologic processes may result in either disorder, depending on whether a growing or nongrowing skeleton is involved.

2. Why is it important to know about osteomalacia and rickets?

In the United States at the beginning of the 20th century, rickets caused by a deficiency of vitamin D was common in urban areas. In the 1920s, it was virtually eliminated by an appreciation of the antirachitic properties of sunlight and the use of cod liver oil (which contains vitamin D). However, with the development of effective treatments for previously fatal diseases (such as chronic renal failure) that affect vitamin D metabolism and with an improved understanding of both vitamin D and mineral metabolism, many additional syndromes with osteomalacia or rickets as a feature have become recognized. In addition, for a significant number of adult women with osteoporosis in the United States, occult vitamin D deficiency may be an unsuspected component of their bone loss.

3. List the causes of osteomalacia and rickets.

The primary abnormality of bone in individuals with osteomalacia or rickets is defective mineralization of bone matrix. The major mineral in bone is hydroxyapatite $[Ca_{10}(PO_4)_6(OH)_2]$. Thus, any disease that limits the availability of calcium (Ca) or phosphorus (P) may result in osteomalacia or rickets. The causes of osteomalacia and rickets fall into three categories: 1) disorders associated with abnormalities of vitamin D metabolism or action that limit the availability of calcium for mineralization of bone; 2) disorders associated with abnormalities of phosphorus metabolism; and 3) a small group of disorders in which there is normal vitamin D and mineral metabolism.

Conditions Associated with Osteomalacia and Rickets

CONDITION	PRIMARY MECHANISM*
Abnormal vitamin D metabolism or action	
• Nutritional deficiency	Vitamin D deficiency
• Malabsorption	Vitamin D deficiency
• Primary biliary cirrhosis	Malabsorption of vitamin D
• Chronic renal disease	Impaired 1α-hydroxylation of 25 hydroxy-vitamin D
• Chronic liver disease	Impaired 25-hydroxylation of vitamin D
• VDDR type I	1α-hydroxylase deficiency
• VDDR type II	Abnormal vitamin D receptor
• Drugs (phenytoin, barbiturates, cholestyramine)	Increased catabolism and/or excretion of vitamin D

Phosphate deficiency or renal phosphate wasting

• Diminished phosphate intake	Phosphate deficiency
• Excessive aluminum hydroxide intake	Increasing binding of intestinal phosphate
• X-linked hypophosphatemic rickets	Renal phosphate transport defect
• Tumor-induced osteomalacia	Renal phosphate transport defect
• Miscellaneous renal tubular defects (RTA, FS)	Renal phosphate transport defect

Normal vitamin D and phosphate metabolism

• Hypophosphatasia	Alkaline phosphatase deficiency
• Drugs (bisphosphonates, fluoride, aluminum)	Inhibition of mineralization or stimulation of matrix synthesis
• Osteogenesis imperfecta	Abnormal bone collagen
• Fibrogenesis imperfecta ossium	Defective bone matrix

*Although only one mechanism for osteomalacia or rickets is given, other mechanisms also may contribute to the bone disease.
VDDR = vitamin D–dependent rickets, RTA = renal tubular acidosis, FS = Fanconi syndrome.

4. Discuss the disease processes that interfere with the metabolism of vitamin D.

The disease processes associated with abnormal vitamin D metabolism or action are best understood with knowledge of the normal vitamin D metabolism. Clinically apparent vitamin D deficiency is rarely seen in the United States except when exposure to sunlight or intake of vitamin D-fortified milk and dairy products is limited. However, the elderly in America are particularly at risk for occult vitamin D deficiency because of 1) an age-related decrease in the dermal synthesis of vitamin D; 2) impaired hepatic and renal hydroxylation of vitamin D; and 3) diminished intestinal responsiveness to 1,25-dihydroxyvitamin D.

Individuals with malabsorption associated with diseases of the small intestine, the hepatobiliary tree, and the pancreas are also at risk for vitamin D deficiency. Celiac disease or sprue, regional enteritis, intestinal bypass surgery, partial gastrectomy, chronic liver disease, primary biliary cirrhosis, and pancreatic insufficiency have been associated with the development of osteomalacia.

Two extremely rare genetic syndromes are also associated with rickets. Vitamin D–dependent rickets (VDDR) type I is associated with an almost complete absence of renal 25-hydroxyvitamin D-1α-hydroxylase activity. VDDR type II is caused by a defective vitamin D receptor, which results in an end-organ resistance to 1,25-dihydroxyvitamin D and a lack of vitamin D action. Anticonvulsant drugs (e.g., phenytoin, phenobarbital) may interfere with the action of 1,25-dihydroxyvitamin D in the peripheral tissues and accelerate hepatic metabolism of this steroid hormone.

5. What conditions associated with abnormalities of phosphate metabolism result in osteomalacia or rickets?

Nutritional phosphate deficiency, decreased intestinal absorption of phosphate due to ingestion of phosphate binders such as aluminum hydroxide, or renal phosphate wasting may result in osteomalacia or rickets. Hypophosphatemic rickets (also called vitamin D–resistant rickets) is a syndrome of renal phosphate wasting and decreased renal synthesis of 1,25-dihydroxyvitamin D. This disorder is the most common inherited form of rickets and is transmitted as an X-linked dominant trait. The abnormal gene for this disorder has been localized to the short arm of the X chromosome.

Tumor-induced osteomalacia is an uncommon syndrome in which usually benign neoplasms (frequently of mesenchymal origin) are found in association with nonfamilial acquired osteomalacia. Such tumors appear to elaborate an as yet unidentified humoral factor that is responsible for renal phosphate wasting and impaired renal production of 1,25-dihydroxyvitamin D observed in this condition. The tumors usually responsible for this dis-

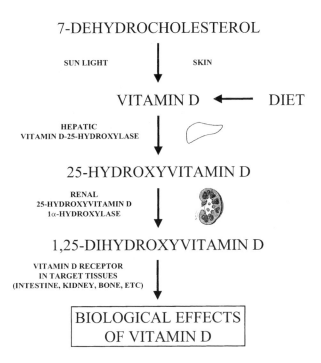

ease include sarcomas, hemangiomas, and giant cell tumors of bone and, rarely, carcinoma of the breast and prostate.

6. How does chronic renal failure cause osteomalacia and rickets?

Chronic renal failure is associated with several bone diseases: osteomalacia or rickets, adynamic bone, osteitis fibrosa cystica (due to longstanding secondary hyperparathyroidism), and a combination of both osteomalacia and osteitis fibrosa cystica, termed mixed renal osteodystrophy. Rickets or osteomalacia is usually a late finding in the course of the kidney disease and is rarely seen before patients begin dialysis. Rickets and osteomalacia are caused by 1) low concentrations of circulating 1,25-dihydroxyvitamin D, 2) aluminum intoxication from aluminum-containing antacids used as phosphate binders or an aluminum-contaminated dialysate, and 3) possibly the chronic metabolic acidosis associated with the renal failure.

7. What clinical findings are associated with osteomalacia and rickets?

In adults, osteomalacia may be asymptomatic. When symptomatic, osteomalacia may present with diffuse skeletal pain (often aggravated by physical activity or palpation), proximal muscle weakness, and sometimes muscle wasting. The muscle weakness often involves the proximal muscles of the lower extremities and may result in a waddling gait and difficulties rising from a chair or climbing stairs. The bone pain is described as dull and aching and is usually located in the back, hips, knees, legs, and at sites of fractures. Fractures may result from only minor trauma.

In children with rickets, because of the impaired calcification of cartilage at the growth plates, additional clinical manifestations are often observed. Especially prominent are widening of the metaphyses (the growth zones between the epiphysis and diaphysis), slowed growth, and various skeletal deformities. The effects of rickets are greatest at sites where the growth of bone is most rapid. Because the rate of growth of the skeleton varies with age, the manifestations of rickets likewise will vary with age. One of the earliest signs of rickets in infants is craniotabes (abnormal softness of the skull). In older infants and young children, thickening of the forearm at the wrist and of the costochondral junctions (also known as the rachitic rosary) may be manifestations of rickets. Harrison's groove, a lateral indentation of the chest wall at the site of attachment of the diaphragm, may also be present. In older children, bowing of the tibia and fibula may be observed. At any age, if the osteomalacia (or rickets) is associated with hypocalcemia, paresthesias of the hands and around the mouth, muscle cramps, positive Chvostek's and Trousseau's signs, tetany, and seizures may also be present.

8. Describe the biochemical findings associated with osteomalacia and rickets.

The laboratory abnormalities associated with osteomalacia or rickets depend on the underlying defect or process causing the bone disease. To understand the biochemical abnormalities observed in conditions associated with the abnormal metabolism of vitamin D, an understanding the body's response to hypocalcemia and knowledge of the vitamin D metabolic pathway is necessary. Thus, in patients with nutritional vitamin D deficiency or malabsorption, the low vitamin D concentrations result in a low-to-low normal serum calcium concentration, which serves as a stimulus for increased secretion of parathyroid hormone (secondary hyperparathyroidism). This hyperparathyroid state in turn causes increased renal excretion of phosphate, low serum phosphate, elevated alkaline phosphatase, and reduced urinary calcium excretion.

Depending on the abnormality of vitamin D metabolism, different vitamin D metabolite patterns may be observed. In nutritional vitamin D deficiency, the 25-hydroxyvitamin D concentrations are low. In VDDR type I, in which there is a deficiency of the renal 25-hydroxyvitamin D-1α-hydroxylase enzyme, normal or increased serum 25-hydroxyvitamin D and low or undetectable serum 1,25-dihydroxyvitamin D concentrations are observed. On the other hand, in VDDR type II, which is caused by a mutation of the vitamin D receptor resulting in resistance of target organs to 1,25-dihydroxyvitamin D, the concentrations of both 25-hydroxyvitamin D and 1,25-dihydroxyvitamin D are elevated.

The hallmarks of the hypophosphatemic osteomalacia syndromes are fasting hypophosphatemia and renal phosphate wasting (as assessed by a decrease in the maximum renal tubular reabsorption of phosphate/glomerular filtration rate [TmP/GFR]). Serum calcium and parathyroid hormone concentrations are usually normal. Inexplicably, serum 1,25-dihydroxyvitamin D concentrations are inappropriately low for the degree of hypophosphatemia, which is normally a stimulus for renal 1α-hydroxylation of 25-hydroxyvitamin D.

The third group of disorders causing osteomalacia and rickets (disorders with normal vitamin D and phosphate metabolism) is associated with few biochemical abnormalities. In patients with congenital hypophosphatasia, an abnormally low serum alkaline phosphatase concentration is usually observed. Serum calcium, 25-hydroxyvitamin D, 1,25-dihydroxyvitamin D, and parathyroid hormone concentrations in patients with this disorder are normal. About one half of patients are hyperphosphatemic due to an increased TmP/GFR. Serum concentrations of calcium and phosphate in fibrogenesis imperfecta ossium are normal, but the serum alkaline phosphatase activity is usually increased.

9. What radiographic findings are associated with osteomalacia and rickets?

The histologic and biochemical abnormalities associated with rickets and osteomalacia are usually found before radiographic abnormalities are observed. The most common radiographic change in patients with osteomalacia is a reduction in skeletal density (generalized osteopenia or osteoporosis). Pseudofractures (also called Looser zones or Milkman fractures) or complete fractures also may be observed. Pseudofractures are straight transverse radiolucent bands ranging from a few millimeters to several centimeters in length, usually perpendicular to the surface of the bones. They are most often bilateral and are particularly common in the femur, pelvis, and small bones of the hands and feet.

Abnormalities, including fraying of the metaphyses of the long bones, widening of the unmineralized epiphyseal growth plates, and bowing of the legs, are observed in children. The skeletal deformities observed in patients with rickets may persist into adulthood.

Patients with osteomalacia may have additional radiographic findings due to secondary hyperparathyroidism. Such findings may include subperiosteal resorption of the phalanges, loss of the lamina dura of the teeth, widening of the spaces at the symphysis pubis and sacroiliac joints, and presence of brown tumors or bone cysts.

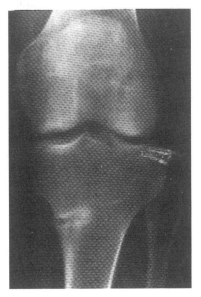

Radiographic evidence of osteomalacia.

10. Discuss the histologic features of osteomalacia.

The two diagnostic bone biopsy features of osteomalacia are the presence of wide osteoid seams and increased mineralization lag time (the time necessary for newly deposited matrix to mineralize). The mineralization lag time is assessed clinically by administration of two short courses of oral tetracycline several weeks apart. Because the tetracycline is deposited at the mineralization front, the lag time may be determined by measuring the distance between the two fluorescent tetracycline bands in the biopsied bone. Depending on the cause of the osteomalacia, hyperparathyroid bone changes also may be seen. Because of the varied clinical signs and symptoms, radiographic findings, and biochemical abnormalities associated with osteomalacia and rickets, none of these tests or findings is pathognomonic. The bone biopsy remains the gold standard in establishing the diagnosis of rickets and osteomalacia. The evaluation of a bone biopsy must be performed by personnel specially trained in the interpretation of bone histology.

11. Describe the therapy for osteomalacia and rickets.

The goal of therapy for patients with osteomalacia and rickets caused by an abnormality of vitamin D metabolism is to correct the hypocalcemia and the deficiency of active vitamin D metabolites by administration of calcium salts and vitamin D preparations. In the United States, vitamin D_2 (ergocalciferol), 25-hydroxyvitamin D (calcifediol), 1,25-dihydroxyvitamin D (calcitriol), and dihydrotachysterol are available. Each of these preparations has a different half-life and potency. The choice and dose of vitamin D preparation are determined by the underlying pathologic defect of vitamin D metabolism. For example, for patients with vitamin D deficiency, a daily dose of 5,000–10,000 IU of ergocalciferol (along with 1 g of elemental calcium) is often sufficient to heal the osteomalacia. In contrast, the treatment of the osteomalacia associated with VDDR type II, which involves profound resistance to the effects of vitamin D, consists of administration of the most potent vitamin D metabolite, 1,25-dihydroxyvitamin D, in doses up to 60 µg/day (an extraordinarily high dose), along with large doses of oral calcium. In severe cases, high-dose intravenous calcium infusions are required to heal the rickets in patients with VDDR type II.

In the treatment of hypophosphatemic rickets, both phosphate supplements and calcitriol are required to heal the bone disease. Tumor removal or irradiation is required to treat tumor-induced osteomalacia.

In chronic renal failure with aluminum-induced osteomalacia, aluminum is removed from the affected bone by treatment with the chelating agent deferoxamine. The osteomalacia can then be treated by calcium together with 1,25-dihydroxyvitamin D. Osteomalacia associated with renal tubular acidosis is treated with vitamin D and bicarbonate to correct the acidosis.

12. What are the complications of treatment with vitamin D_2 or other vitamin D metabolites?

When high doses of vitamin D_2 or one of the potent vitamin D metabolites are used, it is important to monitor carefully for the development of hypercalcemia. Mild hypercalcemia may be asymptomatic. However, severely hypercalcemic patients may complain of anorexia, nausea, vomiting, weight loss, headache, constipation, polyuria, polydipsia, and altered mental status. Impaired renal function, nephrocalcinosis, nephrolithiasis, and even death may eventually ensue. If vitamin D intoxication occurs, all calcium supplements and vitamin D preparations must be discontinued immediately and therapy for hypercalcemia instituted.

BIBLIOGRAPHY

1. Bingham CT, Fitzpatrick LA: Noninvasive testing in the diagnosis of osteomalacia. Am J Med 95:519, 1993.
2. Bliziotes M, Yergey AL, Nanes MS, et al.: Absent intestinal response to calciferols in hereditary resistance to 1,25-dihydroxyvitamin D: Documentation and effective therapy with high-dose intravenous calcium infusions. J Clin Endocrinol Metab 66:294, 1988.
3. Drezner MK. Tumor-induced rickets and osteomalacia. In Favus MJ (e.): Primer on the Metabolic Bone Diseases and Disorders of Mineral Metabolism, 4th ed. New York, Raven Press, 1999, p 331.
4. Drezner MK: Vitamin D–resistant rickets/osteomalacia. Endocrinologist 3:392, 1991.
5. Francis RM, Selby PL. Osteomalacia. Baillieres Clin Endocrinol Metab 11:145, 1997.
6. Glorieux FH. Hypophosphatemic vitamin D-resistant rickets. In Favus MJ (ed): Primer on the Metabolic Bone Diseases and Disorders of Mineral Metabolism, 4th ed. New York, Raven Press, 1999, p 328.
7. Harvey JN, Gray C, Belchetz PE. Oncogenous osteomalacia and malignancy. Clin Endocrinol 37:379, 1992.
8. Klein GL. Nutritional rickets and osteomalacia. In Favus MJ (ed): Primer on the Metabolic Bone Diseases and Disorders of Mineral Metabolism, 4th ed. New York, Raven Press, 1999, p 315.
9. Liberman UA, Marx SJ. Vitamin D–-dependent rickets. In Favus MJ (ed): Primer on the Metabolic Bone Diseases and Disorders of Mineral Metabolism, 4th ed. New York, Raven Press, 1999, p 323.
10. Parfitt AM. Osteomalacia and related disorders. In Avioli LV, Krane SM (eds): Metabolic Bone Diseases and Clinically Related Disorders, 2nd ed. Philadelphia, W.B. Saunders, 1990, p 329.
11. Pitt MJ. Rickets and osteomalacia are still around. Radiol Clin North Am 29:97, 1991.
12. Reichel H, Koeffler HP, Norman AW. The role of the vitamin D endocrine system in health and disease. N Engl J Med 320:980, 1989.
13. Wolinsky-Friedland M.: Drug-induced metabolic bone disease. Endocrinol Metab Clin North Am 24:395. 1995.

13. PAGET'S DISEASE OF BONE

William E. Duncan, M.D., Ph.D.

1. What is Paget's disease of bone?

Paget's disease is characterized by abnormal bone architecture resulting from an imbalance between osteoblastic bone formation and osteoclastic bone resorption. Sir James Paget first described this disease in 1876. Although he called the condition osteitis deformans, we now know that Paget's disease of bone is not an inflammation of bone (osteitis) and only rarely results in deformity.

2. Discuss how Paget's disease is diagnosed.

The diagnosis of Paget's disease is generally based on a combination of clinical manifestations, radiographic signs, and characteristic biochemical changes. Although histologic examination of pagetic bone is diagnostic, a bone biopsy is often unnecessary. Bone biopsy should be performed when the diagnosis of Paget's disease is unclear or when osteogenic sarcoma or metastatic carcinoma must be excluded.

3. What are the clinical manifestations of Paget's disease?

Most patients with Paget's disease are asymptomatic. The diagnosis is often suspected from radiographs done for other reasons or from an unexpected elevation of the serum alkaline phosphatase concentration. The most common symptom of Paget's disease is bone or joint pain. The pain is often described as dull and aching. Other manifestations of Paget's disease, such as headache, bone deformity, skull enlargement, fracture, change in skin temperature over an involved bone, high-output congestive heart failure, and entrapment neuropathies that cause loss of hearing or other neurologic deficits are much less common. Neurologic deficits arise from bony impingement on the brain and cranial nerves exiting from the skull, spinal nerve entrapment, and direct pressure of pagetic vertebrae on the spinal cord. Bony deformity is usually seen in patients with longstanding Paget's disease. Most commonly, the skull, clavicles, and long bones are deformed and exhibit both an increase in size and an abnormal contour. There is speculation that Ludwig Von Beethoven's hearing loss, headaches, and progressive hyperostosis frontalis were the result of longstanding Paget's disease of bone.

Several disorders that are statistically more prevalent in patients with Paget's disease than in unaffected individuals include arthritis, fractures, primary hyperparathyroidism, osteoporosis, thyroid disease, and kidney stones.

Complications Associated with Paget's Disease of Bone

- Bone pain
- Bone deformity
- Secondary arthritis adjacent to pagetic bone
- Neurologic abnormalities
    Spinal stenosis
    Hearing loss and other cranial nerve palsies
    Radiculopathy
- Obstructive hydrocephalus
- Cardiovascular complications
    Increased blood flow to involved bone

Increased cardiac output
Vascular and aortic valve calcifications
- Fracture
- Malignant transformation
- Immobilization hypercalcemia

4. Describe the radiographic abnormalities seen with Paget's disease.

Paget's disease of bone appears to progress through several distinct phases. The first is the early osteolytic phase, in which osteoclastic bone resorption predominates. The osteolytic phase evolves into one marked by both osteoclastic and osteoblastic overactivity. This mixed (or osteoblastic) phase is followed by a less active period of bone remodeling and marked sclerosis. The radiographic appearance of pagetic bone differs with each phase. About 1–2% of patients exhibit a purely lytic phase. The characteristic findings are an advancing wedge-shaped resorption front at either end of the long tubular bones. In the skull, the osteolytic phase is manifested by large circumscribed osteolytic lesions (termed osteoporosis circumscripta). During the mixed phase of the disease, both osteoclastic bone resorption and osteoblastic bone formation may be appreciated on radiographs of involved bones. Evolution of osteolytic lesions into the osteoblastic phase may require years or even decades, during which the affected bone may become sclerotic and enlarged and demonstrate bowing deformities, incomplete transverse fractures (pseudofractures), and even complete fractures. When the skull is involved in the osteoblastic phase, thickening of the calvarium and a patchy increase in bone density may give the skull a "cotton-wool" appearance. In the sclerotic phase, the sclerotic bone changes may be so extensive that they may be confused with metastatic disease. Both metastatic cancer and Paget's disease are common in the elderly and may coexist in the same patient. Thus, the clinician caring for patients with Paget's disease must be alert for evidence of metastatic disease to bone.

The metabolic activity of osteoblastic pagetic bone lesions is most easily assessed by radionuclide scanning. The active pagetic bone lesions avidly take up the technetium-labeled bisphosphonate. Although bone scans are diagnostically less specific than radiographic studies, they will identify approximate 15-30% of pagetic lesions not visualized on X-rays. Conversely, when radiographs demonstrate pagetic involvement but the serum alkaline phosphatase concentration is normal and the bone scan reveals little isotope uptake at those sites, the diagnosis of relatively inactive or "burned out" Paget's disease is most likely. Likewise, predominately lytic bone lesions (such as osteoporosis circumscripta) may not be detected on bone scan. computed tomography and magnetic resonance imaging scans add little to the work-up of patients with uncomplicated Paget's disease.

5. Which bones are involved in Paget's disease?

Paget's disease may be monostotic in about 20% of patients, involving only one skeletal site, or polyostotic, involving several different areas of the skeleton. Common sites of pagetic involvement include the pelvis, hip, spine, skull, tibia, and humerus. Less common sites of involvement (<20% of cases) include the forearm, clavicles, scapulae, and ribs.

6. Discuss the laboratory abnormalities associated with Paget's disease.

The abnormal laboratory values in Paget's disease reflect either increased bone formation or increased bone resorption. Unless a patient with widespread Paget's disease is immobilized, the serum calcium and phosphate concentrations should be normal. The laboratory test that reflects increased osteoblastic function is either the total or bone-specific serum alkaline phosphatase concentration. The serum concentration of osteocalcin, another marker of bone formation, provides little additional information to that supplied by alkaline phosphatase. The serum bone-specific alkaline phosphatase is a more sensitive marker of bone formation than the total alkaline phosphatase and thus may be a useful parameter to follow in the management of monostotic disease. The increased urinary excretion of pyridinium collagen crosslinks (pyridinoline) is a better indicator of increased bone resorption than measurement of the urinary excretion of hydroxyproline. Pyridinoline molecules and the related N- and C-telopeptides of collagen are the most specific components of the bone matrix.

When the Paget's disease is primarily lytic, the alkaline phosphatase concentration may be normal. Otherwise, the serum alkaline phosphatase activity generally parallels the indices of bone resorption. For these reasons, the total serum alkaline phosphatase concentration is the simplest and least expensive laboratory test with which to follow the course and response to treatment of most cases of Paget's disease. Of interest, a markedly elevated alkaline phosphatase concentration (e.g., 10 times the upper limit of normal) is usually associated with pagetic involvement of the skull, whereas widespread disease in the rest of the skeleton without involvement of the skull may be associated with a more modest elevation of serum alkaline phosphatase. In patients with increased total alkaline phosphatase concentrations, liver disease should be excluded because this enzyme is abundant in both liver and bone. If liver-specific tests such as 5¢-nucleotidase, gamma-glutamyl transferase, or the liver alkaline phosphatase isoenzyme are normal, it is likely that the elevated alkaline phosphatase originates from bone.

7. What are the histologic findings in bone affected by Paget's disease?
The early lesions of Paget's disease are characterized by increased numbers of large multinucleated osteoclasts, some containing up to 100 nuclei. In the mixed osteolytic-osteoblastic phase, large numbers of active osteoblasts are seen forming bone at sites of prior osteoclastic bone resorption. The intense osteoblastic reaction in this phase is characterized by bone deposited in a chaotic fashion (the so-called mosaic or woven pattern) rather than in the orderly lamellar pattern of uninvolved bone. The woven bone of Paget's disease is structurally weaker than normal lamellar bone and explains the propensity for pagetic bone to fracture or deform.

8. Who is most likely to have Paget's disease?
The incidence of Paget's disease varies with age, gender, and geographic location. Although Paget's disease may present in younger people, it is most common in patients older than 50 years. Men are more commonly affected than women. (The male-to-female ratio is about 3:2.) Although there is no definite hereditary pattern, a significant number of patients with Paget's disease (12% in one large study) report affected family members. Analyses of large kindreds with Paget's disease suggest that both sporadic and familial forms of the disease exist. Paget's disease is more common in the populations of eastern and northern Europe and in areas where Europeans have immigrated (such as the United States, Australia, New Zealand, and South Africa). Paget's disease is uncommon in Scandinavia, Asia, and Africa and in African-Americans.

9. What is the cause of Paget's disease?
Although the cause of Paget's disease is unknown, the primary defect appears to be an abnormality of the osteoclast. Reports of viral nucleocapsid-like structures in the osteoclasts of active pagetic bone suggest a viral etiology. These nuclear inclusions resemble paramyxovirus nucleocapsids. The measles virus, respiratory syncytial virus, and canine distemper virus have been implicated as etiologic agents. Thus, it appears most plausible that Paget's disease is the late result of a viral infection of bone.

10. What medications are available to treat Paget's disease?
There is no cure for Paget's disease, but several medications are used to decrease the

accelerated rate of osteoclastic bone resorption. The medications used for the treatment of Paget's bone disease include bisphosphonates, calcitonin, plicamycin, and gallium nitrate.

The bisphosphonates available for use in the United States for the treatment of Paget's disease include etidronate (Didronel), alendronate (Fosamax), risedronate (Actonel), tiludronate (Skelid), and pamidronate (Aredia). Several newer bisphosphonates under development such as ibandronate, zoledronate, olpadronate and neridronate have also shown promise as agents for the treatment of this disease. All the available bisphosphonates are orally administered, with the exception of pamidronate, which is an intravenous preparation.

Salmon calcitonin (Calcimar, Miacalcin injection) is a parenteral preparation that requires intramuscular or subcutaneous injection. Salmon calcitonin nasal spray (Miacalcin) is available for the treatment of osteoporosis, but is not effective for treating Paget's disease because of low bioavailability. Resistance to treatment of Paget's disease with salmon calcitonin is usually associated with neutralizing antibody formation. Development of resistance after bisphosphonate therapy has also been reported. However, studies suggest that resistance to one bisphosphonate does not preclude a good response to a second bisphosphonate.

Although not approved for the treatment of Paget's disease, plicamycin (Mithramycin) has occasionally been used with success. Gallium nitrate (Ganite), which is used to treat hypercalcemia, also has some efficacy in the treatment of Paget's disease. However, because of the excellent response of Paget's disease to bisphosphonates, plicamycin and gallium nitrate are rarely used.

After treatment with bisphosphonates, suppression of disease activity is usually prolonged, sometimes lasting for several years, whereas the response to calcitonin or plicamycin is generally short-lived once treatment is discontinued. Thus, for treatment of uncomplicated Paget's disease, an oral bisphosphonate is the agent of choice. Calcitonin should be reserved for patients with primarily lytic disease, for patients in whom a particularly rapid response is required (e.g., patients with high-output cardiac failure or symptomatic disease of the spine), or before elective surgery on pagetic bone. Treatment of symptomatic patients also should include other therapeutic modalities, such as analgesics, nonsteroidal anti-inflammatory drugs, canes, shoe lifts, hearing aids, and surgery.

11. Give the indications for treatment of Paget's disease.

The primary indication for treatment is the presence of symptoms. However, not all symptoms respond to treatment. Bone pain usually responds, as do certain neurologic compression syndromes. In contrast, hearing loss, bony deformities, and mechanically dysfunctional joints are not likely to improve with therapy. Additional indications for treatment of Paget's disease are the prevention of local progression and future complications (see below), planned surgery at a pagetic site, and widespread pagetic involvement in patients in whom prolonged immobilization is anticipated, as immobilization increases the risk for hypercalcemia.

Indications for Treatment of Paget's Disease of Bone

- Symptoms (bone pain, headache, some neurologic abnormalities)
- Osteolytic bone disease
- Active asymptomatic disease in
    Weight-bearing bones
    Areas adjacent to major joints
    Vertebral bodies
    Skull
- Young patients
- Before orthopedic surgery on pagetic bone
- Immobilization hypercalcemia

Treatment of asymptomatic patients with Paget's disease is controversial. However, untreated Paget's disease appears to be progressive with time, and not all asymptomatic patients remain asymptomatic. Thus, many physicians treat patients with osteolytic Paget's disease or asymptomatic patients with active disease involving weight-bearing bones, vertebral bodies, the skull, or areas adjacent to major joints.

12. In asymptomatic patients with Paget's disease, at what concentration of alkaline phosphatase should treatment begin?

The answer to this question is controversial. The level of alkaline phosphatase should be viewed in the context of the radiographic picture. A concentration of alkaline phosphatase only two to three times the upper limit of normal with polyostotic involvement may simply reflect the late "burned-out" phase of the disease. Little benefit results from treatment in these cases. However, the same alkaline phosphatase concentration in a patient with monostotic Paget's disease in a weight-bearing bone or in an area adjacent to a major joint would lead most physicians to consider treatment. In addition, patients with lytic pagetic lesions and normal or near-normal alkaline phosphatase values should also be considered for treatment.

13. When should malignant degeneration be suspected?

One of the most serious complications of Paget's disease is the development of malignant sarcomas in pagetic bone. Such tumors are usually isolated, but 20% may be multicentric. Fortunately, this is a rare complication of Paget's disease, occurring in less than 1% of patients with clinically apparent disease. The tumors are extremely aggressive. Patients with Paget's sarcoma generally survive less than a year. The pelvis and long bones (humerus, femur, and tibia) are the most common sites for sarcomatous transformation. This malignant transformation is usually heralded by the onset of new or worsening bone pain and/or soft tissue swelling. Usually, progressive destruction of pagetic bone is found on radiographs. Less commonly, increasing sclerosis or masses of dense amorphous deposits in bone are suggestive of malignant change. The concentration of serum alkaline phosphatase may rise rapidly in an otherwise previously stable patient. Bone scans usually demonstrate decreased uptake of radionucleotide in the area of the tumor. However, gallium scans show increased uptake in the involved area(s). The tumors are usually osteogenic sarcomas, but fibrosarcomas and chondrosarcomas have also been reported in bone affected by Paget's disease. It is not known whether treatment of Paget's disease lessens the incidence of sarcomatous transformation. A biopsy of the involved bone is usually diagnostic. Other bone neoplasms such as benign giant cell tumors are also associated with Paget's disease, but these tumors do not carry such a grave prognosis.

BIBLIOGRAPHY

1. Altman RD: Long-term follow-up of therapy with intermittent etidronate disodium in Paget's disease of bone. Am J Med 79:583, 1985.
2. Ankrom MA, Shapiro JR: Paget's disease of bone (osteitis deformans). J Am Geriatr Soc 46:1025, 1998.
3. Delmas PD, Meunier PJ: The management of Paget's disease of bone. N Engl J Med 336:558, 1997.
4. Fogelman I, Collier BD, Brown ML: Bone scintigraphy. Part 3: Bone scanning in metabolic bone disease. J Nucl Med 34:2247, 1993.
5. Hadjipavlou A, Lander P, Srolovitz H, Enker IP: Malignant transformation in Paget's disease of bone. Cancer 70:2802, 1992.
6. Hamdy RC: Pharmacologic treatment of Paget's disease. Endocrinol Metab Clin North Am 24:421, 1995.
7. Leach RJ, Singer FR, Roodman GD: The genetics of Paget's disease. J Clin Endocrinol Metab 86:24–28, 2001.

8. Mills BG: Etiology and pathophysiology of Paget's disease—Update. Endocrinologist 7:222, 1997.

9. Papapoulos SE: Paget's disease of bone: Clinical, pathogenetic and therapeutic aspects. Baillieres Clin Endocrinol Metab 11:117, 1997.

10. Proceedings of the Third International Symposium on Paget's Disease. J Bone Mineral Res 14(suppl 2), 1999.

11. Sawin CT: Historical note: Sir James Paget and osteitis deformans. Endocrinologist 7:205, 1997. (Also see page 255 in the same issue for a reproduction of one of James Paget's original articles on osteitis deformans.)

12. Sellars SL: Beethoven's deafness. South Afr Med J 48:1585, 1974.

13. Singer FR: Clinical efficacy of salmon calcitonin in Paget's disease of bone. Calcif Tissue Int 49(suppl 2):87, 1991.

14. Siris ES: Clinical Review—Paget's disease of bone. J Bone Mineral Res 13:1061, 1998.

15. Siris ES: Extensive personal experience—Paget's disease of bone. J Clin Endocrinol Metab 80:35, 1995.

16. Siris ES. Paget's disease of bone. In Favus MJ (ed.): Primer on the Metabolic Bone Diseases and Disorders of Mineral Metabolism, 4th ed. New York, Raven Press, 1999, p 415.

17. Wimalawansa SJ, Gunasekera RD: Pamidronate is effective for Paget's disease of bone refractory to conventional therapy. Calcif Tissue Int 53:237, 1993.

14. HYPERCALCEMIA

Leonard R. Sanders, M.D.

1. What is hypercalcemia? How does protein binding affect the calcium level?

Hypercalcemia is a total serum calcium value above the normal range (8.5–10.5 mg/dL) in the presence of normal serum proteins. Calcium is 50% free (ionized), 40% protein-bound and 10% complexed to phosphate, citrate, bicarbonate, sulfate and lactate. Only elevations in the free calcium are associated with symptoms and signs. Of the protein-bound calcium, about 80% is bound to albumin and 20% to globulins. A decrease or increase in serum albumin of 1 g/dL from 4 gm/dL decreases or increases the serum calcium by 0.8 mg/dL. An increase or decrease in serum globulin by 1 g/dL increases or decreases serum calcium by 0.16 mg/dL. Such protein changes do not affect free calcium and do not cause calcium-related symptoms.

2. How common are hypercalcemia and its main associated conditions?

Hypercalcemia affects 0.5–1% of the general population. The incidence may increase to 3% among postmenopausal women. Primary hyperparathyroidism causes 70% of outpatient and 20% of inpatient cases of hypercalcemia. Cancer-associated hypercalcemia causes 50% of inpatient cases; 10% of patients with malignancy develop hypercalcemia. Together, hyperparathyroidism and cancer cause 90% of all cases of hypercalcemia. About 5–10% of patients with hyperparathyroidism develop nephrolithiasis. Calcium phosphate stones are characteristic of hyperparathyroidism.

3. Describe how mild, moderate and severe hypercalcemia are classified.

First, consider the patient's general health and hypercalcemic symptoms. For example, a patient with renal failure and a serum phosphorus of 8.5 mg/dL may have metastatic calcification with a serum calcium of 10.5 mg/dL. Then correct the serum calcium for the albumin concentration:

$$Ca_{corrected} = Ca_{observed} + [(4.0 - albumin) \times 0.8]$$

With this in mind, a serum calcium of 1.5–3.5 mg/dL above the upper normal limit defines moderate hypercalcemia. Mild hypercalcemia occurs below this range, and severe hypercalcemia, above. Thus, if the upper normal limit for calcium is 10.5 mg/dL, a serum calcium of 12–14 mg/dL is moderate hypercalcemia. A serum calcium of < 12 mg/dL is mild hypercalcemia, and > 14 mg/dL is severe hypercalcemia.

4. What are the signs and symptoms of hypercalcemia?

No symptoms are usually present with mild hypercalcemia (< 12 mg/dL). Moderate or severe hypercalcemia and rapidly developing mild hypercalcemia cause more frequent symptoms and signs. Common symptoms and signs involve (1) the central nervous system (lethargy, stupor, coma, mental changes, psychosis); (2) the gastrointestinal tract (anorexia, nausea, constipation, acid peptic disease); (3) the kidneys (polyuria, nephrolithiasis); (4) the musculoskeletal system (arthralgias, myalgias, weakness); and (5) the vascular system (hypertension). The classic electrocardiographic (EKG) change associated with hypercalcemia is a short Q-T interval. Occasionally, severe hypercalcemia also causes dysrhythmias, ST segment depression, sinus arrest and disturbances in atrioventricular (AV) conduction.

5. Name the sources of serum calcium.

Bone contains 99% of body calcium. Of the remaining 1%, most is intracellular; a small amount is extracellular. Bone calcium approximates 1 kg in young people and 0.5 kg in the elderly. One percent of the skeletal calcium is freely exchangeable with the extracellular fluid. Normal serum calcium is maintained by integrated regulation of calcium absorption, resorption and reabsorption; these processes occur, respectively, in the gut, bone and kidney. The gut absorbs about 30% of dietary calcium; absorption varies from 15–70%, depending on dietary calcium and age. Calcium absorption decreases with age. The kidney reabsorbs 98% of the filtered calcium. A normal dietary calcium intake is 1,000 mg/day. The gut absorbs 300 mg, excretes the remaining 700 mg and secretes an additional 100 mg. The net intestinal excretion is 800 mg/day. The bone exchanges about 500 mg/day with serum, and the kidney excretes 200 mg/day for normal calcium balance.

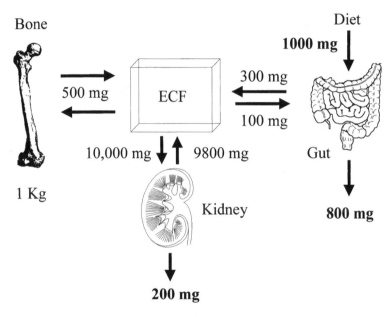

Normal calcium balance.

6. What are the major anatomic and physiologic determinants of serum calcium?

Bone, gut, kidney, liver, skin, parathyroid and thyroid are the main organs affecting serum calcium. They control the serum calcium by regulating serum levels of parathyroid hormone (PTH), 1,25-dihydroxyvitamin D [1,25(OH)$_2$D], calcitonin, phosphate and calcium itself. The parathyroid glands secrete PTH, and the thyroid gland makes calcitonin. Diet, skin, liver and kidney control the synthesis and secretion of 1,25(OH)$_2$D. Vitamin D$_2$ is ingested in the diet, and vitamin D$_3$ is synthesized in the skin. In the liver, 25-hydroxylase hydroxylates both vitamins to form 25-hydroxyvitamin D$_2$ and D$_3$ (25-OHD). Both forms of the vitamin (hormone) circulate, and their biologic activities are the same. In the mitochondria of the proximal renal tubule, 1-alpha-hydroxylase converts 25-OHD to 1,25(OH)$_2$D. All three forms of the vitamin affect calcium metabolism. However, only 1,25(OH)$_2$D is sufficiently potent to have a noticeable effect at physiologic levels. Also located in tubular mitochondria, 24-hydroxylase converts 25-OHD to the second most abundant circulating vitamin D metabolite—24,25-dihydroxyvitamin D [24,25(OH)$_2$D]. There is a relative shift toward more renal production of $24,25(OH)_2D$ when PTH and PO_4 are normal and more production of $1,25(OH)_2D$ when PTH is high and PO_4 is low. The 24-hydroxylation renders $24,25(OH)_2D$ susceptible to oxidation and degradation. Antiresorptive effects of $24,25(OH)_2D$ antagonize the calcium-mobilizing effects of $1,25(OH)_2D$ on bone. When hydroxylated to $1,24,25(OH)_3D$, it increases intestinal calcium absorption. The overall effects of $24,25(OH)_2D$ with limited studies show an association with positive calcium balance and decreased bone resorption. However, studies are too limited to know the true role of $24,25(OH)_2D$; for now its overall role remains unclear.

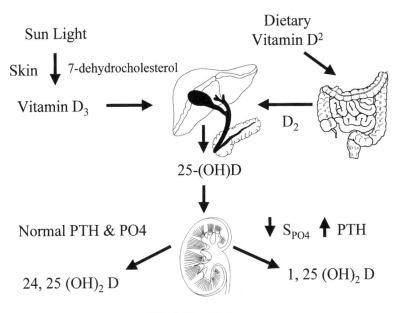

Sun Light

Dietary
Vitamin D^2

Skin   7-dehydrocholesterol

Vitamin D_3

D_2

25-(OH)D

Normal PTH & PO4

$\downarrow S_{PO4}$ $\uparrow$ PTH

24, 25 $(OH)_2$ D

1, 25 $(OH)_2$ D

Vitamin D metabolism.

7. Describe how hormones affect the level of serum calcium.

Both PTH and $1,25(OH)_2D$ provide the main control of serum calcium. Calcitonin may play a role, but its significance is not well defined in humans. PTH and calcitonin affect bone and kidney but have no direct effects on the intestine, whereas $1,25(OH)_2D$ has effects on bone, kidney and intestine. A major effect of $1,25(OH)_2D$ is to increase intestinal absorption of calcium. Both PTH and $1,25(OH)_2D$ increase bone resorption by increasing osteoclast activity. Because osteoclasts have no known receptors for either hormone, PTH and $1,25(OH)_2D$ stimulate osteoclast activity indirectly. PTH enhances the activity of osteoblasts, which secrete factors that stimulate osteoclastic bone resorption, whereas $1,25(OH)_2D$ promotes osteoclast differentiation (promonocytes $\rightarrow$ monocytes $\rightarrow$ macrophages $\rightarrow$ osteoclasts). In addition, $1,25(OH)_2D$ increases calcium transport from bone to blood. Both hormones promote normal bone formation by action on osteoblasts, and $1,25(OH)_2D$ maintains a favorable calcium-phosphate product necessary for normal bone mineralization. Calcitonin inhibits osteoclastic bone resorption, decreases renal tubular reabsorption of calcium and also may enhance osteoblast activity. Other actions and interactions of these hormones on bone, kidney and gut are described later. Estrogen receptors have been identified in osteoblasts and osteoclasts. Estrogens inhibit bone resorption, increase bone growth and modestly lower serum calcium.

8. How do calcium and phosphate interact with the main calcium-regulating hormones?

Interaction of Factors Controlling Serum Calcium

	PTH	1,25(OH)$_2$D	CALCITONIN	CALCIUM	PO$_4$
PTH	—	↑+	+	↑ +	↓ ↑ +
1,25(OH)$_2$D	↓ –	↓ –	+	↑	↑
Calcitonin	+	+	—	↓	↓
Calcium	↓	↓	↑	—	↓
PO$_4$	↑ +	↓	—	↓	

This table summarizes the main factors controlling serum calcium. The arrows show direct actions of factors in the left column on factors in the top row, whereas the plus (+) and minus (–) signs show indirect actions. As a rule, the direct effects predominate as the net effect. Recall that absorption, resorption and reabsorption are the respective effects of gut, bone and kidney. PTH directly stimulates kidney production of 1,25(OH)$_2$D and indirectly enhances renal synthesis of 1,25(OH)$_2$D by its phosphaturic and net hypophosphatemic effect. PTH increases calcium by stimulating bone resorption and distal renal tubular reabsorption. The higher serum calcium stimulates calcitonin secretion. The increased bone resorption also raises serum phosphate. 1,25(OH)$_2$D directly inhibits PTH secretion and renal synthesis of 1,25(OH)$_2$D but stimulates absorption, resorption and reabsorption of both calcium and phosphate, resulting in a net increase in serum calcium and phosphate. The higher serum calcium inhibits synthesis of PTH and 1,25(OH)$_2$D and stimulates secretion of calcitonin. Increased phosphate also inhibits synthesis of 1,25(OH)$_2$D. Calcitonin inhibits resorption and reabsorption of calcium and phosphate. This lowers serum calcium and phosphate, which in turn increases 1,25(OH)$_2$D; the reduced calcium also increases PTH and decreases calcitonin. High calcium inhibits secretion of PTH and renal production of 1,25(OH)$_2$D and stimulates thyroid secretion of calcitonin. By complexing with phosphate, calcium also decreases serum phosphate. Phosphate inhibits renal synthesis of 1,25(OH)$_2$D and complexes with calcium causing a fall in serum calcium that stimulates PTH and inhibits release of calcitonin. Phosphate also directly increases parathyroid production of PTH. Note that 1,25(OH)$_2$D is the only variable listed with direct negative feedback inhibition of its own secretion. The following table summarizes these changes.

Summary of Calcium and Phosphate Control

VARIABLE	DIRECT ACTION
Parathyroid hormone	Increased bone resorption of calcium and phosphate Increased distal renal tubular calcium reabsorption Decreased renal tubular phosphate reabsorption Increased renal production of 1,25(OH)$_2$D Net effect: increased serum calcium and decreased phosphate
1,25-Dihydroxyvitamin D	Increased bone resorption of calcium and phosphate Increased renal reabsorption of calcium and phosphate Increased gut absorption of calcium and phosphate Decreased parathyroid production of PTH Decreased renal production of 1,25(OH)$_2$D Net effect: increased serum calcium and phosphate
Calctonin	Decreased bone resorption of calcium and phosphate Decreased renal reabsorption of calcium and phosphate Decreased gut absorption of phosphate Net effect: decreased serum calcium and phosphate

Summary of Calcium and Phosphate Control (continued)

VARIABLE	DIRECT ACTION
Calcium	Decreases PTH
	Decreases 1,25(OH)$_2$D
	Increases calcitonin
	Decreases phosphate
Phosphate	Increases PTH
	Decreases 1,25(OH)2D
	Decreases calcium

9. What are the main causes of hypercalcemia?

The mnemonic VITAMINS TRAP (Pont, 1989) includes most causes of hypercalcemia:

V	= **V**itamins	**T**	= **T**hiazide diuretics and other drugs (lithium)
I	= **I**mmobilization	**R**	= **R**habdomyolysis
T	= **T**hyrotoxicosis	**A**	= **A**IDS
A	= **A**ddison's disease	**P**	= **P**aget's disease
M	= **M**ilk–alkali syndrome		**P**arenteral nutrition
I	= **I**nflammatory disorders		**P**heochromocytoma
N	= **N**eoplastic-related disease		**P**arathyroid disease
S	= **S**arcoidosis		

10. How do various causes of hypercalcemia increase the serum calcium?

True hypercalcemia results from altered bone resorption, renal tubular reabsorption and gut absorption of calcium. Although the bone (resorption and formation), kidney (reabsorption and excretion) and gut (absorption and secretion) have two major processes involved with mineral metabolism, only resorption, reabsorption and absorption play a significant role in hypercalcemia. An exception to this rule occurs when decreased renal function from renal or prerenal disease impairs calcium filtration and excretion.

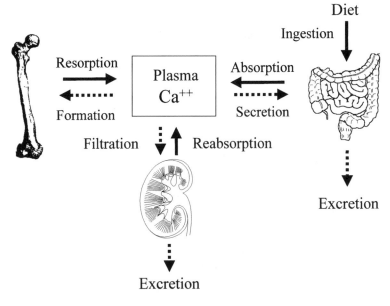

Calcium metabolism.

From the discussions above, one appreciates that mechanisms of hypercalcemia are usually multifactorial. However, most hypercalcemic syndromes have a primary mechanism, as outlined in the table below.

Causes and Mechanisms of Increased Serum Calcium

PRIMARY MECHANISM	CAUSE OF HYPERCALCEMIA
Increased bone resorption	Hyperparathyroidism
	Local metastases
	Humeral hypercalcemia of malignancy
	Thyrotoxicosis
	Pheochromocytoma
	Excessive vitamin A (> 50,000 U/day)
	Immobilization
Increased renal reabsorption or decreased excretion	Milk–alkali syndrome
	Rhabdomyolysis
	Thiazide diuretics
	Familial hypocalciuric hypercalcemia (FHH)
	Renal failure
Increased gut absorption	Excessive vitamin D (usually > 50,000 U/wk)
	Berylliosis
	Candidiasis
	Coccidioidomycosis
	Eosinophilic granuloma
	Histoplasmosis
	Sacroidosis
	Silicone implants
	Tuberculosis
	Inflammatory disorders
	AIDS
	Lymphomas
Unknown causes	Vasoactive intestinal polypeptide-secreting tumor (VIPoma)
	Addison's disease
	Parenteral nutrition
	Theophylline
	Lithium carbonate
	Estrogen and antiestrogens

Increased bone resorption. Malignant tumors cause hypercalcemia primarily by producing humoral or local substances that increase osteoclastic bone resorption. Direct osteolysis by the tumor is now believed to be an unusual cause of hypercalcemia. Increased production of thyroxine (T_4), triiodothyronine (T_3) and interleukin-6 during thyrotoxicosis causes increased bone resorption and hypercalcemia that sequentially decreases PTH secretion, $1,25(OH)_2D$ formation, and intestinal calcium absorption. Pheochromocytomas can coexist with hyperparathyroidism in the multiple endocrine neoplasia type II (MEN II) syndrome; however, pheochromocytomas themselves may also cause hypercalcemia through excessive production of parathyroid hormone-related protein (PTHrP). Immobilization may cause hypercalcemia when associated with hyperparathyroidism, malignancy, young age, Paget's disease of bone, or renal failure. Lithium carbonate increases the set point at which calcium suppresses PTH release and thus causes PTH secretion to persist at higher calcium concentrations.

Increased renal reabsorption or decreased excretion. Hypercalcemia may cause diuresis. The resulting dehydration decreases the glomerular filtration rate (GFR), which increases renal reabsorption of calcium and bicarbonate. In milk–alkali syndrome, alkalosis increases renal reabsorption of calcium, and hypercalcemia increases reabsorption of bicarbonate. Associated renal insufficiency from nephrocalcinosis decreases excretion of calcium. Patients with rhabdomyolysis are often dehydrated and prerenal. The resulting decreased filtration, increased reabsorption and decreased excretion contribute to hypercalcemia. In addition, the injured muscles release calcium and myoglobin. The myoglobin causes renal failure that further increases calcium retention. Posttreatment hypercalcemia from mobilization of precipitated calcium and phosphate is an additional mechanism in rhabdomyolysis. Thiazides decrease intravascular volume, which decreases GFR, increases proximal tubular reabsorption of calcium and concentrates the plasma. These factors increase plasma calcium. Thiazides also directly increase renal distal tubular reabsorption of calcium and may potentiate PTH action on bone. Patients with FHH have a genetically determined increase in PTH secretion and defect in renal excretion in calcium due to an inactivating mutation of the calcium sensor/receptor present on parathyroid and renal tubular cell membranes.

Increased gut absorption. Inflammatory and granulomatous disorders, including sarcoidosis, tuberculosis, coccidioidomycosis, histoplasmosis, candidiasis, eosinophilic granuloma, berylliosis, silicone implants, and certain lymphomas also produce hypercalcemia. In all of these conditions, hypercalcemia is related to excessive production of $1,25(OH)_2D$ by inflammatory or neoplastic tissue with an associated increase in gut absorption of calcium. However, $1,25(OH)_2D$ also acts to increase bone resorption and probably renal calcium reabsorption as well. Milk–alkali syndrome is also associated with increased intestinal absorption of calcium that results from ingestion of excessive amounts of calcium and alkali. The resulting high calcium X phosphate product with associated dehydration may result in nephrocalcinosis and renal failure. The renal failure causes decreased calcium and bicarbonate excretion and worsens hypercalcemia and metabolic alkalosis. These patients present with the classic triad of hypercalcemia, metabolic alkalosis, and renal failure.

11. What are the MEN syndromes?

MEN is associated with three familial syndromes, two of which present with hypercalcemia due to hyperparathyroidism. MEN I or Wermer's syndrome includes the three Ps: pituitary, parathyroid and pancreatic tumors. Hypercalcemia due to hyperparathyroidism is usually the first feature of this syndrome to appear. MEN II has two variants, both of which involve medullary carcinoma of the thyroid (MCT) and pheochromocytoma. Patients with MEN IIa or Sipple's syndrome have MCT, pheochromocytoma and hyperparathyroidism. Patients with MEN IIb have MCT, pheochromocytoma, multiple mucosal neuromas and marfanoid habitus; they usually do not have hyperparathyroidism. Parathyroid tumors in the MEN syndromes are more often bilateral, hyperplastic and malignant in contrast to sporadic hyperparathyroidism. Moreover, anesthesia and surgery can stimulate an undetected pheochromocytoma to cause a hypertension crisis. Thus, patients with suspected MEN II need screening for pheochromocytoma before parathyroid surgery. MCT may cause other endocrine syndromes by secreting excessive adrenocorticotropic hormone (ACTH), antidiuretic hormone (ADH), vasoactive intestinal polypeptide (VIP), prostaglandins, somatostatin, serotonin and other hormones. MEN IIb normally does not present with hypercalcemia. However, pheochromocytoma has been associated with increased production of PTHrP, which may cause hypercalcemia. Thus, a rare patient with MEN IIb may present with hypercalcemia, suggesting hyperparathyroidism. Measurement of PTH and PTHrP levels will differentiate this unlikely possibility.

12. Define familial hypocalciuric hypercalcemia and describe how it is diagnosed.

FHH, also called benign familial hypercalcemia, is due to an autosomal-dominant genetic mutation resulting in a defective calcium sensor/receptor on the membranes of parathyroid and renal tubular cells. FHH is characterized by decreased renal clearance of calcium, normal-to-high serum levels of PTH, mild relative hypermagnesemia, normal or low serum phosphorus and a fractional excretion of calcium (FE_{Ca}) < 1%. In FHH, as in mild primary hyperparathyroidism, PTH is inappropriately high for the level of serum calcium. Therefore, FHH can mimic primary hyperparathyroidism. However, patients with FHH are usually asymptomatic, have no associated complications and require no therapy. In unusual cases, neonates homozygous for the FHH mutation have severe symptomatic hypercalcemia. The clinical importance of FHH is to distinguish it from primary hyperparathyroidism so that invasive procedures such as parathyroidectomy are not done needlessly. Near-total parathyroidectomy does not usually correct the hypercalcemia in FHH. However, total parathyroidectomy causes hypoparathyroidism and hypocalcemia. The most important diagnostic feature of FHH is the combination of a family history of benign hypercalcemia and an FE_{Ca} < 1%. Patients with primary hyperparathyroidism usually have an FE_{Ca} > 2%.

13. Give the likely diagnosis of the following hypercalcemic patient.

An 18-year-old man had a normal screening history and physical exam for college. His physician referred him to an endocrinologist because his screening test showed a serum calcium of 11.3 mg/dL. He is asymptomatic and still has a normal exam. Repeat serum calcium is 11.5 mg/dL. Family history reveals that his mother and brother also have asymptomatic hypercalcemia. Review of his old records shows calcium levels of 10.5–11.8 for at least 2 years. Additional lab tests showed the following values: intact PTH = 70 pg/mL (nL < 60); serum creatinine (Cr) = 1.0 mg/dL; spot urine calcium = 5 mg/dL; and urine Cr = 90 mg/dL. The FE_{Ca} is calculated in the same manner as a fractional excretion of sodium (FE_{Na}), but Ca is substituted for Na, as shown below. Because circulating proteins bind 40% of the calcium and the kidney filters only 60%, the plasma calcium available for filtration is 0.6 × 11.5 = 6.9 mg/dL.

$$FE_{Ca} = [U_{Ca}/P_{Ca}]/[U_{Cr}/P_{Cr}] = [U_{Ca}/P_{Ca}] \times [P_{Cr}/U_{Cr}]$$

$$FE_{Ca} = [5 \text{ mg/dL}/6.9 \text{ mg/dL}] \ 3 \ [1 \text{ mg/dL}/90 \text{ mg/dL}] \ 3 \ 100\% = 0.8\%$$

The FE_{Ca} value for the patient is < 1%, indicating renal absorption of > 99% of the filtered calcium. In the presence of hypercalcemia, this value is clearly abnormal. The FE_{Ca} < 1% supports the diagnosis of FHH. This, plus a family history of benign hypercalcemia and absence of symptoms, signs or complications, is strongly suggestive of FHH. However, to confirm the diagnosis, calculate the FE_{Ca} of the family members. If < 1%, no further workup is needed. As for the FE_{Na} calculation, a fasting morning spot urine sample is sufficient for the FE_{Ca}.

14. Describe the types of drug therapy that are useful in hypercalcemia.

Drug Therapy for Hypercalcemia

THERAPY	DOSE	ROUTE	MONITOR/COMMENT
Saline	250–1,000 mL/hr	IV	Cardiopulmonary function with exam, CVP/PCWP and CXR.
Furosemide	20–80 mg every 2–4 hr or 40 mg/hr CI	IV	Serum and urine electrolytes. Replace K, Mg and PO_4 based on serum levels and urinary losses.
Salmon calcitonin	4–8 IU/kg every 6–12 hr	IM, SC	Allergic reaction. Give a skin test of 1 IU intradermally before treatment.
Prednisone/methyl- prednisolone	20 mg 2–3 times/day	PO/IV	Possible adjunct to calcitonin. Effective in 1,25-D–associated hypercalcemia.
Pamidronate	30–90 mg/week	IV	Infuse over 4–24 hr. Give ½ dose and maximal infusion time in severe renal failure.

Drug Therapy for Hypercalcemia (continued)

THERAPY	DOSE	ROUTE	MONITOR/COMMENT
Etidronate	7.5 mg/kg/day	IV	Infuse over 4 hr as needed each day for 5 days. Give ½ dose in renal failure
Plicamycin	25 µg/kg/day	IV	Infuse over 4 hr as needed every 2–3 days. Avoid in hepatic dysfunction and thrombocytopenia. Monitor CBC, platelets, PT/PTT and liver enzymes.
Gallium nitrate	200 mg/m² BSA/day	IV	Infuse over 24 hr as needed each day for 5 days. Avoid in renal failure. Monitor Cr, PO_4 and CBC.
Neutral sodium phosphate	500–1,000 mg 3 times/ day	PO	Adjunct to other therapy. Avoid if serum $PO_4 > 3.5$ mg/dL.
Dialysis	Low or no calcium dialysate	HD/PD CVVHD	Hypercalcemic crisis or refractory hypercalcemia. Useful in renal failure. Nephrology consultation.
Na or K phosphate (1 mmol phosphate = 31 mg elemental phosphorus)	1–3 mmol phosphate/ hr for 12 hr	IV	Hypercalcemic crisis. Renal and cardiac toxicity and sudden death. Avoid in renal failure and serum $PO_4 > 3$ mg/dL.
Edetate disodium (EDTA)	50 mg/kg/day	IV	Hypercalcemic crisis. Infuse over 3–4 hr. Maximal dose < 3 g/24 hr as needed each day for 5 days. Avoid in renal failure.

CI = continuous infusion; BSA = body surface area; IV = intravenously; IM = intramuscularly; SC = subcutaneously; PO = orally; HD = hemodialysis; PD = peritoneal dialysis; CVVHD = continuous venovenous hemodialysis; CVP = central venous pressure; PCWP = pulmonary capillary wedge pressure; CXR = chest radiograph; Na = sodium; K = potassium; Mg = magnesium; PO_4 = phosphate; CBC = complete blood count; PT = prothrombin time; PTT = partial thromboplastic time; Cr = creatinine.

The preceding table summarizes the current guidelines for drug therapies for hypercalcemia. Most patients with severe hypercalcemia require combined treatment with multiple drugs. The lowest amount and least frequent dose that will achieve and maintain acceptable levels of serum calcium should be given. Most patients with hypercalcemia are dehydrated and require rehydration with normal saline as initial therapy, frequently followed by furosemide. Both therapies increase urinary excretion of sodium and calcium but normalize the serum calcium in < 10% of patients. Saline and diuretic therapy require meticulous monitoring of the patient's blood and urine for volume and electrolyte problems.

Calcitonin, bisphosphonates, plicamycin and gallium nitrate lower serum calcium by inhibiting bone resorption. Calcitonin effectively normalizes serum calcium in 20% of patients within 2–4 hours, and its effects last 2–3 days. Combined use with glucocorticoids arguably prolongs the modest (1–2 mg/dL) hypocalcemic effect for about 1 week. Glucocorticoids probably inhibit synthesis and action of $1,25(OH)_2D$. A single infusion of pamidronate is 90% effective within 48 hours, last 2–8 weeks and is the drug of choice for hypercalcemia of malignancy. Etidronate normalizes the calcium in 40% of patients and requires repeated infusions. Plicamycin is 60% effective, works within 24 hours and lasts up to 1 week. Repeated infusions cause bone marrow and hepatic toxicity that limit its long-term use. Gallium nitrate is 75% effective, requires multiple 24-hour infusions and is nephrotoxic. Oral phosphate is adjunctive therapy in patients with a serum phosphate < 3.5 mg/dL.

Hypercalcemic crisis causes severe cardiac dysrhythmias and neurologic dysfunction.

For extreme emergencies, intravenous (IV) sodium ethylenediamine tetraacetic acid (EDTA) and IV phosphate immediately lower the calcium by chelation and complexation, respectively. Both drugs, however, are dangerous. EDTA may cause severe acute renal failure. Intravenous phosphate may cause metastatic calcification, acute renal failure, cardiac dysrhythmias and death from cardiac arrest. Dialysis against a low- or no-calcium bath can effect immediate lowering of the calcium while other medications take effect. It is of particular benefit in patients with hypercalcemic renal failure and removes chelated calcium EDTA. Dialysis is emergency therapy but probably should be used before IV EDTA or IV phosphate. Mobilization decreases bone resorption. Limiting oral and IV calcium supplements decreasees calcium input.

15. Summarize the mechanism of action of the drugs used to treat hypercalcemia.

Mechanism of Action of Hypercalcemic Drug Therapy

DRUG	MECHANISM OF ACTION
Saline	Dilutes serum calcium by volume expansion. Increases urinary excretion.
Furosemide	Impairs renal calcium reabsorption in Henle's loop and increases urinary flow.
Calcitonin	Binds to receptors on osteoclasts, inhibiting osteoclast activity. Main effect is decreased bone resorption. Also decreases renal reabsorption.
Glucocorticoids	No clear answer. Evidence suggests antagonism of vitamin D and therefore decreased absorption and reabsorption. In tumoral states may be tumorlytic and decrease production of OAFs and vitamin D.
Bisphosphonates	Impair osteoclast differentiation, recruitment, motility and attachment. Incorporate into bone matrix, making the matrix resistant to hydrolysis. Overall effect is decreased bone resorption.
Plicamycin	Inhibits RNA synthesis and is cytotoxic to osteoclasts, decreasing bone resorption.
Gallium nitrate	Adsorbs to and decreases solubility of hydroxyapatite crystale, decreasing bone resorption.
Phosphate	Impairs osteoclastic bone resorption and renal synthesis of 1,25-D. Decreases gut absorption. Increases calcium $\times$ phosphate product and precipitates with calcium in bone, blood vessels and soft tissues.
Edetate disodium	Chelates with calcium cations that are subsequently excreted by the kidney.
Dialysis	Direct removal of calcium from blood.

OAFs = osteoclast-activating factors.
Note: For long-term hypocalcemic effects, drug therapy for hypercalcemia must antagonize one of the three main causes of hypercalcemia: bone resorption, renal reabsorption or gut absorption. All hypercalcemia results from some abnormality in one of the three. Thus, it is good to think about one of these etiologies when choosing drug therapy. As noted, most drug therapy for hypercalcemia impairs bone resorption.

16. What is the mechanism of action and appropriate dose of bisphosphonate therapy?

Bisphosphonates bind tightly to calcified bone matrix and hydroxyapatite crystals, making them less accessible to osteoclasts. Bisphosphonates also impair osteoclast recruitment, differentiation, motility, and attachment to bone, and enhance osteoclast cell death. After binding by bisphosphonates, the bone therefore becomes resistant to resorption by osteoclasts as well as to subsequent mineralization. The bisphosphonate preparations currently available for treatment of hypercalcemia—etidronate (EDHP), pamidronate (APD), and alendronate—are poorly absorbed from the intestine and are effective only when administered intravenously. Pamidronate is the most effective antiresorptive drug available; the usual intravenous dose is 60 or 90 mg for moderate or severe hypercalcemia, respectively. Side effects of pamidronate are unusual, but mild, transient fever may occur. Alendronate has been used in an intravenous dose of 5 mg with effective control of hypercalcemia. However, it is not yet approved for therapy of hypercalcemia and is not available for intravenous use in the US. Zolendronate (intravenously) and risedronate (orally) are also not approved for treatment of hypercalcemia but show promise in clinical trails. Because bisphosphonates are renally excreted, one-half of the recommended dose should be infused over 24 hours for patients with significant renal failure (estimated GFR < 20 ml/min).

17. A 65-year-old woman taking thiazide diuretics presents with altered mentation, nausea, and vomiting. Lab tests show a serum calcium of 18 mg/dL and a creatinine of 4.5 mg/dL. Urine output is marginal. How should her hypercalcemia be managed initially?

Most patients presenting with hypercalcemia of this severity have an underlying malignancy. They are frequently debilitated and have compromised cardiovascular function. Most are dehydrated. Admit her to the intensive care unit. Stop the thiazide diuretic. Order an EKG and chest radiograph. Immediately repeat a sequential multiple analysis-11 (SMA-11), which includes sodium, potassium, chloride, carbon dioxide, blood urea nitrogen, creatinine, glucose, calcium, phosphate, magnesium, and albumin. Place a central line to assess volume status (central venous pressure or pulmonary capillary wedge pressure). Give normal saline at 500–1000 ml/hr, depending on volume status. Give salmon calcitonin, 1 IU intradermally, and check the site after 15–20 minutes. If no wheal or significant erythema develops, give 8 IU/kg salmon calcitonin IM (effective within 2–4 hr). Repeat the IM calcitonin injection every 6 hours. Begin a 60-mg infusion of pamidronate, and continue over 24 hours (maximal dose reduced for renal failure). Once volume is replete, give 20–100 mg IV furosemide every 2–4 hours to maintain urine output at 4–5 L/day. If urine output is not adequate, give 200 mg furosemide IV over 60 minutes, and start 40 mg/hr as a continuous infusion. Replace the urine output with IV normal saline, or alternate with half-normal saline, depending on volume and electrolyte status. Obtain a SMA-11 every 6 hours and a spot urine sample for sodium, potassium, chloride, and creatinine once per day to estimate losses. Replace potassium and magnesium losses as required. If hypercalcemia worsens, CNS function deteriorates or does not improve, or urine output declines, get a nephrology consultation for dialysis. Consider plicamycin at 12.5 mg/kg (dosage reduced for renal failure) if the above measures remain ineffective. Then consider gallium nitrate once serum creatinine is < 2 mg/dl. Obtain a noncontrast CT scan of the head. If possible, because of nephrotoxicity, avoid IV iodinated contrast. Reserve IV EDTA and phosphate for life-threatening, hypercalcemia-induced dysrhythmias.

18. What are calcimimetic drugs and how might they be useful in therapy of hypercalcemia?

Although not yet available for clinical use, calcimimetic drugs are potentially the most useful drugs for treatment of hypercalcemia caused by hyperparathyroidism. These drugs alter the sensitivity of the parathyroid receptor to extracellular calcium and thereby shift the calcium-PTH curve to the left, decrease the responsiveness of parathyroid cells to the stimulatory effects of low extracellular calcium, and increase the sensitivity of parathyroid cells to the suppressive effects of high calcium. The net effect of calcimimetic drugs is a marked reduction in PTH secretion, and a proportionate decrease in PTH induced hypercalcemia.

BIBLIOGRAPHY

1. Brown EM: Familial hypocalciuric hypercalcemia and other disorders with resistance to extracellular calcium. Endocrinol Metab Clin North Am 29:503–522, 2000.
2. Body JJ: Current and future directions in medical therapy: hypercalcemia. Cancer 88(12 suppl): 3054–3058, 2000.
3. Jan de Beur SM, Levine MA: Hypercalcemia. In Bardin CW: Current Therapy in Endocrinology and Metabolism, 6th ed. St. Louis, Mosby, 1997, pp 551–556.

4. Kaye TB: Hypercalcemia. How to pinpoint the cause and customize treatment. Postgrad Med 97:153– 155, 159–160, 1995.
5. Mundy GR: Evaluation and treatment of hypercalcemia. Hosp Pract (off ed) 29:79–86, 1994.
6. Popovtzer MM, Knochel JP, Kumar R: Disorders of calcium, phosphorus, vitamin D, and parathyroid hormone activity. In Schrier RW (ed): Renal and Electrolytes Disorders. Philadelphia, Lippincott-Raven, 1997, pp 241–319.
7. Pont A: Unusual causes of hypercalcemia. Endocrinol Metab Clin North Am 18:753–764, 1989.
8. Rabbani SA: Molecular mechanism of action of parathyroid hormone related peptide in hypercalcemia of malignancy: Therapeutic strategies [review]. Int J Oncol 16(1):197–206, 2000.
9. Reill, RF: The patient with disorders of serum calcium and phosphate. In Schrier RW (ed): Manual of Nephrology. Philadelphia, Lippincott Williams and Wilkins, 2000, pp 62–79.
10. Thakker RV: Multiple endocrine neoplasia type I. Endocrinol Metab Clin North Am 29:541–567, 2000.

15. HYPERPARATHYROIDISM

Leonard R. Sanders, M.D.

1. Define hyperparathyroidism.

Hyperparathyroidism (HPT) is a clinical syndrome causing specific symptoms and signs that result from elevated parathyroid hormone (PTH), PTH-induced bone resorption and hypercalcemia. The three types of HPT are primary, secondary and tertiary.

2. How common is HPT.

The prevalence of HPT is 1/1000; the female-to-male ratio is 2–3:1. The incidence increases with age, and postmenopausal women have an incidence five times higher than the general population.

3. What causes HPT?

Primary hyperparathyroidism is characterized by abnormal regulation of PTH secretion by calcium, resulting in excessive PTH secretion. Although the cause of HPT is not known, increased PTH secretion is due in part to an elevation of the set point and a change in the slope of the calcium-PTH curve, causing relative nonsuppressibility of PTH secretion. Expression of the calcium-sensing receptor protein is reduced in parathyroid adenomas and hyperplasia and may be partly responsible for this relative PTH nonsuppressibility. Most hyperparathyroid patients (85%) have single parathyroid adenomas, 5% have multiple adenomas, 10% have four-gland hyperplasia and << 1% have parathyroid carcinomas. Normal parathyroid glands weigh < 50 mg each. The average weight of parathyroid adenomas is 0.5–5 g; however, they may be > 25 g. The largest reported tumor weighed 120 g.

4. Describe how to diagnose HPT.

Persistent hypercalcemia with increased serum PTH levels makes the diagnosis of HPT. Suspect HPT whenever the patient has documented hypercalcemia. Because symptoms of HPT are nonspecific (see question 7), one must base the diagnosis primarily on laboratory studies. Furthermore, most patients with mild HPT have no specific symptoms or signs. Most cases are suspected after finding an elevated calcium value on routine laboratory screening.

5. How might you make the diagnosis of primary HPT more certain before recommending parathyroidectomy?

Obtain at least three fasting samples for calcium, ideally with no venous occlusion, and two PTH measurements at least several weeks apart. Ensure that the patient has normal renal function. Discontinue any thiazide diuretic for at least 1 week before measurement. Total calcium measurement is sufficient if albumin and total protein are normal. If not, measure ionized calcium, or correct for the protein change. When results are not specific for HPT, other classic laboratory changes may help, including increased chloride (Cl) and decreased phosphate (PO_4) with a Cl/PO4 ratio of > 33, elevated urinary pH (> 6.0) and increased alkaline phosphatase concentrations. Use the immunoradiometric (IRMA) or immunochemiluminometric (ICMA) assays that are specific for intact PTH. Assess PTH-related protein (PTHrP) in any patient with malignancy and hypercalcemia. If assays for intact PTH are borderline or normal but the PTH is inappropriately increased for the level of calcium, consider familial (benign) hypocalciuric hypercalcemia (FHH) and calculate the FE_{Ca}. The FE_{Ca} in FHH should be < 1%. If the FE_{Ca} is low, test family members to confirm the diagnosis. If positive, avoid neck exploration, which will have no effect on reversing the hypercalcemia. Ectopic PTH is rare and need not be considered in the differential unless the patient has clear evidence of malignancy and a negative neck exploration.

6. How does renal failure complicate the diagnosis of HPT?

Renal failure increases serum phosphate and decreases 1,25-dihydroxyvitamin D (calcitriol) levels. Because phosphate directly stimulates and calcitriol directly inhibits PTH secretion, serum PTH levels increase in renal failure. In addition, increased phosphate and decreased calcitriol decrease serum calcium. The resulting absolute or relative hypocalcemia further increases PTH secretion. Symptoms and signs of renal insufficiency may be identical to those of HPT, including lethargy, depression, anorexia, nausea, constipation and weakness. In renal failure, expect an increase in PTH above the normal range due to the stimulatory influences on PTH secretion. In addition, a newly identified molecular form of PTH that does not have the biologic activity of intact PTH-(1-84) accumulates in renal failure and cross-reacts with the intact molecule in the intact two-site assays. For this reason, patients with renal failure may have measured levels of intact PTH > 1.5 times higher than in normocalcemic subjects to maintain physiologic PTH-(1-84) concentrations. Thus, unless overt, the diagnosis of primary HPT may be more difficult in renal failure. Before parathyroidectomy for presumed primary HPT, tissue localization with [99m]technetium-sestamibi scan may be appropriate.

7. Describe the symptoms and signs of primary HPT.

The most important symptoms and signs of moderate-to-severe HPT include the following: neurologic (lethargy, stupor, coma, mental changes, psychosis); gastrointestinal (anorexia, nausea, constipation, acid peptic disease); nephrologic (polyuria, nephrolithiasis); musculoskeletal (arthralgias, myalgias, weakness); and vascular (hypertension). The classic phrase for these features is "stones, bones, abdominal groans and psychic moans." However, health care providers most often discover hypercalcemia unexpectedly on chemistry panels ordered for routine screening or for medical conditions unrelated to HPT. The hypercalcemia is usually mild (< 12 mg/dL) and in more than 80% of patients does not produce specific symptoms or signs. Careful questioning may reveal mild symptoms of weakness, fatigue, headache, depression, anorexia, nausea, vomiting, constipation, polyuria, polydipsia and bone and arthritic pain. These complaints are nonspecific, may not be related to HPT and may or may not improve after parathyroidectomy. Patients with relatively asymptomatic HPT present a difficult therapeutic challenge, and clinicians are not uniformly clear about how to approach their treatment. The relative lack of symptoms associated with the potential for serious complications makes the approach to therapy one of the most controversial in medicine. When clear complaints occur, they are usually related to hypercalcemia. High levels of PTH itself have been a suggested cause of some of the symptoms of HPT. However, no clearly objective data support this association. Currently, the etiology of most mild HPT symptoms remains controversial.

Symptoms, Signs, and Causes of Hyperparathyroidism

SYMPTOMS AND SIGNS	PROBABLE CAUSE
Renal: hypercalciuria, nephrolithiasis, nephrocalcinosis, polyuria, polydipsia and renal insufficiency	PTH stimulates bone resorption, hypercalcemia, bicarbonaturia and phosphaturia, causing decreased tubular responsiveness to antidiuretic hormone (ADH), polyuria, calcium oxalate and phosphate crystallization, nephrocalcinosis and renal insufficiency.

Symptoms, Signs, and Causes of Hyperparathyroidism (Continued)

SYMPTOMS AND SIGNS	PROBABLE CAUSE
Neuromuscular: weakness, myalgia	Prolonged excessive PTH arguably causes direct neuropathy with abnormal nerve conduction velocities (NCV) and characteristic electromyographic (EMG) changes and myopathic features on muscle biopsy.
Neurologic and psychiatric: memory loss, depression, psychoses, neuroses, confusion, lethargy, fatigue and paresthesias	PTH and calcium cause peripheral neuropathy with abnormal NCV and central nervous system damage with abnormal electroencephalographic (EEG) changes.
Skeletal: bone pain, osteitis fibrosa, osteoporosis and subperiosteal skeletal resorption	PTH increases bone resorption and acidosis with subsequent bone buffering and bone loss of calcium and phosphate.
Gastrointestinal: abdominal pain, nausea, peptic ulcer, constipation and pancreatitis	Hypercalcemia stimulates gastrin secretion, decreases peristalsis and increases the calcium-phosphate product with calcium-phosphate deposition and obstruction in pancreatic ducts.
Hypertension	Hypercalcemia causes vasoconstriction and parathyroid hypertensive factor (PHF) may increase blood pressure.
Arthralgia, synovitis, arthritis	HPT is associated with increased crystal deposition from calcium phosphate (paraarticular calcification), calcium pyrophosphate (pseudogout) and uric acid/urate (gout).
Band keratopathy	Calcium-phosphate precipitation in medial and limbic margins of cornea.
Anemia	Unknown.

8. Define parathyroid hypertensive factor.

Although the mechanism is unclear, hypertension is frequently associated with HPT. Parathyroid hypertensive factor (PHF) is a circulating hypertensive factor found in some patients with essential hypertension and noted to be secreted by the parathyroid gland in spontaneously hypertensive rats. Preliminary data show that hypertensive HPT patients positive for PHF before parathyroidectomy have a fall in PHF that correlates with the fall in hypertension after parathyroidectomy. This finding suggests that PHF is secreted by parathyroid tissue in humans and may be associated with the hypertension of HPT in some patients. Data are not available to define the incidence of PHF-associated hypertension in HPT, and its role in essential hypertension is unclear.

9. What is band keratopathy?

Band keratopathy is a classic but unusual sign of HPT characterized by an irregular region of calcium phosphate deposition at the medial and lateral limbic margins of the outer edge of the cornea. The location is believed to be a result of diffusion of carbon dioxide from air-exposed areas of the cornea, leaving an alkaline environment that favors precipitation of calcium phosphate crystals. Band keratopathy occurs only with a high calcium-phosphate product. Diagnosis is made by ophthalmologic slit-lamp examination. It is to be distinguished from arcus senilis, an age-related, linear, concentric gray crescent that is separated from the extreme periphery (limbus corneae) by a rim of clear cornea and that with time completely encircles the cornea.

10. Describe the classic radiographic findings in HPT.

Because most patients are diagnosed early, there are usually no radiographic findings related to HPT. If HPT is prolonged, osteopenia develops. However, the classic radiographic finding is subperiosteal bone resorption along the radial aspect of the middle and distal phalanges and distal clavicles. Salt-and-pepper skull is another classic finding.

11. What is the differential diagnosis of primary HPT?

Because the main abnormality in primary HPT is hypercalcemia, the differential diagnosis initially is hypercalcemia (see Chapter 14). A history and physical exam focused on symptoms and signs (see Question 7) may suggest one of the causes of hypercalcemia. If hypercalcemia is mild and history and physical exam are nonspecific, primary HPT is likely. The two most common causes of hypercalcemia are primary HPT and malignancy. In Humoral hypercalcemia of malignancy the tumor usually produces a PTH-like hormone, PTHrP.

12. Distinguish the three types of HPT.

Parathyroid Hormone and Calcium in Hyperparathyroidism

	PARATHYROID HORMONE	CALCIUM
Primary	Normal ↑	↑
Secondary	↑	↓ Normal
Tertiary	↑ ↑	↑

Primary HPT is idiopathic and results from excessive secretion of PTH in patients with a single adenoma (85%), multiple adenomas (5%), parathyroid hyperplasia (10%) and parathyroid carcinoma (<< 1%). The calcium is high, and PTH is inappropriately normal or high.

Secondary HPT is excessive PTH secretion in response to hypocalcemia, hyperphosphatemia and low levels of calcitriol. All three of these conditions exist in chronic renal failure, the most common cause of secondary HPT. Other causes of hypocalcemia are renal calcium leak, dietary calcium malabsorption and vitamin D deficiency. Hypocalcemia causes parathyroid hyperplasia. Attempting to return the calcium to normal, the enlarged glands secrete excessive PTH. Prolonged hypocalcemia may cause development of autonomous parathyroid function and hypercalcemia.

Spontaneous change from low or normal calcium levels to hypercalcemia marks the transition from secondary to **tertiary HPT**. In tertiary HPT, PTH levels are usually > 10–20 times normal. Occasionally, patients with secondary HPT have hypercalcemia, which usually occurs when hypocalcemic patients with chronic renal failure receive a kidney transplant. The new kidney returns phosphate levels to normal, causing calcium levels to rise. The new kidney also effectively makes $1,25(OH)_2D$ in response to increased PTH and decreased phosphate. Because the parathyroid glands are hyperplastic, basal PTH secretion continues, despite normal-to-high calcium levels. With time, the parathyroid glands involute and the serum calcium returns to normal in the renal transplant patient with secondary HTP. This process may take months and occasionally years. If the increased calcium and PTH fail to correct spontaneously or with calcitriol therapy, the patient has tertiary HPT. Tertiary HPT usually requires resection of at least three and a half parathyroid glands to correct the hypercalcemia.

13. How is humoral hypercalcemia of malignancy (HHM) distinguished from primary HPT?

Hypercalcemia, Primary Hyperparathyroidism and Malignancy

	INTACT PTH	PTHrP	$1,25(OH)_2D$	CALCIUM
Primary hyperparathyroidism	↑	↓	↑	↑
PTHrP malignancy	↓	↑	↓	↑
Non-PTHrP malignancy	↓	↓	↓	↑

The main distinguishing features are the levels of intact PTH, PTHrP and $1,25(OH)_2D$. The classic and most common patterns of these hormones are shown in the table above. Primary HPT usually has elevated levels of intact PTH. PTHrP levels, when measured, are low. Malignancy-associated hypercalcemia, in contrast, has low levels of intact PTH, but 80% of cases have increased levels of PTHrP and 20% have both low intact PTH and PTHrP. Thus, measuring the two hormones distinguishes all three disorders.

PTHrP is a protein with 141 amino acids, whereas PTH has 84 amino acids. The region homologous to PTH is primarily within the first 13 N-terminal amino acids. PTHrP stimulates the same receptors as PTH and has the same biologic effects. However, the two hormones have different effects on levels of $1,25(OH)_2D$, probably because of their differing secretion patterns. Both PTH and PTHrP stimulate receptors that activate renal 1α-hydroxylase. The continuous secretion of PTHrP by malignant tumors probably downregulates these receptors, inhibiting 1α-hydroxylase activity and decreasing $1,25(OH)_2D$ production. Continuous infusion of PTH causes similar decreases in $1,25(OH)_2D$. Secretion of PTH in HPT, in contrast, is intermittent; intermittent secretion avoids downregulation and results in increased $1,25(OH)_2D$. In addition, serum calcium levels are higher in HHM than in HPT. The higher calcium levels further decrease production of $1,25(OH)_2D$. Thus $1,25(OH)_2D$ levels tend to be high in HPT and low in HHM. Traditional associations of primary HPT include mild renal tubular acidosis, hypophosphatemia, hyperchloremia and an increased ratio of chloride to phosphate. Unfortunately, such associations are nonspecific and too insensitive to be of diagnostic use.

14. What PTH assay is most useful in the work-up of hypercalcemia?

Intact PTH has 84 amino acids. Although the first 34 amino acids of the N-terminus contain the full biologic activity of the hormone, intact PTH-(1-84) is the active hormone in vivo. The preferred assays for measurement are the ICMA and IRMA assays for intact PTH; both are highly sensitive and specific. Because of availability, the IRMA is more commonly used. At times, a midmolecule assay for PTH will support the clinical diagnosis of HPT when the ICMA and IRMA assays are both negative.

The teaching that intact PTH and N-terminal PTH assays are not significantly affected by renal failure is generally true, although both assays sometimes reveal false elevations in renal failure, as noted in question 6. The parathyroid glands secrete both intact PTH and C-terminal fragments. The liver then metabolizes intact PTH into its N-terminal and C-terminal fragments and further metabolizes the N-terminal fragments. In renal failure, C-terminal fragments accumulate, whereas intact PTH and N-terminal fragments do not because of rapid hepatic clearance of these molecules. Thus, PTH values measured with intact PTH and N-terminal PTH assays are usually accurate in renal failure patients, but they are falsely elevated when measured with a C-terminal PTH assay.

15. What is parathyroid crisis? How is it treated?

Parathyroid crisis or hypercalcemic crisis caused by HPT results from severe hypercalcemia (usually > 16–18 mg/dL). Patients have usually had HPT and hypercalcemia for years. Most patients are confused. They generally have chronic complications of HPT, including nephrolithiasis and decreased bone density. PTH levels are often > 5–10 times the upper limit of normal. Debilitation, intercurrent illness and associated dehydration may contribute to the severe hypercalcemia due to decreased GFR and calcium retention. Etiologies are the same as for milder cases of HPT, including adenoma, hyperplasia and carcinoma. However, the incidence of multigland hyperplasia and carcinoma may be somewhat higher in patients with parathyroid crisis. Rarely crisis occurs with infarction of a parathyroid adenoma. Most patients are volume-depleted. Thus, the initial treatment is usually normal saline. Overall, emergency treatment targets the severe hypercalcemia (see question 17 of chapter 14). After the patient is stabilized, rule out HHM by measuring PTHrP, because hypercalcemic crisis is much more commonly due to HHM.

CONTROVERSIES

16. What methods best localize the parathyroid tumor in HPT?
Noninvasive localization techniques include high-frequency (7.5–10 MHz) ultrasound, 99mtechnetium pertechnetate and 123iodine (123I) with thallium (20Tl)subtraction scanning, 99mtechnetium-sestamibi scanning, cervical computed tomography or magnetic resonance imaging scanning, and intravenous digital subtraction angiography (IVDSA). Overall, these techniques average 75% sensitivity with false-positive rates of 10–30%. However, 99mtechnetium-sestamibi scanning may be > 80-90% sensitive, specific and accurate and therefore is the procedure of choice when preoperative localization is indicated. Sestamibi scanning is most accurate for localizing parathyroid adenomas and is much less useful in patients with parathyroid hyperplasia. Ultrasonography is usually a complementary test to further localize the PTH-secreting tissue. Invasive techniques include arteriography and selective venous sampling, which have sensitivity rates of 90% and few false-positive results.

17. When should you use preoperative localization of a parathyroid adenoma?
Despite general agreement that reoperative parathyroid surgery requires preoperative localization studies, the following statement by John Doppman in 1986 generally holds true today: "The only localization study indicated in a patient with untreated primary hyperparathyroidism is the localization of an experienced parathyroid surgeon." More than 90–95% of the time, a skilled parathyroid surgeon can localize and remove a parathyroid adenoma without preoperative localization. For this reason, preoperative localization before the first neck exploration for primary HPT is rarely indicated. However, 5–10% of parathyroid adenomas are in aberrant locations, such as within a thyroid lobe, and at times the surgeon will be unsuccessful in finding the parathyroid tumor. Thus, before a second operation localization studies are usually performed.

In addition, there are special circumstances in which the surgeon will request preoperative localization before the initial operation as a "road map" to surgery. One such circumstance is in the patient with renal failure who may have secondary HPT but in whom primary and tertiary HPT are considerations. As noted, patients with renal failure may have a species of PTH that has no biologic activity but cross-reacts with assay specificity for the intact hormone (see question 6). In this setting, PTH as measured by the intact assay will be increased. Depending on the level of calcium and PTH, this increase may suggest primary HPT, although the biolologically intact PTH is actually normal for the level of renal function. Thus, the calcium-PTH relationship may not always allow clear distinction among primary, secondary and tertiary HPT. Because progressive renal insufficiency can be an indication for parathyroidectomy, a localization study may determine whether a clear adenoma or four-gland hyperplasia exists and assist in further management decisions. Preoperative parathyroid localization also may be required in patients with high cardiovascular risk who need limited operative time and patients with unusual cervical anatomy that may compromise the surgical procedure. Preoperative localization has decreased operative time by 50%.

18. Do all hypercalcemic patients with HPT require surgical treatment?
No. The only definitive therapy for HPT is parathyroidectomy. Most clinicians recommend parathyroidectomy for patients with symptoms and signs of hypercalcemia (see question 7) and for asymptomatic patients younger than 50 years or with serum calcium levels > 12 mg/dL. The experienced parathyroid surgeon performs a parathyroidectomy with a 90–95% success rate, < 5% complication rate, little morbidity, rare mortality and brief hospitalization. Unfortunately, not all patients have access to an experienced parathyroid surgeon, and success rates decrease to 70% and operative morbidity increases to > 15% in less experienced hands. Truly symptomatic patients usually improve after parathyroidectomy.

However, most patients with HPT are asymptomatic, remain asymptomatic, and are older than 50 years. Many have increased risks for surgical complications. In addition, no controlled data indicate that mild, asymptomatic HPT causes clinically significant osteoporosis, renal failure or other major complications. Conversely, recent data suggest that mild increases in PTH may increase bone formation and preserve cancellous bone while causing only a modest reduction in cortical bone. Thus, asymptomatic patients with serum calcium levels < 11.5–12 mg/dL do not always require surgery. They do benefit from careful follow-up, increased physical activity, adequate hydration, a normal calcium intake, and estrogen replacement in postmenopausal women. Selected patients may benefit from oral bisphosphonate or phosphate therapy.

The natural history of mild, asymptomatic HPT is unknown and thus many questions remain unanswered. Although recent data suggest long-term stability and no overt clinical complications in patients with mild, asymptomatic disease, a subgroup of these patients develops biochemical progression that meets criteria for parathyroidectomy. For these reasons, long-term medical surveillance and surgery are both acceptable forms of management. Only patients with mild hypercalcemia, no history of life-threatening hypercalcemia, and normal renal and bone status should be medically followed. Unless there are contraindications to or refusal of surgery, the following groups of patients need parathyroidectomy: patients with truly significant symptoms of HPT, patients in whom chronic illness will complicate future management, and patients who will not or cannot comply with long-term follow-up. General indications for parathyroidectomy in symptomatic or asymptomatic patients are summarized in the table below.

Indications for Parathyroidectomy

1. Hypercalcemia > 1.5 mg/dL above the upper normal limit
2. Hypercalciuria > 6 mg/kg ideal body weight/day
3. Truly symptomatic hypercalcemia
4. Decreasing creatinine clearance (< 70% of normal)
5. Decreased and decreasing bone densitometry (> 2 SD)
6. Age < 50 years with mild hypercalcemia
7. Calcium nephrolithiasis

19. How should you monitor patients with asymptomatic HPT who have not had parathyroidectomy?

Make patients aware of the importance and goals of close long-term follow-up and get a commitment from them. Monitor patients for worsening hypercalcemia, renal impairment, renal stones and loss of bone mass. Schedule office visits every 6 months for 2 years until the patient is stable, then yearly for 2 years and finally on an as-needed basis. In the evaluation include questions about symptoms and signs related to HPT, including "stones, bones, abdominal groans and psychic moans." Make sure patients maintain adequate hydration and exercise, avoid thiazide diuretics and excessive calcium input, and alert the primary physician to watch for any medical illness predisposing to dehydration. Add estrogen replacement therapy for postmenopausal women with no contraindications.

Following the Patient with Asyptomatic Hyperparathyroidism

FOLLOW-UP CATEGORY	SPECIFIC TESTING
History	Nephrolithiasis, urinary frequency, arthralgias, neuromuscular weakness, abdominal pain, dyspepsia, depression and personality changes
Physical examination	Hypertension and symptom-focused examination
Laboratory tests	Serum calcium and creatinine; 24-hr urine calcium and creatinine clearance
Radiographs	Kidney, ureter and bladder and bone densitometry

20. Creatinine clearance is important to follow in patients with asymptomatic HPT, yet 24-hour urine collections are inconvenient for patients and often are not done accurately. How can you estimate the creatinine clearance without doing a 24-hour urine collection?

Calculate the clearance using the Cockroft-Gault formula. As long as there are no major fluctuations in weight and the patient is not debilitated, this formula provides an accurate, easy, and reproducible estimate of creatinine clearance (C_{Cr}). If there is doubt, perform the 24-hour urine creatinine clearance. You may do both for comparison at the initial evaluation. The C_{Cr} calculation for men follows:

$$C_{Cr} = (140 - age) \times ideal\ body\ weight\ (kg)/[72 \times serum\ Cr\ (mg/dL)]$$

For women, multiply the above answer by 0.85.

Example: A 60-year-old woman with asymptomatic HPT, serum creatinine of 0.8 mg/dL, weight of 60 kg and average height.

$$C_{Cr} = (140 - 60) \times 60\ kg \times 0.85/(72 \times 0.8\ mg/dL) = 83\ mL/min$$

Because a normal creatine clearance is 100 mL/min and one normally loses 1 mL/min/year after age 40, renal function adjusted for the patient's age is normal. More precise calculations can be made if you calculate ideal body weight as follows:

Ideal body weight for men = 50.0 kg + 2.3 kg per inch over 5 feet tall

Ideal body weight for women = 45.4 kg + 2.3 kg per inch over 5 feet tall

21. How would you estimate the 24-hour urine calcium excretion without doing a 24-hour urine collection?

A good estimate of the 24-hour urine calcium excretion is 1.1 times the calcium-to-creatinine ratio on a random urine specimen. An example in the same patient as in question 20 follows:

U_{Ca} = 20 mg/dL and U_{Cr} = 70 mg/dL   Calcium/creatinine = 20/70 = 0.286 g
1.1 × 286 mg/day = 315 mg/day

Thus, the estimated 24-hour urinary calcium excretion is 315 mg/day. Because normal 24-hour urinary calcium is 4 mg/kg/day or about 240 mg/day in a 60-kg woman, the urinary calcium is elevated, as would be expected in HPT. However, it is not elevated to a degree that requires surgical recommendation in an asymptomatic patient with normal renal function for age. If the estimated 24-hour calcium excretion were repeatedly > 6 mg/kg/day or > 360 mg/day, parathyroidectomy would be a strong consideration.

22. Describe the potential medical approaches to hyperparathyroidism.

Bisphosphonates, phosphate, estrogen and calcimimetics are the main potential medical treatments of HPT. Most of these therapies are aimed at reducing serum calcium levels and inhibiting bone resorption. They are primarily used when patients refuse to have or have contraindications to surgery. These treatments may also be useful in patients who have the rarely encountered parathyroid carcinoma. Bisphosphonates inhibit osteoclastic mediated bone resorption and have been shown to improve bone mass significantly in elderly patients with mild HPT. Oral phosphate precipitates calcium from the extracellular fluid and decreases renal $1,25(OH)_2$ vitamin D formation. Both therapies may reduce serum calcium levels modestly, resulting in an increase in PTH secretion; the clinical consequences of the latter effect, however, are currently unclear. Estrogens (used in postmenopausal patients) decrease bone resorption with minimal changes in serum calcium levels and therefore produce little or no increase in PTH secretion. Although not yet available for clinical use, the potentially most useful drugs for treatment of HPT are calcimimetic agents. These drugs bind to the extracellular calcium sensor/receptor on parathyroid cells and alter their sensitivity to extracellular calcium, shifting the calcium-PTH curve to the left, decreasing parathyroid responsiveness to the stimulatory effects of low extracellular calcium and increasing parathyroid sensitivity to the suppressive effects of high calcium. The net effect of calcimimetics is a reduction of PTH secretion.

BIBLIOGRAPHY

1. Bilezikian JP: Primary hyperparathyroidism: When to observe and when to operate. Endocrinol Metab Clin North Am 29:465–478, 2000.
2. Eigelberger MS, Clark OH: Surgical approaches to primary hyperparathyroidism. Endocrinol Metab Clin North Am 29:479–502, 2000.
3. Hellman P, Carling T, Rask L, Akerstrom G: Pathophysiology of primary hyperparathyroidism. Histol Histopathol 15(2):619–627, 2000.
4. Irvin GL 3rd, Carneiro DM: Management changes in primary hyperparathyroidism. JAMA 284(8): 934–936, 2000.
5. Khan A, Bilezikian J: Primary hyperparathyroidism: pathophysiology and impact on bone. CMAJ 163(2):184–187, 2000.
6. Rossini M, Gatti D, Isaia JG, et al: Effects of oral alendronate in elderly patients with osteoporosis and mild primary hyperparathyroidism. J Bone Min Res 16:113–119, 2001
7. Silverberg SJ: Natural history of primary hyperparathyroidism. Endocrinol Metab Clin North Am 29:451–464, 2000.
8. Siminoski K: Asymptomatic hyperparathyroidism: Is the pendulum swinging back? CMAJ 163(2):173–175, 2000.
9. Strewler GJ: Medical approaches to primary hyperparathyroidism. Endocrinol Metab Clin North Am 29:523–539, 2000.
10. Yudd M, Llach F: Current medical management of secondary hyperparathyroidism. Am J Med Sci 320(2):100–106, 2000.

16. HYPERCALCEMIA OF MALIGNANCY

Michael T. McDermott, M.D.

1. What are the two general categories of hypercalcemia of malignancy?
• Humoral hypercalcemia of malignancy (HHM)
• Local osteolytic hypercalcemia (LOH)

2. What types of cancer are associated with humoral hypercalcemia of malignancy?
Carcinoma of the lung, particularly squamous cell carcinoma, is the most common. Other tumors associated with this disorder include squamous cell carcinomas of the head, neck, and esophagus and adenocarcinomas of the kidney, bladder, pancreas, breast, and ovary.

3. What is the cause of humoral hypercalcemia of malignancy?
HHM results when solid malignancies, both solitary and metastatic, secrete into the circulation one or more substances that cause hypercalcemia. The humoral mediator identified in over 90% of cases is parathyroid hormone–related peptide (PTHrp). Other humoral substances that are occasionally secreted and contribute to the development of hypercalcemia include transforming growth factor alpha (TGFα), tumor necrosis factor (TNF), and various interleukins and cytokines.

4. What is PTHrp?
PTHrp is a protein that has sequence homology with the first 13 amino acids of parathyroid hormone (PTH). Both PTH and PTHrp bind to a common receptor (PTH/PTHrp receptor), resulting in stimulation of bone resorption and inhibition of renal calcium excretion. PTHrp is found in high concentrations in breast milk and amniotic fluid, but it can be detected in almost every tissue in the body; it is increased in the circulation during pregnancy. Its physiologic endocrine function apparently is to govern the transfer of calcium from the maternal skeleton and bloodstream into the developing fetus and into breast milk. As a generalized paracrine factor, it also regulates growth and development of many tissues, most prominently the skeleton and breast.

5. How does PTHrp cause hypercalcemia in patients with cancer?
Elevated circulating levels of PTHrp stimulate generalized bone resorption, flooding the bloodstream with excessive calcium; PTHrp also acts on the kidneys, preventing excretion of the increased calcium load. This combination produces an increase in the serum calcium concentration. Hypercalcemia induces polyuria, which leads to dehydration with impaired renal function, further reducing calcium excretion and leading to a cycle of progressive and eventually life-threatening hypercalcemia.

6. How do you make a diagnosis of humoral hypercalcemia of malignancy?
Hypercalcemia in any patient with a known malignancy should make one suspect this diagnosis. Occasionally, however, a raised serum calcium is the first clue to an underlying cancer. Routine laboratory tests usually reveal hypercalcemia, often associated with low serum albumin levels. The key to the diagnosis is a suppressed serum intact PTH level; this finding reliably excludes hyperparathyroidism, the other leading cause of hypercalcemia. Serum PTHrp levels are nearly always high, but this expensive test is not necessary for diagnosis in most instances. If a patient meeting these diagnostic criteria does not have a known tumor, a careful search for an occult malignancy should be undertaken.

7. What types of cancer are associated with local osteolytic hypercalcemia?

Breast cancer with skeletal metastases, multiple myeloma, and lymphoma are the major cancers associated with LOH.

8. What is the cause of local osteolytic hypercalcemia?

LOH generally occurs when cancer cells are present in multiple sites throughout the skeleton. The pathogenesis involves the elaboration by malignant cells of osteoclast-stimulating factors directly onto the surface of bone. Such factors include PTHrp, lymphotoxin, interleukins, transforming growth factors, prostaglandins, and procathepsin D.

9. How do you make a diagnosis of local osteolytic hypercalcemia?

The diagnosis is fairly straightforward when a patient with one of the above malignancies develops hypercalcemia. In addition to hypercalcemia, patients often have low serum albumin and elevated serum alkaline phosphatase levels. Again, the key is demonstration of a suppressed serum intact PTH, indicating that hyperparathyroidism is not the culprit. Patients without a known malignancy should have a complete blood count, serum and urine protein electrophoresis, and bone scan; if these studies are not informative, a bone marrow biopsy should be performed.

10. Can lymphomas cause hypercalcemia by other mechanisms?

Some lymphomas express 1-alpha hydroxylase activity. This enzyme converts 25-hydroxyvitamin D to 1,25-dihydroxyvitamin D, which then stimulates increased intestinal calcium absorption. This may eventually lead to hypercalcemia, particularly in patients who have reduced renal calcium excretion due to dehydration or intrinsic renal disease.

11. What is the prognosis for patients with hypercalcemia of malignancy?

Because hypercalcemia generally correlates with far advanced disease, the overall prognosis is quite poor. In one study the median survival of patients who developed hypercalcemia was only 30 days. Prognosis for resolution of the hypercalcemia is better, however, because effective treatments are available.

12. How do you treat hypercalcemia of malignancy?

Successful treatment of the underlying malignancy, when possible, is the most effective long-term solution. For the symptomatic patient, however, rapid reduction of serum calcium is indicated. The initial measure in almost all patients should be an intravenous infusion of normal saline to enhance renal calcium excretion. Concomitantly, medication to inhibit bone resorption should be given. The most effective option is pamidronate (60–90 mg IV over 4 hours on the first day and repeated every 2 weeks for maintenance) or etidronate (7.5 mg/kg/day IV over several hours each day for 4–7 days followed by 20 mg/kg/day orally for maintenance). A less effective but more rapidly acting alternative is calcitonin (100–200 units subcutaneously twice daily) plus prednisone (30–60 mg/day). For patients with severe and symptomatic hypercalcemia, the combination of pamidronate and calcitonin is the most reliable way to lower the serum calcium quickly. Refractory hypercalcemia may require treatment with plicamycin (25 µg/kg IV, repeated, if necessary, in 48 hours), gallium nitrate (200 mg/m^2/day IV for 5 days), or hemodialysis.

BIBLIOGRAPHY

1. Bilezikian JP: Management of acute hypercalcemia. N Engl J Med 326:1196–1203, 1992.
2. Grill V, Ho P, Body JJ, et al: Parathyroid hormone related protein: Elevated levels in both humoral hypercalcemia of malignancy and hypercalcemia complicating metastatic breast cancer. J Clin Endocrinol Metab 73:1309–1315, 1991.

3. Hortobagyi GN, Theriault RL, Porter L, et al: Efficacy of pamidronate in reducing skeletal complications in patients with breast cancer and lytic bone metastases. N Engl J Med 335:1785–1791, 1996.
4. Mundy GR, Guise TA: Hypercalcemia of malignancy. Am J Med 103:134–145, 1997.
5. Nussbaum SR, Younger J, Vandepol CJ, et al: Single dose intravenous therapy with pamidronate for the treatment of hypercalcemia of malignancy: Comparison of 30, 60, and 90 mg doses. Am J Med 95: 297–304, 1993.
6. Ralston SH, Gallacher SJ, Patel U, et al: Cancer associated hypercalcemia: Morbidity and mortality. Clinical experience in 126 treated patients. Ann Intern Med 112:499–504, 1990.
7. Singer FR, Ritch PS, Lad TE, et al: Treatment of hypercalcemia of malignancy with intravenous etidronate. A controlled multicenter study. Arch Intern Med 151:471–476, 1991.
8. Stewart AF, Broadus AE: Parathyroid hormone related proteins: Coming of age in the 1990's. J Clin Endocrinol Metab 71:1410–1414, 1990.
9. Wimalawansa SJ: Optimal frequency of administration of pamidronate in patients with hypercalcemia of malignancy. Clin Endocrinol 41:591–595, 1994.
10. Wimalawansa SJ: Combined therapies with calcitonin and corticosteroids, or biphosphonate, for treatment of hypercalcemia of malignancy. J Bone Miner Metab 15:160–154, 1997.

17. HYPOCALCEMIA

Reed S. Christensen, M.D.

1. Define hypocalcemia.

Hypocalcemia is the state in which the serum calcium level drops below the normal range of 8.5–10.5 mg/dl (2.1–2.5 mmol/L) despite correction for serum albumin, to which calcium is bound. Calcium levels are corrected for hypoalbuminemia by adding 0.8 mg/dl to the serum calcium level for every 1.0 g/dl that the albumin level is below 4.0 g/dl. The adjusted level of serum calcium correlates with the level of ionized calcium, which is the physiologically active form of serum calcium.

2. What is the normal level of serum ionized calcium?

Approximately 50% of serum calcium is bound to albumin, other plasma proteins, and related anions, such as citrate, lactate, and sulfate. Of this, 40% is bound to protein and 10–13% is attached to anions. The remaining 50% is unbound, giving a normal ionized calcium level of 1.0–1.15 mmol/L.

3. What factors other than albumin influence the levels of serum ionized calcium?

Serum pH influences levels of ionized calcium by causing decreased binding of calcium to albumin in acidosis and increased binding in alkalosis. As an example, respiratory alkalosis, which is seen in hyperventilation, causes a drop in the level of serum ionized calcium. A shift of 0.1 pH unit is associated with an ionized calcium change of 0.04–0.05 mmol/L. Increased levels of chelators, such as citrate, also may lower the levels of ionized calcium, as does heparin.

4. How is calcium regulated?

Three hormones maintain calcium homeostasis: parathyroid hormone (PTH), vitamin D, and calcitonin. PTH acts in three ways to raise serum calcium levels: (1) it stimulates osteoclastic bone resorption; (2) it increases conversion of 25-hydroxyvitamin D to 1,25-dihydroxyvitamin D (calcitriol) and thereby increases intestinal calcium absorption; and (3) it increases renal reabsorption of calcium. Vitamin D is obtained through the diet or is formed in the skin in the presence of ultraviolet light. Vitamin D is converted to 25-hydroxyvitamin D in the liver and finally to 1,25-dihydroxyvitamin D, the most active form of vitamin D, in the kidney. 1,25 Dihydroxyvitamin D acts directly on intestinal cells to increase calcium absorption. Calcitonin, which is produced by the C-cells of the thyroid, decreases the level of serum calcium by suppressing osteoclast activity in bone. The interplay of these hormones maintains calcium levels within a very narrow range in a normal individual.

5. What are the major causes of hypocalcemia?

The etiology of hypocalcemia must be considered in relation to the level of serum albumin, the secretion of PTH, and the presence or absence of hyperphosphatemia. The potential for multiple causes of hypocalcemia is due to the multiple organ and hormonal regulatory systems involved in calcium homeostasis. Initially hypocalcemia may be approached by looking for failure in one or more of these systems. The systems primarily involved are the parathyroid glands, bone, kidney, and liver.

Clinical Entity	Mechanism
Hypoparathyroidism	Decreased PTH production
Hypomagnesemia	Decreased PTH release
Pseudohypoparathyroidism	PTH ineffective at target organ
Liver disease	Decreased albumin production
	Decreased 25-hydroxyvitamin D production
	Drugs that stimulate 25-hydroxyvitamin D metabolism
Renal disease	Renal calcium leak
	Decreased 1,25-dihydroxyvitamin D production
	Elevated serum phosphate (PO_4) from decreased PO_4 clearance
	Drugs that increase renal clearance of calcium
Bone disease	Drugs suppressing bone resorption
	"Hungry bone syndrome"—recovery from hyperparathyroidism or hyperthyroidism
Phosphate load	Endogenous: tumor lysis syndrome, hemolysis, rhabdomyolysis
	Exogenous: phosphate-containing enemas and laxatives, phosphorus burns
Other illness	
Pancreatitis	Sequestration of calcium in the pancreas
Toxic shock syndrome	
Other critical illness	Decreased PTH production or PTH resistance

6. What laboratory tests are clinically useful in distinguishing among the causes of hypocalcemia?

In the evaluation of an individual patient, many causes can be excluded on the basis of history and physical examination. The following table summarizes the laboratory findings in conditions for which these values define the diagnosis.

Differential Diagnosis of Laboratory Evaluation of Hypocalcemia

	CALCIUM	PHOSPHATE	PTH	25-VITAMIN D	1,25-VITAMIN D
Hypoparathyroidism	↓	↑	↓	Normal	↓
Pseudohypoparathyroidism	↓	↑	↑	Normal	↓ or Normal
Liver disease	↓	↓	↑	↓	↓ or Normal
Renal disease	↓	↑	↑	Normal	↓ or Normal

7. What are the neurologic and psychological symptoms of hypocalcemia?

Hypocalcemia may present with numbness, tingling, muscle cramps, and fasciculations. Psychiatric symptoms of irritability, paranoia, depression, psychosis, and organic brain syndrome may also develop. Subnormal intelligence also has been reported with hypocalcemia. Individuals may be unaware of symptoms because of their gradual onset and may realize an abnormality only when their sense of well-being improves with treatment. Neurologic symptoms may progress to tetany and seizures. Seizures occur because of a lowered seizure threshold that reveals underlying epilepsy or as "cerebral tetany" (see below), which is not a true seizure.

Chvostek's and Trousseau's signs are useful in detecting hypocalcemia. Chvostek's sign is a facial twitch elicited by tapping over the zygomatic arch. Trousseau's sign is forearm spasm induced by inflation of an upper arm blood pressure cuff for up to 3 minutes. It is important to note that 4–25% of normal individuals have a positive response.

Calcifications of basal ganglia may occur in the small blood vessels of that region. These occasionally may cause extrapyramidal signs but usually are asymptomatic. Of note, 0.7% of routine computed tomographic (CT) scans of the brain show calcification of the basal ganglia.

8. In hypocalcemia, how does cerebral tetany differ from a true seizure?

Cerebral tetany is manifested by generalized tetany without loss of consciousness, tongue biting, incontinence, or postictal confusion. Anticonvulsants may relieve the symptoms, but because they enhance 25-hydroxyvitamin D catabolism, they also may worsen the hypocalcemia.

9. How does hypocalcemia affect cardiac function?

Calcium is involved in cardiac automaticity and is required for muscle contraction. Hypocalcemia can therefore result in arrhythmias and reduced myocardial contractility. This decrease in force of contraction may be refractory to pressor agents, especially those that involve calcium in their mechanism of action. Beta blockers and calcium channel blockers, which decrease calcium availability to intracellular processes, can exacerbate cardiac failure. The Q-T interval is prolonged with low serum calcium, and, although the relationship is variable, the calcium level correlates moderately well with the interval from the Q-wave onset to the peak of the T-wave.

10. What are the potential ophthalmologic findings in hypocalcemia?

Papilledema may occur with subacute and chronic hypocalcemia. Patients are most often asymptomatic, and the papilledema usually resolves with normalization of the serum calcium level. If symptoms develop or if papilledema does not resolve when the patient is normocalcemic, a cerebral tumor and benign intracranial hypertension must be excluded. Optic neuritis with unilateral loss of vision occasionally develops in hypocalcemic patients. Lenticular cataracts also may occur with longstanding hypocalcemia but usually do not increase in size once hypocalcemia is corrected.

11. With what autoimmune disorders is hypocalcemia sometimes associated?

Hypoparathyroidism may result from autoimmune destruction of the parathyroid glands. This disorder has been associated with adrenal, gonadal, and thyroid failure as well as with alopecia areata, vitiligo, and chronic mucocutaneous candidiasis. This combination of conditions, each associated with organ-specific autoantibodies, has been termed the autoimmune polyglandular syndrome, type 1.

12. Hypocalcemia is frequently encountered in intensive care settings. What are the potential causes?

Low total serum calcium levels, found in 70–90% of intensive care patients, result from multiple causes. Hypoalbuminemia is one major cause. In addition, administration of anionic loads (i.e., citrate, lactate, oxalate, bicarbonate, phosphate, ethylenediaminetetraacetic acid [EDTA], and radiographic contrast) may lower serum ionized calcium levels by chelation, as noted above. Parathyroid failure and decreased vitamin D synthesis are also believed to play a role. Underlying disease states and malnutrition frequently contribute as well. The inflammatory response associated with sepsis appears to induce some degree of resistance to the biologic effects of PTH. Furthermore, rapid blood transfusion with citrate ion as a preservative and anticoagulant therapy may transiently decrease ionized calcium by 14–40%. Because of all the above factors, it is recommended that ionized serum calcium rather than total serum calcium be measured in patients with severe illness.

13. Hypercalcemia is not unusual in patients with cancer. What conditions may lead to hypocalcemia in this patient group?

- Tumor lysis syndrome with hyperphosphatemia is associated with hypocalcemia because of the formation of intravascular and tissue calcium-phosphate complexes.
- Multiple chemotherapeutic agents, such as vincristine/prednisone-16 (VP-16), and antibiotics, such as amphotericin B and aminoglycosides, may induce hypomagnesemia, which leads to hypocalcemia. Hypomagnesemia impairs calcium homeostasis by reducing secretion of PTH and by causing resistance to PTH in skeletal tissue.
- Thyroid surgery and neck irradiation may cause hypoparathyroidism transiently or permanently.
- Medullary carcinoma of the thyroid and pheochromocytoma may secrete calcitonin and on rare occasions cause hypocalcemia.

14. What drugs may cause hypocalcemia?

Phenobarbital, phenytoin, primidone, rifampin, and glutethimide increase hepatic metabolism of 25-hydroxyvitamin D and may thereby cause hypocalcemia. Aminoglycosides, diuretics (furosemide), and chemotherapeutic agents that induce renal magnesium wasting, and laxatives or enemas that create a large phosphate load, also may be associated with hypocalcemia. Ketoconazole, isoniazid, heparin, fluoride, bisphosphonates, foscarnet, and glucagon may also induce hypocalcemia by a variety of mechanisms.

15. Which vitamin D metabolite is best for assessing total body vitamin D stores, 25-hydroxyvitamin D or 1,25-dihydroxyvitamin D?

The serum level of 25-hydroxyvitamin D best reflects the total body stores of vitamin D, because conversion to 1,25-dihydroxyvitamin D is tightly controlled. The level of serum 1,25-dihydroxyvitamin D is maintained despite significant vitamin D depletion since secondary hyperparathyroidism stimulates increased conversion of 25-hydroxyvitamin D to 1,25-dihydroxyvitamin D in this situation.

16. How is hypocalcemia treated?

Asymptomatic hypocalcemia requires supplementation with oral calcium and vitamin D derivatives to maintain the serum calcium level at least in the range of 7.5–8.5 mg/dl. When the serum calcium level falls acutely to a level at which the patient is symptomatic, intravenous administration is recommended. The dose of calcium depends on the amount of elemental calcium present in a given preparation. Approximately 90 mg of elemental calcium can be given intravenously as a bolus for a hypocalcemic emergency, followed by an infusion of 0.5–2.0 mg/kg/hr.

Elemental Calcium Contents of Commonly Used Preparation

PREPARATION	ORAL DOSE	ELEMENTAL CALCIUM
Calcium citrate	950 mg	200 mg
Citracal		
Calcium acetate	667 mg	169 mg
PhosLo		
Calcium carbonate		
Tums	500 mg	200 mg
Tums Ex	750 mg	300 mg
Oscal	625 mg	250 mg
Oscal 500	1250 mg	500 mg
Calcium 600	1500 mg	600 mg
Titralac (suspension)	1000 mg/5 ml	400 mg

INTRAVENOUS AGENT	VOLUME	ELEMENTAL CALCIUM
Calcium chloride	2.5 ml of 10% solution	90 mg
Calcium gluconate	10 ml of 10% solution	90 mg
Calcium gluceptate	5 ml of 22% solution	90 mg

17. When is treatment with 1,25 dihydroxyvitamin D (calcitriol) indicated?

Under normal conditions, 25-hydroxyvitamin D is converted to 1,25-dihydroxyvitamin D (calcitriol) in the kidney under the stimulatory influence of PTH. Two conditions can therefore make the body unable to produce adequate amounts of calcitriol: hypoparathyroidism and renal failure. Since calcitriol is essential for normal intestinal calcium absorption, oral calcitriol (Rocaltrol) supplementation is indicated in patients who have either hypoparathyroidism or chronic renal failure. The usual dose of calcitriol is 0.25–1.0 µg/day, given along with sufficient oral calcium to maintain the serum calcium level within the desired range. If calcitriol is unavailable, these patients must be given large doses of vitamin D (50,000–100,000 units/day), since vitamin D has very weak biologic activity. All patients receiving any form of vitamin D or calcitriol must be monitored regularly for the development of hypercalciuria (urine calcium > 300 mg/day) and hypercalcemia.

BIBLIOGRAPHY

1. Bringhurst FR, Demay MB, Kronenberg HM: Hypocalcemic disorders. In Wilson JD (ed): Williams Textbook of Endocrinology, 9th ed. Philadelphia, WB Saunders, 1998, pp 1185–1192.
2. Cada DL (ed): Drug Facts and Comparisons. St. Louis, Facts and Comparisons, 1997, p 11a.
3. Lebowitz MR, Moses AM: Hypocalcemia. Semin Nephrol 12:146–158, 1992.
4. Lind L: Hypocalcemia and parathyroid hormone secretion in critically ill patients. Crit Care Med 28:93–98, 2000.
5. McEvoy G (ed): Calcium salts. In AHFS Drug Information. Bethesda, MD, American Society of Hospital Pharmacists, 1996, pp 1862–1863.
6. Olinger ML: Disorders of calcium and magnesium metabolism. Emerg Med Clin North Am 7: 795–822, 1989.
7. Potts JT: Hypocalcemia. In Fauci AS (ed): Principles of Internal Medicine, 14th ed. New York, McGraw-Hill, 1998, pp 2241–2247.
8. Shane E: Hypocalcemia: Pathogenesis, differential diagnosis and management. In Favus MJ (ed): Primer on the Metabolic Bone Diseases and Disorders of Mineral Metabolism, 4th ed. Philadelphia, Lippincott Williams & Wilkins, 1999, pp 223–226.
9. Zaloga GP: Hypocalcemia in critically ill patients. Crit Care Med 20:251–262, 1992.

18. NEPHROLITHIASIS

Leonard R. Sanders, M.D.

1. Define hypercalciuria, kidney stones, renal calculi, nephrolithiasis, urolithiasis, renal lithiasis and nephrocalcinosis.

Hypercalciuria is urinary excretion of > 300 mg/day of calcium in men and > 250 mg/day in women. A more accurate definition is urinary calcium excretion > 4 mg/kg ideal body weight/day in either sex. **Kidney stones, renal calculi, nephrolithiasis, urolithiasis** and **renal lithiasis** are synonymous terms that define the clinical syndrome of formation and movement of stones in the urinary collecting system. Renal calculi are abnormally hard, insoluble substances that form in the renal collecting system. Nephrocalcinosis is deposition of calcium salts in the renal parenchyma.

2. Who is at risk of developing kidney stones?

Two to 4 percent of the United States population is at risk of developing one stone, 50–60% have recurrence within 5–10 years. Stones occur most commonly between ages 18 and 45 and two or three times more commonly in men than women. However, the gap between men and women has narrowed in recent years. The cause of the increase in kidney stones in women is not clear. It may represent changes in diet (increased calcium and protein intake), exercise (dehydration) or other causes. Anyone with a family history of stones is also at high risk, as are people with autosomal dominant polycystic kidney disease and medullary sponge kidney. Others at risk are those with urine volume < 2 L/day, dietary sodium < 2 g/day, hypercalciuria, hyperoxaluria, hyperuricosuria, hypocitraturia, hypomagnesiuria and high protein intake.

3. Describe the composition and approximate frequency of most kidney stones.

There are six major types of stones: mixed calcium oxalate and phosphate (40%), calcium oxalate (30%), calcium phosphate (10%), struvite (magnesium ammonium phosphate) (10%), uric acid (7%), and cystine (2%). On rare occasions, kidney stones may form from xanthine. By epitaxy, triamterene and uric acid may serve as substrates for calcium oxalate stone formation.

4. What are the main causes of nephrolithiasis?

The most common causes of nephrolithiasis are the various types of idiopathic hypercalciuria: absorptive hypercalciuria type I, type II and type III (renal phosphate leak) and renal hypercalciuria. Other causes include primary hyperparathyroidism, hyperoxaluric calcium nephrolithiasis, hyperuricosuric calcium nephrolithiasis, hypocitriaturic calcium nephrolithiasis, hypomagnesiuric calcium nephrolithiasis, infection stones, gouty diathesis, renal tubular acidosis, cystinuria, and the newly identified *Nanobacteria*. Patients with idiopathic nephrolithiasis make up 10–20% of stone formers and have no identifiable cause after routine work-up.

5. Describe the conditions associated with both renal stone disease and hypercalciuria.

Calcium-containing stones account for 70–80% of all kidney stones. About 40–50% of calcium stone formers have hypercalciuria. Most of these patients (40%) have idiopathic hypercalciuria. About 5% have primary hyperparathyroidism, and 3% have renal tubular

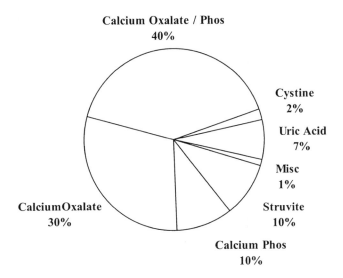

Frequency of renal stones.

acidosis. Other causes of hypercalciuria include excessive dietary vitamin D, excessive calcium and alkali intake, sarcoidosis, Cushing's syndrome, hyperthyroidism, Paget's disease
of bone and immobilization.

6. What are the most important causes of normocalciuric calcium nephrolithiasis?

The most important and most common causes of normocalciuric calcium nephrolithiasis
are hypocitraturia (50%), hyperuricosuria (25%), hyperoxaluria (10%) and urinary stasis (5%).

7. Describe the process of renal stone formation.

Initially, urinary crystallization or precipitation of sparingly soluble salts and acids
occurs. Nucleation follows as the initial crystals and urinary matrix ions form a stable
framework for crystal enlargement through growth and aggregation. Once sufficiently large,
the crystals become trapped in a narrow portion of the urinary collecting system. The
trapped particles then serve as a nidus or focus for further growth and development of the
stone. Usually stones originate in the renal papilla. Once formed, the stone may detach,
move distally and cause obstruction. Common sites for obstruction are the ureteropelvic
junction, mid-ureter and ureterovesical junction.

8. Discuss the pathophysiologic factors that influence formation of renal stones.

Renal stones do not form without quantitative or qualitative imbalances of stone precursors, inhibitors or promoters. Hereditary or acquired defects may cause such imbalances. The
main pathogenic factors for stone formation include supersaturation of stone precursors,
appropriate physicochemical conditions, deficiency of stone-formation inhibitors and possibly
excess of stone-formation promoters. The driving force to crystallization is supersaturation
with mineral precursors such as calcium oxalate. Recent studies show that calcium oxalate
crystals bind to an ionic, sialic acid–containing glycoproteins on the apical surface of renal
tubular epithelial cells, allowing them to be retained by the tubule potentially for further
growth. Known inhibitors of stone formation include citrate, nephrocalcin, glycosaminoglycans and uropontin, all of which inhibit epithelial cell adhesion and internalization of calcium
oxalate crystals. This may be one means by which inhibitors prevent renal stone formation.

Other factors that increase stone formation include urinary stasis (medullary sponge kidney), decreased flow (obstruction), increased urine ammonium (infection), dehydration (concentrated urine) and level of urinary acidity (renal tubular acidosis). Renal tubular acidosis promotes stone formation by causing hypercalciuria, hypocitraturia and alkaline urine.

9. What are the main chemical precursors of renal stones?

Relatively high concentrations of salt and acid solutes are the main determinants of crystalluria and stone formation. Calcium oxalate is most common and is supersaturated in normal urine to four to five times its solubility. Other precursors are calcium phosphate (hydroxyapatite) and calcium phosphate monohydrate (brushite). Uric acid, cystine, struvite (magnesium ammonium phosphate) and mucoprotein are undersaturated stone precursors. Drugs, such as ascorbic acid (conversion to oxalate) and triamterene (nidus for stone formation), also may promote renal stone formation.

10. List the main inhibitors of renal stone formation and describe how they work.

Inhibitors include urinary citrate, pyrophosphate, nephrocalcin, magnesium, glycosaminoglycans, Tamm-Horsfall protein and uropontin. Most inhibitors bind crystal precursors, thus improving solubility, and impair precipitation, nucleation, crystal growth or aggregation. Inhibitors also compete with stone precursor minerals such as calcium oxalate for binding to the apical surface of epithelial cells. Thus, the precursors are less likely to become established as a focus for crystallization and stone growth.

11. What is nephrocalcin? What role does it play in formation of renal stones?

Nephrocalcin is an anionic protein produced by the proximal renal tubule and the loop of Henle. It normally inhibits the nucleation, crystal growth and aggregation phases of stone formation. However, nephrocalcin isolated from many stone formers has defective structure and function and is found in the matrix of many calcium stones. Thus, nephrocalcin may have a dual role in stone formation. When normal, it acts as an inhibitor of stone formation. When abnormal, it may act as a promoter by binding calcium and forming a nidus for crystallization.

12. Describe the promoters of renal stone formation.

Promoters of renal stone formation are poorly characterized but are believed to be primarily urinary mucoproteins and glycosaminoglycans. Under certain conditions, promoters enhance the formation of renal stones.

13. Summarize the basic determinants of serum calcium.

In the serum, calcium is 40% protein-bound, 10% complexed and 50% ionized. The three sources of serum calcium are intestinal absorption, bone resorption and renal reabsorption. Intestinal calcium absorption is a variable proportion of the intake (15–70%); renal calcium reabsorption is a variable portion of the filtered load (95–99.5%). The net flux of calcium from bone varies, depending on changes in the intestines and kidney. Under normal physiologic conditions, flux of calcium into and out of bone is the same. Parathyroid hormone (PTH) and vitamin D control the normal bone, gastrointestinal and renal handling of calcium. The figure below summarizes normal daily calcium balance.

14. How does the kidney handle calcium?

The ionized and complexed portions of serum calcium are filterable. Thus, about 60% of the serum calcium is filtered by the glomerulus. The kidney reabsorbs 97–98% of the filtered calcium. Calcium reabsorption is passive throughout the nephron. The proximal convoluted tubule (PCT) reabsorbs 60%; the loop of Henle, 30%; and the distal nephron, about 10%. In the PCT, calcium is passively reabsorbed with water and other solutes. In the loop

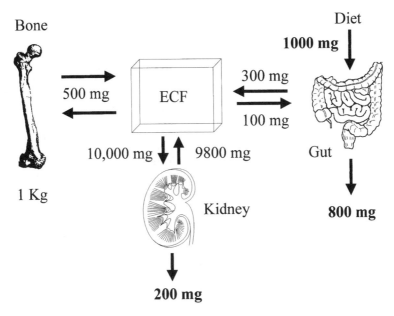

Normal calcium balance.

of Henle and the distal nephron, passive calcium reabsorption depends on favorable electrochemical gradients linked to active transport of sodium (Na) and potassium (K). Because K^+ is recycled to the lumen in the loop of Henle, passive Na-K-2Cl transport generates a positive potential difference that enhances calcium transport. Therefore, inhibition of Na-K-2Cl transport by furosemide depresses calcium transport and increases urinary calcium. On the other hand, inhibition of Na transport by thiazides in the distal convoluted tubule makes the interior of the cell more electronegative and enhances calcium entry (reabsorption). PTH also may impair sodium entry in the distal nephron and increase calcium absorption by enhancing calcium channel activity.

15. Calculate the normal filtered and excreted load of calcium per day.

The serum calcium is normally 10 g/dL. The kidney filters complexed and free calcium, which makes up 60% of the total or 6 mg/dL. The normal glomerular filtration rate (GFR) = 120 mL/min. Thus, the filtered load of calcium of 6 mg/100 mL × 120 mL/min × 1440 min/day = 10,368 mg/day. Because the kidney reabsorbs 98% of the filtered calcium, only 2% is excreted. Thus, normally the kidney excretes about 200 mg of calcium/day. The calculation is as follows:

$$10,368 \text{ mg/day} \times 0.02 = 207 \text{ mg/day}$$

If the excreted calcium increases to 5%, the urinary calcium increases to 500 mg/day.

16. How do serum calcium and dietary sodium affect hypercalciuria?

Normal mechanisms of calcium homeostasis prevent hypercalcemia by increasing urinary calcium excretion. Thus, any nonrenal elevation in serum calcium causes increased filtered calcium and increased urinary calcium. Increased sodium delivery to the loop of Henle and the distal tubule also increases urinary calcium. In normal people, urinary calcium excretion increases about 1 mmol/day (40 mg/day) for each 100 mmol/day (100 mEq/day) increase in Na^+ excretion. Thus, the Ca^{2+}/Na^+ excretion ratio is about 40 mg/100 mEq. In hypercalciuric stone formers, the Ca^{2+}/Na^+ excretion ratio increases to 2 mmol/100 mmol or about 80 mg/100 mEq. In the steady state, the amount of dietary sodium input equals the urinary sodium output. Thus, increasing dietary sodium by 100 mEq (2300 mg) increases urinary Ca^{2+} by 80 mg. Increased dietary sodium causes volume expansion; increased GFR; decreased proximal reabsorption of sodium, calcium and water; and increased distal delivery and excretion. Increased distal delivery also impairs calcium reabsorption in the loop of Henle. Thus, restricting dietary sodium is important for decreasing urinary calcium excretion.

17. Discuss the etiology and pathophysiology of idiopathic hypercalciuria.

Idiopathic hypercalciuria (IH) is a heterogeneous disorder associated with elevated urinary calcium due to one of two major pathophysiologic mechanisms: intestinal hyperabsorption of calcium (absorptive hypercalciuria) or decreased renal tubular reabsorption of calcium (renal hypercalciuria or renal leak). Absorptive hypercalciuria (AH) may result from a primary gut abnormality causing hyperabsorption (rare), from increased gut responsiveness to calcitriol or from increased serum levels of calcitriol. AH types I and II (AH-I and AH-II) are associated with sequentially increased gut absorption of calcium, increased serum calcium, increased filtered calcium, relatively decreased PTH, decreased renal calcium reabsorption and increased urinary calcium excretion. Because many AH-I patients and some AH-II patients have decreased bone mass, there is some evidence that suggests increased bone resorption as contributing to a mild increase in serum calcium, subsequent increased urinary calcium filtration and increased hypercalciuria. AH-I and AH-II appear to have autosomal-dominant inheritance and occur in 30–50% of calcium stone formers. A third subtype, AH-III, results from increased levels of calcitriol caused by a renal phosphate leak that sequentially causes urinary loss of phosphate, decreased serum phosphate, increased renal calcitriol production, increased gut absorption of calcium, increased serum calcium and hypercalciuria. AH-III is unusual and is treated effectively with oral phosphates.

Renal hypercalciuria results from a primary renal calcium leak due to impaired tubular reabsorption of calcium, which causes increased urinary calcium loss, decreased serum calcium, increased PTH, increased calcitriol, increased bone resorption and increased gut absorption. Question 28 distinguishes the various forms of idiopathic hypercalciuria.

18. What causes hyperoxaluria? Why is it important in nephrolithiasis?

Normally, 14% of urinary oxalate comes from dietary absorption. The remainder comes in equal amounts from metabolism of glyoxylate and ascorbic acid. Hereditary hyperoxaluria is a rare autosomal recessive disorder caused by increased oxidation of glyoxylate to oxalate. However, enteric hyperoxaluria caused by small bowel resection, bypass or inflammation is clinically more important.

Small bowel disease may cause bile salt and fat malabsorption. The resulting increase in intestinal concentrations of bile salts damages colonic mucosa, increases its permeability and increases oxalate absorption. The increased fatty acids are negatively charged and bind calcium and magnesium. Free calcium and magnesium in the gut normally bind oxalate and limit its absorption. Once bound by fatty acids, however, calcium and magnesium are no longer available to complex with oxalate, leaving more free oxalate for intestinal absorption. The net effect is increased oxalate absorption and hyperoxaluria. Remember that oxalate is primarily absorbed in the colon. Thus patients with small bowel disease and an ileostomy usually will not have hyperabsorption of oxalate.

Low-calcium diets with less calcium for binding oxalate presumably cause an increased incidence of calcium stones for the same reason. Excessive dietary oxalate also leads to hyperoxaluria. Although ethylene glycol ingestion and methoxyflurane anesthesia increase urinary excretion of oxalate crystals, there are no documented associations with calcium oxalate stones. Ascorbic acid in doses > 2 g/day may promote calcium oxalate stones. Because hyperoxaluria causes calcium oxalate supersaturation more potently than calcium, it is a powerful stimulus for calcium oxalate stone formation. Normal urinary oxalate is < 45 mg/day.

19. Describe hyperuricosuria contributes to renal stones.

About 25% of patients with symptomatic tophaceous gout develop uric acid stones. Excessive urinary uric acid (> 600 mg/day) supersaturates the urine, crystallizes and forms uric acid stones. However, most uric acid stone formers do not have gout, hyperuricemia or hyperuricosuria. All do have a low urinary pH, < 5.5, which promotes uric acid stone formation.

Approximately 25% of calcium stone formers have hyperuricosuria. Uric acid crystals may form a nidus for calcium phosphate and calcium oxalate deposition or interfere with inhibitors, resulting in increased calcium stone formation. This disorder is called hyperuricosuric calcium nephrolithiasis and is characterized by normal serum calcium, urinary uric acid > 600 mg/day, urine pH > 5.5 and recurrent calcium stones.

20. How does urinary pH relate to renal stones?

Because uric acid has a pKa of 5.5, acid urine shifts the equilibrium so that the concentration of uric acid is greater than the concentration of sodium urate. The Henderson-Hasselbalch equation for uric acid and sodium urate defines this equilibrium as follows:

$$pH = 5.5 + \log ([urate] \div [uric\ acid])$$

A urine pH of 6.5 is 1.0 pH unit higher than the pKa for uric acid. At this urine pH, only 10% will be in the form of uric acid and about 90% in the form of sodium urate. Because uric acid is 100 times less soluble than urate, uric acid stones are more likely to form in acid urine. This equilibrium is so important that uric acid stones virtually never develop unless the urinary pH is < 5.5. Cystine stones are also more likely in acid urine, whereas calcium phosphate (brushite) stones usually form only in alkaline urine and calcium oxalate stones may develop in either.

21. Describe the conditions causing low levels of urinary citrate.

Patients with hypocitraturia excrete < 320 mg/day. Idiopathic hypocitraturia occurs in < 5% of patients with calcium stones, and secondary hypocitraturia may occur in 30%. Citrate is freely filtered by the glomerulus, and 75% is reabsorbed by the PCT. Little citrate is secreted. Most secondary causes of hypocitraturia decrease urinary citrate by increasing proximal renal tubular reabsorption, leaving less available for urinary excretion. Secondary causes of low citrate include dehydration, metabolic acidosis, hypokalemia, thiazide diuretics, carbonic anhydrase inhibitors, magnesium depletion, renal tubular acidosis and diarrhea. Diarrhea also causes direct gastrointestinal loss of citrate and magnesium.

22. Discuss the role of diet in the formation of kidney stones.

The high animal protein intake of the average American diet (1–1.5 g/kg/day) may increase both sulfate and uric acid in the urine. High levels of sulfate provide an acid load that decreases urinary pH and citrate excretion. Thus, increased sulfate and uric acid may act as cofactors in the formation of calcium oxalate and uric acid stones. High sodium intake increases urinary calcium as discussed in question 16. High calcium intake, recommended for prevention or treatment of osteoporosis, may lead to hypercalciuria or at least higher urinary concentrations of calcium. However, low calcium intake decreases oxalate binding in the gut and increases oxalate absorption and urinary oxalate. High dietary oxalate increases calcium oxalate crystalluria. The table below lists common foods rich in oxalate, and the reference provides a more detailed list.

Selected High-Oxalate Foods

FRUITS	VEGETABLES	OTHER
Rhubarb	Leafy dark greens	Roasted coffee
Raspberries	Spinach	Ovaltine
Blueberries	Mustard greens	Tea
Blackberries	Collard greens	Cocoa
Gooseberries	Cucumbers	Chocolate
Strawberries	Green beans	Nuts
Fruit cocktail	Beets	Peanuts
Tangerines	Sweet potatoes	Wheat germ
Purple grapes	Summer squash	Baked beans
Citrus peel	Celery	Tofu

Adapted from Renal diseases and disorders. In Nelson JK, Moxness KE, Jensen MD, Gastineau CF (eds): Mayo Clinic Diet Manual, 7th ed. St. Louis, Mosby, 1994.

23. What are the presenting symptoms and signs of renal stones?

Renal stones may be asymptomatic and found as incidental radiologic findings. They also may present as a dull ache in the posterior flank. However, the classic symptom of renal stones is excruciating and intermittent pain. The pain starts in the posterior lumbar area and then radiates anteroinferiorly into the abdomen, groin, genital region and medial thigh. Symptoms of nausea, vomiting, sweating and general prostration may occur. Intense pain may last several hours and be followed by dull flank pain. The patient with renal colic appears acutely ill and restless and moves from side to side, attempting to relieve the pain. Fever, chills and hematuria may be present. Physical examination shows tenderness and guarding of the respective lumbar area. Deep palpation worsens the patient's discomfort, but rebound tenderness is absent. Urinary tract infection may be present. Obstruction, if present, is usually unilateral. Clinical evidence of renal failure is usually absent.

24. Outline the general diagnostic approaches to the patient with kidney stones.

Present, past and family histories provide important clues to diagnosis. Attention should be directed to ascertaining a previous history of stone disease in the patient and family. Drug history should include the use of triamterene and vitamins A, C and D. Dietary history should include fluid intake and sources of excessive calcium, salt, oxalate, uric acid and protein. Physical exam is generally not helpful except during acute disease, as outlined in question 23. Urinalysis should focus on pH, hematuria, pyuria, bacteriuria and crystalluria. Acid urine suggests uric acid or cystine stones. Recurrent infections and alkaline urine suggest struvite stones. Kidney, ureter and bladder radiographs, intravenous pyelography (IVP), computed tomography (CT) scan and ultrasound may be helpful (see question 27). During an acute stone episode, the patient should strain all urine and save the stone if passed. The only means of definitive diagnosis is crystallographic analysis of the stone.

If this is the patient's first stone, there is no continued pain and the stone is < 5 mm, careful follow-up for several months is acceptable, as outlined in question 32. Ninety percent of stones < 5 mm will pass spontaneously. If the patient has continued symptoms, if the stone is > 1 cm or if obvious obstruction is present, consult a urologist and plan for a more extensive work-up. A 1-cm stone is not likely to pass spontaneously. Besides an IVP, patients with microscopic and macroscopic hematuria may need urology consultation and cytoscopy, depending on age and history. Questions below cover specific issues about additional laboratory and radiographic work-up.

25. Describe the clinical significance of urinalysis in patients with renal stones.

Most stone formers have macroscopic or microscopic hematuria. The remainder of the urinalysis is usually normal. Crystals are normally absent in freshly voided urine. Therefore, crystals seen in microscopic examination of warm, freshly voided urine suggest the diagnosis. However, most urine specimens cool before examination, and crystals may form in normal urine with time and cooling. Thus, most crystalluria has little clinical significance. An exception is the presence of cystine crystals, which are diagnostic of cystinuria. Persistently acidic urine (pH < 5.5–5.0) suggests uric acid or cystine stones. Uric acid renal stones never form unless the urine pH is acid. Persistently alkaline urine (pH > 7.5–8) and recurrent urinary tract infection strongly suggest struvite stones. Struvite stones never form unless the urine pH is alkaline. The patient may use nitrazine paper to help follow the response to therapy. However, accurate measurement of urine pH with a pH meter is important for diagnosis. For accurate pH measurement, the patient should collect the urine in a chilled container, seal it and keep it on ice. The urinary pH should be measured with a pH meter within 24 hours. Collection under oil is not necessary.

26. What are the characteristics of urinary crystals in patients with renal stones?
  Calcium oxalate monohydrate crystals may be dumbbell-shaped, needle-shaped or oval, with the latter resembling red blood cells. Calcium oxalate dihydrate crystals are pyramid-shaped and have an envelope appearance. Calcium phosphate crystals are too small for standard light microscopic resolution and look like amorphous debris. Uric acid crystals also usually resemble amorphous debris. However, uric acid crystals have a characteristic yellow-brown color. The less common uric acid dihydrate crystals may be rhomboid-shaped or resemble the six-sided diamonds on a deck of cards. Any of these crystals may be found in normal urine; their presence is not diagnostic of disease. However, the presence of cystine crystals always means cystinuria. Cystine crystals are flat, hexagonal plates resembling benzene rings. Unlike benzene rings, however, the rings of cystine crystals may have equal or unequal sides. Struvite (magnesium ammonium phosphate) crystals are rectangular prisms that resemble coffin lids.

27. How do radiographic tests help to evaluate patients with renal stones?
  A radiograph of the **kidney, ureter, and bladder (KUB)** should be obtained for all stone formers. The KUB shows calcium stones but does not differentiate the type. KUB with tomograms or a digitally enhanced KUB better localizes and identifies renal stones. Calcium oxalate stones are usually small, dense and circumscribed. Cystine stones are faint, soft and waxy. Struvite stones are irregular and dense. Uric acid stones are radiolucent and not seen on KUB.
  IVP should be performed on all symptomatic patients who have not passed the stone and on patients who have passed the stone but continue to have symptoms and hematuria or have multiple stones on KUB. IVP localizes stones in the urinary tract and shows the degree of obstruction and renal function. If needed during pregnancy, a limited IVP (KUB + 10-min postcontrast film) may be appropriate. A radiolucent obstruction on IVP suggests a uric acid stone. Before ordering IVP, make sure that the patient has normal serum creatinine and no allergy to radiocontrast media.
  Ultrasonography does not detail the anatomic location of small stones. However, it is often helpful in managing renal stone disease because it may give size and location of larger stones, is sensitive for diagnosing obstructive uropathy and provides a noninvasive means of monitoring for development of new stones or changes in size.
  Non-contrast Helical CT scanning is the most sensitive procedure for localizing renal stones and may be required to rule out uroepithelial malignancy. CT urography may identify the location of an obstruction stone.
  Magnetic resonance imaging (MRI) has been used for evaluation of nephrolithiasis, but is less available, more costly, and not as sensitive, specific or accurate as CT scanning.

28. Distinguish among the various forms of idiopathic hypercalciuria (IH).

IH involves four primary syndromes: AH types I, II and III and renal hypercalciuria (RH). They have the following features:

Forms of IH

LAB VALUE	AH-I	AH-II	AH-III	RH
Serum calcium	Normal	Normal	Normal	Normal
Serum phosphorus	Normal	Normal	↓	Normal
Serum intact parathyroid hormone	Normal	Normal	Normal	↑
24-hr urinary calcium (1-g calcium diet)	↑	↑	↑	↑
Urine calcium/creatinine (1-g calcium load	↑	↑	↑	↑
24-hr urinary calcium (400-mg calcium diet)	↑	Normal	↑	↑
Fasting urinary calcium (mg/dL glomerular filtration rate)	Normal	Normal	↑	↑

Serum phosphorus is low in AH-III because of a primary renal phosphate leak. Intact PTH is high in RH because the primary defect is decreased renal tubular calcium reabsorption, which causes relative hypocalcemia and stimulates PTH. All patients have high 24-hour urinary calcium on a 1-g calcium diet and a high urine calcium/creatinine (Ca/Cr) ratio after a 1-g calcium load. AH-II normalizes 24-hr urine calcium on a restricted calcium diet (400 mg/day) because the absorptive excess is not as severe. However, the 24-hr urine calcium during calcium restriction remains high in AH-I, AH-III and RH. It remains high in AH-I because of marked hyperabsorption of calcium; in AH-III, because hypophosphatemia decreases renal tubular reabsorption of calcium; and in RH, because decreased renal tubular reabsorption is the primary defect.

Low serum phosphorus is < 2.5 mg/dL on an 800 mg/day phosphorus diet. High 24-hr urinary calcium is > 4 mg/kg ideal body weight. Normal 24-hr urinary calcium on a 400 mg/day calcium restriction is < 200 mg/day. Normal fasting urine calcium is < 0.11 mg/100 mL GFR. Normal urine Ca/Cr is < 0.20 after a 1-g oral load of calcium. Occasionally, the above work-up varies in the same patient, overlaps in different categories and may not change initial therapy. For these reasons, most clinicians do not differentiate the various forms of IH. However, complicated stone disease probably requires the above thorough evaluation.

29. Which medications are useful for treating the various stone-forming conditions?

Oral Drug Therapy for Renal Stones

DISORDER	DRUG	DOSAGE
Absorptive type I	Hydrochlorothiazide	25–50 mg twice daily
	Potassium citrate	10–30 mEq 3 times/day
	Cellulose sodium phosphate	5 g 1–3 times/day with meals
	Magnesium gluconate	1–1.5 g twice daily and as needed
Absorptive type II	Hydrochlorothiazide	25–50 mg/day as needed
Renal phosphate leak	Neutral sodium phosphate	500 mg 3 times/day
Renal hypercalciuria	Hydrochlorothiazide	25–50 mg twice daily
Hypocitraturia	Potassium citrate	10–30 mEq 3 times/day
Hyperuricosuria	Potassium citrate	10–30 mEq 3 times/day
Hyperuricosuria	Potassium citrate	10–30 mEq 3 times/day
	Allopurinol	200–600 mg/day

Oral Drug Therapy for Renal Stones (continued)

DISORDER	DRUG	DOSAGE
Enteric hyperoxaluria	Potassium citrate	10–30 mEq 3 times/day
	Magnesium gluconate	1–1.5 g twice daily
	Calcium citrate	950 mg 4 times/day
	Calcium carbonate	250–500 mg 4 times/day
	Cholestyramine	4 g 3 times/day
	Pyridoxine	100 mg/day
Cystinuria	Potassium citrate	10–30 mEq 3 times/day
	α-Mercaptopropionylglycine	250–500 mg 4 times/day
	D-Penicillamine	250–500 mg 4 times/day
	Pyridoxine	50 mg/day
Struvite stones	Acetohydroxamic acid	250 mg 2–4 times/day

Note: Dosages are estimated ranges and not absolute recommendations. Each drug must be adjusted according to the patient's tolerance. Use the lowest dosage necessary to attain the desired effect and avoid side effects. Always use drug therapy in addition to appropriate dietary changes and fluid input. Potassium citrate is better tolerated in lower dosages taken three times a day. However, twice-daily dosing may improve compliance. Potassium citrate is often required to correct thiazide-induced hypokalemia and hypocitraturia. Also see question 34.

30. What therapy is appropriate in all stone formers?

Increase water intake to increase urine output to > 2 L/day. Restrict dietary sodium to 2 g/day and protein to 0.8–1 g/kg ideal body weight/day. Decrease animal protein and avoid excessive calcium, oxalate and vitamin C.

CONTROVERSIES

31. Discuss which patients with renal stones need a thorough metabolic evaluation.

Metabolically active stones enlarge, recur, are multiple and are associated with passage of gravel. Patients with metabolically active stones; patients with presumed cystine, uric acid or struvite stones; and patients requiring chronic drug therapy for symptomatic stone disease need a thorough metabolic evaluation. Metabolically active stones recur in about 30% of first-time stone formers and > 50% of recurrent stone formers. Such patients require drug therapy. The most common drug therapies for mephrolithiasis are thiazide diuretics and potassium citrate (see question 29). Because most patients respond to this therapy, some physicians empirically treat with one or both of these drugs. However, therapy for renal stone disease is lifelong. Thiazides can cause hyponatremia, hypokalemia, hypocitraturia, dehydration, hyperuricemia, gout, hyperglycemia and hypersensitivity reactions. Furthermore, patients may have combined defects that will be missed or complicated by therapy without at least one metabolic work-up. Finally, potassium citrate is expensive. For these reasons, perform a basic work-up for all stone formers before starting lifelong therapy. The work-up may improve selection of therapy by revealing several defects that promote stone formation.

32. What is the best initial approach to patients with nephrolithiasis?

The patient with a first kidney stone needs only a limited work-up. If not yet done, advise saving any stone passed for analysis. Focus the history and physical exam on risk factors for nephrolithiasis, including low fluid intake; excessive intake of vitamins C, D and A; excessive dietary oxalate; history of chronic diarrhea; inflammatory bowel disease; and other factors outlined in question 24. If the patient has no obvious risk factors by history and physical exam, perform a limited evaluation. Order a chemistry panel that includes serum sodium, potassium, chloride, carbon dioxide, blood urea nitrogen, creatinine, glucose, calcium, phosphorus, albumin, magnesium and uric acid. In addition, order urinalysis, KUB and baseline ultrasound and repeat the serum calcium. If pH is high on urinalysis, perform a urine culture. Consider a spot urine for determination of the Ca/Cr ratio. Depending on symptoms, repeat the renal ultrasound every 6–12 months and initiate therapy outlined in question 30.

If stones become metabolically active, the patient has recurrent symptoms, or history, physical exam or lab tests reveal a possible etiology (e.g., hyperuricemia, cystinuria), perform more extensive testing directed at the etiology. Additional testing in such patients includes repeating the serum chemistry panel and performing a 24-hour urine for creatinine, sodium, calcium, phosphorus, magnesium, oxalate, citrate and uric acid. Some laboratories require acidifying the urine to measure oxalate and citrate and alkalinizing the urine to measure uric acid. This protocol requires three separate 24-hr urine collections for the one evaluation. However, current methods allow accurate measurement of all factors with one sample. Talk to the lab director to implement the procedure that is most time- and cost-effective. If results agree with the clinical impression, begin therapy according to the results. Because diet and other factors may cause the results to change, most experts suggest at least two 24-hr urine collections before starting lifelong therapy.

33. How should patients with complicated renal calculi be further evaluated?

Further testing depends on the severity of the stone disease and the response to initial therapy. Always attempt to analyze the stone if not yet done. If the patient has failed initial medical therapy and the diagnosis of stone etiology remains in question, repeat the baseline tests and determine serum intact PTH and 1,25-dihydroxyvitamin D. For recurrent calcium stone formers, perform further tests as follows. After an overnight fast with nothing by mouth but distilled water, tests should be done to determine values for serum calcium and creatinine and 2-hr urine excretion of calcium and creatinine. This should be followed by a 4-hr urine sample for calcium and creatinine after giving 1 g of elemental calcium orally. From these measurements, the fasting urinary calcium can be calculated in mg/dL GFR (normal = < 0.11), and the absorption of calcium can be estimated by calculating the urinary Ca/Cr ratio (normal = < 0.20). See below for formulas These measurements may identify the cause of hypercalciuria (see question 28).

$$\text{Fasting urinary calcium (g/dL GFR)} = U_{Ca} \text{ (mg)} \times P_{Ca} \text{ (mg/dL)}/U_{Cr} \text{ (mg/dL)}$$

$$\text{Urinary Ca/Cr ratio after calcium load} = U_{Ca} \text{ (mg)}/U_{Cr} \text{ (mg)}$$

One week before the fast and calcium-load test, prescribe a new diet of 400 mg calcium, 100 mEq sodium and 50 mg oxalate with continued hydration with 2–3 L of water/day. An easy way to provide the 1-g load of elemental calcium in a readily absorbable form is as 1.5 oz of liquid calcium glubionate (115 mg elemental calcium/5 cc). Calculation is as follows:

$$100 \text{ mg} \times 5 \text{ cc}/115 \text{ mg} \times 1 \text{ oz}/30 \text{ cc} = 1.45 \text{ or about } 1.5 \text{ oz}$$

34. Describe some pitfalls in the drug therapy of nephrolithiasis.

Alkalinization of the urine is recommended for treatment of uric acid stones to increase the urinary pH (0.6–7.0) and thereby increase solute solubility. However, the use of sodium bicarbonate increases urinary excretion of sodium and thus of calcium. The increased urinary calcium and the epitaxy effects of hyperuricemia may increase calcium stone formation. Potassium citrate (30–90 mEq in two or three divided doses) beneficially increases urinary pH and citrate but does not have the negative effects of increasing urinary sodium or calcium. Potassium citrate often is the only therapy necessary if hyperuricosuria is mild (< 800 mg/day). However, allopurinol may be needed if uric acid stones continue or hyperuricemia is more severe.

Cellulose sodium phosphate (CSP) binds calcium and magnesium in the gut, decreasing absorption of both. CSP s recommended for patients with AH-I; however, these patients often have osteopenia. By binding calcium, CSP may worsen osteopenia and also increase urinary oxalate. Furthermore, by binding magnesium it may cause hypomagnesemia. These effects increase the tendency to renal stones. Therefore, in patients with AH-I, thiazides and potassium citrate should be tried first. CP should be reserved for refractory stone disease, and magnesium should be replaced as required. Thiazide therapy initially causes increased bone mass in such patients, but over time this beneficial effect may decrease. For this reason, patients need periodic monitoring of bone mass. Neutral sodium phosphate, 500 mg three times a day, effectively lowers urinary calcium and has no negative effects on urinary citrate. Phosphate may be tried if patients are refractory to other therapy.

In patients with AH-II, calcium restriction to 400–500 mg/day may decrease or correct the hypercalciuria. However, a low calcium diet is not beneficial in the treatment of calcium oxalate stones. The low dietary calcium decreases calcium binding of oxalate in the gut. This causes increased oxalate absorption that may increase urinary oxalate excretion and calcium oxalate stone formation. Furthermore, low calcium intake may contribute to osteopenia and subsequent bone fractures. Thus, calcium should not normally be restricted in these patients.

Thiazide diuretics are a clear choice for therapy of renal hypercalciuria because they increase proximal (indirectly) and distal (directly) tubular reabsorption of calcium. Data show that the increased reabsorpion of calcium is a persistent effect. Therefore, the drug is beneficial for long-term therapy. Thiazide diuretics at doses of 50 mg two times a day and lower cause hypokalemia and hypocitraturia. Use potassium citrate as needed to correct these deficiencies. Urine values should be measured after 2–6 months of therapy to assess effects, depending on the patient's symptoms and response. Adjust the thiazide dose as necessary to lower urinary calcium and avoid adverse effects.

35. What is the best thiazide diuretic to use in patients with nephrolithiasis?

Any thiazide diuretic decreases urinary excretion of calcium by increasing proximal and distal tubular resorption. Options include hydrochlorothiazide, 25–50 mg one to three times a day; trichlormethiazide, 2–4 mg/day; indapamide, 2.5–5 mg/day; and chlorthalidone, 25–50 mg/day. All may have problems with potassium wasting. Hypokalemia causes intracellular acidosis, increases citrate lyase (which increases intracellular citrate metabolism) and increases the renal tubular cell luminal-membrane sodium-citrate cotransporter. All three processes enhance citrate reabsorption and cause hypocitraturia. Potassium citrate is reasonable replacement therapy for patients developing hypokalemia and hypocitraturia. Avoid triamterene because of its potential pathogenetic role in stone formation. However, 5–10 mg/day of amiloride is reasonable therapy because it has no known stone-forming effects and directly increases calcium reabsorption in the cortical collecting tubule.

36. Define resorptive hypercalciuria.

RH refers to hypercalciuria resulting from increased bone resorption. The classic cause is primary hyperparathyroidism. However, any cause of RH, including malignancy or primary or secondary increases in calcitriol or PTH, may be associated with resorptive hypercalciuria. Treatment is directed at the underlying cause. Of note, calcium phosphate stones are more likely to be associated with hyperparathyroidism.

37. How would you treat an asymptomatic patient with a renal stone 1–2 cm in size?

Unless they are specifically contraindicated, apply the therapeutic options in question 30. Most urologists treat symptomatic patients with calcium stone 1–2 cm in size in the renal pelvis or a significant proximally obstructing stone (0.6–2 cm) with extracorporeal shock-wave lithotripsy. The asymptomatic patient is a toss-up. Each expert has an opinion based on the experience of the local medical community. Specifics of stone location, duration and overall patient health are also important in the decision. Metabolically active asymptomatic stones (see question 31) probably should also be treated. Nephrology and urology consultations are appropriate. Other forms of lithotripsy include percutaneous ultrasonic lithotripsy and endoscopic ultrasonic lithotripsy. The two most common techniques for intracorporeal lithotripsy are pulsed dye laser and electrohydraulic lithotripsy. If the stone is > 3 cm, lithotripsy usually fails. The initial approach to patients with stones of this size is percutaneous nephrolithotomy. Open lithotomy is now unusual. Stones 2–3 cm in size are in a gray area, and therapy depends on the patient's overall status and the wishes and experiences of the patient, primary physician and urologist.

38. Describe the role of bacteria in nephrolithiasis.

It is well known that urea-splitting organisms are associated with an elevated urinary pH and struvite stones. Bacterial urease, usually from *Proteus* species, causes chemical changes in the urine that result in struvite stone formation. Recent work has suggested an infectious origin for other stones. *Nanobacteria* are small intracellular bacteria found in human kidney stones. The *Nanobacteria* make a calcium oxalate shell and then shed it into the urine. This calcium oxalate shell or the bacteria with the surrounding shell may act as a nidus for stone formation.

BIBLIOGRAPHY

1. Bushinsky DA: Nephrolithiasis. J Am Soc Nephrol 9(5):917–924, 1998.
2. Goldfarb DS, Coe FL: Prevention of recurrent nephrolithiasis. Am Fam Physician 60(8):2269–2276, 1999.
3. Kramer G, Klingler HC, Steiner GE: Role of bacteria in the development of kidney stones. Curr Opin Urol 10(1):35–38, 2000.
4. Lieske JC, Deganello S, Toback FG: Cell-crystal interactions and kidney stone formation. Nephron 81(suppl 1):8–17, 1999.
5. Marangella M, Vitale C, Bagnis C, et al: Idiopathic calcium nephrolithiasis. Nephron 81(suppl 1): 38–44, 1999.
6. Martini LA, Wood RJ: Should dietary calcium and protein be restricted in patients with nephrolithiasis? Nutr Rev 58(4):111–117, 2000.
7. Scheinman SJ: Nephrolithiasis. Semin Nephrol 19(4):381–388, 1999.
8. Wasserstein AG: Nephrolithiasis: acute management and prevention. Dis Mon 44(5):196–213, 1998.
9. Zheng W, Denstedt JD: Intracorporeal lithotripsy. Update on technology. Urol Clin North Am 27(2):301–313, 2000.

Note: The entire issue of *Seminars in Nephrology*, Volume 16, number 5 (Sept), 1996, is devoted to a review of all aspects of nephrolithiasis.

III. Pituitary and Hypothalamic Disorders

19. PITUITARY INSUFFICIENCY

William J. Georgitis, M.D., FACP

CAUSES

1. What causes pituitary insufficiency?

Pituitary insufficiency (hypopituitarism) results from pituitary, hypothalamic, or parasellar diseases that disrupt the normal function of the hypothalamic-pituitary unit by displacement, infiltration, or destruction. Pituitary insufficiency represents failure of the gland to make adequate amounts of one or more of the following anterior pituitary hormones or posterior pituitary hormones.

Adenohypophysis	Neurohypophysis
Growth hormone (GH)	Anti-diuretic hormone (ADH)
Prolactin (PRL)	Oxytocin (OXT)
Corticotropin (ACTH)	
Thyrotropin (TSH)	
Luteinizing hormone (LH)	
Follicle-stimulating hormone (FSH)	

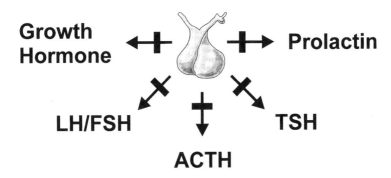

Pituitary insufficiency (hypopituitarism).

2. What happens to anterior pituitary hormones when the pituitary stalk is completely severed?

Serum levels of all the anterior pituitary hormones that are secreted in response to hypothalamic releasing hormones decline; this includes TSH, LH, FSH, GH, and ACTH. In contrast, prolactin levels rise. This response, which is unique among adenohypophysial hormones, results from the loss of the inhibitory effect of hypothalamic dopamine on lactotropes.

3. What disorders adjacent to the pituitary or hypothalamus can cause pituitary dysfunction?

Extrasellar diseases include meningiomas, chordomas, craniopharyngiomas, optic nerve gliomas, carotid aneurysms, sphenoid sinus mucoceles, nasopharyngeal carcinomas, and pineal dysgerminomas.

4. What is a craniopharyngioma?

Craniopharyngioma is a squamous cell tumor that arises from Rathke's pouch remnants. It is the most common tumor in the region of the hypothalamus and pituitary in children but is relatively less common in adults. Two thirds are suprasellar, and one third extend into or are confined within the sella. Most are cystic, but some contain both cystic and nodular components. The cyst fluid is characteristically viscous and yellow-brown in color, resembling motor oil. Calcification of the rim of the tumor, resembling an eggshell, can be a useful radiographic sign. This is best demonstrated with computed tomography. Calcifications are present in 75% of children but in only 35% of adults. Surgery is indicated for both treatment and pathologic confirmation.

5. Describe the clinical presentation of a pineal dysgerminoma.

This tumor can grow to involve the hypothalamus and disrupt both posterior and anterior pituitary function. Patients often present with a combination of gonadal dysfunction and polyuria with polydipsia. Thus, there is anterior hypopituitarism and posterior hypopituitarism represented by secondary hypogonadism and neurogenic diabetes insipidus.

6. What is pituitary apoplexy?

Apoplexy means loss of consciousness followed by paralysis. Classic pituitary apoplexy is an acute life-threatening event characterized by severe headache and collapse with evidence of pituitary hemorrhage. An expanding hemorrhagic mass arising most often from an infarcted pituitary adenoma may compress parasellar structures, including cranial nerves coursing through the adjacent cavernous sinuses. Ocular paralysis and ptosis from involvement of the third, fourth, and sixth cranial nerves as well as facial nerve involvement contribute the component of paralysis necessary to meet the general definition of apoplexy. Anterior pituitary insufficiency is common following pituitary apoplexy. Posterior pituitary functions are almost always preserved. Most patients recover spontaneously. Subacute forms of pituitary necrosis occur in patients with diabetes mellitus and sickle-cell disease. Radiologic evidence of pituitary infarction, whether sudden and catastrophic in presenting signs and symptoms or silent, always deserves a comprehensive functional evaluation.

7. Is primary empty sella syndrome frequently associated with symptomatic pituitary dysfunction?

No. Primary implies that the "empty" sella is not the end result of infarction, surgical removal, or irradiation of a tumor. Some believe that this disorder is a normal anatomic variant or perhaps results from a congenital defect in the diaphragm covering the sella. The sella is not, in fact, empty. It is totally or partially filled with cerebrospinal fluid. Furthermore, the pituitary gland is present but tends to be flattened against the walls of the sella. The prevalence of hypopituitarism with signs of symptomatic dysfunction in primary empty sella is probably less than 10%.

8. What is Sheehan's syndrome? How common is it?

Sheehan's syndrome is an acquired form of empty sella syndrome due to ischemic pituitary necrosis generally following delivery of a child complicated by severe blood loss and hypotension. Thirty percent of women suffering postpartum hemorrhage and vascular collapse eventually may demonstrate a spectrum of anterior pituitary insufficiency from mild to severe. Failure to lactate sufficiently to nurse a baby followed by persistent amenorrhea postpartum is a feature of this syndrome. If secondary adrenal insufficiency accompanies secondary hypogonadism, loss of adrenal and ovarian androgenic steroid dependent axillary and pubic hair may also appear.

DIAGNOSIS

9. Do presenting features of pituitary insufficiency differ between children and adults?

In childhood, a signal of hypopituitarism is failure to grow normally. In adolescents, abnormalities in sexual maturation may be the sentinel features. Failure to achieve puberty or arrest in sexual maturation may indicate pituitary malfunction. Puberty spans many years and occurs at a time when patients often change providers from pediatricians to family practioners and internists. Signs of pituitary insufficiency can easily be overlooked. In adults, symptoms and signs of hypogonadism dominate the clinical picture. Hypogonadism may easily go unsuspected in postmenopausal women or elderly men, since older patients often fail to complain about declining sexual function or desire. Such complaints also lack specificity for hypopituitarism because they are so prevalent in the elderly. Features of hypothyroidism and adrenal insufficiency also may appear insidiously.

10. Is there an easy way to tell if the sella turcica is enlarged?

If a dime (diameter = 16 mm) fits within the sella on lateral skull films, enlargement of the sella turcica is probably present. The most common cause for this finding is a pituitary adenoma. Pituitary tumors comprise 10–15% of intracranial neoplasms and are present in 6–23% of pituitary glands carefully inspected at autopsy. Carcinoma of the pituitary is extremely rare and appears mainly as case reports rather than series in the medical literature. Metastases to this anatomic region from primary tumors elsewhere in the body are also rare and more often involve the highly vascular hypothalamus, presenting most commonly with features such as secondary hypopituitarism and diabetes insipidus.

11. What tests should be considered for hypopituitary patients?

The evaluation should include assessment of anterior pituitary hormones, radiographic imaging by computed tomography or magnetic resonance imaging to assess anatomy, and formal visual fields testing. The tests for anterior pituitary function usually include serum levels of testosterone (men), estradiol (women), LH, FSH, thyroxine (T_4), TSH, prolactin, GH (children), and cortisol (before and after intravenous ACTH administration). Nocturia, polyuria, or polydipsia suggests the need to test for adequacy of vasopressin secretion by performing a water deprivation test.

12. What is the Houssay phenomenon?

Houssay, an Argentinian Nobel laureate, showed improvement in the diabetes of pancreatectomized dogs following hypophysectomy. He and other investigators subsequently demonstrated the diabetogenic actions of pituitary extracts. The clinical relevance of the Houssay phenomenon sometimes appears in diabetic patients who demonstrate diminishing insulin requirements in the presence of hypopituitarism. The diabetic patient with recurrent serious hypoglycemic episodes leading to major reductions in medications may have acquired hypopituitarism with resultant deficiencies of the insulin counterregulatory factors GH and cortisol. To further understand the significance of hormones counterregulatory to insulin in carbohydrate metabolism, consider that the diabetes secondary to GH excess in acromegaly also may improve or resolve after pituitary surgery, pituitary apoplexy, or octreotide therapy.

13. What characteristics of adrenal insufficiency are present in ACTH-deficient patients?

Nonspecific symptoms, such as fatigue and weight loss, are often encountered with ACTH deficiency. In women, axillary and pubic hair may diminish or disappear. Serum sodium levels tend to be low, but potassium remains normal. Features of glucocorticoid deficiency are usually not as severe as those seen with primary adrenal failure.

14. What is the difference between primary and secondary hypothyroidism?

Hypothyroidism is primary when the thyroid gland itself fails. Elevation of the serum TSH level is the most sensitive and specific test for the diagnosis of primary hypothyroidism because TSH levels increase as the thyroid's secretion of T_4 declines. In secondary (or central) hypothyroidism, thyroid hormone deficiency is secondary to loss of TSH secretion by the pituitary gland or TRH production by the hypothalamus. Symptoms and signs are similar to those seen in primary hypothyroidism but are generally milder. Even patients with massive pituitary tumors may not have obvious features of hypothyroidism. Laboratory tests abnormalities, like the symptoms and signs, are more subtle than those in primary hypothyroidism. TSH levels are often in the normal range but may be low whereas serum T_4 levels are decreased.

Several defects explain the decline in thyroid hormone secretion in secondary hypothyroidism. TSH pulsatility in patients with pituitary macroadenomas is often abnormal,l as depicted in the figure. Both TSH pulse frequency and amplitude are decreased, resulting in loss or diminution of the normal nocturnal surge in TSH secretion. Circulating TSH molecules are also abnormal, having higher molecular weights than TSH molecules produced in normal individuals. Failure to remove sugar moieties during post-translational processing by the Golgi apparatus appears to be the responsible mechanism. These higher molecular weight forms of TSH show decreased ability to stimulate thyroid hormone secretion by thyrocytes in bioassays.

15. What cortisol level is consistent with adrenal insufficiency?

Morning serum cortisols less than 10 μg/dl or ACTH-stimulated cortisol levels below 20 μg/dl are consistent with adrenal insufficiency. Plasma ACTH levels, when assayed properly, are elevated in primary adrenal insufficiency but are normal or low in secondary (central) adrenal insufficiency.

16. Is secondary adrenal insufficiency as common as gonadotropin deficiency in patients with pituitary tumor?

No. The frequency of deficiency among the anterior pituitary hormones at the time of diagnosis of a pituitary tumor presents a spectrum of prevalence with GH > LH/FSH > TSH > ACTH. Prolactin deficiency rarely is recognized clinically. Posterior pituitary dysfunction with diabetes insipidus is so infrequent that its presence should suggest diseases primarily of hypothalamic or pineal origin, and OXT deficiency is not usually considered at all. Most patients with pituitary adenomas have surprisingly intact anterior pituitary function before treatment and usually acquire hypopituitarism only after surgical or radiation treatment. This is even true for most macroadenomas. The search for medical therapies as alternatives to ablation by surgery and radiation for pituitary tumors continues with a focus on preservation or restoration of normal pituitary function.

TREATMENT

17. Is life expectancy altered by hypopituitarism?

All-cause mortality in patients with hypopituitarism is significantly increased approximately 1.7-fold. Women tend to fare worse than men, with observed/expected death ratios of 2.3 compared with 1.5, respectively. The increase is suspected to be due to vascular disease events but is probably multifactorial. Age and gonadal status appear to be independent risk factors, with hypogonadal patients having a better prognosis than eugonadal hypopituitary patients.

18. Are health-related costs greater for patients with hypopituitarism?

A Swedish endocrine unit reported that hypopituitary patients have almost 2-fold higher direct health-related costs per annum. They also have 2- fold more claim disability pensions and take a 1.6-fold greater number of sick days than the general population. None of the studied populations were on somatotropin replacement.

19. What is the most important hormone deficiency to identify and treat in patients with anterior pituitary disease?

Inadequate cortisol secretion is the most important to identify and treat. Acute adrenal insufficiency may be life-threatening.

20. Why is aldosterone deficiency generally absent in hypopituitarism?

Secretion of aldosterone is regulated primarily by the renin-angiotensin axis, and therefore aldosterone secretion is normal in patients with hypopituitarism. However, hyponatremia may still be a clue to hypopituitarism because it may result from either thyroid hormone or glucocorticoid deficiency and will be corrected with appropriate thyroid hormone and/or glucocorticoid replacement therapy.

21. Is anterior pituitary hormone deficiency always a commitment to life-long replacement?

Yes, in most cases, but there are important exceptions. Primary hypothyroidism sometimes causes significant pituitary hyperplasia with hyperprolactinemia and may present as amenorrhea-galactorrhea in women or as impotence and impaired libido in men. Dramatic reduction of pituitary size, normalization of serum prolactin levels, and resolution of the hypogonadism usually occur with thyroid replacement. Hypopituitarism from hemochromatosis, an inherited disorder of iron storage, has also improved with therapy directed at the underlying disorder. Another example is seen in certain patients with pituitary macroadenomas. Mild elevations in serum prolactin and deficiencies of other anterior pituitary hormones, especially ACTH, sometimes resolve immediately after surgical excision of the tumor.

22. When one hormone deficiency in hypopituitarism is diagnosed, why is it important to define whether other hormone deficiencies are present?

Replacement with thyroid hormone alone in a patient with coexistent adrenal deficiency may precipitate an acute adrenal crisis. Furthermore, vasopressin deficiency may be masked by adrenal insufficiency. After glucocorticoid replacement, central diabetes insipidus may appear and require specific treatment with a vasopressin analogue.

23. What is the treatment of pituitary insufficiency?

The treatment of pituitary insufficiency consists of replacing the hormones normally made by the pituitary gland or by the endocrine glands regulated by the anterior pituitary hormones. Thus, patients with hypopituitarism are usually treated with replacement doses of thyroid hormone, glucocorticoids, and sex steroids. Patients with diabetes insipidus are treated with a vasopressin preparation. The medications and doses commonly used to treat patients with hypopituitarism are listed at the end of the next chapter.

24. Who should receive growth hormone treatment?

Treatment is indicated for children with short stature, open epiphyses, and documented congenital or acquired GH deficiency. Evidence is also accumulating that adults with growth hormone deficiency may benefit from growth hormone replacement, although the cost effectiveness of this intervention is an unsettled issue.

BIBLIOGRAPHY

1. Arafah B: Reversible hypopituitarism in patients with large nonfunctioning pituitary adenomas. J Clin Endocrinol Metab 62:1173–1179, 1986.
2. Bates AS, Van't Hoff W, Jones PJ, Clayton RN: The effect of hypopituitarism on life expectancy. J Clin Endocrinol Metab 81:1169–1172, 1996.
3. Cummings DE, Merriam GR: Age-related changes in growth hormone secretion: Should the somatopause be treated? Semin Reprod Endocrinol 17:311–325,1999.
4. Ehrnborg C, Hakkaart-Van Roijen L, Jonsson B, et al: Cost of illness in adult patients with hypopituitarism. Pharmacoeconomics 17:621–628, 2000.
5. Gama R, Smith MJ, Wright J, Marks V: Hypopituitarism in primary haemochromatosis; recovery after iron depletion. Postgrad Med J 71:297–298,1995.
6. Hazouard E, Piquemal R, Dequin PF, et al: Severe non-infectious circulatory shock related to hypopituitarism. Intensive Care Med 25?865–868 , 1999.
7. Lurie SN, Doraiswamy PM, Husain MM, et al: In vivo assessment of pituitary gland volume with magnetic resonance imaging: The effect of age. J Clin Endocrinol Metab 71:505–508,1990.
8. Schmidt DN, Wallace K: How to diagnose hypopituitarism. Learning the features of secondary hormonal deficiencies. AD—Allegheny University of the Health Sciences, Philadelphia, USA. Postgrad Med 104:77–87, 1998.
9. Vance ML: Hypopituitarism. N Engl J Med 330:1651–1662, 1994.
10. Webb SM, Rigla M, Wagner A, et al: Recovery of hypopituitarism after neurosurgical treatment of pituitary adenomas. J Clin Endocrinol Metab 84:3696–700, 1999.

20. NONFUNCTIONING PITUITARY TUMORS

Michael T. McDermott, M.D.

1. Name the functioning pituitary tumors.

Prolactin-secreting tumors, growth hormone–secreting tumors, corticotropin (ACTH)–secreting tumors, thyrotropin (TSH)–secreting tumors, and gonadotropin (FSH/LH)–secreting tumors are the major functioning pituitary neoplasms. Some tumors secrete a mixture of hormones.

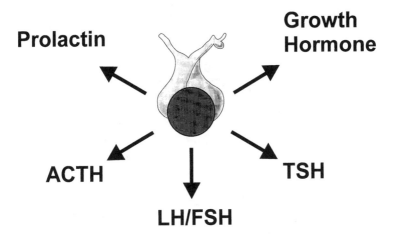

Functioning pituitary tumors.

2. What is a nonfunctioning pituitary tumor?

A nonfunctioning pituitary tumor arises from cells of the pituitary gland but does not secrete clinically detectable amounts of a pituitary hormone. These tumors are usually benign adenomas.

3. What is the alpha subunit?

The alpha subunit is a component of 3 pituitary hormones: TSH, LH, and FSH. Each of these hormones consists of a common alpha subunit and a specific beta subunit (TSH beta, LH beta, and FSH beta). The alpha and beta subunits normally combine before the intact hormone is secreted into the circulation. Some nonfunctioning pituitary tumors actually synthesize and secrete measurable amounts of the free alpha subunit, which may therefore serve as a tumor marker.

4. What other lesions can resemble nonfunctioning pituitary tumors?

Tumors that are not of pituitary origin may be found within the sella turcica; examples include metastatic carcinomas, craniopharyngiomas, meningiomas, and neural tumors. Nonneoplastic Rathke's pouch cysts, arterial aneurysms, and infiltrative diseases of the pituitary, such as sarcoidosis, histiocytosis, tuberculosis, lymphocytic hypophysitis, and hemochromatosis, also may be seen in this location.

5. Differentiate between a microadenoma and a macroadenoma.

A pituitary microadenoma is less than 10 mm in its largest dimension, whereas a macroadenoma is 10 mm or larger. A macroadenoma may be contained entirely within the sella turcica or may have extrasellar extension.

6. Which structures may be damaged by growth of a pituitary tumor outside the sella turcica?

Pituitary tumors that grow superiorly may compress the optic chiasm and pituitary stalk. Tumors that grow inferiorly may erode into the sphenoid sinus. Laterally they may invade the cavernous sinuses and compress cranial nerves III, IV, and VI or the internal carotid artery. Anterior and posterior growth may erode the bones of the tuberculum sellae and dorsum sellae, respectively.

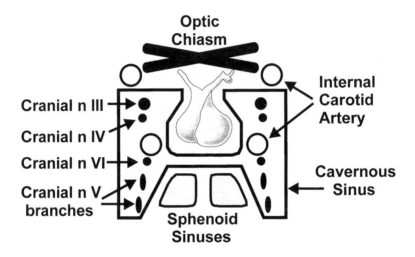

Pituitary fossa.

7. What are the clinical features of nonfunctioning pituitary tumors?

Many nonfunctioning pituitary tumors are asymptomatic and are discovered incidentally during cranial imaging procedures performed for other reasons. This is true of both microadenomas (< 10 mm) and macroadenomas (≥ 10 mm). Nonfunctioning pituitary tumors that cause symptoms are usually large space-occupying macroadenomas that compress nearby neurologic and/or vascular structures. Common clinical manifestations include headaches, visual field defects, visual loss, and extraocular nerve palsies. Pituitary insufficiency also may result from destruction of the remaining normal pituitary tissue.

8. What anatomic evaluation is necessary for a pituitary tumor?

Magnetic resonance imaging (MRI) or computed tomography (CT) of the pituitary gland and parasellar regions often allows a precise diagnosis and determines the presence and extent of extrasellar invasion. Visual field testing helps to assess function of the optic chiasm and tracts. Angiography may be needed in some cases to rule out the presence of an aneurysm.

9. What evaluation is necessary to determine that a pituitary tumor is nonfunctioning?

A thorough history and physical examination must be performed to detect any signs or symptoms of overproduction of pituitary hormones. Hormone testing should include measurement of serum prolactin, insulin-like growth factor 1 (IGF-1), thyroid-stimulating hormone (TSH), free thyroxine (free T_4), luteinizing hormone (LH), follicle-stimulating hormone (FSH), testosterone (men), estradiol (women), and 24-hour urinary free cortisol excretion. Serum alpha subunit, when available, is also helpful.

10. Does an elevated level of serum prolactin mean that a tumor is functioning?
No. Secretion of prolactin is negatively regulated by hypothalamic inhibitory factors, such as dopamine, which reach the anterior pituitary gland through the pituitary stalk. Stalk compression from a nonfunctioning tumor can impair dopamine delivery and thus increase the release of prolactin from the normal pituitary gland. The serum prolactin concentration rarely exceeds 100 ng/ml in such cases, whereas it is usually much higher with prolactin-secreting tumors.

11. What is the primary treatment for a nonfunctioning pituitary tumor?
Asymptomatic microadenomas can be managed with observation by serial imaging studies. Asymptomatic macroadenomas ($\geq$ 1 cm) should be considered for surgical removal, although serial observation is an option if the tumor does not grow and does not cause significant patient anxiety.

The treatment of choice for symptomatic tumors is transsphenoidal surgery, in which access to the pituitary gland is gained through the sphenoid sinus. Radiation therapy may be used if surgery is contraindicated or not desired. Medications such as bromocriptine are rarely helpful.

12. Is postoperative radiation therapy recommended for incompletely resected tumors?
Older literature, primarily from uncontrolled studies, suggests that postoperative radiation therapy is beneficial. Currently, however, most experts advise radiation only for large tumor remnants that compress vascular or neural structures. Many centers are now utilizing stereotactic rather than conventional radiotherapy in these situations in order to deliver a greater focused radiation dose to neoplastic tissue with less radiation exposure to surrounding structures. Residual disease of lesser severity may be monitored with imaging studies and not treated unless growth occurs.

13. What endocrine complications occur in the immediate postoperative period?
Transient diabetes insipidus (vasopressin deficiency) manifested by high-volume urine output is common in the first few days. It may be followed by a short period (1–2 days) of water intoxication (vasopressin excess) causing hyponatremia. Both conditions result from reversible trauma and/or edema of the neurohypophysis, where vasopressin is stored. Fluid balance and serum electrolytes, therefore, must be closely monitored. Secondary adrenal insufficiency is of little immediate concern because high-dose dexamethasone is often given to prevent cerebral edema, but it may sometimes become apparent after dexamethasone is stopped. Deficiencies of other pituitary hormones do not tend to be an early postoperative problem if levels of these hormones were normal preoperatively.

14. What is the management of postoperative diabetes insipidus and water intoxication?
Mild postoperative diabetes insipidus can be managed with isovolumetric, isotonic fluid replacement. More severe cases should be treated with aqueous vasopressin, 5 units subcutaneously every 4–6 hours, or with desmopressin (DDAVP), .25–.5 ml (1–2 µg) bid intravenously or subcutaneously, until urine volumes become normal. If hyponatremia develops, vasopressin must be reduced or stopped and free water intake restricted. If diabetes insipidus persists beyond 1 week, patients may be switched to intranasal DDAVP, .1–.2 ml once or twice daily, or oral DDAVP tablets, .1–.4 mg daily.

15. What endocrine problems may occur during long-term follow-up?

Deficiency of one or more pituitary hormones may develop weeks, months, or years after treatment, especially if radiation was given. The only major concern in the first month is adrenal insufficiency. Accordingly, during this time one should question the patient about symptoms suggesting this disorder and, if they are present, obtain a morning cortisol level. If the cortisol level is low, begin hydrocortisone replacement and retest the patient in 3–6 months with an ACTH stimulation test. At that time, serum free T_4, TSH, LH, FSH, testosterone (men) and estradiol (women) should also be checked and replacement therapy should be initiated for any identified hormone deficiencies. It is recommended that these tests then be monitored at 6 months, 1 year, and annually thereafter.

16. What is the long-term management of pituitary insufficiency?

Deficiency	Replacement Regimen
Adrenal insufficiency	Hydrocortisone, 20 mg a.m., 10 mg p.m.
Hypothyroidism	Levothyroxine, 1.6 µg/kg/day
Hypogonadism, men	Depo-testosterone, 200 mg intramuscularly q 2 weeks
	Androderm patch, 5–7.5 mg q day
	Testoderm TTS patch, 5–10 mg q day
	Androgel, 5–10 G q day
Hypogonadism, women	Premarin, .625–1.25 mg q day or days 1-25
	Estratabs, .625–1.25 mg q day or days 1-25
	Estrace, 0.5–1.0 mg q day or days 1-25
	Estraderm patch, .05–.10 mg patch twice a week
	Vivelle patch, .05–.10 mg patch twice a week
	Climara patch, .05–.10 mg patch once a week
	PremPro, .625/2.5 mg or .625/5.0 mg q day
	CombiPatch, .05/.14 mg or .05/.25 mg patch twice a week
	Provera*, 2.5 mg q day or 5–10 mg days 15-25
Diabetes insipidus	DDAVP nasal spray, .1–.2 ml q day or BID
	DDAVP tablets, .1–.4 mg q day or BID

*Used daily or cyclically in a woman with an intact uterus

17. What are the clinical features of pituitary carcinomas?

Pituitary carcinomas, which are extremely rare, expand rapidly and cause mass effects. Some secrete hormones causing endocrine syndromes similar to those seen with adenomas. Metastatic disease to the central nervous system, cervical lymph nodes, liver, and bone is commonly associated.

18. What is the treatment of pituitary carcinoma?

Transsphenoidal surgery is the primary therapy, followed by postoperative radiation. No significant use of chemotherapy has been reported for pituitary carcinoma.

19. What is the prognosis for pituitary carcinoma?

The mean survival is approximately 4 years.

20. Which cancers metastasize to the pituitary gland?

Metastatic disease to the pituitary gland occurs in approximately 3–5% of patients with widely disseminated carcinoma. The most commonly reported primary tumors are of the breast, lung, kidney, prostate, liver, pancreas, and nasopharynx, plasmacytoma, sarcoma, and adenocarcinoma of unknown primary site.

BIBLIOGRAPHY

1. Arafah BM, Kailani SH, Nekl KE, et al: Immediate recovery of pituitary function after transsphenoidal resection of pituitary macroadenomas. J Clin Endocrinol Metab 79:348–354, 1994.

2. Arafah BM, Prunty D, Ybarra J, et al: The dominant role of increased intrasellar pressure in the pathogenesis of hypopituitarism, hyperprolactinemia, and headaches in patients with pituitary adenomas. J Clin Endocrinol Metab 85:1789–1793, 2000.

3. Branch CL Jr, Laws ER Jr: Metastatic tumors of the sella turcica masquerading as primary pituitary tumors. J Clin Endocrinol Metab 65:469–474, 1987.

4. Bulow B, Attewell R, Hagmar L, et al: Postoperative prognosis in craniopharyngioma with respect to cardiovascular mortality, survival, and tumor recurrence. J Clin Endocrinol Metab 83:3897–3904, 1998.

5. Freda PU, Wardlaw SL: Diagnosis and treatment of pituitary tumors. J Clin Endocrinol Metab 84:3859–3866, 1999.

6. Gittoes NJL: Review: Current perspectives on the pathogenesis of clinically non-functioning pituitary tumours. J Endocrinol 157:177–186, 1998.

7. Kaltsas GA, Mukherjee JJ, Plowman PN, et al: The role of cytotoxic chemotherapy in the management of aggressive and malignant pituitary tumors. J Clin Endocrinol Metab 83:4233–4238, 1998.

8. Katznelson L, Alexander JM, Klibanski A: Clinically nonfunctioning pituitary adenomas. J Clin Endocrinol Metab 76:1089–1094, 1993.

9. King JT Jr, Justice AC, Aron DC: Management of incidental pituitary microadenomas: A cost-effectiveness analysis. J Clin Endocrinol Metab 82:3625–3632, 1997.

10. Klibanski A, Zervas NT: Diagnosis and management of hormone-secreting pituitary adenomas. N Engl J Med 324:822–831, 1991.

11. Molitch ME: Evaluation and treatment of the patient with a pituitary incidentaloma. J Clin Endocrinol Metab 80:3–6, 1995.

12. Mountcastle RB, Roof BS, Mayfield RK, et al: Case report: Pituitary adenocarcinoma in an acromegalic patient: Response to bromocriptine and pituitary testing: A review of the literature on 36 cases of pituitary carcinoma. Am J Med Sci 298(2):109–118, 1989.

13. Mukherjee JJ, Islam N, Kaltsas G, et al: Clinical, radiological and pathological features of patients with Rathke's cleft cysts: Tumors that may recur. J Clin Endocrinol Metab 82:2357–2362, 1997.

14. Pernicone PJ, Scheithauer BW, Sebo TJ, et al: Pituitary carcinoma: A clinicopathological study of 15 cases. Cancer 79:804–812, 1997.

15. Shimon I, Melmed S: Management of pituitary tumors. Ann Intern Med 129:472–483, 1998.

16. Shin JL, Asa SL, Woodhouse LJ, et al: Cystic lesions of the pituitary: Clinicopathological features distinguishing craniopharyngioma, Rathke's cleft cyst, and arachnoid cyst. J Clin Endocrinol Metab 84:3972–3982, 1999.

17. Wilson CB: Extensive personal experience: Surgical management of pituitary tumors. J Clin Endocrinol Metab 82:2381–2385, 1997.

21. PROLACTIN-SECRETING PITUITARY TUMORS

Virginia Sarapura, M.D.

1. Describe the normal control of prolactin secretion. How is it altered in prolactin-secreting tumors?

There are multiple factors that affect prolactin secretion (see figure). However, the principal influence on prolactin secretion is tonic inhibition by dopamine input from the hypothalamus. For this reason, pituitary stalk interruption leads to increased serum levels of prolactin. Prolactin inhibition is mediated by the interaction of dopamine with receptors of the D2 subtype on pituitary lactotroph membranes. This interaction activates the inhibitory G-protein, leading to decreased adenylate cyclase activity. In prolactin-secreting pituitary adenomas, a monoclonal population of cells autonomously produces prolactin, escaping the normal physiologic input of dopamine from the hypothalamus. In almost all cases, responsiveness to a pharmacologic dose of dopamine is maintained.

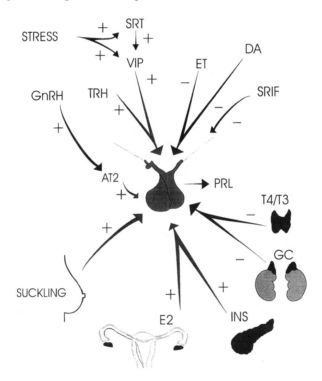

2. What are the normal levels of serum prolactin? Are they different in men and women? What levels are seen in patients with prolactin-secreting tumors?

The normal serum prolactin level is < 15 or 20 ng/ml, depending on the laboratory. Women tend to have slightly higher levels than men, probably because of estrogen stimulation of prolactin secretion. In patients with prolactin-secreting tumors, the levels are usually > 100 ng/ml but may be as low as 30–50 ng/ml if the tumor is small. A level > 200 ng/ml is almost always indicative of a prolactin-secreting tumor.

3. What are the physiologic causes of an elevated prolactin level that need to be considered in the differential diagnosis of prolactin-secreting tumors? What levels can be reached under these circumstances?

The most important physiologic states in which prolactin is found to be elevated are pregnancy and lactation. During the third semester of pregnancy, the prolactin level may reach 200–300 ng/ml and then gradually decreases during the first months postpartum despite continued lactation. Prolactin levels are also elevated during sleep, strenuous exercise, stress, and nipple stimulation. In these cases, the elevation is mild, below 50 ng/ml.

4. List the abnormal causes of an elevated serum prolactin level other than a prolactin-secreting tumor. State the mechanism underlying the abnormal prolactin production. What are the typical levels of serum prolactin associated with each cause?

Causes of Elevated Levels of Serum Prolactin

CAUSES	MECHANISM	PROLACTIN LEVEL

1. Pituitary stalk interruption
  Trauma
  Surgery
  Pituitary, hypothalamic,
   or parasellar tumors
  Infiltrative disorders of
   the hypothalamus
	Interference with the hypothalamic-
	pituitary pathways, which usually
	causes hypopituitarism; prolactin
	levels increase because the tonic
	inhibition of prolactin secretion is
	interrupted
		Usually 30–50 ng/ml, rarely
		above 100 ng/ml

2. Pharmacologic agents
  Phenothiazines
  Tricyclic antidepressants
  Alpha-methyldopa
  Metoclopramide
  Cimetidine
  Estrogens
	Specific interference with dopamin-
	ergic input to the pituitary gland
		Usually 30-50 ng/ml, rarely
		above 100 ng/ml

3. Hypothyroidism	Increased TRH that stimulates- prolactin release	Usually 30–50 ng/ml

4. Renal failure and
  liver cirrhosis
  in chronic renal failure
	Decreased metabolic clearance
	 of prolactin
		Usually 30–50 ng/ml; some-
		times as high as 150 ng/ml

5. Intercostal nerve stimulation
  Chest wall lesions
  Herpes zoster
	Mimicking of the stimulation
	caused by suckling
		Usually 30–50 ng/ml

TRH = thyrotropin-releasing hormone.

5. Is medical treatment available for prolactin-secreting tumors? What is the mode of action?

Medical treatment with dopamine agonists has been available for about 20 years. The most commonly used drug is bromocriptine; cabergoline was approved in 1997 by the Food and Drug Administration for this indication. Pergolide and hydergine are also available but are not yet approved specifically for treatment of prolactin-secreting tumors. These medications are highly effective in reducing both the prolactin level and tumor size. The mode of action is as follows: dopamine agonists bind to the pituitary-specific D2 dopamine receptors on the cell membrane of prolactin-secreting cells, decreasing intracellular levels of cyclic adenosine monophosphate (cAMP) and Ca^{2+}. This results in inhibition of the release and synthesis of prolactin. An increase in cellular lysosomal activity causes involution of the rough endoplasmic reticulum and Golgi apparatus. The action of dopamine agonists on D1 dopamine receptors in the brain causes side effects of nausea and dizziness.

6. What is galactorrhea? Do most patients with prolactin-secreting tumors present with this symptom?

Galactorrhea is the discharge of milk from the breast not associated with pregnancy or lactation. Although a typical symptom of prolactin-secreting tumors, it may be absent in up to 50% of women and is uncommon in men. In men, galactorrhea may be seen in conjunction with gynecomastia when decreased gonadal function results in a low ratio of testosterone to estrogen.

7. Why do men with prolactin-secreting tumors often present with more advanced disease than do women?

The major symptoms of elevated prolactin levels in men are decreased libido and impotence. These symptoms may be ignored or attributed to psychological causes. Many years may go by before an evaluation is sought, often when the patient develops headaches and visual field defects related to the mass effect of the tumor. Women are more likely to seek evaluation early in the disease process, when infertility or menstrual irregularities prompt an evaluation of their hormonal status. In addition, recent studies suggest that large tumors are biologically different and may be so from their onset.

8. What is the imaging technique of choice when a prolactin-secreting tumor is suspected? Why?

Magnetic resonance imaging (MRI) of the pituitary with a contrast agent such as gadolinium is the imaging technique of choice in the evaluation of pituitary tumors. In particular, discrimination of small tumors is enhanced. Computed tomographic scanning allows better visualization of bone structures, such as the floor of the sella, in cases of large tumors. However, the relationship of the tumor to other soft tissue structures, such as the cavernous sinuses and carotid arteries, is better visualized with MRI. Skull radiographs and tomograms are not helpful.

9. If a prolactinoma is left untreated, what is the risk of tumor enlargement?

Many longitudinal studies agree that progression of the disease is rare and occurs at a slow pace. This is particularly true of small prolactin-secreting tumors, less than 5% of which will enlarge. There is no reliable way to predict which patients will show progression. Spontaneous resolution, attributed to necrosis, has also been described in some patients.

10. Bone metabolism is altered when prolactin levels are elevated. What is the mechanism for this effect?

Elevated prolactin levels suppress the hypothalamic-pituitary-gonadal axis by interference with the secretion of gonadotropin-releasing hormone (GnRH) in the hypothalamus. The resulting decrease in circulating levels of estrogen or testosterone causes a corresponding decrease in osteoblastic bone formation and an increase in osteoclastic bone resorption.

11. If a woman with a prolactin-secreting tumor becomes pregnant while on medical treatment, should the treatment be continued? Should she be allowed to breast-feed her infant?

Even though many studies have found that maternal treatment with dopamine agonists is safe to the fetus, it is recommended that the drug be stopped as soon as pregnancy is diagnosed. The risk of tumor re-expansion is low: < 5% for small prolactin-secreting tumors and 15–35% for large tumors. Assessment of symptoms, particularly headaches, and visual field tests, should be done monthly; any evidence of tumor re-expansion should prompt the reinstitution of treatment. Breast-feeding does not appear to add significant risk for these patients, but close follow-up should be continued.

12. What is the consequence of altered bone metabolism? Is it reversible?

The consequence is a decrease in bone mineral density and progression to osteoporosis. Studies suggest that normalization of the prolactin level restores bone density in most but not all patients, particularly those affected at an early age prior to the development of peak bone mass.

13. How long does it take for medical treatment to reduce the serum prolactin level? To reduce the size of the tumor?

The onset of action of dopamine agonists is rapid, and because prolactin has a serum half-life of 50 minutes, a decrease in the prolactin level may be noted in 1–2 hours. However, normalization of the prolactin level may take weeks or months, with the maximal decrease usually seen by 3 months. A reduction in tumor size may be apparent within the first 48 hours and may be demonstrated by improvement in the visual fields. Tumor shrinkage of at least 50% is usually evident by 3 months. Maximal shrinkage, however, is not usually observed until after 6–12 months of treatment.

14. How long is medical treatment of prolactin-secreting tumors required? Why?

In general, life-long treatment is required, because prolactin levels rise and tumors re-expand when treatment is interrupted, suggesting that the effect is mostly cytostatic. Recent reports, however, suggest that about 20% of cases may be cured after 2–5 years of treatment, and some evidence suggests a cytolytic effect of dopamine agonists.

15. When is surgical removal of a prolactin-secreting tumor indicated? When is radiotherapy indicated?

With the availability of dopamine agonists, surgery has become a secondary choice in the treatment of prolactin-secreting tumors, particularly since the long-term surgical cure rate for large tumors is only 25–50%. The principal indications for surgical treatment of a prolactin-secreting tumor are intolerance or resistance to dopamine agonists and acute hemorrhage into the tumor. A CSF leak due to erosion of the floor of the sella turcica is another indication for surgical debulking and repair. Radiotherapy has been rarely utilized because hypopituitarism is a common side effect. This complication is of critical concern, particularly in patients under treatment for infertility. However, radiotherapy may be a useful adjunct in patients who need additional treatment after surgery and who do not tolerate dopamine agonists. Some experts advocate the use of radiotherapy 3 months before attempting pregnancy in women with large tumors in order to avoid tumor re-expansion during pregnancy. The development of new stereotactic radiosurgical techniques, such as the gamma-knife, may improve outcomes and minimize radiation side effects.

BIBLIOGRAPHY

1. Biller BMK: Guidelines for the diagnosis and treatment of hyperprolactinemia. J Reprod Med 44:1075, 1999.
2. Colao A, et al: Prolacinomas in adolescents: Persistent bone loss after 2 years of prolactin normalization. Clin Endocrinol 52:319, 2000.
3. Freda PU, et al: Long-term treatment of prolactin-secreting macroadenomas with pergolide. J Clin Endocrinol Metab 85:8, 2000.
4. Klibanski A, Greenspan SL: Increase in bone mass after treatment of hyperprolactinemic amennorrhea. N Engl J Med 315:542, 1986.
5. Klibanski A, Zervas NT: Diagnosis and management of hormone-secreting pituitary adenomas. N Engl J Med 324:822, 1991.
6. Kovacs K, Stefaneanu L, Horvath E, et al: Effect of dopamine agonist medication on prolactin-secreting pituitary adenomas: A morphological study including immunocytochemistry, electron microscopy and in situ hybridization. Virchows Arch A Pathol Anat 418:439, 1991.

7. Molitch ME: Prolactinoma. In Melmed S (ed): The Pituitary. Oxford, Blackwell Science, 1995, p 443.
8. Thorner MO, Perryman RL, Rogol AD, et al: Rapid changes of prolactinoma volume after withdrawal and reinstitution of bromocriptine. J Clin Endocrinol Metab 153:480, 1981.
9. Verhelst J, et al: Cabergoline in the treatment of hyperprolactinemia: A study of 455 patients. J Clin Endocrinol Metab 84:2518, 1999.
10. Xu RK, et al: Pituitary prolactin-secreting tumor formation: Recent developments. Biol Signals Recept 9:1, 2000.

22. GROWTH HORMONE–SECRETING PITUITARY TUMORS

Mary H. Samuels, M.D.

1. What is the normal function of growth hormone in children and adults?

In children, growth hormone is responsible for linear growth. In children and adults, growth hormone has many effects on intermediary metabolism, including protein synthesis and nitrogen balance, carbohydrate metabolism, lipolysis, and calcium homeostasis.

2. How are levels of growth hormone normally regulated?

Pituitary secretion of growth hormone is regulated by two hypothalamic hormones: stimulatory growth hormone–releasing hormone (GHRH) and inhibitory somatostatin. Secretion of growth hormone is also affected by adrenergic and dopaminergic hormones as well as by other central nervous system factors.

3. Does growth hormone directly affect peripheral tissues?

No. Many (although not all) effects of growth hormone are mediated by another hormone called somatomedin-C or insulin-like growth factor type 1 (IGF-1). IGF-1 is made by the liver and other organs in response to stimulation by growth hormone. IGF-1 feeds back to the pituitary gland and suppresses growth hormone secretion. Unlike growth hormone, IGF-1 has a long half-life in plasma, and thus plasma levels of IGF-1 are helpful in the diagnosis of growth hormone abnormalities.

4. What are the clinical features of excessive production of growth hormone in children?

In children who have not yet undergone puberty and whose long bones still respond to growth hormone, excessive growth hormone causes accelerated linear growth. The result is gigantism.

5. What are the clinical features of excessive production of growth hormone in adults?

In adults, excessive growth hormone causes acromegaly. The pathologic and metabolic effects include the following:

1. Periosteal formation of new bone, leading to overgrowth of the maxillary and mandibular bones, frontal bossing, and nasal bone and laryngeal hypertrophy (causing deepening of the voice)
2. Hypertrophy of joint cartilage and osseous overgrowth, leading to osteoarthritis and carpal tunnel syndrome
3. Soft tissue hypertrophy, leading to enlargement of hands and feet
4. Cardiac abnormalities, including hypertension and left ventricular hypertrophy
5. Hypertrophy of other organs, including sweat glands (excessive sweating and unpleasant odor), skin (skin tags), and tongue and upper airway (obstruction and sleep apnea).
6. Hypogonadism
7. Diabetes mellitus or impaired glucose tolerance
8. Colonic polyps and increased risk of colon cancer

6. What is the single best clue when examining a patient suspected of having acromegaly?

An old driver's license picture or other old photographs provide the best clues. Patients with acromegaly are often unaware of the gradual disfigurement due to the disease or attribute it to aging. Comparing serial photographs can help to establish the diagnosis as well as date its onset.

7. From what do patients with acromegaly die?

The mortality from untreated or inadequately treated acromegaly is about double the expected rate in healthy subjects matched for age. Major causes of death include hypertension, cardiovascular disease, diabetes, pulmonary infections, and cancer.

8. In patients with acromegaly, are skin tags all over the neck and chest a relevant finding?

There appears to be an association between multiple skin tags and colonic polyps in acromegaly. Therefore, the patient should undergo careful colonoscopic screening for polyps and colon cancer. However, even patients without active disease or skin tags may be at risk for colonic neoplasia and probably should be screened regularly.

9. The husband of the patient with acromegaly complains that he cannot sleep because his wife snores so loudly. Is this relevant?

Sleep apnea occurs in up to 80% of patients with acromegaly. It can be due to soft tissue overgrowth of the upper airway or to altered central respiratory control. Sleep apnea may contribute to morbidity and mortality in acromegaly by producing hypoxia and pulmonary hypertension.

10. How is the diagnosis of acromegaly or gigantism made?

Two main biochemical tests may confirm excessive secretion of growth hormone:

1. Plasma levels of growth hormone in the fasting state and after administration of oral glucose. Some patients with acromegaly have extremely elevated fasting levels of growth hormone, and further testing is not necessary. Most patients, however, have growth hormone levels that are only mildly elevated or overlap with levels in healthy subjects. Therefore, the diagnosis is usually made by measuring growth hormone levels after a glucose tolerance test. Healthy subjects suppress growth hormone levels after glucose, whereas patients with acromegaly show no suppression or an increase in growth hormone levels.

2. Plasma levels of IGF-1. Because plasma levels of IGF-1 are independent of food intake, samples can be drawn any time of day. In adults, acromegaly is essentially the only condition that causes elevated IGF-1 levels. In children, IGF-1 levels are more difficult to interpret, because growing children normally have higher levels than adults.

11. Once the biochemical diagnosis of acromegaly or gigantism is made, what is the next step?

Excessive secretion of growth hormone is almost always due to a benign pituitary tumor. Therefore, the next step is to obtain a radiologic study of the pituitary gland. The optimal study is magnetic resonance imaging (MRI) with special cuts through the pituitary gland. If MRI is not available, the best alternative study is a CT scan with special cuts through the pituitary gland.

12. What causes growth hormone-secreting pituitary tumors?

Growth hormone–secreting pituitary tumors have been shown to be monoclonal, suggesting that a spontaneous somatic mutation is a key event in neoplastic transformation of somatotrophs. Further studies have clarified the nature of the mutation in some growth hormone tumors that appear to have an altered stimulatory subunit (G_S) of the G-proteins that regulate adenylate cyclase activity. In a mutated cell, alterations in the G_S subunit cause autonomous adenylate cyclase activity and elevated secretion of growth hormone. However, the mutant G_S is found only in a subset of patients with acromegaly. The mechanism of growth hormone regulation and tumor growth may differ in other patients with acromegaly.

13. Are other endocrine syndromes possible in patients with acromegaly or gigantism?

Of course. Otherwise, acromegaly and gigantism would not be endocrine disorders. Three endocrine syndromes include acromegaly:

1. **Multiple endocrine neoplasia type 1 (MEN-1).** This autosomal dominant familial syndrome includes parathyroid hyperplasia (leading to hypercalcemia), pituitary tumors (secreting growth hormone or other pituitary hormones), and gut tumors (secreting gastrin, insulin, or other gut hormones). Therefore, when evaluating patients with acromegaly, check calcium levels (almost all patients with MEN-1 have hypercalcemia) and ask about symptoms of peptic ulcer disease or hypoglycemia.

2. **McCune-Albright syndrome.** McCune-Albright syndrome, which occurs mostly in girls, includes polyostotic fibrous dysplasia, café-au-lait spots, sexual precocity, and hyperfunction of multiple endocrine glands, including at times excessive secretion of growth hormone.

3. **Carney's complex.** Carney's complex is an inherited, autosomal dominant disease of multicentric tumors in many organs. Tumors include cardiac myxomas, pigmented skin lesions, pigmented nodular adrenal dysplasia (causing Cushing's syndrome), myxoid fibroadenomas of the breast, testicular tumors, and growth hormone–secreting pituitary adenomas.

14. Do other tumors besides pituitary tumors make growth hormone and cause acromegaly or gigantism?

Yes. Rare tumors of the pancreas, lung, ovary, and breast may produce growth hormone. However, only one patient has been reported to develop clinical acromegaly from ectopic growth hormone production (from a pancreatic tumor).

15. Do tumors ever cause acromegaly or gigantism by making excessive GHRH?

Yes. Over 50 cases of GHRH production by various tumors have been described. These tumors occur in the lung, gastrointestinal tract, or adrenal glands and cause acromegaly by stimulating pituitary secretion of growth hormone. The clinical and biochemical features of acromegaly in such patients are indistinguishable from those of acromegaly due to a pituitary adenoma. Pituitary enlargement also occurs as a result of hyperplasia of somatotrophs. Some patients have had inadvertent transsphenoidal surgery before the correct diagnosis was made. Therefore, the plasma level of GHRH should be measured in any acromegalic patient with an extrapituitary abnormality or with hyperplasia on pituitary pathology.

16. If MRI of the pituitary confirms a tumor in the acromegalic patient, what issues other than the metabolic effects of excessive growth hormone should be considered?

Three other issues should be considered in any patient with a pituitary tumor:

1. Is the tumor making any other pituitary hormones besides growth hormone? For example, many growth hormone-secreting tumors also produce prolactin; rare tumors also make thyroid-stimulating hormone or other pituitary hormones. In patients with acromegaly, prolactin levels should be measured as well as other hormones when clinically indicated.

2. Is the tumor interfering with the normal function of the pituitary gland? Specifically, what is the patient's thyroid, adrenal, and gonadal function? Does the patient have diabetes insipidus? It is important to diagnose and treat pituitary insufficiency before ther-

apy for the excessive secretion of growth hormone, especially if the patient is scheduled for surgery.

3. Is the tumor causing effects owing to its size and location? Possible effects include headache, visual field disturbances, and extraocular movement abnormalities. Formal visual fields examination should be carried out in patients with large pituitary tumors.

17. How big are growth hormone–secreting pituitary tumors?

Growth hormone–secreting tumors vary considerably in size, but most are larger than 1 cm in diameter when diagnosed (i.e., macroadenomas). Tumor size is an important issue because it determines success rates of treatment.

18. How should acromegaly or gigantism be treated?

The treatment of choice for growth hormone–secreting tumors is transsphenoidal surgery by an experienced neurosurgeon. Most patients with microadenomas are cured, and larger tumors are debulked. Significant reduction in growth hormone levels and improvement in symptoms typically follow surgery, even when further treatment is required.

19. What if surgery does not cure the patient?

If transsphenoidal surgery is not curative, there are two additional treatment options, often used together:

1. **Radiotherapy.** Conventional radiation therapy of growth hormone–secreting tumors causes a gradual decline in growth hormone levels over many years. Stereotactic "radiosurgery" has been applied to pituitary tumors, including acromegaly. Stereotactic radiosurgery consists of applying a highly concentrated high-energy radiotherapy beam to the tumor, and it appears to be more effective and to work more quickly than conventional radiotherapy for pituitary tumors. However, stereotactic radiosurgery still takes months to years to work. Therefore, although it is not a good initial choice, radiotherapy is often used after surgery for additional control of the residual tumor. Many patients eventually develop hypopituitarism from radiotherapy.

2. **Octreotide.** Most growth hormone-secreting tumors have somatostatin receptors and respond to exogenous somatostatin with decreases in growth hormone levels. The development of octreotide, a long-acting analogue of somatostatin, was a major advance in the treatment of acromegaly. Given as injections 2 or 3 times/day, octreotide leads to markedly decreased levels of growth hormone in most acromegalic patients. It also causes tumor shrinkage in some patients. However, it does not cure acromegaly; stopping the drug usually leads to increases in growth hormone levels and tumor regrowth. Therefore, octreotide must be given indefinitely or while waiting for radiation to take effect. Recently, long-acting depo forms of octreotide have been developed, so most patients can be treated with an injection every 28 days, rather than 2–3 times per day.

20. What are the side effects of octreotide?

Gastrointestinal side effects are common, including abdominal bloating, mild diarrhea, nausea, and flatulence. The incidence of gallstones may be increased with octreotide, and therefore patients should be monitored with serial ultrasonography of the gallbladder.

21. How can one tell whether a patient has been cured of acromegaly?

The criteria for cure of acromegaly are somewhat controversial. Older studies defined cure as a random growth hormone level below 5 μg/L. More recent studies have shown that this criterion is inadequate, because patients with low levels of growth hormone may still have acromegaly. Therefore, more rigorous criteria have been developed. Note that even these more rigorous criteria are under revision as new growth hormone assays become available, and as long-term data on tumor recurrence and mortality are collected. The following are commonly used current criteria for cure:

1. Fasting growth hormone level < 5 ng/ml
2. Growth hormone levels < 1 ng/ml following oral glucose
3. Normal level of IGF-1

22. The patient has undergone transsphenoidal surgery for acromegaly and now has normal postoperative fasting levels of growth hormone, suppressed levels of growth hormone following oral glucose, and a normal level of IGF-1. How should the patient be followed?

It appears that the patient is cured, but growth hormone tumors can slowly regrow over years. At the least, measurements of growth hormone and/or IGF-1 should be repeated every 6–12 months. Some physicians also repeat a pituitary MRI at yearly intervals. The patient also needs monitoring for colonic neoplasia at regular intervals. In addition, one needs to assess whether the surgery damaged normal pituitary function by determining the patient's thyroid, adrenal, gonadal, and posterior pituitary function. Finally, the effects of surgery on visual fields should be assessed, especially if the patient had preoperative defects.

23. The patient asks which symptoms and physical abnormalities will improve after cure is confirmed. What is the appropriate answer?

Most soft tissue changes improve, including coarsening of facial features, increased size of hands and feet, upper airway hypertrophy, carpal tunnel syndrome, osteoarthritis, and excessive sweating. Hypertension, cardiovascular disease, and diabetes also improve. Unfortunately, bony overgrowth of the facial bones does not regress after treatment.

24. For bonus points, name an actor with acromegaly and the movie in which he starred.

Andre the Giant starred in "The Princess Bride."

BIBLIOGRAPHY

1. Ezzat S, Melmed S: Are patients with acromegaly at increased risk for neoplasia? J Clin Endocrinol Metab 72:245–249, 1991.
2. Feek CM, McLelland J, Seth J, et al: How effective is external pituitary radiation for growth hormone-secreting pituitary tumors? Clin Endocrinol 20:401–408, 1984.
3. Freed PU, Wardlaw SL. Primary medical treatment for acromegaly. J Clin Endocrinol Metab 83:3031–3033, 1998
4. Grunstein RR, Ho KY, Sullivan CE: Sleep apnea in acromegaly. Ann Intern Med 115:527–532, 1991.
5. Hansen J, Tsalikian E, Beaufrere B, et al: Insulin resistance in acromegaly: Defects in both hepatic and extrahepatic insulin action. Am J Physiol 250:E269–E273, 1986.
6. Klibanski A: Further evidence for a somatic mutation theory in the pathogenesis of human pituitary tumors. J Clin Endocrinol Metab 71:1415A–1415C, 1990.
7. Lim MJ, Barkan AL, Buda AJ: Rapid reduction of left ventricular hypertrophy in acromegaly after suppression of growth hormone hypersecretion. Ann Intern Med 117:719–726, 1992.
8. Melmed S, Ho K, Klibanski A, et al: Recent advances in pathogenesis, diagnosis, and management of acromegaly. J Clin Endocrinol Metab 80:3395–3402, 1995.
9. Newman CB, Melmed S, Snyder PJ, et al: Safety and efficacy of long term octreotide therapy of acromegaly: Results of a multicenter trial in 103 patients—a Clinical Research Center study. J Clin Endocrinol Metab 80:2768–2775, 1995.
10. Sano T, Asa SL, Kovacs K: Growth hormone–eleasing hormone–producing tumors: Clinical, biochemical, and morphological manifestations. Endocrinol Rev 9:357–373, 1988.

23. GLYCOPROTEIN-SECRETING PITUITARY TUMORS

Robert C. Smallridge, M.D.

1. What are glycoprotein hormones?

Of the four glycoprotein hormones, three are produced in the pituitary gland: luteinizing hormone (LH), follicle-stimulating hormone (FSH), and thyrotropin (TSH). Chorionic gonadotropin (CG) is produced in the placenta. Glycoprotein hormones are composed of two noncovalently bound subunits. The alpha subunit (α-SU) is similar among all four hormones. In contrast, the beta subunit (β-SU) is unique both immunologically and biologically for each hormone; these subunits are identified as LHβ, FSHβ, TSHβ, and βCG.

2. What are the types of glycoprotein-secreting pituitary tumors? What clinical syndromes do they produce?

Gonadotropinomas secrete one or more of the following: LH, FSH, LHβ, FSHβ, or α-SU. They usually do not cause endocrine symptoms but, because of their large size, often produce neurologic symptoms. Thyrotropinomas secrete TSH and cause hyperthyroidism. They also secrete α-SU.

3. Do pituitary tumors secrete only a single hormone?

No. Many tumors make two or more hormones or subunits. In some circumstances, sufficient quantities of multiple hormones are secreted to produce clinical symptoms characteristic of several syndromes within the same patient.

4. Under what circumstances should a TSH-secreting tumor be considered?

In any patient with suspected hyperthyroidism, an increased serum free thyroxine (T_4) or free T_4 index, and, most importantly, a detectable serum TSH using a second- or third-generation assay, a TSH-secreting tumor should be considered.

5. A patient has an increased level of serum total T_4 and a detectable or elevated level of serum TSH. Describe the differential diagnosis.

Transient

1. Exogenous
   L-thyroxine (L-T_4) therapy (noncompliant patient who took L-T_4 on the day blood was drawn)
   Other drugs (amiodarone, ipodate, amphetamines)
2. Endogenous (subgroup of nonthyroidal illness)
   Acute psychiatric illness
   Acute liver disease

Permanent

1. Binding protein disorders
   Excessive thyroxine-binding globulin (TBG)
   Abnormal thyroxine-binding prealbumin (TBPA) (transthyretin)
   Familial dysalbuminemic hyperthyroxinemia (FDH)
   T_4 autoantibody
   TSH heterophile antibody (requires separate cause for T_4 elevation)

2. Inappropriate TSH secretion
Resistance to thyroid hormone (generalized, central)
Pituitary tumor

6. What tests are useful in the differential diagnosis of the patient with an elevated serum total T_4 and a detectable or elevated serum TSH?

The history and physical examination usually rule out medications and nonthyroidal medical or psychiatric conditions as the cause. The most important laboratory test is the free T_4 measurement. A normal free T_4 strongly suggests that the patient has one of the binding protein disorders. An elevated free T_4, in contrast, generally narrows the differential to two disorders: a thyroid hormone resistance syndrome or a TSH-secreting pituitary tumor. Consistent with the elevated free T_4 levels, clinical thyrotoxicosis is commonly present in patients with either condition. One should confirm the abnormal test results in a second laboratory prior to initiating a work-up for these uncommon disorders.

7. How can one distinguish between the hyperthyroid patient with thyroid hormone resistance and the patient with a pituitary tumor?

TSH tumors secrete α-SU in excess of the whole TSH molecule. The molar ratio of serum α-SU to TSH is greater than unity (i.e., α/TSH > 1.0) in more than 80% of patients with TSH tumors, but it is almost always normal in persons with thyroid hormone resistance. Assessment with thyrotropin-releasing hormone (TRH; protirelin) is also helpful. Fewer than 20% of patients with a pituitary tumor have a 2-fold or greater increase in serum TSH after administration of TRH, whereas almost all patients with resistance respond briskly to TRH. If a tumor is suspected after both tests are completed, a magnetic resonance imaging (MRI) scan of the pituitary gland should be obtained. Most TSH tumors (about 90%) are macroadenomas (i.e., ≥ 10 mm in size). Most microadenomas (< 10 mm) are also visualized, but on rare occasions it has been necessary to perform sampling of inferior petrosal sinus blood to localize the tumor. Dynamic MRI scan or somatostatin receptor scintigraphy (octreoscan) is also useful.

8. How is an α/TSH molar ratio calculated?

TSH values are expressed as μU/ml (or mU/L). One must know the bioactivity and convert these units to ng/ml, the units of α-SU. Furthermore, the molecular weight of the subunit is only half the molecular weight of the whole TSH molecule; this fact also must be considered in calculating the molar ratio. From a practical standpoint, the following formula can be used:

$$\text{Molar ratio} = [\alpha\text{-SU (ng/ml)/TSH (}\mu\text{U/ml)}] \times 10$$

9. Name the various therapeutic options for managing TSH-secreting tumors and their likelihood of success.

Pituitary ablation is the treatment of choice. However, surgery alone has been curative in only 33% of cases; surgery followed by external beam irradiation has slightly better results. Now that tumors are identified earlier, surgical cures may improve. Too few patients have been treated with radiation therapy alone to assess its efficacy.

Several medical therapies known to suppress TSH secretion have been tried. Bromocriptine has met with limited success. Dexamethasone reduces serum TSH, but the side effects of steroids make it untenable for long-term treatment. The somatostatin analogue octreotide reduces TSH in more than 90% of cases, reduces T_4 in almost all cases, reduces tumor size in 52%, and may improve visual symptoms. Although octreotide is not recommended as primary therapy, it has a promising adjunctive role.

Thyroid gland ablation (with surgery or [131]iodine) should never be used as primary therapy. It does nothing to control TSH secretion. In fact, there is theoretical concern that thyroid ablation may enhance pituitary activity and growth.

10. Do all patients with an enlarged pituitary gland and an elevated level of serum TSH have thyrotropinomas?

No. Patients with longstanding hypothyroidism may develop pituitary hyperplasia, producing a pseudotumor (see figure). The pituitary mass can extend into the suprasellar region and cause visual field defects. Serum T_4 is always low, and shrinkage of the enlarged gland usually occurs with L-T_4 replacement therapy. No patient should undergo pituitary gland surgery without a preoperative measurement of serum T_4 and TSH.

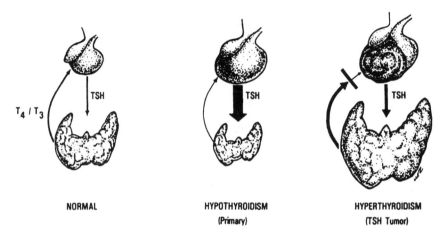

NORMAL   HYPOTHYROIDISM (Primary)   HYPERTHYROIDISM (TSH Tumor)

Schema of the pituitary-thyroid axis in normal persons and in patients with thyrotropin (TSH)-secreting pituitary tumors. On the left is the appropriate feedback loop in euthyroid individuals, with the width of the arrows representing the normal serum concentration of TSH and thyroxine (T_4). The middle figure depicts a small thyroid gland due to primary hypothyroidism. The low T_4 levels result in markedly increased secretion of TSH and, in some patients, a generalized hyperplasia of the anterior pituitary gland. On the right is an autonomous pituitary tumor secreting GSH. Serum TSH levels may vary greatly but in all cases are sufficiently biologically active to increase levels of serum T4 above normal. The elevated T_4 level has little, if any, ability to suppress tumor function. (From Smallridge RC: Thyrotropin-secreting tumors. Endocrinol Metab Clin North Am 16:765, 1987, with permission.)

11. What clinical features raise suspicion of a TSH-secreting pseudotumor?

Of greatest importance, almost all patients have symptoms of hypothyroidism. As mentioned, the serum T_4 concentration is always low. The underlying abnormality is usually autoimmune thyroiditis, which is predominantly a disease of women. Indeed, approximately 80% of reported cases of pituitary enlargement with hypothyroidism were in women. In contrast, only 55% of true TSH tumors have occurred in women. In children, precocious puberty may occur. Thyroid antibodies are present in more than 75% of cases with pseudotumor, compared with about 10% of patients with TSH tumors that produce hyperthyroidism.

12. Does the presence of abnormal visual fields help to distinguish between patients with pituitary hyperplasia due to primary hypothyroidism and patients with TSH-secreting tumors?

No. Abnormal visual fields have been reported in 28% of patients with pituitary hyperplasia compared with 42% of patients with tumors. In contrast, patients with thyroid hormone resistance have normal vision.

13. Does family history provide any clues in distinguishing these disorders?

In pseudotumor from thyrotroph hyperplasia, the family history may be positive for the presence of autoimmune diseases (e.g., thyroiditis, Graves' disease, type 1 diabetes mellitus, rheumatoid arthritis, lupus erythematosus, Sjögren's syndrome, vitiligo, Addison's disease, pernicious anemia). In TSH tumors, family history is of no use. Most cases of generalized thyroid hormone resistance are familial with autosomal dominant inheritance (i.e., 50% of the family have the biochemical abnormalities).

14. Which hormones are elevated in the serum of patients with gonadotroph adenomas?

Serum FSH is increased much more often than LH. An increase in α-SU is not specific for gonadotrophs, because it may also derive from thyrotrophs. Furthermore, an α/LH (or FSH) molar ratio has not been clinically useful.

15. What are the presenting symptoms of patients with gonadotropinomas?

Gonadotropinomas usually do not cause an endocrine disorder from excessive hormone production. They are large, with substantial extrasellar growth. Many patients are identified because of visual impairment due to impingement by the tumor on the optic chiasm. Headaches, diplopia, and pituitary apoplexy also occur. Endocrine symptoms are usually due to deficiencies of other pituitary hormones created by the mass effect of the large tumor.

16. When gonadotropin levels are elevated, how can one distinguish clinically between a gonadotroph adenoma and primary hypogonadism?

This distinction can be difficult, especially in women, because their levels of LH and FSH increase after menopause. This is probably why most gonadotroph adenomas have been recognized in men. Historically, men with such tumors experienced a normal puberty and may have fathered children. On examination, their testicular size may be normal. In contrast, men with hypogonadism may have had abnormal pubertal development or a history of testicular injury; the testes are small.

17. What laboratory tests are helpful?

In primary hypogonadism, both FSH and LH are increased, whereas FSH is elevated but LH is usually normal in patients with gonadotropinomas. When LH is high in men with gonadotropinomas, testosterone also is high rather than low, as in hypogonadism. Of interest, for unexplained reasons about one third of patients with a tumor have an anomalous rise in serum FSH or LHβ when given a TRH injection. An MRI scan of the pituitary reveals a large tumor. Occasionally, a patient with longstanding hypogonadism may have some degree of pituitary enlargement.

18. How are gonadotropinomas treated?

Pituitary surgery is the treatment of choice. Although complete cure is often impossible, substantial reduction in tumor size and hormone secretion is common. Reduced hormone secretion provides a convenient marker for monitoring recurrence of tumor; an abrupt increase in FSH or α-SU should prompt a repeat imaging study. Radiotherapy is often given after surgery in the hope of delaying tumor recurrence.

19. Is medical therapy effective?

Agonist analogues of gonadotropin-releasing hormone (GnRH) reduce secretion from normal gonadotrophs. Unfortunately, they usually have the opposite effect on gonadotropinomas. An antagonist analogue (Nal-Glu-GnRH) has effectively reduced serum FSH in a small group of men with gonadotropinomas but did not reduce tumor size. Bromocriptine has reduced hormone levels in an occasional patient, whereas octreotide has reduced a-SU and improved visual fields in certain patients.

20. Are pituitary tumors malignant?

Pituitary carcinomas are rare, but a small number have been reported for active tumors secreting the following hormones: adrenocorticotropic hormone (ACTH), prolactin, and growth hormone. One case of a TSH-secreting pituitary carcinoma has been reported.

BIBLIOGRAPHY

1. Beck-Peccoz P, Brucker-Davis F, Persani L, et al: Thyrotropin-secreting pituitary tumors. Endocr Rev 17:610–638, 1996.
2. Burch HB: Abnormal thyroid function tests in euthyroid persons. In Becker KL (ed.): Principles and Practice of Endocrinology and Metabolism. Philadelphia, JB Lippincott, 1996, pp 323–332.
3. Gancel A, Vuillermet P, Legrand A, et al: Effects of a slow-release formulation of the new somato-statin analogue lanreotide in TSH-secreting pituitary adenomas. Clin Endocrinol 40:421–428, 1994.
4. Katznelson L, Oppenheim DS, Coughlin JF, et al: Chronic somatostatin analog administration in patients with α-subunit-secreting pituitary tumors. J Clin Endocrinol Metab 75:1318–1325, 1992.
5. Klibanski A, Zervas NT: Diagnosis and management of hormone-secreting pituitary tumors. N Engl J Med 324:822–831, 1991.
6. Lamberts SWJ, Krenning EP, Reubi J-C: The role of somatostatin and its analogs in the diagnosis and treatment of tumors. Endocr Rev 12:450–482, 1991.
7. McGrath GA, Goncalves RJ, Udupa JK, et al: New technique for quantitation of pituitary adeno-noma size; use in evaluating treatment of gonadotroph adenomas with a gonadotropin-releasing hormone agonist. J Clin Endocrinol Metab 76:1363-1368, 1993.
8. Refetoff S, Weiss RE, Usala SJ: The syndromes of resistance to thyroid hormone. Endocr Rev 14:348– 399, 1993.
9. Smallridge RC, Czervionke LF, Fellows DW, et al: Corticotropin- and thyrotropin-secreting pitu-itary microadenomas: Detection by dynamic magnetic resonance imaging. Mayo Clin Proc 75: 521-528, 2000.
10. Smallridge RC: Thyrotropin-and gonadotropin-producing tumors. In Korenman SG, Molitch ME (eds.): Atlas of Clinical Endocrinology. Vol. IV: Neuroendocrinology and Pituitary Disease. Philadelphia, Blackwell Science, 2000, pp 95–113.
11. Smallridge RC: Thyroid function tests. In Becker KL (ed.): Principles and Practice of Endocrinol-ogy and Metabolism. Philadelphia, JB Lippincott, 1996, pp 299–306.
12. Smallridge RC: Thyrotropin-secreting tumors. In Mazzaferri EL, Samaan NA (eds.): Endocrine Tumors. Boston, Blackwell, 1993, pp 136–151.
13. Snyder PJ: Gonadotroph adenomas. In Mazzaferri EL, Samaan NA (eds.): Endocrine Tumors. Boston, Blackwell, 1993, pp 152–166.
14. Snyder PJ: Gonadotroph adenomas. J Clin Endocrinol Metab 80:1059–1061, 1995.
15. Young WF, Scheithauer BW, Kovacs KT, et al: Gonadotroph adenoma of the pituitary gland: A clinicopathologic analysis of 100 cases. Mayo Clin Proc 71:649–656, 1996.

24. CUSHING'S SYNDROME

Mary H. Samuels, M.D.

1. What is the normal function of cortisol in healthy subjects?

Cortisol and other glucocorticoids have many effects as physiologic regulators. They increase glucose production, inhibit protein synthesis and increase protein breakdown, stimulate lipolysis, and affect immunologic and inflammatory responses. Glucocorticoids are important for maintenance of blood pressure and form an essential part of the body's response to stress.

2. How are cortisol levels normally regulated?

Secretion of cortisol from the adrenal glands is stimulated by the pituitary hormone adrenocorticotropin (ACTH). Secretion of ACTH, in turn, is stimulated by the hypothalamic hormones corticotropin-releasing hormone (CRH) and vasopressin (ADH). Cortisol feeds back to the pituitary and hypothalamus to suppress levels of ACTH and CRH. Under basal (nonstress) conditions, cortisol is secreted with a pronounced circadian rhythm, with higher levels early in the morning and low levels late in the evening. Under stressful conditions, secretion of CRH, ACTH, and cortisol increases and the circadian variation is blunted. Because of the wide variation in cortisol levels over 24 hours and appropriate elevations during stressful conditions, it may be difficult to distinguish normal from abnormal secretion. Many biochemical tests have been devised to diagnose pathologic hypercortisolemia, but none has proved completely accurate. For this reason, the evaluation of a patient with suspected Cushing's disease is often complex and confusing.

3. What are the clinical symptoms of excessive levels of cortisol?

1. Obesity, especially central (truncal) obesity, with wasting of the extremities, moon facies, supraclavicular fat pads, and buffalo hump
2. Thinning of the skin, with facial plethora, easy bruising, and violaceous striae
3. Muscular weakness, especially proximal muscle weakness and atrophy
4. Hypertension, atherosclerosis, congestive heart failure, and edema
5. Gonadal dysfunction and menstrual irregularities
6. Psychologic disturbances (e.g., depression, emotional lability, irritability, sleep disturbances)
7. Osteoporosis and fractures
8. Increased rate of infections and poor wound healing

Some manifestations of Cushing's syndrome are common but nonspecific, whereas others are less common but quite specific. These findings are listed below in order of decreasing frequency.

Clinical Features of Cushing's Syndrome

SIGN/SYMPTOM	SENSITIVITY (%)	SPECIFICITY (%)
Hypokalemia ($K^+ < 3.6$)	25	96
Ecchymoses	53	94
Osteoporosis	26	94
Weakness	65	93
Diastolic blood pressure (>105 mmHg)	39	83
Red or violaceous striae	46	78

Continued on following page

Clinical Features of Cushing's Syndrome (Continued)

SIGN/SYMPTOM	SENSITIVITY (%)	SPECIFICITY (%)
Acne	52	76
Central obesity	90	71
Hirsutism	50	71
Plethora	82	69
Oligomenorrhea	72	49
Generalized obesity	3	38
Abnormal glucose tolerance	88	23

4. A patient presents with a history of obesity, hypertension, irregular menses, and depression. Does she have excessive production of cortisol?

Excessive cortisol is highly unlikely. Although the listed findings are consistent with glucocorticoid excess, they are nonspecific; most patients with such findings do *not* have Cushing's syndrome. A few symptoms and signs of glucocorticoid excess are more specific, although they do not occur in every patient with Cushing's syndrome: spontaneous ecchymoses, purple (not pale) striae, proximal muscle weakness, osteoporosis, and hypokalemia. Any of these findings should immediately raise suspicion of excessive production of glucocorticoids.

5. The patient also complains of excessive hair growth and has increased terminal hairs on the chin, along the upper lip, and on the upper back. Is this finding relevant?

Hirsutism is a common, nonspecific finding in many female patients. However, it is also consistent with Cushing's syndrome. If it is due to Cushing's syndrome, hirsutism is a complication not of excessive glucocorticoids but of excessive production of androgen by the adrenal glands under ACTH stimulation. Thus, hirsutism in a patient with Cushing's syndrome is a clue that the disorder is due to excessive production of ACTH. (The only other condition associated with excessive production of glucocorticoids and androgen is a malignant adrenal tumor, which is usually obvious on presentation.)

6. The patient also has increased pigmentation of the areolae, palmar creases, and an old surgical scar. Are these findings relevant?

Hyperpigmentation is a sign of elevated production of ACTH and related peptides by the pituitary gland. It is uncommon (but possible) in Cushing's syndrome due to benign pituitary tumors, because levels of ACTH do not usually rise high enough to cause hyperpigmentation. It is more common in the ectopic ACTH syndrome, because ectopic tumors produce more ACTH and other peptides. The combination of Cushing's syndrome and hyperpigmentation may be bad news.

7. What is the cause of death in patients with Cushing's syndrome?

Patients with Cushing's syndrome have a markedly increased mortality rate, usually from cardiovascular disease or infections.

8. What are the causes of Cushing's syndrome?

Cushing's syndrome is a nonspecific name for any source of excessive glucocorticoids. There are four main causes:

1. **Exogenous glucocorticoids.** Patients who receive glucocorticoids for inflammatory or autoimmune diseases (e.g., asthma, rheumatoid arthritis, systemic lupus erythematosus, dermatitis) invariably develop Cushing's syndrome over time. Other patients surreptitiously ingest glucocorticoids and also develop Cushing's syndrome. Such patients may be quite difficult to diagnose.

2. **Pituitary Cushing's syndrome.** This entity, called Cushing's disease, is due to a benign pituitary adenoma that secretes excessive ACTH.

3. **Ectopic production of ACTH.** Of the two varieties of ectopic production of ACTH, one is due to malignant tumors, usually of the lung. Patients present with obvious metastatic tumor, weight loss, hypertension, hypokalemia, and hyperpigmentation. The second type is due to more slowly growing tumors called carcinoids. Patients with carcinoid tumors that produce ACTH may appear identical to patients with pituitary Cushing's disease on clinical examination and biochemical testing. Thus, the differential diagnosis between pituitary tumor and carcinoid tumor in a patient with Cushing's syndrome may be difficult.

4. **Adrenal causes of Cushing's syndrome.** Both benign and malignant adrenal tumors can produce excessive glucocorticoids and cause Cushing's syndrome. Benign adrenal adenomas clinically resemble other types of Cushing's syndrome; hirsutism is absent, however, because the tumor produces only cortisol without producing androgens. Malignant adrenal carcinomas causing Cushing's syndrome usually present with obvious widespread tumor in the abdomen and have a poor prognosis. In addition, unusual types of adrenal Cushing's syndrome are associated with multiple adrenal nodules, discussed below.

Causes of Cushing's Syndrome and Their Relative Frequency

ACTH-DEPENDENT (80%)	ACTH-INDEPENDENT (20%)
Pituitary (85%)	Adrenal adenoma (> 50%)
Corticotroph adenoma	Adrenal carcinoma (< 50%)
Corticotroph hyperplasia (rare)	Micronodular hyperplasia (rare)
Ectopic ACTH syndrome (15%)	Macronodular hyperplasia (rare)
Oat cell carcinoma (50%)	Exogenous glucocorticoids (common)
Foregut tumors (35%)	Therapeutic
Bronchial carcinoid	Factitious (rare)
Thymic carcinoid	
Medullary thyroid carcinoma	
Islet cell tumors	
Pheochromocytoma	
Other tumors (10%)	
Ectopic CRH (< 1%)	

9. Of the various types of Cushing's syndrome, which is the most common?

Overall, exogenous Cushing's syndrome is most common. It rarely presents a diagnostic dilemma, because the physician usually knows that the patient is receiving glucocorticoids. Of the endogenous causes of Cushing's syndrome, pituitary Cushing's disease accounts for at least 70% of cases. Ectopic secretion of ACTH and adrenal tumors cause approximately 15% of cases each.

10. Do age and gender matter in the differential diagnosis of Cushing's syndrome?

Of patients with Cushing's disease (pituitary tumors) 80% are women, whereas the ectopic ACTH syndrome is more common in men. Therefore, in a male patient with Cushing's syndrome, the risk of an extrapituitary tumor is increased. The age range in Cushing's disease is most frequently 20–40 years, whereas ectopic ACTH syndrome has a peak incidence at 40–60 years. Therefore, the risk of an extrapituitary tumor in an older patient with Cushing's syndrome is increased.

11. The patient with obesity, hypertension, irregular menses, depression, and hirsutism looks like she may have Cushing's syndrome. What should you do?

The single best screening test for excessive production of cortisol is a 24-hour urine collection for urinary free cortisol and creatinine. If the patient can collect her urine for 24 hours, the test should be ordered. Another widely used screening test is the overnight low-dose dexamethasone suppression test. The patient takes 1 mg of dexamethasone at 11 PM and measures her serum cortisol level at 8 AM the next morning. In healthy subjects with intact hypothalamic-pituitary-adrenal function, dexamethasone (a potent glucocorticoid that does not react with the cortisol assay) suppresses production of CRH, ACTH, and cortisol. Patients with Cushing's syndrome of any cause should not suppress cortisol production (serum cortisol remains > 5 mg/dl) when given 1 mg of dexamethasone.

Unfortunately, the overnight dexamethasone suppression test is not foolproof. Occasional patients with Cushing's disease suppress cortisol levels with dexamethasone, and many patients without Cushing's syndrome will not, particularly those with other acute or chronic illnesses, depression, or alcohol abuse. All of these diseases activate the hypothalamic-pituitary-adrenal axis because of stress and make the patient resistant to dexamethasone suppression. In fact, because Cushing's syndrome is so rare, a nonsuppressed cortisol level after dexamethasone is more likely to be a false-positive result rather than truly indicating the presence of Cushing's syndrome. Because of such difficulties in the initial screening tests for Cushing's syndrome, patients may require repeated screening and evaluation over time.

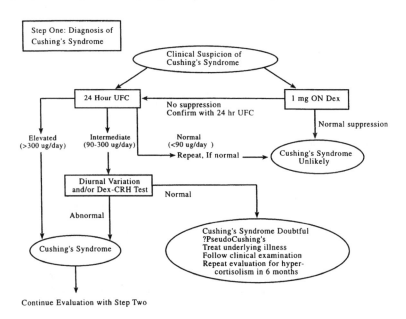

Diagnosis of Cushing's syndrome

12. The patient has an elevated 24-hour urinary level of free cortisol, and serum cortisol levels are not suppressed after overnight 1-mg dexamethasone administration. What do you do?

It looks like the patient has Cushing's syndrome. However, it is still possible that the patient has other reasons for her symptoms and elevated cortisol levels. It can be very difficult to distinguish mild or moderate Cushing's syndrome from stress-induced hypercortisolism, especially in patients who have active medical or psychiatric illnesses. The distinction between true Cushing's syndrome and pseudo-Cushing's syndrome (stress-induced hypercortisolemia) depends on the clinical suspicion and degree of elevation of the cortisol levels. In general, a 24-hour urine free cortisol level of greater than 300 μg is diagnostic of true Cushing's syndrome in the absence of severe stress. Lesser elevations of urine free cortisol may require confirmatory tests for the presence of Cushing's syndrome. The best confirmatory test is somewhat controversial, but two that are commonly used are loss of diurnal variation in plasma cortisol levels and the dexamethasone-CRH test. These tests are best administered and interpreted by experienced endocrinologists, since the results can be skewed if the tests are not performed properly.

Assuming that the patient really has Cushing's syndrome, rather than stress-induced hypercortisolemia, the next step is to determine whether she has ACTH-dependent or ACTH-independent disease. This distinction is made by measuring plasma levels of ACTH. Measurements should be repeated a number of times, because secretion of ACTH is variable.

13. The patient's ACTH level is "normal." Was the original suspicion of Cushing's syndrome incorrect?

No. Normal levels of ACTH are a common finding in pituitary-dependent Cushing's disease. A normal or slightly elevated ACTH level is the usual finding in ACTH-secreting pituitary adenomas. More marked elevations of ACTH levels suggest ectopic secretion of ACTH, although small carcinoid tumors also have normal or mildly elevated levels of ACTH. Suppressed ACTH levels, in contrast, suggest an adrenal tumor.

14. What happened to the 2-day low-dose and high-dose dexamethasone tests for the differential diagnosis of Cushing's syndrome?

The 2-day low-dose and high-dose dexamethasone suppression tests were once widely used in attempts to distinguish pituitary, ectopic, and adrenal causes of Cushing's syndrome. Although they are still performed, the results are often confusing, and rates of both false-positive and false-negative results are high. Therefore, these tests to some extent have been supplanted by more accurate ACTH assays, the overnight high-dose dexamethasone test, and CRH stimulation tests.

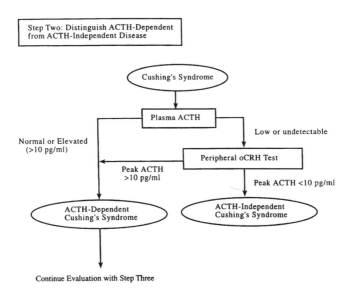

Distinguishing ACTH-dependent from ACTH-independent disease.

15. After diagnosis of ACTH-dependent Cushing's syndrome, what is the next step?

Because the most common site of excessive secretion of ACTH is a pituitary tumor, radiologic imaging of the pituitary gland is the next step. The best study is high-resolution MRI with thin cuts through the pituitary gland. A chest radiograph should also be obtained at this point in case the patient has a carcinoid tumor large enough to be seen on plain film.

16. The pituitary MRI in the patient with ACTH-dependent Cushing's syndrome is normal. Is the next step a search for carcinoid tumor, under the assumption that the pituitary is not the source of excessive ACTH?

Not so fast. At least one half of pituitary MRI or CT scans are negative in proven pituitary-dependent Cushing's syndrome, because most corticotroph adenomas are tiny and may not be visible on MRI or CT.

17. The pituitary MRI shows a 3-mm hypodense area in the lateral aspect of the pituitary gland. Is it time to call the neurosurgeon?

Again, not so fast. This finding is nonspecific and occurs in many healthy people. It may or may not be related to Cushing's syndrome. The odds are good that the patient has a pituitary tumor, but the MRI does not prove so. The MRI is diagnostic in Cushing's syndrome only if it shows a large tumor.

18. So what is the next step?

One option is to proceed directly to pituitary surgery, because a patient with an abnormal MRI has a 90% chance of having an ACTH-secreting pituitary tumor. To achieve 100% diagnostic certainty, the best test to distinguish a pituitary source from an ectopic source of ACTH is bilateral simultaneous inferior petrosal sinus sampling (IPSS) for ACTH levels. Catheters are advanced through the femoral veins into the inferior petrosal sinuses, which drain the pituitary gland. Blood samples are obtained through the catheters and assayed for ACTH levels. If ACTH levels in the petrosal sinuses are significantly higher than those in

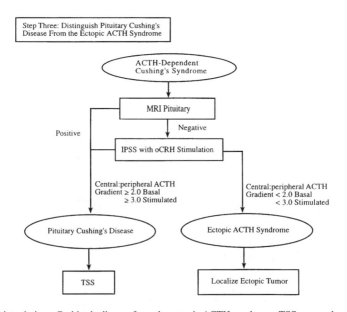

Distinguishing pituitary Cushing's disease from the ectopic ACTH syndrome. TSS, transsphenoidal surgery.

peripheral blood samples, the pituitary gland is the source of excessive ACTH. If there is no gradient between petrosal sinus and peripheral vein levels of ACTH, the patient probably has a carcinoid tumor somewhere else in the body. The accuracy of the test is further increased if ACTH responses to injection of exogenous CRH are measured, because pituitary tumors increase secretion of ACTH in response to CRH. Bilateral inferior petrosal sinus sampling should be performed ideally by experienced invasive radiologists or neuroradiologists at referral centers.

19. Inferior petrosal sinus sampling shows no gradient in ACTH levels. Now what?

Start the search for a carcinoid tumor. Because the most likely location is the lung, a CT scan or MRI of the lungs should be ordered. If the results are negative, a CT scan or MRI of the abdomen should be ordered, because carcinoids also occur in the pancreas, intestinal tract, and adrenal glands.

20. Inferior petrosal sinus sampling shows a marked central-to-peripheral gradient in ACTH levels. Now what?

Transsphenoidal surgery should be scheduled with an experienced neurosurgeon who is comfortable examining the pituitary for small adenomas. ACTH levels from the right and left petrosal sinuses obtained during the sampling study may tell the neurosurgeon in which side of the pituitary gland the tumor is likely to be found, but this information is not 100% accurate.

21. What if surgery is unsuccessful?

If transsphenoidal surgery does not cure a patient with Cushing's disease, alternative therapies must be tried, because patients with inadequately treated hypercortisolism have increased morbidity and mortality rates. Of the various options after failed surgery, none is ideal:

1. Reevaluate the evidence for a pituitary source for ACTH. If necessary, repeat the petrosal sinus sampling (although this is more difficult after surgery). If the pituitary is in fact the source, repeat surgery should be considered, including the option of total hypophysectomy. Even tumors so tiny that they cannot be seen by surgeons are removed with total hypophysectomy.

2. Consider treating the patient with ketoconazole, which blocks adrenal steroidogenesis. It does not cure the underlying tumor but improves the patient's metabolic status and may buy time for further studies or radiation therapy. However, most patients do not respond to ketoconazole over the long haul.

3. Consider pituitary radiotherapy, which eventually leads to control of cortisol levels in many patients with Cushing's disease. Because radiotherapy may take years to work, it is not a good initial option.

4. Consider bilateral adrenalectomy. This was the preferred treatment for Cushing's syndrome until transsphenoidal surgery was shown to be effective and much safer. It is still an option in a patient with the devastating clinical consequences of Cushing's syndrome in whom a pituitary tumor cannot be found.

22. What is the main drawback to bilateral adrenalectomy in patients with Cushing's disease?

One drawback is the extensive nature of the surgery, which leads to high levels of morbidity and a lengthy postoperative recuperative period. This problem has been addressed recently by performing adrenalotomy via a laparoscopic approach, which is easier on the patient. However, the main drawback is the development of Nelson's syndrome in up to 30% of patients after adrenalectomy. Nelson's syndrome is the appearance, sometimes years after adrenalectomy, of an aggressive corticotroph pituitary tumor.

23. What are the correct diagnostic and treatment options for patients with ACTH-independent (adrenal) Cushing's syndrome?

Such patients usually have either an adrenal adenoma or an adrenal carcinoma. Once consistent suppression of ACTH levels is confirmed, an adrenal CT scan should be ordered. A mass is almost always present, and surgery should be planned. If the mass is obviously cancer, surgery may still help in debulking the tumor and improving the metabolic consequences of hypercortisolemia.

24. The patient has ACTH-independent Cushing's syndrome, but instead of a solitary adrenal mass, the adrenal glands have multiple nodules. What is the underlying condition?

A number of disease processes cause adrenal Cushing's syndrome with multiple adrenal masses:

1. **Primary pigmented nodular adrenal dysplasia (PPNAD).** In recent years, descriptions of a syndrome of ACTH-independent Cushing's syndrome due to bilateral small pigmented adrenal nodules has appeared. Clinical symptoms usually occur during the second decade of life (earlier than in other causes of Cushing's syndrome). The disease may be sporadic or familial. Careful radiologic and pathologic studies reveal unilateral or bilateral adrenal nodularity, with nodule sizes ranging from tiny to 3 cm. Most are deeply pigmented and appear black or brown on cut section. PPNAD may be an autoimmune disease caused by production of adrenal-stimulating immunoglobulins. Patients with PPNAD should undergo bilateral adrenalectomy, which is curative.

2. **Carney complex.** In 1985 Carney at the Mayo Clinic noted an association between PPNAD and cardiac myxomas in a few patients. His resulting description has since been named the Carney complex. This entity is an inherited, autosomal dominant disease of multicentric tumors in many organs, including cardiac myxomas, pigmented skin lesions, PPNAD, myxoid fibroadenomas of the breast, testicular tumors, growth hormone-secreting pituitary adenomas, and peripheral nerve lesions.

3. **Macronodular adrenal hyperplasia.** With the advent of high-resolution CT scans, some patients with Cushing's syndrome are seen to have bilateral adrenal nodules, ranging in size from 0.5 to 7 cm. This entity, distinct from PPNAD and called macronodular adrenal hyperplasia (MAH), presents with variable biochemical and radiologic findings. MAH probably represents a heterogeneous group of patients with varying degrees of adrenal autonomy. The hypothesis underlying the development of MAH is that longstanding stimulation by ACTH leads to formation of adrenal nodules and that some of the nodules may become autonomous. Treatment must be individualized for each patient with MAH; the most important decision is whether the patient still has ACTH-dependent disease.

4. **McCune-Albright syndrome (polyostotic fibrous dysplasia).** McCune-Albright syndrome is characterized by polyostotic fibrous dysplasia, café-au-lait pigmentation of the skin, and multiple endocrinopathies. The most common endocrine disorders include sexual precocity and pituitary adenomas that secrete growth hormone. In a few cases, autonomous adrenal hyperfunction and Cushing's syndrome have been described; adrenal pathology is characterized by nodular hyperplasia and formation of adenomas.

25. What happens to the hypothalamic-pituitary-adrenal axis after a patient undergoes successful removal of an ACTH-secreting pituitary adenoma or a cortisol-secreting adrenal adenoma?

The axis is suppressed, and the patient develops clinical adrenal insufficiency, unless he or she is given gradually decreasing doses of exogenous glucocorticoids for a time after surgery.

26. What would be the most likely diagnosis if the original patient had all the signs of Cushing's syndrome but *low* urinary and serum levels of cortisol?

The most likely scenario is that the patient is surreptitiously ingesting a glucocorticoid that gives all the findings of glucocorticoid excess but is not measured in the cortisol assay. The patient and family members should be questioned about possible access to medications, and special assays can measure the different synthetic glucocorticoids.

27. A patient has all the findings of Cushing's syndrome and elevated 24-hour urinary levels of free cortisol. One month later, however, she no longer has clinical signs of Cushing's syndrome. Repeat urine free cortisol is now normal. What is happening?

There are two possibilities: (1) the patient is intermittently ingesting a glucocorticoid that is measured in the cortisol assay (exogenous Cushing's syndrome), or (2) she has a rare corticotroph tumor that is only intermittently active (periodic hormonogenesis).

28. Do tumors ever cause Cushing's syndrome by making excessive CRH?

Yes. Occasionally patients who undergo transsphenoidal surgery for a presumed corticotroph adenoma have corticotroph hyperplasia instead. At least some of these cases are secondary to ectopic production of CRH from a carcinoid tumor in the lung, abdomen, or other location. Therefore, levels of serum CRH should be measured in patients with Cushing's syndrome and corticotroph hyperplasia. If the levels are elevated, a careful search should be performed for possible ectopic sources of CRH.

BIBLIOGRAPHY

1. Findling JW, Doppman JL: Biochemical and radiologic diagnosis of Cushing's syndrome. Endocrinol Metab Clin North Am 23:511–538, 1994.
2. Graham KE, Samuels MH: Recent advances in the evaluation of Cushing's Syndrome. Endocrinologist 8:425–35, 1998
3. Limper AH, Carpenter PC, Scheithauer B, Staats BA: The Cushing syndrome induced by bronchial carcinoid tumors. Ann Intern Med 117:209–214, 1992.
4. Loli P, Berselli E, Tagliaferri M: Use of ketoconazole in the treatment of Cushing's syndrome. J Clin Endocrinol Metab 63:1365–1371, 1986.
5. Melby JC: Therapy of Cushing's disease. A consensus for pituitary microsurgery. Ann Intern Med 109:445–456, 1988.
6. Moore TJ, Dluhy RG, Williams GH, Cain JP: Nelson's syndrome: Frequency, prognosis, and effect of prior pituitary irradiation. Ann Intern Med 85:731–734, 1976.
7. Oldfield EH, Doppman JL, Nieman LK, et al: Petrosal sinus sampling with and without corticotropin-releasing hormone for the differential diagnosis of Cushing's syndrome. N Engl J Med 325:897–905, 1991.
8. Orth DN: Differential diagnosis of Cushing's syndrome. N Engl J Med 325:957–959, 1990.
9. Samuels MH: Cushing's syndrome associated with corticotroph hyperplasia. Endocrinologist 3: 242– 247, 1993.
10. Samuels MH, Loriaux DL: Cushing's syndrome and the nodular adrenal gland. Endocrinol Metab Clin North Am 23:555–569, 1994.
11. Trainer PJ, Besser M: Cushing's syndrome: Therapy directed at the adrenal gland. Endocrinol Metab Clin North Am 23:571–584, 1994.
12. Yanovski JA, Cutler GB: Glucocorticoid action and the clinical features of Cushing's syndrome. Endocrinol Metab Clin North Am 23:487–510, 1994.

25. DISORDERS OF WATER METABOLISM

Leonard R. Sanders, M.D.

1. List the abbreviations used to discuss disturbances of water metabolism.

Common Abbreviations

P_{Na}	Plasma sodium concentration
U_{Na}	Urine sodium concentration
P_{osm}	Plasma osmolality
U_{osm}	Urine osmolality
TBW	Total body water
ECF	Extracellular fluid
ICF	Intracellular fluid
*ADH	Antidiuretic hormone
*AVP	Arginine vasopressin
ANP	Atrial natriuretic peptide
SIADH	Syndrome of inappropriate antidiuretic hormone secretion
DI	Diabetes insipidus
ECV	Effective circulating volume
C_{osm}	Osmolar clearance
Q_B	Blood flow
P	Pressure
R	Resistance
CO	Cardiac output
SV	Stroke volume
PVR	Peripheral vascular resistance
SVR	Systemic vascular resistance
V_1 receptor	Vasopressin 1 receptor
V_2 receptor	Vasopressin 2 receptor

Other Abbreviations

ISF	Interstitial fluid
IVF	Intravascular fluid
PCT	Proximal convoluted tubule
LOH	Loop of Henle
DCT	Distal convoluted tubule
CCT	Cortical collecting tubule
EVP	Effective vascular pressure
RAAS	Renin-angiotensin-aldosterone system
EC	Effective circulation
ABP	Arterial blood pressure
TBV	Total blood volume

*ADH and AVP are the same hormone.
P_X or U_X (where X is any substance) represents the plasma or urine **concentration** of that substance.
C_X is the clearance of that substance. Collecting tubule = collecting duct.

2. What is the water composition of the human body?

Water composition of the body depends on age, sex, muscle mass, body habitus, and fat content. Various body tissues have the following water percentages: lungs, heart, and kidneys (80%); skeletal muscle and brain (75%); skin and liver (70%); bone (20%); and adipose tissues (10%). Clearly, people with more muscle than fat will have more water. Generally, thin people have less fat and more water. Men are 60% and women, 50% water by weight. Older people have more fat and less muscle. The average man and woman older than 60 yr are made up of 50% and 45% water, respectively. Most discussions of TBW consider a man who is 60% water, weighs 70 kg, and is 69 inches (175 cm) tall.

Water as a Percent of Body Weight

BODY HABITUS	INFANT	MAN	WOMAN
Thin	80	65	55
Medium	70	60	50
Obese	65	55	45

3. Where is water located within the body?

TBW equals water located inside (ICF) and outside the cells (ECF). TBW is 60% of body weight; ICF and ECF water are 40% and 20%, respectively, of body weight. The ECF contains both interstitial (15%) and intravascular water (5%). Thus, in a 70-kg man, TBW = 42 L, ICF water = 28 L, and ECF water = 14 L. The interstitial water is 10.5 L and intravascular (plasma) water 3.5 L. Therefore, of the TBW, two-thirds is ICF and one-third is ECF. Of the ECF, about one-fourth is IVF and three-fourths is ISF. Tight regulation of the relatively small volume of IVF (plasma) maintains blood pressure and avoids symptomatic hypovolemia and congestive heart failure. Normal plasma is 93% water and 7% proteins and lipids. TBV is only a small portion of the ECF, and arterial volume is only 15% of TBV. Although arterial volume is small, its integrity is most important for maintaining the effective circulation and preventing abnormalities of water balance.

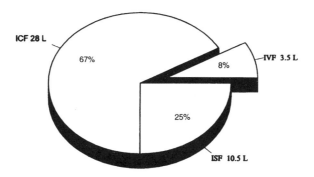

Distribution of body water.

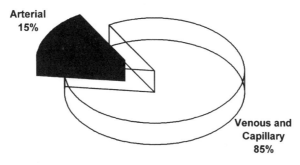

Total blood volume.

4. What is transcellular water? What is its importance?

Transcellular water (TCW) is that water formed by cellular transport activities and located in various ducts and spaces throughout the body. This water includes cerebrospinal fluid and aqueous humor; secretions in the sweat, salivary, and lacrimal glands; and secretions in pancreas, liver, biliary, gastrointestinal, and respiratory tracts. TCW carries secretions to specific sites for enzymatic and lubricant activity and is normally quite small. In disease states, excess or deficiency of TCW can cause dysfunction. Excess TCW formation may decrease ECV, stimulate ADH and aldosterone release, and cause retention of salt and water.

5. What controls distribution of body water?

With few exceptions (e.g., ascending LOH and distal nephron), water moves freely across cell membranes, depending on tonicity. Because tonicity depends on impermeable solutes such as sodium (Na), disorders of water metabolism are reflected by changes in solute concentrations. In addition to changes in water distribution, changes in TBW, blood volume, and ECV also affect overall water balance. A thorough understanding of disorders of water metabolism requires a clear understanding of changes in P_{Na}, P_{osm}, and ECV.

6. What is ECV?

That arterial volume required to maintain a **normal baroreceptor pressure** that is appropriate for a given level of vascular resistance. ECV is also called effective arterial blood volume (EABV). By inducing changes in baroreceptor tone, alterations in ECV have a major impact on water balance. Low ECV brings about renal salt and water retention, whereas high ECV causes renal salt and water loss. Depending on the patient's water intake, these changes may produce significant hyponatremia. Maintaining normal ECV maintains circulatory homeostasis by stabilizing neurohumoral changes that would be altered with changes in ECV.

7. How do baroreceptors affect ECV?

Baroreceptors are the major sensors of changes in ECV. However, their main role is to maintain normal pressure (not volume) at the level of the baroreceptor sensors located primarily in the carotid sinus, aortic arch, atria, pulmonary veins, and afferent renal arterioles. These anatomic locations are important because perfusion to these areas affects the three main effectors of circulatory homeostasis: brain, heart, and kidneys.

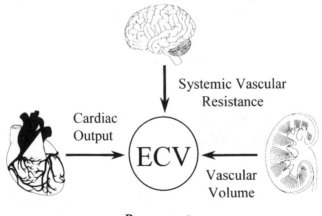

Baroreceptors

Components of effective circulation.

8. How does vascular pressure as sensed by the baroreceptors relate to effective circulating volume and hyponatremia?

$$P = Q_B \times R$$
$$Q_B = P/R$$
$$ABP = CO \times PVR$$
$$ABP = HR \times SV \times PVR$$

The above formulas define pressure, flow, and resistance. To maintain functional vascular integrity, tissues must receive adequate Q_B. Superficially, the first two formulas suggest that volume is unimportant for tissue perfusion. However, volume is contained within flow, because $Q_B = CO$ and $CO = HR$ (heart rate) $\times$ SV (stroke volume).

Baroreceptors sense changes in pressure and, in response, alter their tone. Alteration in tone sends impulses via the vagus and glossopharyngeal nerves to the nucleus tractus solitarius. Acting through central nervous system (CNS) connections, these nerves buffer changes in the cardiovascular system and have been called the buffer nerves. Increased vascular pressure increases baroreceptor tone that inhibits tonic discharge of vasoconstrictor nerves and stimulates vagal cardiac nerves. The net result is decreased ABP from vascular dilation, bradycardia, and **renal loss of salt and water**. A decrease in effective vascular pressure reduces baroreceptor stimulation, causing an increase in ABP from vascular constriction, increased cardiac rate, and **renal retention of salt and water**.

Because baroreceptors sense changes in pressure, the focus probably should change more to pressure than volume. A more appropriate term to describe what is meant by ECV is **EVP**. Arterial pressure clearly has a major role in maintaining the effective circulation. However, decreases in venous pressure (via arterial stretch receptors) initiate vasopressin (ADH) release and renal sodium and water retention often before arterial pressure has changed enough to take part. Furthermore, venous pressure and volume are major determinants of cardiac output and thereby ABP. Thus, changes in both the venous and arterial systems participate in maintaining vascular homeostasis.

A drop in the ECV or EVP reduces atrial, aortic, carotid, and renal baroreceptor tone, decreasing tonic inhibition of hormone release and thereby increasing renin, aldosterone, angiotensin II, and ADH secretion. ANP and urodilatin (ANP-like hormone made in the kidney) decrease. These alterations enhance renal Na and water retention. If the patient receives free water, these changes may lead to hyponatremia. It is important to remember that hyponatremia cannot develop unless the patient retains more water than is excreted. Decreased ECV/EVP predisposes to water retention, but the patient must receive free water to develop hyponatremia.

9. Define osmolality and tonicity and outline their effects on water movement.

Osmolality is the **concentration** of active particles in a kilogram of water. Osmolality of a substance is the concentration of the substance in a liter of water divided by its molecular weight. Tonicity = effective osmolality—the osmotic pressure caused by dissolved particles restricted to one side of the cell membrane. Because Na and glucose (in insulin deficiency) are restricted to the ECF, they account for normal tonicity and are called effective osmols. Mannitol, sorbitol, glycerol, and glycine are also effective osmols. Because urea freely crosses cell membranes and distributes evenly in TBW, changes in urea change osmolality but not tonicity. Therefore, urea is an ineffective osmol. Ethanol and methanol are other ineffective osmols.

Water will always move across cell membranes from lower to higher osmolality until osmolality on both sides is equal. Accordingly, **ICF osmolality will always equal ECF osmolality**. Because plasma is part of the ECF, the following is always true: **ICF osmolality = ECF osmolality = P_{osm}**. Clinical changes in osmolality are usually due to changes in TBW or the movement of water between the ICF and ECF.

10. What formulas are useful in evaluating osmolality and tonicity?
ECF osmolality = $2P_{Na}$ + glucose/18 + blood urea nitrogen (BUN)/2.8
Normal osmolality = 2 (140) + 90/18 + 14/2.8 = 280 + 5 + 5 = 290 mOsm/kg
ECF tonicity (effective osmolality) = $2P_{Na}$ + glucose/18
Normal tonicity = 2(140) + 90/18 = 280 + 5 = 285 mOsm/kg

However, the normal range for P_{Na} is 135–146 mEq/L. After substitution, the normal range for P_{osm} is 280–295 mOsm/kg and normal tonicity is 275–290 mOsm/kg. Correction factors for other effective solutes (osmols) are mannitol/18, sorbitol/18, and glycerol/9. Correction factors for other ineffective solutes (osmols) are ethanol/4.6 and methanol/3.2.

11. A 75-year-old woman presents with confusion but no focal neurologic signs. She has type II diabetes. Blood pressure is 110/54 mmHg. Pulse is 96 beats per minute. Neck veins are not visualized in the supine position. $P_{glucose}$ = 900 mg/dL, P_{Na} = 135 mEq/L, plasma creatinine = 3.0 mg/dL, BUN = 50 mg/dL, U_{Na} = 40 mEq/L, urine SG = 1.012, and ketones equals 3+. Describe her fluid and volume status.
Glucose remains in the ECF because of insulin deficiency. Glucose increases ECF tonicity, and increased tonicity pulls water from the ICF to the ECF, concentrating the ICF and diluting the ECF until ICF and ECF osmolalities are equal. The osmotic pressure of 900 mg/dl glucose (900/18 = 50 mOsm/kg) is the driving force for water movement from ICF to ECF. Water movement from ICF to ECF dilutes the ECF and decreases P_{Na}. Each 100 mg/dl rise in $P_{glucose}$ above 100 mg/dl decreases the P_{Na} by 1.6 mEq/L. In this patient, the predicted decrease in P_{Na} = [(900 – 100)/100 × 1.6] = 13 mEq/L. The predicted P_{Na} would be 140 – 13 = 127 mEq/L. P_{Na} of 135 suggests further water loss from osmotic diuresis. The P_{osm} of [2(135) + 900/18 + 56/2.8] 340 mOsm/kg is compatible with hyperosmolar coma. Because this woman has decreased TBW and volume, you might expect her to be prerenal and the U_{Na} to be low and the U_{osm} high. However, osmotic diuresis caused by urine glucose, ketones, and urea increases urinary Na and water, making U_{Na} and U_{osm} less useful markers of dehydration.
A good rule of thumb is that U_{osm} approximates 35 × the last two digits of the urine specific gravity. By this rule, her U_{osm} approximates [12 × 35] 420 mOsm/kg. Postural vital signs are not given, but **flat neck veins in the supine position are usually due to intravascular volume depletion.** Rapid lowering of her glucose to 100 mg/dL will rapidly decrease P_{osm}, shift water to the ICF, increase P_{Na} by 13 mEq/L, and potentially cause cardiovascular collapse and cerebral edema. Thus, therapy is normal saline to replace volume and judicious lowering of $P_{glucose}$ with intravenous insulin.

12. How do P_{Na} and total body potassium relate to TBW?
The following formulas are useful in understanding the relationship of P_{Na}, plasma potassium (P_K), total body sodium and potassium [Na^+ + K^+], and TBW. [Na^+ + K^+] estimates total body solute.
1. $P_{Na} \cong$ total body [Na^+ + K^+]/TBW
2. TBW $\propto$ [Na^+ + K^+]/P_{Na}
3. $P_{Na} \propto P_{osm} \propto$ [total body osmolality] $\propto$ [total body solutes] $\propto$ 1/TBW

Thus, P_{Na} is proportional to total body Na plus K and inversely proportional to TBW. From these equations and factors outlined in questions 9 and 10, P_{Na} is a convenient surrogate to help one estimate plasma water, TBW, P_{osm}, total body osmolality, and total body solute. An increase or decrease in total plasma Na particles can proportionately change the P_{Na}. However, in clinical medicine, **changes in P_{Na} usually reflect changes in plasma water.** When P_{Na} is high, plasma water is low. When P_{Na} is low, plasma water is high.

Although 98% of K^+ is intracellular, P_{Na} is proportional to total body K^+, and infusions of Na^+ or K^+ will increase P_{Na}. This occurs as follows. In hypokalemia, the infused K^+ enters cells. To preserve electroneutrality, Na^+ leaves cells or chloride (Cl^-) enters. ECF water follows K^+ and Cl^- into cells due to increased osmolality. Both mechanisms increase P_{Na}. Hypokalemic patients infused with equal amounts of KCl or NaCl will have equal increases in P_{Na}. Thus, addition of KCl to isotonic saline makes hypertonic saline, and infusion of saline with too much KCl may correct hyponatremia too rapidly. (See question 35.)

13. Describe the input and output of water.
TBW is a balance of input (including endogenous production) and output. In an average adult, input approximates 1600 mL (liquids), 700 mL (foods), and 200 mL (metabolic oxidation of carbohydrate and fat) for a total of 2500 mL/day. Average water losses are 1500 mL (kidneys), 500 ml (skin [400 mL evaporation and 100 ml perspiration]), 300 mL (lung – respiration), and 200 mL from the gastrointestinal tract (stool) for a total of 2500 mL/day. Large losses of water (increased output) occur with excessive sweating, respiration (exercise), burns, diarrhea, vomiting, and diuresis. Decreased water input occurs when defects in thirst alter mental or physical function (especially in the elderly) and prevent access to water.

14. A 35-year-old schizophrenic is admitted to the hospital because of excessive urine output. U_{osm} = 70 mOsm/kg. P_{osm} = 290 mOsm/kg. 24-hr urine output = 12 L/day. How much free water is being excreted each day?
Free water clearance (C_{H_2O}) is the amount of solute free water excreted per day. Osmolar clearance is the amount of urine excreted per day that contains all the solute that is isosmotic to plasma. When the urine is hypotonic to plasma, the total urine volume consists of two components. One part free of solute (C_{H_2O}), and the other contains all the solution that is isosmotic to plasma (C_{osm}). To measure how much of the urine is pure (free) water, calculate the free water clearance. To do so, you need to know the osmolar clearance (C_{osm}) and the urine volume (V). The formula for clearance of any substance (including osmols) is always the same:

$$C = UV/P$$

where C is the volume of plasma cleared of the substance per unit time, U is the urinary concentration of the substance, P is the plasma concentration of the substance, and V is the total urinary volume per unit time. The calculations for this patient follow:

1. $V = C_{osm} + C_{H_2O}$
2. $C_{H_2O} = V - C_{osm}$
3. $C_{osm} = U_{osm} V/P_{osm}$
4. C_{osm} = (70 mOsm/kg × 12 L/day)/290 mOsm/kg = 2.9 L/day or about 3 L/day
5. $C_{H_2O} = V - C_{osm}$ = [12 L/day – 3 L/day] = 9 L/day

By manipulating formula 2, another means of calculating free water clearance follows:

1. $C_{H_2O} = V [1 - U_{osm}/P_{osm}]$
2. C_{H_2O} = 12 L/day [1 – 70/290] = 9 L/day

Thus, the patient's daily urine output contains 9 L/day of pure (free) water and 3 L/day that is isotonic to plasma. This information does not distinguish primary polydipsia from DI. However, the relatively high P_{osm} of 290 suggests DI.

15. Another patient has P_{osm} = 280 mOsm/kg, P_{Na} = 130 mEq/L, U_{osm} = 600 mOsm/kg, U_{Na} = 130 mmol/L, U_K = 60 mmol/L, and urine volume = 1 L/day. How much free water is being excreted each day?
Urine is hypertonic to plasma if the $U_{osm} > P_{osm}$ or the $U_{Na+K} > P_{Na}$. Urine hypertonic to plasma contains two parts. The volume that would be required to contain all solute and

remain isosmotic to plasma is the osmolar (C_{osm}). The volume of free water that was removed from the isotonic glomerular filtrate to make $U_{osm} > P_{osm}$ or the $U_{Na+K} > P_{Na}$ is T^{CH_2O} (negative free water clearance). There are two ways to calculate free water clearance. One method uses osmolality as in question 14. The other uses electrolytes (Na and K). Electrolyte free water clearance more accurately estimates free water clearance and negative free water clearance, especially when urine contains large numbers of nonelectrolyte osmolites, such as urea, that increase osmolality unrelated to free water clearance. To calculate electrolyte free water clearance, use the urinary concentrations of Na and K and the plasma Na. Because $[U_{Na} + U_K] > P_{Na}$ [(130 + 60) > 130], the *net* urinary excretion of free water is negative, and therefore free water clearance is negative. Calculations for osmolar and electrolyte free water clearance in the above patient follow:

Calculations for classic osmolar (negative) free water clearance:

1. $V = C_{osm} - T^{CH_2O}$
2. $T^{CH_2O} = C_{osm} - V$
3. $C_{osm} = 1$ L/day [600/280] = 2.14 L/day
4. $T^{CH_2O} = 2.14$ L/day $- 1$ L/day = 1.4 L/day

By manipulating formula 2, another means of calculating negative free water clearance follows:

1. $T^{CH_2O} = V [U_{osm}/P_{osm} - 1]$
2. $T^{CH_2O} = 1$ L/day [600/280 $- 1$] = 1.14 L/day

Calculations for electrolyte (negative) free water clearance

1. $T^{CH_2O} = C_{[Na + K]} - V$
2. $C_{[Na + K]} = [U_{Na+K}/P_{Na} \times V]$
3. $C_{[Na + K]} = [190$ mEq/L/130 mEq/L $\times 1$ L/day] = 1.46 L/day
4. $T^{CH_2O} = 1.46$ L/day $- 1$ L/day = 0.46 L/day

Thus, the patient's kidneys add (by water reabsorption) a net of 460–1140 mL of free water to plasma each day. With a low P_{osm}, it is usually inappropriate to retain water in excess of output. This finding suggests the syndrome of inappropriate ADH (SIADH). Volume depletion, adrenal insufficiency, and hypothyroidism must be excluded before the diagnosis of SIADH can be made.

16. What are the normal limits of urine output?

Water intake and osmotic products of metabolism determine the usual daily output of urine. On a normal diet, a normal adult must excrete 800–1000 mOsm of solute per day. The range of normal renal concentrating function is 50–1200 mOsm/kg. Based on this fact, the obligate water excretion varies from 0.8–20 L/day. The calculations are as follows:

1000 mOsm/1200 mOsm/kg = 0.8 L/day at maximal concentration
1000 mOsm/50 mOsm/kg = 20 L/day at maximal dilution

Note that higher solute loads (e.g., dietary) require more water excretion. Thus, low solute intake (starvation) with high water intake predisposes to water retention and water intoxication. This combination exists in binge beer drinkers, in whom the solute load may be only 300 mOsm/day. By similar calculations, the range of urine output would drop to 0.25–6 L/day in such patients.

As a consequence of aging, elderly patients lose glomerular filtration rate (GFR), concentrating ability, and diluting ability. Thus, an 80-year-old woman may have a normal (for age) renal-concentrating range of 100–700 mOsm/kg. However, maximal U_{osm} in the elderly may be as low as 350 mOsm/kg. The woman's average diet may generate only 600 mOsm/day. Her normal range of urine output would then be 0.9–6.0 L/day. If her dietary intake fell to 300 mOsm/day, her maximal urine output would fall to 3 L/day. Given free access to water and a thiazide diuretic, which impairs urinary dilution, she could easily become water intoxicated and hyponatremic. The mechanism of hyponatremia in beer potomania and the "tea and toast diet" is low total osmolar intake and relatively increased water intake. The decreased osmotic load for excretion limits the amount of water excreted.

17. What are the main factors controlling water metabolism?

Thirst, hormonal, and renal mechanisms are tightly integrated for control of water metabolism.

18. What are the stimuli of thirst?

Osmoreceptors in the organum vasculosum of the anterior hypothalamus control thirst. Increasing plasma tonicity stimulates thirst at a threshold about 5 mOsm/kg higher than that which stimulates ADH release. However, oropharyngeal receptors are also important in thirst regulation. A dry mouth increases thirst. Drinking and swallowing water decrease thirst even without changing P_{osm}. As with ADH release, volume depletion and resulting afferent baroreceptor input increase thirst. Increased angiotensin II from volume depletion is also an important stimulus. Of interest is an unusual idiosyncratic effect of angiotensin-converting enzyme inhibitors to cause central polydipsia and increased ADH release and thereby hyponatremia.

19. What hormonal mechanisms are involved in control of body water?

Supraoptic and paraventricular nuclei in the hypothalamus respond to changes in osmolality and volume by increasing or decreasing ADH secretion. ADH and other hormones, including ANP, aldosterone, prostaglandins, and angiotensin II, as well as neurohumoral influences, control renal excretion and retention of salt and water. The kidney also produces its own ANP-like hormone called urodilatin. However, ADH remains the most important influence on water retention and excretion.

ADH has a short half-life of 15–20 minutes and is metabolized in the kidney and liver. It attaches to its V_2 receptors on the basolateral membrane of the principal cells of the cortical and medullary collecting tubules and activates cyclic adenosine monophosphate (cAMP). The increased cyclic adenosine monophosphate activates protein kinase, causing intracellular water channels called aquaporins to insert into the luminal membrane. Water moves from the lumen through these channels down an osmotic gradient and into the cell and interstitium (reabsorption). Of the nine known aquaporin (AQP) isoforms, at least six are present in the kidney. The collecting duct has high concentrations of AQP-2 (AQP2) that serve as the major target for ADH regulation of renal water reabsorption. Inherited and acquired abnormalities of AQP2 expression and targeting cause some cases of nephrogenic diabetes insipidus. Conversely, increased AQP2 expression and/or targeting may be responsible for water retention in some conditions such as pregnancy and congestive heart failure. Although V_2 is the major ADH receptor, 20% of ADH receptors in the collecting tubular cells are V_1 receptors. When ADH activates V_1 receptors, it stimulates prostaglandin E_2 and prostacyclin synthesis. These prostaglandins oppose the antidiuretic effects of ADH. Because the ADH-stimulated V_1 receptors are activated only at very high ADH levels, this short negative feedback loop opposes excessive ADH action.

20. What are the major conditions that influence ADH secretion?

ADH functions to maintain osmotic and volume homeostasis. Secretion starts at an osmotic threshold of 280 mOsm/kg and increases proportionately to further rises in tonicity. A 1–2% increase in osmolality stimulates ADH secretion, whereas a 10% drop in vascular volume is required for the same effect. By acting on carotid sinus, aortic, and atrial barore-ceptors, increased ECV raises the osmotic threshold for ADH secretion; in contrast, decreased ECV lowers this threshold. Severe volume depletion and hypotension may com-pletely override the hypoosmotic inhibition of ADH secretion. This finding has been called the **law of circulating volume**. In severe volume depletion and hypotension, ADH secretion continues despite low osmolality, thereby worsening the hyponatremia. Nausea, pain, and stress, as seen postoperatively, are also potent stimuli of ADH release and may produce life-threatening hyponatremia if excessive free water is given. This consideration is especially important if drugs that potentiate release or action of ADH are given.

Major causes of ADH secretion: hyperosmolality, hypovolemia, nausea, pain, stress, human chorionic gonadotropin as in pregnancy, nicotine (possibly by nausea), hypo-glycemia, (corticotropin-releasing hormone [CRH]/ADH release), CNS infections, CNS tumors, vascular catastrophes (thrombosis, hemorrhage), and ectopic ADH of malignancy (carcinomas of lung [oat cell and bronchogenic], duodenum, pancreas, ureter, bladder, and prostate and lymphoma). ADH secretion may be increased by any major pulmonary disor-der, including pneumonia, tuberculosis, asthma, atelectasis, cystic fibrosis, positive pressure ventilation, and adult respiratory distress syndrome. Human immunodeficiency virus infec-tion may have the multifactorial role of causing CNS dysfunction, pulmonary disease, and malignancy. Excessive exogenous ADH or desmopressin acetate (DDAVP) in patients with diabetes insipidus directly increases ADH effect. Oxytocin also has significant ADH activ-ity in the large doses used to induce labor.

Drugs that stimulate ADH secretion: morphine, carbamazepine, clofibrate, intra-venous cyclophosphamide, vincristine, haloperidol, amitriptyline, thioridazine, and bromo-criptine. Because psychosis itself may cause SIADH, one must question the true ADH stim-ulatory effect of the listed antipsychotic drugs.

Drugs that enhance ADH effect on the kidneys: chlorpropamide, tolbutamide, carba-mazepine, acetaminophen, nonsteroidal antiinflammatory drugs, and intravenous cyclophosphamide.

Major inhibitors of ADHsecretion: Hypoosmolality, hypervolemia, ethanol, pheny-toin, and vasoconstrictors (baroreceptor effect).

Drugs that decrease ADH effect on the kidneys: demeclocycline, lithium, acetohexa-mide, tolazamide, glyburide, propoxyphene, amphotericin, methoxyflurane, colchicine, vin-blastine, prostaglandin E_2, and prostacyclin.

21. How does the kidney handle salt and water?

In order for the kidney to control for excess or deficiency of water intake, there must be a normal GFR allowing the delivery of isotonic fluid to the LOH; separation of solute from water in the ascending limb of the LOH, DCT, and cortical connecting segment; and normal action of ADH to allow controlled reabsorption or excretion of water in the cortical and medullary collecting tubules (CCT and MCT). Because normal GFR is 125 ml/min, the normal kidneys filter 180 L of plasma each day. Because the normal urine output is 1.5–2.0 L/day, the kidneys reabsorb 99% of the water and salt.

The $3Na^+$-$2K^+$-ATPase pump located on the basolateral membrane provides the energy for solute reabsorption **throughout the nephron**. Solute is usually reabsorbed from the tubular lumen by carrier proteins that do not require additional active transport processes. However, active transport of Na and K by the $3Na^+$-$2K^+$-ATPase pump establishes osmotic, electrical, and chemical gradients necessary for solute reabsorption. For this reason, solute reabsorption may be said to occur by secondary active transport. The kidneys reabsorb water passively along an osmotic concentration gradient established by solute reabsorption. The PCT reabsorbs **65%** of filtered Na and water isotonically. The LOH receives 35% of the glomerular filtrate, and the descending limb reabsorbs **25%** of this filtrate isotonically. The ascending limb, however, is impermeable to water. The Na^+-K^+-2Cl carrier on the luminal membrane of the thick ascending limb removes Na, K, and Cl from the tubular lumen. This causes net reabsorption of Na and Cl, but Krecycles to the lumen for reuse. As in the proximal tubule, the $3Na^+$-$2K^+$-ATPase active pump on the basolateral membrane transports intracellular Na and Cl to the medullary interstitium, forming the osmotic gradient for passive Na^+-K^+-2Cl carrier transport.

The overall process **directly dilutes the urine and forms a hypertonic medullary interstitium necessary for ADH-induced urinary concentration**. Urea reabsorption from the MCT further increases the interstitial tonicity. The osmolality of the filtrate leaving the ascending limb is about 100–150 mOsm/kg, whereas the osmolality of the medullary interstitium may be as high as 1200 mOsm/kg. **Ten percent** of filtered Na and water enters the DCT. The DCT and connecting segment reabsorb about 5% of the filtered NaCl, further diluting the urine. However, like the ascending LOH, the distal tubule and connecting segment are impermeable to water. The final volume delivered to the CCT is about **10%** of the initial glomerular filtrate and has an osmolality of 100 mOsm/kg. The collecting tubule reabsorbs all but **1%** of the remaining filtrate. In the absence of ADH, this fluid (about 18 L/day) would be lost in the urine and cause marked dehydration. However, in the presence of ADH, the collecting duct becomes permeable to water and the final urine output is reduced to 1.5–2.0 L/day.

22. What are the consequences and causes of decreased renal excretion of water?

Any reduction in water excretion predisposes to **hyponatremia** and **hypoosmolality**. Conditions that impair GFR, delivery of tubular fluid to the distal nephron, or ability of the distal nephron to separate solute from water or that increase the permeability of the collecting tubule to water will impair water excretion. Such conditions include renal failure, decreased ECV, diuretics (thiazides>>loop), and excessive ADH.

23. How do hypothyroidism and adrenal insufficiency cause hyponatremia?

Hypothyroidism decreases cardiac output and ECV. Adrenal insufficiency causes volume depletion, decreased blood pressure, and decreased cardiac output, all of which reduce ECV. The decreased ECV lowers GFR, which reduces delivery of filtrate to the distal nephron and enhances proximal tubular water reabsorption. Decreased ECV also stimulates secretion of ADH, further promoting water reabsorption. CRH and ADH are cosecreted from the same neurons in the paraventricular nuclei of the hypothalamus and both hormones work synergistically to release adrenocorticotropic hormone from the anterior pituitary. Cortisol then feeds back negatively at the hypothalamus and pituitary to inhibit the release of both CRH and ADH. Therefore, cortisol itself directly increases ADH levels to further enhance water reabsorption. Although hyponatremia may occur with both primary and secondary adrenal insufficiency, it occurs more commonly in primary adrenal insufficiency. This emphasizes the importance of aldosterone deficiency in the pathogenesis of the hyponatremia; aldosterone deficiency directly causes salt wasting and volume depletion and thus indirectly increases ADH secretion. All of these events combined with continued water intake strongly contribute to the resulting hyponatremia.

24. What plasma sodium concentrations are a cause for concern?

The severity of hyponatremia or hypernatremia depends on the rapidity of development. Patients with a P_{Na} of 115 mEq/L or 165 mEq/L may not show any clinical abnormalities if they develop the problem over days to weeks. However, both conditions may produce major neurologic dysfunction if they develop over hours to days. As a rule, however, sodium concentrations of 120–155 mEq/L are not usually associated with symptoms. P_{Na} outside these limits and occasionally rapidly developing disturbances within these limits may be of major concern.

25. What causes the symptoms and signs of increased or decreased TBW?

The main symptoms and signs of too much (decreased P_{Na}) or too little (increased P_{Na}) TBW result from brain swelling or contraction. If changes in TBW occur more rapidly than the brain can adapt, symptoms and signs will occur. The severity of the symptoms and signs depends on the degree and rapidity of the TBW change. Once the adaptation occurs, correcting the disturbance in body water too rapidly may be more deleterious than the initial disturbance.

26. What are the symptoms and signs of hyponatremia? Hypernatremia?

Hyponatremia: headache, confusion, muscle cramps, weakness, lethargy, apathy, agitation, nausea, vomiting, anorexia, altered levels of consciousness, seizures, depressed deep tendon reflexes, hypothermia, Cheyne-Stokes respiration, respiratory depression, coma, and death.

Hypernatremia: weakness, irritability, lethargy, confusion, somnolence, muscle twitching, seizures, respiratory depression, paralysis, and death.

27. How does the brain adapt to changes in TBW?

Brain adaptation to hyponatremia. Because ICF and ECF osmolality must always be equal, developing hyponatremia immediately shifts water into the brain, increasing intracranial pressure. The increased intracerebral pressure (ICP) causes loss of NaCl into the cerebrospinal fluid. Over the next several hours there is also loss of intracellular potassium and over the next few days loss of organic solute. These changes return the brain volume to normal. However, if severe hyponatremia occurs too rapidly, there is not enough time for cerebral adaptation. Brain edema occurs, further increasing intracranial pressure; the brain herniates and the patient dies.

Brain adaptation to hypernatremia. Because brain water is part of TBW, it immediately adapts to changes in P_{osm}. With acute hypernatremia and increased P_{osm}, an immediate shift of water out of the brain decreases ICP. The decreased ICP promotes movement of cerebrospinal fluid with NaCl into the brain ECF, partially correcting volume. Within hours, further brain adaptation occurs, increasing ICF K^+, Na^+, and Cl^-. The resulting increase in osmolality pulls water from the ECF and restores about 60% of the brain volume. Over the next several days, the brain accumulates organic solutes (osmolites), previously called idiogenic osmoles, that return the brain volume to a near-normal level. These solutes include glutamine, taurine, glutamate, myoinositol, and phosphocreatine. If the brain has no time to adapt to rapidly developing hypernatremia, it will shrink, retract from the dura, and tear vessels, causing intracranial hemorrhage, increased ICP, compressive injury, herniation, and death.

28. How should you approach the patient with hyponatremia?

Hyponatremia occurs in >3% of hospitalized patients. Hyponatremia always means too much ECF water relative to sodium. Because total body volume ∝ total body Na, a thorough assessment of the patient's volume status will allow rational selection of therapy. Patients with flat neck veins and postural changes in blood pressure and pulse (standing blood pressure decreases >20/10 mmHg and pulse increases >20 per minute) are invariably saline (isotonic NaCl)-depleted. Patients with distended neck veins and edema are saline-overloaded. Always direct treatment at correcting the underlying disorder. If patients have lost saline, give them saline. If they have retained too much water, restrict their water. If they have retained too much salt and water but more water than salt, restrict their salt and water but water more than salt. Sounds simple—and it is.

The difficulty is remembering the importance of and performing an **initial thorough volume assessment**. Assess the patient's volume by looking at neck veins, postural signs, and edema. At times, the best clinician cannot get a good assessment of ECV, and central monitoring with a Swan-Ganz catheter is sometimes necessary. Get an initial weight and assess weight daily. Continue assessment of postural signs as needed. Initially, obtain P_{osm}, general chemistry panel (Na, K, Cl, CO_2, Cr, BUN, glucose, albumin, Ca, Mg), and urinary Na, Cl, Cr, and fractional excretion of sodium. Approach therapy as outlined below.

Approach to Hyponatremia

CONDITION	POSTURAL SIGNS	EDEMA	U_{Na}	TREATMENT
Renal saline loss	Yes	No	>20	Give isotonic saline
Nonrenal saline loss	Yes	No	<10	Give isotonic saline
Water excess	No	No	>20	Restrict water
Na and water excess	No	Yes	<10	Restrict water > salt
Na and water excess	No	Yes	>20	Restrict water > salt

Because P_{Na} is usually measured with ion-selective electrodes, artifactual lowering of the P_{Na} is now unusual. If your lab does not use ion-selective electrodes, marked hyperlipidemia or hyperproteinemia may produce pseudohyponatremia. Notwithstanding, measured P_{osm} will differentiate these disorders. Because P_{osm} measures the osmotic activity of plasma water and because plasma water excludes lipids and proteins contribute little to P_{osm}, the measured P_{osm} will be essentially normal in pseudohyponatremia.

Causes of Hyponatremia

PATHOPHYSIOLOGY	ASSOCIATED CONDITIONS
Renal saline loss	Diuretics
	Primary adrenal insufficiency
	Renal tubular acidosis
	Salt-losing nephritis
Nonrenal saline loss	Vomiting
	Diarrhea
	Pancreatitis, rhabdomyolysis, burns
Water excess	Syndrome of inappropriate ADH secretion
	Secondary adrenal insufficiency
	Hypothyroidism
Saline excess with decreased ECV	Congestive heart failure
	Cirrhosis
	Nephrotic syndrome
Saline excess without decreased ECV	Acute renal failure
	Chronic renal failure

Note: Hyponatremia always means too much plasma water relative to sodium. Volume assessment is crucial. Volume loss = saline loss. Volume excess = saline excess. Water excess usually means normal saline volume but an excess in water sufficient to produce a mild excess of volume that stimulates baroreceptor activity.

29. How should you characterize, diagnose, and manage the patient with SIADH?

Hyponatremia is the tipoff to SIADH. Approach the patient as in question 28. It is important to establish normovolemia by physical examination. Then measure P_{osm}, U_{osm}, P_{Na}, U_{Na}, and U_K. Finally, exclude pituitary, adrenal, and thyroid dysfunction before diagnosis. Confirmatory criteria of SIADH include P_{Na} (<135 mEq/L), low P_{osm} (<280 mOsm/kg), U_{osm} > 100 mOsm/kg, U_{Na} > 40 mEq/L, and $[U_{Na} + U_K] > P_{Na}$. Patients with SIADH are usually said to have normal volume status. However, they actually have excessive TBW. Unlike excessive saline that is limited to ECF, excessive water distributes two-thirds to the ICF and one-third to the ECF. Thus the ECF excess is minor and not usually perceptible by clinical examination. Nonetheless, patients with SIADH have mildly increased ECV that is sensed by the kidney. The kidney increases GFR, which causes a low uric acid, BUN, and creatinine. The increased ECV also increases ANP, which, with the increased GFR, promotes natriuresis. These are the classic findings in SIADH. Obviously SIADH does not protect against dehydration and other conditions that can obscure the classic presentation. For example, a patient with ectopic ADH from lung cancer may present with dehydration from diarrhea and lack of water intake from debilitation. In this instance, the U_{Na} and U_{Cl} may be less than 10 mEq/L.

Initially, treat SIADH with water restriction. If the patient has marked symptoms, treat for symptomatic hyponatremia. (See question 36.) Also attempt to correct the underlying abnormality. (See question 20.) If the patient has unresectable cancer and water restriction (500–1500 ml/day) is not tolerated, give demeclocycline, 600–1200 mg/day, or lithium carbonate, 600–1200 mg/day, in two to four divided doses. Because lithium carbonate can cause neurologic, cardiovascular, and other toxicities, avoid it unless demeclocycline is contraindicated. Demeclocycline may cause severe renal failure in patients with cirrhosis. Thus, it is contraindicated in patients with cirrhosis and severe liver disease.

30. What are the four patterns of SIADH?

The table below summarizes the four SIADH patterns according to responses of ADH to P_{osm}.

PATTERN	CHARACTERISTICS	FREQUENCY (%)
Type I	**Erratic ADH secretion** with no predictable relationship to P_{osm}	20
Type II	**Reset osmostat** with normal relationship of ADH to P_{osm} but a lower threshold for ADH release (e.g., 250–260 mOsm/kg)	35
Type III	**ADH leak with selective loss of ADH suppression** and continued secretion when P_{osm} is low but normal suppression and secretion when P_{osm} is normal	35
Type IV	**ADH-dissociated antidiuresis** at low P_{osm} with appropriately low or undetectable ADH (possibly from increased renal sensitivity to ADH or unknown ADH-like substance)	10

31. Define polyuria and list the main causes.

Polyuria is a urine output greater than 2.5–3.0 L/day. Four main disorders cause polyuria: psychogenic polydipsia (psychosis), dipsogenic diabetes insipidus (defect in thirst center), central neurogenic DI (defect in ADH secretion), and nephrogenic DI (defect in ADH action on the kidney). All forms of DI may be partial or complete. Polyuria also may occur from osmotic diuresis in such conditions as diabetes (glucose), recovery from renal failure (urea), and intravenous infusions (saline, mannitol). See question 20 for drugs and conditions that decrease ADH secretion and action. Causes of acquired nephrogenic DI include chronic renal disease, electrolyte abnormalities (hypokalemia and hypercalcemia), drugs (lithium, demeclocycline), sickle cell disease (damaged medullary interstitium), diet (increased water and decreased solute—beer, starvation), inflammatory or infiltrative renal disease (multiple myeloma, amyloidosis, sarcoidosis), and others.

32. How do you distinguish polyuric patients with the various forms of DI from excessive water drinking?

If the diagnosis of polyuria is not clear from the history and initial lab tests, perform a water restriction test (WRT). Other names for the WRT are dehydration test and water deprivation test. The test may take 6–18 hr depending on the initial state of hydration. Perform the WRT as follows:

1. Admit mildly polyuric patients to the ward and more severely polyuric patients to the intensive care unit. Start the test at 10:00–11:00 PM for mildly polyuric patients and at 6:00 AM for more severely polyuric patients.

2. Measure **baseline** weight, P_{osm}, P_{Na}, P_{BUN}, $P_{glucose}$, U_{volume}, U_{osm}, U_{Na}, and U_K. Measure **hourly** weight and U_{osm}.

3. Allow no food or water.
4. Watch the patient closely for signs of dehydration and surreptitious water drinking.
5. End the WRT when U_{osm} has not increased more than 30 mOsm/kg for three consecutive hours and P_{osm} has reached 295–300 mOsm/kg or the patient has lost 3–5% of body weight. If weight loss exceeds 5% of body weight, further dehydration is unsafe.
6. At P_{osm} of 295–300 mOsm/kg, endogenous ADH levels should be 3–5 pg/mL, and the kidney should respond with maximal urinary concentration.
7. Repeat all baseline tests toward and at the end of the WRT.
8. Give 5 units of aqueous AVP or 2 µg of DDAVP subcutaneously.
9. Repeat the baseline tests at 30, 60, and 120 minutes.
10. Calculate U_{osm}/P_{osm} and $[U_{Na} + U_K]/P_{Na}$ as a check on measured U_{osm}/P_{osm}.

The table below summarizes the expected results of the WRT. The WRT stimulates maximal endogenous release of ADH by increasing P_{osm} and evaluates the concentrating ability of the kidney by measuring U_{osm}. Giving exogenous ADH allows evaluation of the renal concentrating response to ADH if dehydration-induced ADH production was impaired. Save frozen baseline and end-test plasma to measure ADH if results are equivocal. Expected values for P_{ADH} are ≤ 0.5 pg/mL for P_{osm} ≤280 mOsm/kg and ≥ 5pg/mL for P_{osm} ≥295 mOsm/kg.

Values Before and After Water Restriction

	PRE P_{OSM}	PRE P_{Na}	POSTU_{OSM}/P_{OSM}	POST U_{OSM}/P_{OSM} + ADH	POST P_{ADH}
Normals	NL	NL	>1	>1 (<10%)	↑
PPD/DDI	↓	↓	>1	>1 (<10%)	↑
CCDI	↑	↑	<1	>1 (>50%)	–
PCDI	↑	↑	>1	>1 (10–50%)	↓
CNDI	↑	↑	<1	<1 (<10%)	↑↑
PNDI	↑	↑	>1	>1 (<10%)	↑↑

PPD/DDI = psychogenic polydipsia/dipsogenic DI; CCDI = complete central DI; PCDI = partial central DI; CNDI = complete nephrogenic DI; and PNDI = partial nephrogenic DI. Relative to the normal range, the down and up arrows, respectively, mean low or low normal and high or high normal values for P_{osm}, P_{Na}, and P_{ADH}. Recall that when U_{osm} > P_{osm}, there is antidiuresis and the kidney is retaining free water. The same is true when $[U_{Na} + U_K]$ > P_{Na}, and these tests are more easily obtainable. When U_{osm} < P_{osm} or $[U_{Na} + U_K]$ < P_{Na}, there is net loss of free water with little net clinical ADH effect. The percent in parentheses indicates the percentage change in U_{osm} (not the U_{osm}/P_{osm} ratio) after 5 units of subcutaneous aqueous vasopressin.

33. What are the expected plasma ADH concentrations and urinary osmolality in polyuric patients after water restriction?

Expected plasma ADH concentrations and urinary osmolality (U_{osm}) after water restriction depend on the cause of polyuria. After water restriction, ADH concentrations and Uosm values are as follows: **normals**, ADH >2 pg/ml and U_{osm} >800 mOsm/kg; **complete central DI**, ADH undetectable and Uosm <300 mOsm/kg; **partial central DI**, ADH <1.5 pg/mL and Uosm 300–800 mOsm/kg; **nephrogenic DI**, ADH >5 pg/mL and Uosm 300–500 mOsm/kg; and **primary polydipsia**, ADH <5 pg/mL and Uosm >500 mOsm/kg.

34. How should you approach the patient with hypernatremia?

Problems of hypernatremia uncommon compared with hyponatremia and occur in < 1% of hospitalized patients. Loss of water, not gain of Na, usually causes hypernatremia. However, unless patients have an abnormality of thirst or do not have access to water, they usually maintain near-normal P_{Na} by drinking water in proportion to losses. As in question 28, assess the patient's volume status. Once lab studies are obtained, approach the patient per the following table. If the patient has polyuria, also include the approach in questions 31 and 32.

Approach to Hypernatremia

CONDITIONS CAUSING HYPERNATREMIA	POSTURAL SIGNS	EDEMA	U_{NA}	U_{osm}	TREATMENT
Renal Na and H_2O loss	Yes	No	>20	↓–	Hypotonic saline
Nonrenal Na and H_2O loss	Yes	No	<10	↑	Hypotonic saline
Sodium excess	No	No	>20	↑–	Diuretics and water
Renal H_2O loss	No	No	VAR	↓↑–	Water
Nonrenal H_2O loss	No	No	VAR	↑	Water

VAR = variable, ↑ = hypertonic, ↓ = hypotonic, – = isosmotic.

Causes of Hypernatremia

PATHOPHYSIOLOGY	ASSOCIATED CONDITION
Low total body sodium and water with water loss > sodium loss	Renal sodium and water loss
	Osmotic diuretics
	Loop diuretics
	Renal disease
	Postobstructive diuresis
	Osmotic diarrhea
	Vomiting
	Nonrenal sodium and water loss
	Sweating
	Diarrhea
	Burns
High total body sodium	Hyperaldosteronism
	Cushing's syndrome
	Excessive intake of NaCl or $NaHCO_3$
	Hypertonic saline and bicarbonate
	Hypertonic dialysis
Normal total body sodium with excessive water loss	Renal water losses
	Central diabetes insipidus
	Nephrogenic diabetes insipidus
	Nonrenal sodium and water loss
	Increased sensible loss
	No access to water

Note: Hypernatremia always means too little plasma water relative to sodium. With access to water, hypernatremia usually does not occur or is mild. However, unattended patients who are too old, too young, or too sick may not have adequate access to water, and hypernatremia may be severe.

35. How should you diagnose and manage the patient with diabetes insipidus?

DI is a syndrome of excessive water loss by the kidney due to decreased ADH (central DI) or renal resistance to ADH effect (nephrogenic DI). Therefore, the hallmark of DI is polyuria. As in questions 31 and 32, first distinguish primary polydipsia from DI and identify the DI as central or nephrogenic. Then give water to prevent dehydration until the evaluation suggests definitive therapy. A patient with DI will probably self-treat with water unless there is a thirst deficit or the patient has no access to water. An example is a 70-year-old woman who noted the onset of polyuria and polydipsia a week before admission. She increased water intake but then developed the flu and could not hold down liquids. Family brought her to the hospital. Her P_{Na} was 150 mEq/L. Her weight was 60 kg. Her evaluation showed breast cancer metastatic to the brain. Her water deficit is as follows:

$$\text{Water deficit} = [(\text{observed } P_{Na} - \text{normal } P_{Na})/\text{normal } P_{Na}] \times \text{TBW}$$

$$= [(P_{Na} - 140)/140] \times \text{TBW} = [(150 - 140)/140] \times 0.5 \times 60 \text{ kg} = 2 \text{ L deficit in TBW}$$

Treat the polyuria and the underlying cause if possible. If not, just treat the polyuria. If the diagnosis is central DI, as in this case, desmopressin acetate is the therapy of choice. DDAVP has an antidiuretic-to-pressor ratio of 2000:1 compared with AVP's ratio of 1:1. The usual initial dose is 5–20 μg intranasally. If this dosage is insufficient, 5–20 μg may be given twice daily. DDAVP is now available in nasal spray, rhinal tube, and injectable forms. Important underlying causes of central DI include idiopathic (autoimmune) disease, primary tumors (craniopharyngioma), metastatic tumors (breast, lung, leukemia), infections (viral), vascular disorders (aneurysm), granulomas (sarcoidosis), drugs (clonidine), head trauma, and cranial or pituitary surgery.

Treat nephrogenic DI with 12.5–25.0 mg hydrochlorothiazide one to two times a day to decrease ECV, enhance proximal nephron water reabsorption, and increase medullary interstitial osmolality. Other therapies that increase U_{osm} by ADH-independent mechanisms include low sodium and protein diet, amiloride, and nonsteroidal anti-inflammatory drugs (e.g., indomethacin). By preventing sodium and lithium entry into the tubular cell, amiloride is particularly useful in lithium carbonate-induced DI. Since Nephrogenic DI may be incomplete, a trial of DDAUP described above for central DI may be beneficial.

CONTROVERSIES

36. How quickly should you correct states of water excess or deficiency?
The main concern of therapy is to prevent devastating neurologic complications. Understanding brain adaptation to changes in TBW, as outlined in question 27, emphasizes the need for urgent therapy in the symptomatic patient. There are three useful rules in treating disturbances of water (measured by changes in P_{Na}):

1. Return the P_{Na} to normal at the relative speed that it became abnormal. If the change in P_{Na} was slow (days), correct it slowly (days). If the change was rapid (minutes to hours), correct it rapidly (minutes to hours).
2. If there are no symptoms of water or Na imbalance (see question 26), there is no immediate urgency. If there are symptoms, there is an urgency. Question 27 outlines the brain adaptations to altered tonicity that may cause devastating changes in brain volume. These adaptations also cause the patient's symptoms. Thus, symptoms should drive the clinician to correct the altered tonicity rapidly.
3. The degree of P_{Na} correction should be **toward normal** not **to** normal (until symptoms abate).

Example. A 34-year-old woman presents 12 hr after discharge following cholecystectomy. She has headache, confusion, muscle cramps, weakness, lethargy, agitation, nausea, and vomiting but was asymptomatic at discharge. P_{Na} was 110 mEq/L. By this history, hyponatremia developed rapidly and was symptomatic. Treatment is intensive care unit admission and administration of 3% saline and furosemide at rates sufficient to increase P_{Na} 1.5–2.0 mEq/L/hr for 2–4 hours based on symptom resolution. Measure hourly P_{Na}, U_{Na}, and U_K to follow progress and guide therapy. Once serious signs and symptoms improve, decrease the rate of correction to 0.5–1.0 mEq/hr until symptoms further improve or the P_{Na} is 120 mEq/L. Unless patient symptoms dictate otherwise, attempt to avoid a net increase in $P_{Na} > 12$ mEq/L/day and 18–20 mEq/L over 2 days. For chronic hyponatremia without symptoms, the appropriate rate of correction is 0.5 mEq/L/hr with similar net daily increases in P_{Na}. Acute symptomatic hyponatremia requires expeditious correction of the P_{Na} because the symptomatic patient has cerebral edema caused by "normal" brain-cell solute content that pulls water into the brain. Acutely raising P_{Na} increases ECF tonicity, pulls water out of the swollen brain, and reduces the brain volume toward normal. Conversely, the patient with chronic asymptomatic hyponatremia has adapted by loss of brain solute and has near-normal brain volume. Increasing this patient's P_{Na} too rapidly (>0.5 mEq/L/hr) will shrink the brain and predispose to the osmotic demyelination syndrome (previously called central pontine myelinolysis). The risks of not correcting acute symptomatic hyponatremia include increased cerebral edema, seizures, coma, and death. Outlined below are calculations of water excess and how much NaCl will correct the P_{Na} of the patient in the example to 120 mEq/L.

$$\text{Water excess} = [(\text{normal } P_{Na} - \text{observed } P_{Na})/\text{normal } P_{Na}] \times \text{TBW}$$
$$= [(140 - 110)/140] \times 0.5 \times 60 \text{ kg} = 0.21 \times 30 \text{ L} = 6.3 \text{ L excess in TBW}$$

$$\text{Na}^+ \text{ deficit} = (\text{desired } P_{Na} - \text{observed } P_{Na}) \times \text{TBW} = (120 - 110) \times 0.5 \times 60 \text{ kg}$$
$$= 10 \text{ mEq/L} \times 30 \text{ L} = 300 \text{ mEq Na}$$

Knowing the sodium deficit is useful clinically because it can be replaced at a controlled rate to improve the hyponatremia. The Na^+ in 3% saline is 513 mEq/L:

$$300 \text{ mEq Na}^+/513 \text{ mEq/L} = 0.585 \text{ L}$$

Thus, assuming no Na or water loss, giving 585 mL of 3% saline will correct the P_{Na} to 120 mEq/L. Make a similar calculation for the amount of 3% saline to infuse over 3–4 hours to increase the P_{Na} by 6 mEq/L. The answer is 350 ml. Use P_{Na}, U_{Na}, and U_K to estimate loss and gain of sodium and water during therapy.

The same concepts of **speed, symptoms,** and **degree of P_{Na} correction** apply in opposite osmotic directions for hypernatremia.

37. How do frequent measurements of urinary Na and K help with hyponatremia therapy?

Initial assessments for sodium repletion, as outlined in question 36, do not account for urinary water and electrolyte losses that may alter the expected P_{Na} response to therapy. Therefore, replacement of urinary losses allows more accurate correction of P_{Na}. Measure the U_{Na+} and U_{K+} and urine volume every 1–2 hr, and replace urine volume with saline of appropriate strength. For example, if the urinary volume was 100 ml/hr, the $U_{Na+} = 43$ mEq/L, and the $U_{K+} = 35$ mEq/L, the sum of $U_{Na+} + U_{K+} = 78$ mEq/L at 100 ml/hr. In this case, replacing urinary losses with 0.45% saline (77 mEq/L NaCl) intravenously at 100 ml/hr will prevent major deviations in P_{Na} from the value calculated. This replacement fluid should be given in addition to that calculated to correct the P_{Na}. KCl replacement depends on serum potassium. Replace potassium to correct the serum K to normal, remembering that potassium replacement will increase P_{Na}. Therefore, decrease the replacement Na by the amount of K given. Some evidence also suggests that hypokalemia may predispose to osmotic demyelination. Therefore, correcting serum potassium may decrease this risk.

38. What are vasopressin receptor antagonists and how might they change the future of hyponatremia therapy?

The conventional treatment of hyponatremia is water restriction or saline administration. In the future, vasopressin receptor antagonists that are selective for the V_2 (antidiuretic) receptor will provide more effective therapy for hyponatremia. These agents are now being tested in humans and produce a selective water diuresis with no effect on Na and K excretion. The term *aquaretic drugs* (aquaretics) has been coined for these medications to highlight their different mechanism of action compared with the saluretic diuretic furosemide. They will prove beneficial in SIADH and in hyponatremic patients with congestive heart failure and cirrhosis. By blocking ADH effect, rapid correction of hyponatremia may occur; therefore, judicious monitoring of P_{Na} changes are important to prevent excessively rapid correction of the serum sodium concentration.

39. What is the appropriate P_{Na} correction factor for hyperglycemia?

The standard correction factor is a 1.6 mEq/L decrease in P_{Na} for each 100 mg/dl increase in plasma glucose concentration above 100 mg/dL. For glucose values greater than 400 mg/dL, recent data suggest a correction factor as high as a 4.0 mEq/L decrease in P_{Na} for each 100 mg/dL increase in plasma glucose and an average correction factor of 2.4 mEq/L.

BIBLIOGRAPHY

1. Adrogue HJ, Madias NE: Hyponatremia. N Engl J Med. 342(21):1581–1589, 2000.
2. Adrogue HJ, Madias NE: Hypernatremia. N Engl J Med 342(20):1493–1499, 2000.
3. Berl T, Schrier RW. The patient with hyponatremia and hypernatremia. In Schrier RW (ed): Manual of Nephrology, 5th ed. Philadelphia, Lippincott Williams & Wilkins, 2000, pp 21–36.
4. Fall PJ: Hyponatremia and hypernatremia. A systematic approach to causes and their correction. Postgrad Med 107(5):75–82, 179, 2000.
5. Hillier TA, Abbott RD, Barrett EJ: Hyponatremia: evaluating the correction factor for hyperglycemia. Am J Med 106(4):399–403, 1999.
6. Kugler JP, Hustead T: Hyponatremia and hypernatremia in the elderly. Am Fam Physician 61(12):3623–3630, 2000.
7. Mayinger B, Hensen J: Nonpeptide vasopressin antagonists: A new group of hormone blockers entering the scene. Exp Clin Endocrinol Diabetes 107(3):157–165,1999.
8. Nielsen S, Kwon TH, Christensen BM, et al.: Physiology and pathophysiology of renal aquaporins. J Am Soc Nephrol 10(3):647–663, 1999.
9. Oster JR, Singer I: Hyponatremia, hyposmolality, and hypotonicity: Tables and fables. Arch Intern Med 159(4):333–336,1999
10. Singer I, Oster JR, Fishman LM: The management of diabetes insipidus in adults. Arch Intern Med 157(12):1293–1301, 1997.

26. DISORDERS OF GROWTH

Philip Zeitler, M.D., Ph.D., and Robert H. Slover, M.D.

1. What is normal growth velocity for children?

The normal growth increment in the first 6 months of life is 16–17 cm, and in the second 6 months about 8 cm. Growth in the second year of life is just over 10 cm, whereas it is about 8 cm in the third year and 7 cm in the fourth year. During the fifth through tenth years (until puberty), growth averages 5–6 cm/year. Some children may experience a transient period of slow growth just prior to the onset of puberty, followed by the pubertal growth spurt that reaches a maximum of 11–13 cm/year. In girls, the growth spurt occurs early in puberty (breast Tanner stage II), but is later in boys (pubic hair Tanner stage III–IV, testicular volume 12–15 ml).

2. What are the tools used to define growth in children?

First and most essential to the detection of growth abnormalities is the ability to obtain accurate and reproducible measurements. Accuracy in measurement requires the availability of appropriate equipment, as well as proper positioning of the patient. At all ages, children should be measured at *full stretch* with a straight spine, since this is the only position that will be reproducible. They should be shoeless and hair decorations or braids may need to be removed. In infants and children up to age 2 years, supine length is measured, ideally using a box-like structure with a headboard and a movable footplate. Accurate measurement of an infant requires two people, with one holding the head against the headboard while the other straightens the legs and places the ankles at 90 degrees against the movable foot plate. In children 2 years of age and older, standing height is measured, most accurately by a stadiometer with a rigid headboard, footplate, and backboard. The child stands against the backboard, with heels, buttocks, thoracic spine, and head touching. The measurer exerts upward pressure on the patient at the angle of the jaw to bring the spine into full stretch, and the headboard is lowered until it touches the top of the head. A counter reads the measurement. If this device is not available, the child should stand against a wall in the same position as used for a stadiometer. A right angle is moved downward to touch the top of the head, and a mark is made and measured. Scales with floppy arms are unreliable. Weight and (when appropriate) head circumference should be recorded.

The second tool is the growth curve, and all measurements should be plotted rather than just recorded as a number in the chart. Despite being low-tech, a carefully constructed and up-to-date growth curve is critical to the recognition of growth abnormalities. Furthermore, the more points that are plotted on the curve, the greater the understanding of the child's growth. Thus, efforts should be made to obtain growth measurements at all patient contacts, since routine well-child visits are infrequent during the middle childhood years when growth abnormalities are most common. Errors in plotting of growth points are a frequent cause of erroneous growth abnormalities. Common errors include plotting the wrong height, not plotting at the exact chronologic age, and use of an inappropriate growth chart. A number of growth charts are available, and consideration should be given to the appropriate chart for a particular patient. In particular, the clinician should be aware of the difference between charts for plotting supine length (the 0–36 month charts in common use) and those for stature (the 2–18 year charts). Since a patient measured supine will be longer than the same patient standing up, the charting of a standing patient on a supine chart will give the erroneous impression of decreased growth velocity. Growth charts are also available for a variety of ethnic groups and common syndromes, and their use should be considered when appropriate.

A careful history is critical to understanding a child's growth and should include birth history, birth weight, developmental milestones, presence of chronic illnesses or long-term medications, history of surgery or trauma, current symptoms, parental heights, and timing of parental puberty. Physical examination should focus on signs of chronic illness, as well as physical evidence of a syndrome.

Finally, a bone-age film can provide important information about skeletal and (by implication) physical maturity. A radiograph of the left hand and wrist is obtained in children over 2 years of age, and maturation of epiphyseal centers is compared with available standards.

3. What is the most important factor in identifying abnormal growth curve?

An abnormal growth velocity for age generally distinguishes growth abnormalities from normal growth variants. Although there are many causes of short stature, including genetic and ethnic inheritance, short normal children grow normally, whereas children with a problem will have an abnormal growth velocity. For example, a 5th percentile child growing with a normal growth velocity is less worrisome than the child who has fallen from the 90th to the 75th percentile, even though the latter child is taller than the former. Growth velocity abnormalities may, however, be subtle.

4. What are the causes of abnormal growth in children?

Abnormalities in growth are most frequently either due to normal growth variants or are a consequence of underlying chronic medical illness, either recognized or unrecognized. Hormonal causes are less frequent. Causes of poor growth include:

1. Normal growth variants
   a. Familial short stature
   b. Constitutional delay of growth and puberty
2. Syndromes
   a. Down syndrome
   b. Prader-Willi syndrome
   c. Turner syndrome
   d. Noonan syndrome
   e. Other chromosomal abnormalities
3. Poor growth due to non-endocrine disease and treatments
   a. Malnutrition
   b. Pulmonary disease
      1. Cystic fibrosis
      2. Asthma
   c. Cardiac disease
   d. Rheumatologic disease
   e. Gastrointestinal disease
      1. Crohn's disease
      2. Inflammatory bowel disease
   f. Neurologic disease
      1. Ketogenic diet
      2. Stimulant medications
   g. Renal disease
   h. Anemia
   i. Neoplasia
   j. Chronic glucocorticoid use
4. Endocrine disease (see below)

Example 1: 7-year-old girl with height of 110 cm

Height age = 5 years, 3 months
Bone age = 7 years

Father's height = 65 in (165 cm)
Mother's height = 62 in (157 cm)

Corrected midparental height (± 1 SD) =
155 ± 5 cm

Predicted adult height = 60 in

The child has a predicted adult height within
genetic potential and a bone age equal to
chronologic age. She has genetic or familial
short stature.

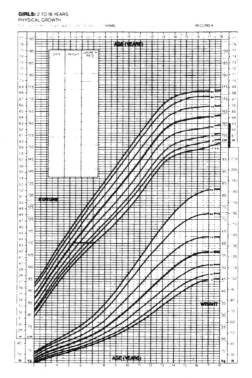

Example 2: 7-year-old girl with height of 110 cm

Height age = 5 years, 3 months
Bone age = 5 years

Father's height = 70 in (178 cm)
Mother's height = 66 in (168 cm)

Corrected midparental height (± 1 SD) =
1675 ± 5 cm

The child is growing below the fifth percentile, but extrapolation of her growth to
adult height gives a final height below
genetic potential. Clearly her height cannot
be attributed to genetic short stature alone.

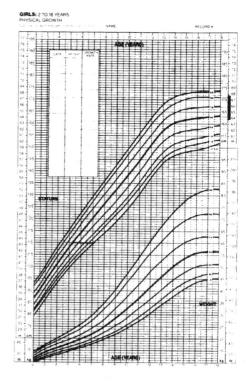

5. Using the tools of growth curve, bone age, and height, how does one distinguish between familial (genetic) short stature and other causes?

Children with familial short stature grow at a normal velocity but below the normal curve. However, such children grow within their expected target height percentile, i.e., they are as tall as expected for their genetic potential. A simple formula helps to determine whether a child's size is explained by parental heights: add the parents' heights in cm; add 13 cm if the child is male, or subtract 13 cm if the child is female; and then divide by two. The resulting "midparental height" ± 5 cm gives a rough target range for adult height. If the child's projected height (by extrapolation of the growth curve) falls within this range, the likelihood is high that current height may be explained by genetic factors. In such children, bone age approximately equals chronologic age. For example, a 5-year-old whose height is below the third percentile, but whose growth has traced a line parallel to the third percentile and projects within the parental target range and whose bone age is also 5 years, may reasonably be expected to have familial short stature. Conversely, if the projected height falls below the predicted range, other factors *may be* involved in the short stature. See examples 1 and 2.

6. Other than familial short stature, what is the most common etiology of short stature?

Constitutional delay of growth (constitutional short stature), which affects up to 2% of children, is characterized by short stature and delayed bone age and represents a normal growth pattern simply shifted to a later age. Affected children typically have a period of subnormal growth between 18 and 30 months of age followed by normal growth velocity throughout the remainder of childhood. In accord with the delayed developmental pattern, bone age is delayed. The continuing growth delay also results in a delay in pubertal development and physical maturity. Such children (usually boys) often have a family history of a similar growth pattern and may have a more dramatic deceleration of growth velocity before

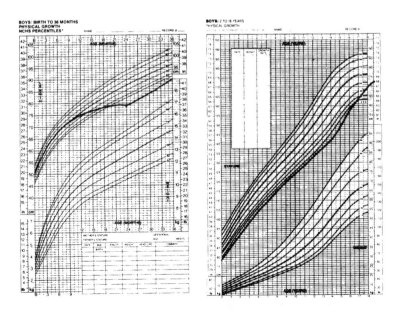

Constitutional delay of growth. Subnormal velocity during second year of life followed by normal velocity through childhood and a prolonged growth period with eventual achievement of normal adult height.

Example: 6-year-old boy

Height age = 3 years, 6 months
Bone age = 3 years, 9 months
Normal velocity
Predicted adult height = 68½ in

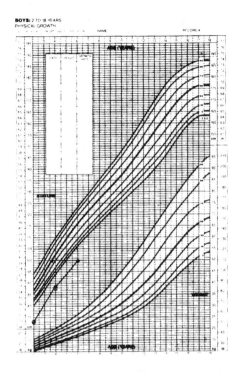

entering puberty than normal children. They complete their growth at a later age, ending at normal adult height within expected genetic potential.

7. How is the diagnosis of constitutional delay of growth made?

The following elements may allow one to feel comfortable with the diagnosis of constitutional delay of growth:

1. Short stature.
2. A period of poor growth in the second year followed by a normal growth velocity.
3. Delayed bone age.
4. Height prediction appropriate for family—this can be roughly determined by plotting the current height at the patient's bone age and following the resulting percentile to adult height. In constitutional delay, this will lead to a projected height within the parental target range.
5. Positive family history, delayed dentition, and delayed puberty in adolescence.

The diagnosis of constitutional delay of growth based on the above criteria does not need further laboratory support. See example above.

8. What is the effect of testosterone therapy on boys with constitutional delay of growth?

Short-term testosterone therapy for boys with constitutional delay (75–100 mg/month of long-acting testosterone esters given for 6 months, starting at bone age 12.5 years) accelerates growth and stimulates pubertal development without compromising final adult height or advancing bone age. Clinically the boys experience pubertal changes, including genital enlargement (but not testicular growth), growth of pubic and axillary hair, deepening of voice, body odor, and acne. Not surprisingly, there are fairly typical personality changes as well.

9. Name the endocrine causes for short stature in children in order of prevalence.

1. Hypothyroidism—congenital or acquired
2. Growth hormone deficiency
3. Glucocorticoid excess—iatrogenic or endogenous (less common)
4. Pseudohypoparathyroidism

10. Describe the etiologies of growth hormone deficiency.

Idiopathic growth hormone deficiency affects as many as 1:10,000–15,000 children. It is sporadic in the great majority of cases, but a handful of hereditary cases have been reported, some with specific deletions of the growth hormone gene. The other important underlying causes are listed below:

1. Congenital
   a. Septo-optic dysplasia
   b. Ectopic posterior pituitary with hypopituitarism
   c. Pituitary aplasia
   d. Growth hormone gene deletion
   e. Biologically inactive growth hormone
2. Trauma
   a. Accidental
   b. Non-accidental (child abuse)
3. Iatrogenic
   a. Surgery
   b. Radiation
4. Infectious and infiltrative diseases
   a. Sarcoidosis
   b. Tuberculosis
   c. Histiocytosis
5. Vascular
6. Psychosocial disorders
   a. Depression
   b. Maternal deprivation
7. Tumors of the hypothalamus and pituitary
   a. Craniopharyngioma, glioma, pinealoma, hamartoma, neurofibroma, prolactinoma
8. End-organ resistance
   a. Laron dwarfism (growth hormone receptor dysfunction)
   b. Malnutrition

11. How is growth hormone deficiency diagnosed?

The diagnosis of growth hormone deficiency is primarily a clinical one, aided by laboratory support, rather than a diagnosis based on definitive testing. Most important is choosing the appropriate patient. Children with subnormal growth should be evaluated for growth hormone deficiency only after a thorough search fails to reveal any other etiology for growth delay. In most cases, evaluation should begin with the measurement of serum insulin-like growth factor 1 (IGF-1). IGF-1, previously known as somatomedin C, is a growth hormone– dependent protein that is produced in most target tissues in response to growth hormone and mediates some, but not all, of the effects of GH. Serum IGF-1 reflects production of the protein by the liver and is thought to give an indirect indication of growth hormone secretion. Because levels of IGF-1 remain constant during the day, unlike levels of growth hormone, measurement of this protein provides an attractive approach to initial screening. In general, concentrations of IGF-1 are reduced in growth hormone deficiency, though the sensitivity is limited. Thus, a low IGF-1 (<2 SD from the mean for age) is 70–80% predictive of failing more rigorous tests of growth hormone secretion. Conversely, normal levels of IGF-1 are reassuring, but do not rule out partial growth hormone deficiency in the appropriate clinical context.

Poor nutrition, chronic disease, and hypothyroidism influence IGF-1 levels. Furthermore, they vary with age and values must be compared with appropriate age- and pubertal stage–specific norms available from performing laboratories. Below the age of 6, values are quite low and the overlap between normal and GH-deficient renders the test highly insensitive. Other GH-dependent proteins currently under consideration as indirect screens for GH deficiency include IGF-binding protein 3 (minimal variation with age, less affected by nutri-

Example: 14½-year-old boy with growth hormone deficiency treated from age 9.

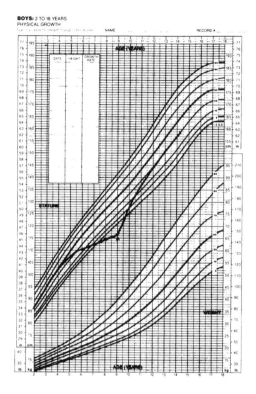

BOYS: 2 TO 18 YEARS
PHYSICAL GROWTH

tional state), IGF-binding protein 2 (rises in the presence of GH deficiency), and ALS (acid labile subunit).

Because secretion of growth hormone is episodic, random levels are not helpful for the formal diagnosis of deficiency. Rather, growth hormone is measured in response to a series of stimuli. Normal children typically respond to stimulation with growth hormone levels above 10 ng/ml and may have levels as high as 30 ng/ml. Failure to respond to all tests with a value greater than 10 ng/ml is consistent with the diagnosis of classic growth hormone deficiency. Criteria for the diagnosis of partial growth hormone deficiency and for the entity known as neurosecretory dysfunction (normal pituitary response to stimuli, but low IGF-1 suggesting endogenous secretion is impaired) are less well established. For results to have meaning, the child must be euthyroid, with no underlying chronic disease or psychosocial deviation. A variety of pharmacologic agents that stimulate growth hormone secretion are available, and there is currently no consensus on which agents are optimal. At least two tests are generally performed, because a patient may fail to respond to one agent on a given day but respond on another. All tests require an overnight fast.

12. How is idiopathic growth hormone deficiency treated?

Children with growth hormone deficiency have been successfully treated for over 30 years. Currently, growth hormone is available through recombinant DNA technology, and the majority of children are treated with 6–7 daily shots/week at a total weekly dose of approximately 0.30 mg/kg administered subcutaneously. Because the effect of growth hormone wanes after several years of therapy, it is common to see dramatic catch-up growth (~10–12 cm/year) in the first year or two of therapy, followed by velocities ranging from normal to 1.5 times normal in subsequent years. Throughout therapy, levels of thyroid hormone as well as other pituitary hormones must be monitored closely.

13. What is the prognosis for adult height in treated children with idiopathic growth hormone deficiency?

Although nearly all treated children reach an adult height significantly better than predicted before therapy is initiated, many do not reach their predicted genetic potential. Children diagnosed and treated at an earlier age have a better height prognosis than do those whose therapy is initiated later. Similarly, the more mature the skeleton at diagnosis, the poorer the final outcome.

14. When is growth hormone therapy discontinued?

In children with idiopathic growth hormone deficiency, the point of diminishing benefit of therapy correlates with skeletal maturity rather than chronologic age or duration of therapy. Therapy often is discontinued at a bone age of 15 years (96% growth) to 16 years (98% of growth) in boys and 14 years (98% of growth) in girls. However, these practices are undergoing some change as the indications for treatment of growth hormone deficiency in adulthood become clarified. It can be anticipated that some patients with severe growth hormone deficiency will require life-long hormonal replacement.

15. What other syndromes are considered indications for growth hormone therapy?

Turner syndrome (45 XO or mosaic variants) in girls is commonly associated with short stature independent of the reduction in height caused by gonadal failure. It has become common practice to treat affected girls with growth hormone or with combinations of growth hormone and estrogen or oxandrolone. Prader-Willi syndrome is associated with short stature, severe obesity, and behavioral abnormalities. Recent studies indicate that growth hormone can improve body composition, strength, and performance of daily activities, and growth hormone has been approved by the FDA for these patients.

16. What is the prognosis for girls with Turner syndrome treated with growth hormone?

Girls with Turner syndrome generally demonstrate a significant increase in predicted adult height, with an average increase of 8.8 cm. The overall effectiveness of therapy, like that in growth hormone deficiency, is dependent on the age at initiation, the bone age at initiation, and the duration of treatment. In addition to increasing final height, growth hormone therapy in Turner syndrome normalizes height in younger girls, so that estrogen replacement therapy can be initiated at an age similar to that of the patient's peers.

17. What are the other indications for growth hormone therapy?

Growth hormone therapy is currently indicated for growth hormone deficiency, Turner syndrome, Prader-Willi syndrome, and chronic renal insufficiency prior to transplant. The latter three indications do not require demonstration of growth hormone deficiency. In addition, the use of growth hormone in a variety of other situations, including other syndromes, chronic glucocorticoid use, intrauterine growth retardation, and renal insufficiency after transplant, is under investigation.

18. What are the potential risks of human growth hormone therapy?

The side effects of growth hormone therapy can be divided into three categories:
1. Common, but clinically unimportant: salt/water retention presenting as transient peripheral edema, headache, joint aches, and stiffness.
2. Uncommon, but potentially clinically important: pseudotumor cerebri, slipped capital femoral epiphysis, glucose intolerance. These are most common in children being treated with Turner syndrome and chronic renal failure.
3. Rare and theoretical, but of questionable clinical relevance: Worldwide. about 35 patients receiving human growth hormone have developed leukemia. For the most

part, these children were already at risk for development of leukemia because of previous treatment with chemotherapy or radiation. The actual increased risk for leukemia and whether this risk is increased also for patients with idiopathic growth hormone deficiency remains unclear because of the small numbers of patients involved. Concerns have also been raised about the potential for growth hormone to promote recurrence in brain tumor patients. No study to date has indicated that recurrence rates are indeed higher in growth hormone–treated patients.

19. Should short children without growth hormone deficiency be treated with growth hormone?

This question continues to be intensely controversial among pediatric endocrinologists. Certainly this group represents by far the largest number of short children. Short-term studies involving small cohorts have demonstrated a consistent increase in growth velocity with growth hormone therapy in children in whom no secretory abnormality could be demonstrated. Bone ages did not advance disproportionately. Again, growth response was greatest in the first year of therapy and declined in the second year. Several small studies have followed children to final height and have disagreed on the overall effectiveness of therapy.

One of the problems in determining the effect of growth hormone in "normal" short children is the difficulty discussed previously in determining who is truly growth hormone– deficient. Because our ability to definitively define normal growth hormone function is limited, we have a problem in determining that a short child is growth hormone–sufficient beyond reasonable doubt. A consensus is slowly emerging among pediatric endocrinologists that short children growing with an abnormal growth velocity and/or with predicted adult height well outside the parental target range merit a trial of growth hormone therapy. Conversely, short children growing normally and within their parental target are unlikely to benefit significantly.

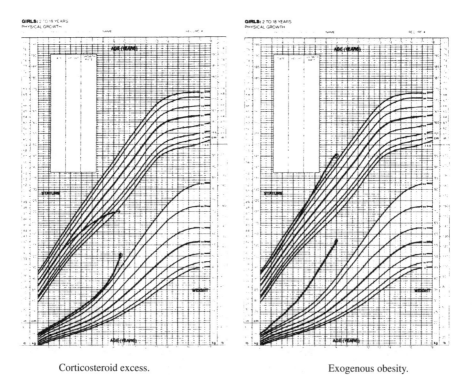

Corticosteroid excess.   Exogenous obesity.

20. How does the pattern of growth in children with excessive glucocorticoids differ from the pattern in children with exogenous obesity?

Glucocorticoid excess, whether iatrogenic (common) or intrinsic (rare), results in impairment of linear growth. The mechanism relates to direct glucocorticoid metabolic actions, including increased protein catabolism, decreased lipolysis, and a decline in collagen synthesis. Glucocorticoids also reduce growth hormone effects by suppressing the pulsatile release of growth hormone from the pituitary gland and the production of IGF-1 at the target organ. The net result is that children with steroid excess are frequently short. They also have an increased weight-to-height ratio and appear obese. Children with exogenous obesity, on the other hand, generally show accelerated linear growth; thus they seem not only obese but also tall for their age.

21. What conditions are associated with excessive growth in childhood?

In contrast to the large number of conditions that delay or suppress growth, relatively few conditions result in overgrowth. The most common, other than genetic tall stature, is constitutional advanced growth. As expected, affected children have advanced bone age, accelerated growth, and early puberty.

Growth hormone excess (pituitary gigantism) is rare in children but causes tall stature rather than the bony overgrowth seen in adults (acromegaly), since the growth plates are open. Growth hormone excess is diagnosed by demonstrating elevated random levels of growth hormone that are not suppressed during a standard glucose tolerance test, as well as extremely high levels of IGF-1.

Syndromes associated with large size and rapid growth include the following:

1. Genetic factors
2. Constitutional advanced growth
3. Klinefelter's syndrome (47 XXY): tall stature, small testes, delay of puberty
4. Connective tissue disorders
   a. Marfan's syndrome: tall stature, arachnodactyly, joint laxity, lens displacement
   b. Stickler's syndrome
5. Growth hormone excess (pituitary gigantism)
6. Soto's syndrome (cerebral gigantism): macrocephaly, progressive macrosomia, dilated ventricles, retardation, advanced bone age
7. Hyperthyroidism
8. Androgen excess
   a. Precocious puberty
   b. Congenital adrenal hyperplasia
   c Androgen-producing tumor
9. Estrogen excess
   a. Precocious puberty
   b. Congenital adrenal hyperplasia
   c. Estrogen-producing tumor
10. Obesity
11. Beckwith-Wiedemann syndrome: macroglossia, umbilical hernia, hypoglycemia, macrosomia in infancy
12. Homocystinuria: arachnodactyly, retardation, homocystine in urine

BIBLIOGRAPHY

1. Binder G, Schwarze CP, Ranke MB: Identification of short stature caused by SHOX defects and therapeutic effect of recombinant human growth hormone. J Clin Endocrinol Metab 85:245–249, 2000.
2. Cohen MM Jr: Overgrowth syndromes: an update. Adv Pediatr 46:441–491, 1999.

3. Juul A, Bernasconi S, Chatelain P, et al: Diagnosis of growth hormone (GH) deficiency and the use of GH in children with growth disorders. Horm Res. 51:284–299, 1999.
4. Kelnar CJ, Albertsson-Wikland K, Hintz RL, et al: Should we treat children with idiopathic short stature? Horm Res. 52:150–157, 1999.
5. Myers SE, Carrel AL, Whitman BY, Allen DB: Sustained benefit after 2 years of growth hormone on body composition, fat utilization, physical strength and agility, and growth in Prader-Willi syndrome. J Pediatr. 137:42–49, 2000.
6. Pasquino AM, Pucarelli I, Roggini M, Segni M: Adult height in short normal girls treated with gonadotropin-releasing hormone analogs and growth hormone. J Clin Endocrinol Metab 85: 619–622, 2000.
7. Rosenfeld RG: Disorders of growth hormone and insulin-like growth factor secretion and action. In Sperling MA (ed): Pediatric Endocrinology. Philadelphia, WB Saunders, 1996, pp 117–169
8. Sas TC, de Muinck Keizer-Schrama SM, Stijnen T, et al: Normalization of height in girls with Turner syndrome after long-term growth hormone treatment: Results of a randomized dose-response trial. J Clin Endocrinol Metab. 84:4607–4612, 1999.
9. Zachmann SS, Prader A: Short term testosterone treatment at bone age of 12 to 13 years does not reduce adult height in boys with constitutional delay of growth and adolescence. Helv Pediatr Acta 42:21, 1987.

27. GROWTH HORMONE USE AND ABUSE

Robbie J. Rampy, M.D., and Homer J. LeMar, Jr., M.D..

1. What is growth hormone?

Growth hormone (GH) is a peptide produced and secreted by the anterior pituitary gland. It is the most abundant hormone in the human pituitary gland. Growth hormone secretion is stimulated by growth hormone–releasing hormone (GHRH) and inhibited by somatostatin, both from the hypothalamus. Another major regulator of growth hormone production is insulin-like growth factor–1 (IGF-1), which acts at the pituitary to directly inhibit growth hormone production and at the hypothalamus to inhibit the production of GHRH and to stimulate somatostatin. Humans produce growth hormone throughout their lifetime. Growth hormone production increases at puberty and decreases with aging at an average rate of 14% per decade beyond age 40.

2. What does growth hormone do?

As the name implies, growth hormone stimulates both linear growth and growth of internal organs. Several prominent effects on protein, lipid, and carbohydrate metabolism are also induced. When endogenously secreted or exogenously administered, acute growth hormone effects include increased nitrogen retention, amino acid uptake, and protein synthesis by liver and muscle; increased glucose uptake and utilization by muscle; and antagonism of the lipolytic effect of catecholamines on adipose tissue. Additionally, there are increases in cardiac muscle mass and cardiac output at rest and during maximal exercise, in plasma volume and red cell mass, in bone turnover and bone mineral density, in collagen turnover in nonskeletal sites including tendons, and in rates of sweating and thermal dispersion during exercise. With chronic administration, growth hormone reduces glucose utilization, enhances lipolysis, and continues to increase lean body mass. This may result in an overall change in body composition.

3. Does growth hormone exert all of its effects directly?

No. Many of the effects are mediated by insulin-like growth factor-1 (IGF-1), which is also called somatomedin C. Growth hormone stimulates the production of IGF-1 in peripheral tissues, particularly the liver.

4. How do abnormalities of growth hormone secretion affect health?

Excessive growth hormone secretion during childhood results in gigantism. Robert Wadlow, "the Alton giant," reached a height of just over 8 feet 11 inches and wore size 37AA shoes. Excessive growth hormone production after epiphyseal closure results in acromegaly. Deficiency of growth hormone production in childhood results in short stature (see Chapter 26). Growth hormone deficiency in adults, frequently unrecognized in the past, has been more thoroughly studied in recent years. This disorder most often results from surgery and/or radiation therapy used to treat various types of pituitary tumors. Growth hormone deficiency in adults can result in decreased muscle force, strength, and lean body mass; decreased bone density; decreased extracellular water; increased adiposity; reduced cardiac function; and diminished exercise performance. Patients have reduced aerobic capacity and strength levels and often complain of lethargy and fatigue. Their quality of life is diminished, manifested by depression, anxiety, mental fatigue, and decreased self-esteem and life fulfillment. Excessive intra-abdominal fat is associated with an increased risk of cardiovascular disease, which is the predominant cause of mortality in these patients.

5. Where do we get the growth hormone used therapeutically?

From 1958 to 1985, growth hormone was available only from the pituitaries of human cadavers. Since 1985, biosynthetic growth hormone preparations have allowed production of much larger quantities of growth hormone and markedly improved availability. A requirement for bioassays has become a Food and Drug Administration requisite to substantiate biologic activity among different preparations. The bioassays could be replaced by in vitro binding assays using growth hormone receptors derived from molecular techniques.

6. Besides availability, what problem was associated with growth hormone derived from human cadavers?

Creutzfeldt-Jakob disease, an uncommon, rapidly progressive, and fatal spongiform encephalopathy, has been reported from iatrogenic transmission through human cadaver pituitary tissue. Because of the high cost of recombinant growth hormone, some athletes are purchasing cadaveric-derived growth hormone. More than 30 young adults who had received human cadaver pituitary products have died of this disease, and at least 60–70 cases of Creutzfield-Jakcob disease have been identified in recipients.

7. How is growth hormone used medically?

For several years the only approved indication for growth hormone therapy was treatment of short stature in children with growth hormone deficiency. Recently, growth hormone was also approved for treatment of short stature associated with Turner syndrome and progressive chronic renal insufficiency in children, for wasting in patients with AIDS, and for replacement therapy in growth hormone–deficient adults. Growth hormone has other potential uses: (1) Prader-Willi syndrome; (2) Noonan syndrome; (3) Russell-Silver syndrome; (4) chondrodysplasia in children; (5) short stature associated with intrauterine growth retardation; (6) steroid-induced growth suppression; (7) short stature associated with myelomeningocele; (8) any severe wasting state (e.g., wounds, burns, cancer); (9) normal aging; (10) non–islet-cell tumor hypoglycemia; (11) gonadal dysgenesis; (12) Down syndrome; and (13) short stature associated with neurofibromatosis.

8. How does growth hormone help growth hormone–deficient adults?

The apparent beneficial effects in deficient adults are an increase in muscle mass and function, reduction of total body fat mass, increased plasma volume and improved peripheral blood flow. Reductions in serum total and LDL cholesterol, reduction in diastolic blood pressure, and a trend toward reduction in systolic blood pressure have also been documented. In addition, an improvement in psychological well-being and quality of life can occur with growth hormone replacement. Growth hormone also has beneficial effects on bone metabolism and skeletal mass.

9. What are the therapeutic doses of growth hormone? How is it administered?

The recommended doses in North America for children are from 0.175 mg/kg/week to 0.35 mg/kg/week in growth hormone deficiency, 0.35 mg/kg/week for impaired growth of chronic renal insufficiency, and 0.375 mg/kg/week for Turner syndrome. The dose can be divided into twice-weekly, thrice-weekly, or daily regimens. Daily injections appear to give greater growth velocity than less frequent administration. Currently, the appropriate adult replacement dose appears to be 0.006 mg/kg/day with a maximal dose of 0.0125 mg/kg/day. Growth hormone is administered by subcutaneous injection.

10. Why is growth hormone used as an ergogenic aid by athletes? How is abuse detected?

Athletes have used growth hormone in an effort to improve performance. Supraphysiologic doses of growth hormone have been shown to increase lean body mass and to reduce body fat in trained athletes. To date, there is no reliable way to detect growth hormone use by athletes. During the 2000 Summer Olympics in Sydney, Australia, commentators discussed the use of drugs among athletes and noted the difficulty in growth hormone detection. Detection presents a number of unique problems, in that endogenous growth hormone is secreted naturally in a pulsatile manner, and increased random measurements could reflect a spontaneous peak in secretion, especially when stimulated by acute exercise. In addition, exogenous growth hormone is not distinguishable from endogenous hormone. Furthermore, the release of growth hormone may be affected by nutritional supplements used frequently by athletes. The International Olympic Committee and The European Union have established a collaborative study group to examine the possibility of developing a test to differentiate exogenous growth hormone from endogenous growth hormone secretion in athletes. Most other banned ergogenic drugs, such as anabolic steroids, are difficult to hide from sophisticated assays.

11. How prevalent is growth hormone use among athletes?

The prevalence is not known because abuse is currently undetectable, but there has been an increase in reported growth hormone abuse by athletes over the last decade. There have been several reported recent seizures of growth hormone found in athletes' luggage. The well-publicized seizures of recombinant growth hormone from Chinese swimmers at the World Championships in Perth, Australia, and from Tour de France cyclists in 1998 suggest use at an elite level. Use is probably not as extensive as with anabolic-androgenic steroids. One limiting factor is the expense. Even a 1-month supply may cost several thousand dollars, depending on doses. In addition, some athletes who have tried growth hormone have reportedly been disappointed with the results.

12. What are the adverse effects of the therapeutic use of growth hormone?

Fluid retention causing edema and carpal tunnel syndrome are common in adults but not in children. Pseudotumor cerebri has been reported in children; this is most common in children with renal disease, although it has also been observed in children with growth hormone deficiency and in girls with Turner syndrome. Growth hormone therapy is associated with an increased risk of slipped capital femoral epiphysis in the same three groups of children. Children with growth hormone deficiency due to deletion of the growth hormone gene may develop antibodies to growth hormone with secondary growth deceleration. This phenomenon is rare in other children. Elderly men may develop gynecomastia. Arthralgias and myalgias are also common (5–41%) in adults. Carbohydrate intolerance and diabetes are theoretical problems but appear to be unusual and limited mostly to people with risk factors. No data support an increased risk of nonleukemic extracranial neoplasms with therapeutic growth hormone use. To date, more than 50 cases of leukemia have been reported in growth–hormone treated patients, but it is limited to patients with risk factors or syndromes associated with the development of leukemia. Other potential side effects include prepubertal gynecomastia, pancreatitis, behavioral changes, worsening of neurofibromatosis, scoliosis and kyphosis, and hypertrophy of tonsils and adenoids. All patients receiving growth hormone treatment must be regularly monitored for potential side effects.

13. What adverse effects occur in athletes using growth hormone?

Little is known about side effects of growth hormone use in athletes. One may speculate that athletes use higher than therapeutic doses and for prolonged periods. Chronic abuse of supraphysiologic doses of growth hormone may lead to features of acromegaly, including coarsening of the facial features, osteoarthritis, irreversible bone and joint deformities, increased vascular, respiratory and cardiac abnormalities, hypertrophy of other organs, hypogonadism, diabetes mellitus, abnormal lipid metabolism, increased risk of breast and colon cancer, and muscle weakness due to myopathy. Clearly, in this scenario the risk to athletes is potentially high.

BIBLIOGRAPHY

1. Allen DB: Safety of human growth hormone therapy: Current topics. J Pediatr 128(Suppl):S8–S13, 1996.
2. Azcona C, Preece MA, Rose SJ, et al: Growth response to rhIGF-I 80 μg/kg twice daily in children with growth hormone insensitivity syndrome: Relationship to severity of clinical phenotype. Clin Endocrinol 51: 787–792, 1999.
3. Blethen SL: Monitoring growth hormone treatment: Safety considerations. Endocrinologist 6: 369–374, 1996.
4. Bouillanne O, Raenfray M, Tissandier O, et al: Growth hormone therapy in elderly people: An age delaying drug? Fundament Clin Pharmacol 10:416–430, 1996.
5. Hintz RL: Current and potential therapeutic uses of growth hormone and insulin-like growth factor I. Endocrinol Metab Clin North Am 25:759–773, 1996.
6. Hurel SJ, Koppiker N, Newkirk, J, et al: Relationship of physical exercise and ageing to growth hormone production. Clin Endocrinol 51: 687–691, 1999.
7. Jenkins PJ: Growth hormone and exercise. Clini Endocrinol 50:683–689, 1999.
8. Kemp SF: Growth hormone therapeutic practice: Dosing issues. Endocrinologist 6:231–237, 1996.
9. Murray RD, Skillicorn CJ, Howell SJ, et al: Influences on quality of life in GH deficient adults and their effect on response to treatment. Clini Endocrinol 51: 565–573, 1999.
10. Reiter EO, Rosenfeld RG: Normal and aberrant growth. In Wilson: Williams Textbook of Endocrinology, 9th ed. Philadelphia, WB Saunders, 1998, pp 1427–1507.
11. Rodrigues-Arnao J, Jabbar J, Fulcher K, et al: Effects of growth hormone replacement on physical performance and body composition in GH deficient adults. Clin Endocrinol 51: 53–60, 1999.
12. Russell-Jones DL, Weissberger AJ: The role of growth hormone in the regulation of body composition in the adult. Growth Regul 6:247–252, 1996.
13. Thorner MO, Vance ML, Laws ER Jr, et al: The anterior pituitary. In Wilson:Williams Textbook of Endocrinology, 9th ed. Philadelphia, WB Saunders, 1998, pp 249–340.
14. Wallace JD, Cuneo RC: Growth hormone abuse in athletes: A review. Endocrinologist 10:175–184, 2000
15. Zachwieja JJ, Yarasheski EK: Does growth hormone therapy in conjunction with resistance exercise increase muscle force production and muscle mass in men and women qged 60 years or older? Physical Therapy 79:76–81, 1999

IV. Adrenal Disorders

28. PRIMARY ALDOSTERONISM

Arnold A. Asp, M.D.

1. What is primary aldosteronism?

Primary aldosteronism is a generic term for a group of disorders in which excessive production of aldosterone by the zona glomerulosa of the adrenal cortex occurs independently of normal renin-angiotensin stimulation. These primary disorders of the adrenal system are distinct from forms of secondary hyperaldosteronism due to excessive renin, such as renal artery stenosis. The five clinical entities comprising primary aldosteronism include solitary aldosterone-producing adenoma (APA), bilateral hyperplasia of the zona glomerulosa (also known as idiopathic hyperaldosteronism or IHA), primary adrenal hyperplasia, adrenal carcinoma, and glucocorticoid-remediable aldosteronism.

The terms "aldosteronism" and "hyperaldosteronism" are used interchangeably in the literature. This chapter uses the most common designation for each disorder.

2. How common are these disorders?

The most common manifestation of hyperaldosteronism is hypertension. It is estimated that 0.05–2.0% of the hypertensive population may have primary aldosteronism.

3. What are the common clinical manifestations of primary aldosteronism?

Aldosterone normally acts at the renal distal convoluted tubule to stimulate reabsorption of sodium ions (Na^+) as well as secretion of potassium (K^+) and hydrogen ions (H^+) and at the cortical and medullary collecting ducts to cause direct secretion of H^+. Excess secretion of aldosterone in primary aldosteronism results in hypertension, hypokalemia, and metabolic alkalosis; hypomagnesemia can also develop. Spontaneous hypokalemia (< 3.5 mEq/L) occurs in 80% of cases of primary aldosteronism; the remaining patients develop hypokalemia within 3–5 days of initiation of liberal sodium intake (150 mEq/day). Most symptoms cited by patients are manifestations of hypokalemia: weakness, muscle cramping,

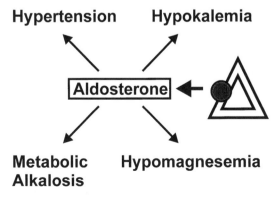

Primary aldosteronism.

paresthesias, headaches, palpitations, polyuria, and polydipsia. Glucose intolerance due to insulinopenia occurs in approximately 25% of patients.

4. When and in whom is primary aldosteronism most common?

This group of disorders affects more women than men and occurs most commonly in the third through fifth decades of life.

5. What is the most common form of primary aldosteronism?

Of the five causes mentioned in question 1, solitary aldosterone-producing adenomas (APAs) are most common, accounting for up to 65% of cases in most series. APAs are small (< 2 cm), occur more commonly in the left adrenal gland, and are composed of zona glomerulosa cells, zona reticularis cells, and hybrid cells with characteristics of both layers. Adenomas produce greater amounts of aldosterone than do other forms of aldosteronism; consequently, the degree of hypertension and the extent of biochemical abnormalities tend to be more severe. APAs also secrete excess 18-hydroxycorticosterone (18-OHB), an immediate precursor of aldosterone produced by hydroxylation of corticosterone; this facilitates the biochemical diagnosis. APAs demonstrate partial autonomy of function, secreting aldosterone in response to stimulation by corticotropin (ACTH) but not by angiotensin II. Aldosterone synthesis by these tumors, therefore, parallels the normal circadian rhythm of ACTH secretion, with the highest serum aldosterone concentrations occurring in the mornings and the lowest in the evenings. APAs are also known as Conn's syndrome.

6. What is the second most common cause of primary aldosteronism?

Idiopathic hyperaldosteronism (IHA), also known as bilateral adrenal glomerulosa hyperplasia, makes up approximately 30% of cases of primary aldosteronism. IHA is characterized by bilateral hyperplasia (diffuse and focal) of the zona glomerulosa layer of both adrenal glands. Because both glands appear to be hyperstimulated, the presence of a circulating secretagogue has been postulated. The most likely cause, however, is a supranormal sensitivity of the zona glomerulosa in affected adrenal glands to physiologic concentrations of angiotensin II. Aldosterone is produced in smaller amounts in IHA than in APA; therefore, the degree of hypertension, hypokalemia, hypomagnesemia, and metabolic alkalosis is less dramatic. Serum aldosterone levels tend to increase during upright posture, perhaps owing to increased sensitivity to angiotensin II.

7. How commonly does adrenal cancer cause primary aldosteronism?

The literature reports fewer than 20 cases. The tumors are very large (> 6 cm) and usually have metastasized by the time of diagnosis.

8. What is primary adrenal hyperplasia?

In this seemingly rare clinical entity (which may be more commonly recognized in the future), the zona glomerulosa of one adrenal gland becomes hyperplastic and histopathologically resembles unilateral IHA. Biochemically, however, such cases more closely resemble APA and respond to surgical resection.

9. What is glucocorticoid-remediable aldosteronism?

In this rare cause of aldosteronism, production of mineralocorticoid is stimulated solely by ACTH. The disorder is inherited in an autosomal-dominant fashion. Although there are fewer than 100 cases reported in 17 kindreds, the syndrome illustrates important aspects of the genetic control of steroid synthesis. Humans possess two mitochondrial 11 β-hydroxylase isoenzymes that are responsible for cortisol and aldosterone synthesis (designated CYP11B1 and CYP11B2). Both are encoded on chromosome 8. CYP11B1, which is responsible for conversion of 11-deoxycortisol to cortisol, is expressed only in the zona reticularis. CYP11B2, which is responsible for the conversion of corticosterone to aldosterone, is expressed only in the zona glomerulosa. CYP11B1 activity is stimulated by ACTH, whereas CYP11B2 is stimulated by angiotensin II or hypokalemia.

Glucocorticoid-remediable aldosteronism results from a heritable mutation that causes the fusion of the promoter region of the CYP11B1 gene with the structural region of the CYP11B2 gene. The resulting chimeric gene responds to ACTH with overproduction of aldosterone as well as precursors 18-hydroxycortisol and 18-oxocortisol. These metabolites of the cortisol C-18 oxidation pathway are biochemical markers that facilitate identification of affected kindreds. Excessive secretion of aldosterone may be inhibited by administration of glucocorticoids that suppress secretion of ACTH by the pituitary.

10. How are patients screened for primary aldosteronism?

The diagnosis of primary aldosteronism is based on the demonstration of inappropriately elevated levels of plasma aldosterone (PA) with concomitantly suppressed plasma renin activity (PRA). Unfortunately, there is no single specific and sensitive screening test. Hypokalemia (K<3.5 mEq/L) is often the first clue.

One method of screening the hypertensive, hypokalemic patient is to discontinue diuretics, beta blockers, and inhibitors of angiotensin-converting enzyme (ACE) for at least 2 weeks. Prazosin may be used to control hypertension. The patient is allowed to consume at least 150 mEq of sodium daily, and potassium supplements are administered to maintain the serum potassium > 3.5 mEq/L. Then, while the patient assumes an upright posture, blood samples for assessment of PA and PRA are drawn. A 24-hour urine collection for aldosterone also should be collected. A ratio of PA (in ng/dl) to PRA (in ng/ml/hr) that exceeds 20 raises the possibility of primary aldosteronism. Because 12% of patients may have PA:PRA ratios lower than 20, review of the urinary aldosterone value is helpful. Urinary excretion of aldosterone (18-monogluconide) that exceeds 20 mg/day is also suggestive of primary aldosteronism.

11. How is the diagnosis of primary aldosteronism confirmed?

Several diagnostic schemas may be used to confirm the diagnosis of primary aldosteronism. The following protocol not only confirms the diagnosis but also aids in identification of the specific disorder.

The patient is instructed to consume at least 150 mEq of sodium each day of the week before testing. Ample potassium supplements are given to ensure a serum potassium level greater than 3.5 mEq/L. The patient is then admitted in the evening and remains recumbent overnight. At 8:00 AM, levels of PA, PRA, and 18-OHB are determined while the patient is supine. The patient then assumes an upright posture and/or ambulates for 4 hours, after which levels of PA and PRA are again determined.

In normal and essential hypertensive patients, a high sodium diet suppresses PA, whereas upright posture for 4 hours stimulates PRA. In patients with primary aldosteronism, excessive sodium does not suppress synthesis of aldosterone; supine levels of PA at 8:00 AM exceed 15 ng/dl. Because excessive aldosterone in such patients causes intravascular expansion, PRA is undetectable (< 1 ng/ml/hr) and remains suppressed despite 4 hours of upright posture. An unsuppressed PA with a concomitant unstimulated PRA confirms the diagnosis of primary aldosteronism.

Some centers rely on a saline-loading procedure rather than a high-salt diet to assess suppression of aldosterone. In this test, 2 liters of saline solution are administered intravenously over 4 hours. PRA, PA, and 18-OHB are determined at the beginning, and PRA and PA at the conclusion of the test. As in the previous test, patients with primary aldosteronism should demonstrate undetectable levels of PRA, whereas PA should exceed 15 ng/dl before and after saline loading.

Differentiation of APA from IHA is also possible with the above data. APAs produce greater amounts of aldosterone and can be stimulated by ACTH. Patients with APA, therefore, have greater PA levels at 8:00 AM, and these levels decrease over the ensuing 4 hours as normal secretion of ACTH diminishes. Patients with IHA, on the other hand, have somewhat lower levels of PA at 8:00 AM, and they experience increase with upright ambulation. Finally, APAs produce large amounts of 18-OHB; levels > 100 μg/dl occur only in APA and primary adrenal hyperplasia.

12. Is it important to differentiate APA from IHA?

Yes. APA is amenable to surgical resection of the involved adrenal gland, whereas IHA is usually treated medically.

13. Does computed tomography (CT) or magnetic resonance imaging (MRI) aid in differentiation?

To a limited extent, both localizing procedures may aid in identifying the cause of primary aldosteronism. A large APA may be discernible on high-resolution CT, which at some institutions can identify adenomas as small as 5 mm. MRI at present performs as well as CT in identifying APA but involves higher cost and longer scan time. The diagnostic accuracy of MRI or CT in preoperatively localizing an APA is approximately 70–85%. Neither modality is able to differentiate IHA from a small APA. Adrenal carcinoma, a rare cause of excessive aldosterone, is easily identified with either modality.

14. Are other localizing tests of help if CT or MRI fails to identify an APA when biochemical data indicate the presence of an adenoma?

Yes. The least invasive is a radionuclide test with NP-59 (6b-^{131}I-iodomethyl-19-norcholesterol). In this procedure, supraphysiologic doses of dexamethasone are administered to the patient for 7 days in an attempt to suppress adrenal cortical activity. NP-59, which is incorporated into steroid molecules by the adrenal cortex, is then administered to the patient on the fourth day of the procedure. The patient is imaged under a γ-camera. If an APA is present, NP-59 is concentrated within the tumor, which becomes visible on the scan. IHA does not visualize. Accuracy of the procedure is approximately 70%.

A more accurate, but hazardous, localizing procedure to differentiate a normal adrenal gland from one containing an adenoma is adrenal venous sampling. In this procedure, catheters are introduced into the left and right adrenal veins and the inferior vena cava. Levels of PA are determined from these sites, along with concomitant levels of cortisol. APAs produce large amounts of aldosterone; the normal concentration of PA is 100–400 ng/dl, whereas APAs may generate concentrations of 1,000–10,000 ng/dl. The ratio of PA produced on the affected side vs. the unaffected side always exceeds 10:1. Cortisol levels are determined to ensure that the adrenal veins are properly catheterized. Therein is the difficulty with adrenal venous sampling. Collection of aldosterone and cortisol from the left adrenal gland is relatively simple, because the venous effluent drains directly into the left renal vein. The venous flow from the right adrenal, however, flows directly into the inferior vena cava. Catheterization of the right adrenal vein is difficult because of the few angiographic landmarks. Contrast material used to localize the right adrenal gland can cause corticomedullary hemorrhage during the procedure (10% incidence). Overall, the procedure is 90% accurate in localizing APA.

15. How is the patient with APA managed?

The patient undergoes screening tests, as described in question 10. The diagnosis of primary aldosteronism is confirmed with salt loading, as described in question 11. Levels of aldosterone are elevated but decline during the course of ambulation. 18-OHB exceeds 100 μg/dl. All such findings indicate the probability of APA. If the patient is fortunate, CT scan reveals a unilateral adenoma. If an APA is not visible on CT or if the physician is concerned about a concomitant incidental nonfunctioning adenoma, NP-59 radionuclide imaging is appropriate, or adrenal venous sampling may be performed by an experienced angiographer.

After the APA is localized, unilateral adrenalectomy is performed. Laparoscopic resection is now widely available and may be preferable to the "standard" posterior approach. One year postoperatively, 70% of patients are normotensive. By the fifth postoperative year, only 53% remain normotensive. Normal potassium balance tends to be permanent.

16. Do all patients with APA require surgery?

Although surgical resection is preferred, patients who have other comorbid conditions that preclude surgery may be successfully treated medically as described in the next question.

17. How is a patient with IHA managed?

The patient undergoes screening and confirmatory tests, as described in questions 10 and 11. Concentrations of aldosterone are elevated but continue to rise with ambulation over 4 hours. Levels of 18-OHB are less than 100 μg/dl. CT fails to reveal unilateral enlargement of the adrenals. NP-59 imaging fails to visualize an adenoma. Adrenal venous sampling fails to lateralize. After the diagnosis of IHA is made, the patient is scrupulously sequestered from surgical colleagues.

Pharmacologic therapy is quite effective. The agent of choice is spironolactone (50–200 mg twice daily), a competitive inhibitor of aldosterone. Hypokalemia corrects dramatically, whereas hypertension responds after 4–8 weeks. Unfortunately, spironolactone also inhibits synthesis of testosterone and peripheral action of androgens, causing decreased libido, impotence, and gynecomastia in men. In patients intolerant of spironolactone, amiloride (5–15 mg twice daily) corrects hypokalemia within several days. A concomitant antihypertensive agent is usually necessary to reduce blood pressure. Success also has been reported in cases of IHA treated with calcium channel blockers (calcium is involved in the final common pathway for production of aldosterone) and ACE inhibitors (IHA appears to be sensitive to low concentrations of angiotensin II).

18. How is a patient with primary adrenal hyperplasia (PAH) managed?

During evaluation, these rare cases appear to be APA. Screening and confirmatory tests, as described in questions 10 and 11, seemingly indicate an APA. Levels of 18-OHB exceed 100 μg/dl. Localizing tests are consistent with APA, and patients usually undergo surgical resection of a nodular hyperplastic gland. The diagnosis is made retrospectively, but surgery is curative.

19. How is a patient with glucocorticoid-remediable aldosteronism managed?

This disorder is discussed in question 9. Therapy with low doses of dexamethasone (0.75 mg/day) or any of the agents used for therapy of IHA (see question 17) may be effective.

BIBLIOGRAPHY

1. Artega E, Klein R, Biglieri EG: Use of the saline infusion test to diagnose the cause of primary aldosteronism. Am J Med 79:722–728, 1985.
2. Biglieri EG, Shambelin M, Hirai J, et al: The significance of elevated levels of plasma 18-hydroxy-corticosterone in patients with primary aldosteronism. J Clin Endocrinol Metab 49:87–91, 1979.
3. Blevins LS, Wand GS: Primary aldosteronism: An endocrine perspective. Radiology 184: 599–600, 1992.
4. Blumenfeld JD, Sealey JE, Schlussel Y, et al: Diagnosis and treatment of primary hyperaldosteronism. Ann Intern Med 121:877–885, 1994.

5. Bornstein SR, moderator: Adrenocortical tumors: recent advances in basic concepts and clinical management. Ann Intern Med 130: 759–771, 1999.
6. Dluhy RG, Lifton RP: Glucocorticoid-remediable aldosteronism. J Clin Endocrinol Metab 84: 4341–4344, 1999.
7. Fardella CE, Mosso L, Gomez-Sanchez C, et al: Primary hyperaldosteronism in essential hypertensives: Prevalence, biochemical profile, and molecular biology. J Clin Endocrinol Metab 85: 1863–1867, 2000.
8. Ghose RP, Hall PM, Bravo EL: Medical management of aldosterone-producing adenomas. Ann Intern Med 131:105–108, 1999.
9. Jossart GH, Burpee SE, Gagner M: Surgery of the adrenal glands. Endocrinol Metab North Am 29:57–68, 2000.
10. Liftin RP, Dluhy RG, Powers M, et al: A chimaeric 11-hydroxylase/aldosterone synthetase gene causes glucocorticoid-remediable aldosteronism and human hypertension. Nature 355:262–265, 1992.
11. Melby JC: Diagnosis of hyperaldosteronism. Endocrinol Metab Clin North Am 20:247–255, 1991.
12. Sohaib SA, Peppercorn PD, Allen C. et al: Primary hyperaldosteronism (Conn syndrome): MR imaging findings. Radiology 214:527–531, 2000.
13. Vallotton MB: Primary aldosteronism. Part I: Diagnosis of primary hyperaldosteronism. Clin Endocrinol 45:47–52, 1996.
14. Vallotton MB: Primary aldosteronism. Part II: Differential diagnosis of primary hyperaldosteronism and pseudoaldosteronism. Clin Endocrinol 45:53–60, 1996.
15. White PC: Disorders of aldosterone biosynthesis and action. N Engl J Med 331:250–258, 1994.
16. White PC, Curnow KM, Pascoe L: Disorders of steroid 11-hydroxylase isoenzymes. Endocrine Rev 15:421–438, 1994.
17. Young WF, Hogan MJ, Klee GG, et al: Primary aldosteronism: Diagnosis and treatment. Mayo Clin Proc 65:96–110, 1990.

29. PHEOCHROMOCYTOMA

Arnold A. Asp, M.D.

1. What is a pheochromocytoma?

A pheochromocytoma is an adrenal medullary tumor composed of chromaffin cells and capable of secreting biogenic amines and peptides, including epinephrine, norepinephrine, and dopamine. Such tumors arise from neural crest–derived cells, which also give rise to portions of the central nervous system and the sympathetic (paraganglion) system. Because of this common origin, neoplasms of the sympathetic ganglia, such as neuroblastomas, paragangliomas, and ganglioneuromas, may produce similar amines and peptides.

2. How common are pheochromocytomas?

Pheochromocytomas are relatively rare. Data from the Mayo Clinic indicate that pheochromocytomas occur in 1–2/100,000 adults/year; autopsy data from the same institution reflect an incidence of 0.3%. The incidence of pheochromocytoma from other countries, such as Japan, is lower: 0.4 cases/million/year.

3. Where are the tumors located?

Nearly 90% of tumors arise within the adrenal glands, whereas approximately 10% are extra-adrenal and therefore classified as paragangliomas. Sporadic, solitary pheochromocytomas are located more commonly in the right adrenal gland, whereas familial forms (10% of all pheochromocytomas) are bilateral and multicentric. Bilateral adrenal tumors raise the possibility of multiple endocrine neoplasia 2A or 2B (MEN-2A or MEN-2B) syndromes (see Chapter 54). Paragangliomas occur most commonly within the abdomen but also have been described along the entire sympathetic paraganglia chain from the base of the brain to the testicles. The most common locations for paragangliomas are the organ of Zuckerkandl, the aortic bifurcation, and the bladder wall; the mediastinum, heart, carotid arteries, and glomus jugulare bodies are less common locations.

4. Can pheochromocytomas metastasize?

Yes. Demonstration of a metastatic focus in tissue normally devoid of chromaffin cells is the only accepted indication that a pheochromocytoma is malignant. Metastasis occurs in 3–14% of cases. The most common sites of metastases include regional lymph nodes, liver, bone, lung, and muscle.

5. What is the rule of 10s for pheochromocytomas?

Approximately 10% are extra-adrenal, 10% are bilateral, 10% are familial, and 10% are malignant.

6. What are the common clinical features of a pheochromocytoma?

The signs and symptoms of a pheochromocytoma are variable. The classic triad of sudden severe headaches, diaphoresis, and palpitations carries a high degree of specificity (94%) and sensitivity (91%) for pheochromocytoma in a hypertensive population. The absence of all three symptoms reliably excludes the condition. Hypertension occurs in 90–95% of cases and is paroxysmal in 25–50% of these. Orthostatic hypotension occurs in 40% because of hypovolemia and impaired arterial and venous constriction responses. Tremor and pallor also may be accompanying signs, whereas flushing is uncommonly encountered. Other symptoms include anxiety and constipation.

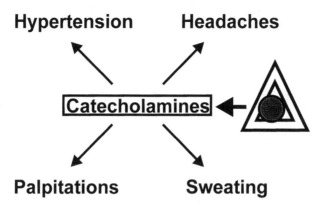

Classic manifestations of pheochromocytoma.

7. What are some of the nonclassic manifestations of pheochromocytomas?

Signs and symptoms of other endocrine disorders may dominate the presentation of a pheochromocytoma. Tumors have been reported to elaborate corticotropin (ACTH) with resultant manifestations of Cushing's syndrome and hypokalemic alkalosis. Vasoactive intestinal peptide has been produced in several cases, resulting in severe diarrhea. Hyperglycemia, owing to catecholamine-associated antagonism of insulin release, and hypercalcemia, as a result of adrenergic stimulation of the parathyroid glands or elaboration of parathyroid hormone–related peptide (PTHrP), also have been encountered. Lactic acidosis may be observed as a result of catecholamine-associated decrements in tissue oxygen delivery with concomitant increases in oxygen utilization.

Cardiovascular manifestations of pheochromocytomas include arrhythmias and catecholamine-induced congestive cardiomyopathy. Atrial and ventricular fibrillations commonly result from precipitous release of catecholamines during surgery or from therapy with tricyclic antidepressants, phenothiazines, metoclopramide, and naloxone. Although cardiogenic pulmonary edema may result from cardiomyopathy, noncardiogenic pulmonary edema also may occur as a result of transient pulmonary vasoconstriction and increased capillary permeability. Finally, seizures, altered mental status, and cerebral infarctions may occur as a result of intracerebral hemorrhage or embolization.

8. What do pheochromocytomas elaborate?

Most pheochromocytomas secrete norepinephrine. Tumors that produce epinephrine are more commonly intra-adrenal, because the extra-adrenal sympathetic ganglia do not contain phenylethanolamine-N-methyltransferase (PNMT), which converts norepinephrine to epinephrine. Dopamine is most commonly associated with malignant tumors.

9. Why is the blood pressure response among patients with pheochromocytomas so variable?

Blood pressures vary so widely among patients with pheochromocytomas for several reasons:

1. The tumors elaborate different biogenic amines. Epinephrine (EPI), a beta-adrenergic stimulatory vasodilator that causes hypotension, is secreted by some intraadrenal tumors, whereas norepinephrine (NE), an alpha stimulatory vasoconstrictor that causes hypertension, is produced by most intraadrenal and all extra-adrenal tumors.

2. Tumor size indirectly correlates with concentrations of plasma catecholamines. Large tumors (> 50 g) manifest slow turnover rates and release catecholamine degrada-

tion products, whereas small tumors (< 50 g) with rapid turnover rates elaborate active catecholamines.

3. Tissue responsiveness to ambient concentrations of catecholamines does not remain constant. Prolonged exposure of tissue to increased plasma catecholamines causes down-regulation of alpha$_1$-receptors and tachyphylaxis. Plasma catecholamine levels, therefore, do not correlate with mean arterial pressure.

10. How is a pheochromocytoma diagnosed?

The diagnosis depends on the demonstration of excessive amounts of catecholamines in plasma or urine or degradation products in urine. The most widely used tests involve measurement of urinary metanephrine (MN), normetanephrine (NMN), vanillylmandelic acid (VMA), and free catecholamines produced in a 24-hour period. The ability of such tests to differentiate pheochromocytomas from essential hypertension varies among institutions: for VMA, sensitivity is 28–56% and specificity is 98%; for MN and NMN, sensitivity is 67–91% and specificity is 100%; and for free catecholamines, sensitivity is 100% and specificity is 98%. Many groups advocate 24-hour urinary levels of MN and catecholamines as good screening tests. Yield is improved when urine is collected after a paroxysmal episode of symptoms.

Direct measurement of plasma catecholamines (NE and EPI), collected from an indwelling venous catheter at rest, may contribute to diagnostic accuracy of timed urine assays. Levels greater than 2000 pg/ml are abnormal and suggestive of pheochromocytoma, whereas levels less than 500 pg/ml are normal and levels of 500–2000 pg/ml are equivocal.

11. What conditions may alter the above diagnostic tests?

Older assays for VMA were sensitive to dietary vanillin and phenolic acids, requiring patients to restrict their intake of such substances. High-pressure liquid chromatography assays have eliminated most false-positive results due to diet and drugs. The following list includes some of the more common drugs and conditions that may obfuscate the diagnosis of pheochromocytoma:

Drugs that alter metabolism of catecholamines:
Reduce plasma and urine concentrations: alpha$_2$ agonists, calcium channel blockers (chronic), angiotensin-converting enzyme inhibitors, bromocriptine
Decrease VMA and increase catecholamines and MN: methyldopa, monoamine oxidase inhibitors
Increase plasma or urine catecholamines: alpha$_1$ blockers, beta blockers, labetalol
Produce variable changes in any test: phenothiazines, tricyclic antidepressants, levodopa

Interfering medications:
Decrease MN: methylglucamine in radiocontrast agents
Decrease urinary catecholamines: methenamine mandelate
Decrease VMA: clofibrate
Increase VMA: nalidixic acid

Miscellaneous conditions:
Stimulation of endogenous catecholamines: physiologic stress (ischemia, exercise), drug withdrawal (alcohol, clonidine), vasodilator therapy (nitroglycerin, acute administration of calcium channel blockers)
Exogenous catecholamines: appetite suppressants, decongestants

12. What other biochemical tests are available?

Cases in which screening tests are equivocal may warrant a clonidine suppression test. This test employs a centrally acting alpha$_2$ agonist that, in patients without a pheochromocytoma, suppresses neurogenically mediated release of catecholamines through the sympathetic nervous system. Blood samples to assess plasma catecholamines (NE and EPI) are drawn through an indwelling venous catheter; clonidine, 0.3 mg, is administered orally; and plasma catecholamines are sampled again at 1, 2, and 3 hours. Plasma catecholamines decrease to less than 500 pg/ml in patients with essential hypertension but exceed this level in patients with pheochromocytomas.

The glucagon stimulation test has been proposed for patients in whom clinical features are highly suggestive of a pheochromocytoma, but whose plasma catecholamines are < 1000 pg/ml. After an intravenous bolus of 1–2 mg of glucagon, patients with pheochromocytomas manifest a 3-fold increase in levels of plasma catecholamines (at least > 2000 pg/ml) and a rise in blood pressure of at least 20/15 mmHg. The hazard associated with increased blood pressure can be attenuated by pretreatment with calcium channel or alpha-adrenergic blockade. This test is used less frequently than the clonidine suppression test.

Chromogranin A is a soluble protein stored with NE and released from catecholamine storage vesicles. Chromogranin A may be elevated by pheochromocytomas as well as by other neuroendocrine tumors.

13. How are pheochromocytomas localized?

The majority of tumors are larger than 3 cm, rendering them detectable by computed tomographic (CT) or magnetic resonance imaging (MRI) studies. CT, with special attention to the adrenal glands and pelvis, is advocated as the initial localizing procedure (97% are intra-abdominal). Many also recommend MRI as an adjunctive localizing modality. Advantages of MRI include the lack of radiation exposure and the characteristic hyperintense image on T_2-weighted scans. The hyperintense image allows definition of tumor size, differentiation from vascular structures, and identification of unsuspected metastases. Scintigraphic localization with m-(^{131}I) iodobenzylguanidine (MIBG) may also reveal unsuspected metastases. MIBG is actively concentrated by sympathomedullary tissue and is subject to interference by drugs that block reuptake of catecholamines (tricyclic antidepressants, guanethidine, labetalol). Performance criteria of each localizing procedure are depicted below:

	CT (%)	MRI (%)	MIBG (%)
Sensitivity	98	100	78
Specificity	70	67	100
Positive predictive value	69	83	100
Negative predictive value	98	100	87

14. How are pheochromocytomas treated?

Surgical resection is the only definitive therapy. Preoperative preparation with alpha blockade reduces the incidence of intraoperative hypertensive crisis and postoperative hypotension. The most commonly used agent is phenoxybenzamine, a long-acting, noncompetitive antagonist (10–20 mg 2–3 times/day, advanced to 80–100 mg/day), or prazosin, a short-acting antagonist (1 mg 3 times/day, advanced to 5 mg 3 times/day). Therapy may be limited by hypotension, tachycardia, and dizziness. Goals of therapy include blood pressure < 160/90, an electrocardiogram free of ST- or T-wave changes over 2 weeks before surgery, and no more than one premature ventricular contraction/15 min. Opinions about the duration of preparation vary between 7 and 28 days before surgery. Beta blockade to control tachycardia is added only after alpha-adrenergic blockade has been instituted to prevent unopposed alpha stimulation. Other agents used in the preoperative period include labetalol or calcium channel blockers. Intraoperative hypertension associated with tumor manipulation may be controlled with either phentolamine or nitroprusside. Postoperative hypotension may be minimized by preoperative volume expansion with crystalloid.

15. How are malignant pheochromocytomas treated?

Although evidence of malignancy may be discovered at the time of surgery, metastases from slow-growing pheochromocytomas may remain unapparent for several years. Therapy is rarely curative, because the tumors respond poorly to radiotherapy and chemotherapy; treatment is therefore palliative. Surgical debulking is the therapy of choice, followed by use of alpha-methyltyrosine. This drug is a "false" catecholamine precursor that inhibits tyrosine hydroxylase (the rate-limiting enzyme in catecholamine synthesis) and reduces excessive production of catecholamines. Combination chemotherapy with cyclophosphamide, vincristine, and adriamycin may slow tumor growth, as may ablation with MIBG. Unfortunately, neither of these therapeutic measures has resulted in prolonged survival. Prognosis, however, is not dismal; cases of 20-year survival have been reported, and the 5-year survival rate with malignant pheochromocytomas is 44%.

16. Which medical conditions are associated with pheochromocytomas?

MEN-2A: hyperparathyroidism, medullary carcinoma of the thyroid, pheochromocytoma

MEN-2B: medullary carcinoma of the thyroid, marfanoid habitus, pheochromocytoma

Carney's triad: paragangliomas, gastric epithelial leiomyosarcomas, benign pulmonary chondromas (females), and Leydig cell tumors (males)

Neurofibromatosis: café-au-lait spots in 5% of patients with pheochromocytoma; 1% of patients with neurofibromatosis have pheochromocytomas

Von Hippel–Lindau syndrome: retinal and cerebellar hemangioblastomas; as many as 10% may have pheochromocytomas

BIBLIOGRAPHY

1. Bravo EL: Evolving concepts in the pathophysiology, diagnosis and treatment of pheochromocytoma. Endocrine Rev 15:356–368, 1994.
2. Bravo EL: Pheochromocytoma: New concepts and future trends. Kidney Int 40:544–566, 1991.
3. Bravo EL, Tarazi RC, Fouad FM, et al: Clonidine-suppression test. A useful aid in the diagnosis of pheochromocytoma. N Engl J Med 305:623–626, 1981.
4. Francis IR, Gross MD, Shapiro B, et al: Integrated imaging of adrenal disease. Radiology 187: 1–13, 1992.
5. Golub MS, Tuck ML: Diagnostic and therapeutic strategies in pheochromocytoma. Endocrinologist 2:101–105, 1992.
6. Jossart GH, Burpee SE, Gagner M: Surgery of the adrenal glands. Endocrinol Metab North Am 29:57–68, 2000.
7. Krane NK: Clinically unsuspected pheochromocytomas: Experience at Henry Ford Hospital and a review of the literature. Arch Intern Med 146:54–57, 1986.
8. Prys-Roberts C: Phaeochromocytoma—recent progress in management. Br J Anaesth 85:44–57, 2000.
9. Sheps SG, Jiang N, Klee GG, van Heerden JA: Recent developments in the diagnosis and treatment of pheochromocytoma. Mayo Clin Proc 65:88–95, 1990.
10. Sjoberg RS, Simcic K, Kidd GS: The clonidine suppression test for pheochromocytoma. A review of its utility and pitfalls. Arch Intern Med 152:1193–1197, 1992.
11. Wittles RM, Kaplan EL, Roizen MF: Sensitivity of diagnostic and localization tests for pheochromocytoma in clinical practice. Arch Intern Med 160:2521–2524, 2000.

30. ADRENAL MALIGNANCIES

Michael T. McDermott, M.D.

1. What types of cancer occur in the adrenal glands?
Carcinomas may arise in the adrenal cortex (adrenocortical carcinomas) or the adrenal medulla (malignant pheochromocytomas). They also may metastasize to the adrenals from other primary sites.

2. Do adrenocortical carcinomas produce hormones?
Approximately 50–70% of adrenocortical carcinomas secrete steroid hormones, whereas 30–50% are nonfunctioning.

3. What are the clinical features of functioning adrenocortical carcinomas?
Functioning adrenocortical carcinomas secrete aldosterone, cortisol, or androgens—alone or in combination. Excessive aldosterone (Conn's syndrome) causes hypertension and hypokalemia. Overproduction of cortisol results in the development of Cushing's syndrome. Excessive androgen secretion causes hirsutism and virilization in women and abnormal precocious puberty in children but is often asymptomatic in men.

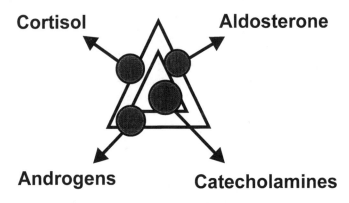

Functioning adrenal tumors.

4. What are the clinical features of nonfunctioning adrenocortical carcinomas?
Nonfunctioning adrenocortical carcinomas present clinically as abdominal or flank pain or as an adrenal mass discovered incidentally during an imaging procedure.

5. What clues are most suggestive that an adrenocortical tumor is malignant?
Malignancy is most strongly suggested by elevated urinary excretion of 17-ketosteroids, tumor size greater than 6 cm, and evidence of locally invasive or metastatic disease to the liver or lungs. However, the diagnosis of malignancy is frequently not suspected until the tumor is examined histologically after its removal.

6. What is the treatment for an adrenocortical carcinoma?
The treatment of choice is surgery. Mitotane, an adrenal cytotoxic agent, has produced

partial or complete tumor regression, reduced production of adrenal hormones, and improved survival in nonrandomized, noncontrolled trials. The combination of mitotane with etoposide, cisplatin and doxorubicin has shown some promise, but responses to chemotherapy have, in general, been disappointing.

7. What is the prognosis for patients with adrenocortical carcinoma?
The mean survival is about 15 months. The 5-year survival rate is approximately 20–35%. Prognosis is improved by younger patient age, smaller tumor size, localized disease, and complete tumor resection, and in nonfunctioning tumors.

8. How often are pheochromocytomas malignant?
Approximately 10–15% of pheochromocytomas are malignant.

9. What are the clinical features of a malignant pheochromocytoma?
Most pheochromocytomas cause hypertension, headaches, sweating, and palpitations; they are diagnosed by the finding of increased urinary excretion of vanillylmandelic acid (VMA), metanephrine, or catecholamines or by elevated levels of plasma catecholamines. Malignant pheochromocytomas usually do not differ clinically at presentation from those that are benign.

10. What clues suggest that a pheochromocytoma is malignant?
Malignancy is most strongly suggested by disproportionately increased urinary excretion of dopamine and/or homovanillic acid (HVA), tumor size greater than 6 cm, and evidence of extra-adrenal spread, usually to the lymph nodes, liver, lungs, or bones. The malignant character of some tumors may be missed, even histologically, and not become apparent until metastatic disease appears.

11. What is the treatment for a malignant pheochromocytoma?
Surgery is the treatment of choice. Alpha-adrenergic blocking agents, such as phenoxybenzamine and prazosin, are given preoperatively to control blood pressure and to replete intravascular volume. For patients with unresectable tumors, these drugs and alpha-methyltyrosine, an inhibitor of catecholamine synthesis, are also effective long-term therapy. Cyclophosphamide, vincristine, dacarbazine, and I-131 metaiodobenzylguanidine (MIBG) may cause partial regression of residual tumors.

12. What is the prognosis for malignant pheochromocytoma?
The 5-year survival rate for malignant pheochromocytoma is 40–45%.

13. What tumors metastasize to the adrenal glands?
The vascular adrenal glands are a frequent site of bilateral metastatic spread from cancers of the lung, breast, stomach, pancreas, colon, and kidney and from melanomas and lymphomas.

14. What is the clinical significance of metastatic disease to the adrenal glands?
Acute adrenal crisis is rare. However, up to 33% of patients may have subtle adrenal insufficiency manifested by nonspecific symptoms and an inadequate cortisol response (serum cortisol level < 20 mg/dl) to the ACTH (Cortrosyn) stimulation test. Patients often experience improvement in well-being when given physiologic glucocorticoid replacement.

15. How should the incidentally discovered adrenal mass be evaluated?
Incidental adrenal masses should be evaluated for evidence of hormone secretion and malignancy. Plasma aldosterone and renin, serum testosterone and dehydroepiandrosterone

sulfate (DHEAS), and 24-hour urinary excretion of cortisol, VMA, metanephrine, and catecholamines should be measured. Size is the greatest predictor of cancer; masses < 6 cm are rarely malignant.

16. How should the incidentally discovered adrenal mass be managed?
Nonfunctioning masses > 6.0 cm and all hormone-secreting tumors should be removed surgically. Some experts recommend a size cutoff of 4.5 cm for surgery. Smaller masses should be reassessed in 3–6 months, then annually, and removed if growth occurs or if excess hormone secretion develops.

BIBLIOGRAPHY

1. Berruti A, Terzolo M, Pia A, et al: Mitotane associated with etoposide, doxorubicin, and cisplatin in the treatment of advanced adrenocortical carcinoma. Cancer 83:2194–2200, 1998.
2. Demeure MJ, Somberg LB: Functioning and nonfunctioning adrenocortical carcinoma: Clinical presentation and therapeutic strategies. Surg Oncol Clin North Am 7:791–805, 1998.
3. Freeman DA: Adrenal carcinoma. Curr Ther Endocrinol Metab 6:173–175, 1997.
4. Grinspon SK, Biller BMK: Laboratory assessment of adrenal insufficiency. J Clin Endocrinol Metab 79:923–931, 1994.
5. Gross MD, Shapiro B: Clinically silent adrenal masses. J Clin Endocrinol Metab 77:885–888, 1993.
6. Harrison LE, Gaudin PB, Brennan MF: Pathologic features of prognostic significance for adrenocortical carcinoma after curative resection. Arch Surg 134:181–185, 1999.
7. Luton J-P, Cerdas S, Billaud L, et al: Clinical features of adrenocortical carcinoma, prognostic factors, and the effect of mitotane therapy. N Engl J Med 322:1195–1201, 1990.
8. Oelkers W: Adrenal insufficiency. N Engl J Med 335:1206–1212, 1996.
9. Ross NS, Aron DC: Hormonal evaluation of the patient with an incidentally discovered adrenal mass. N Engl J Med 323:1401–1405, 1990,
10. Schteingart DE: Treating adrenal cancer. Endocrinologist 2:149–257, 1992.
11. Schulick RD, Brennan MF: Long-term survival after complete resection and repeat resection in patients with adrenocortical carcinoma. Ann Surg Oncol 6:719–726, 1999.
12. Tritos NA, Cushing GW, Heatley G, Libertino JA: Clinical features and prognostic factors associated with adrenocortical carcinoma: Lahey Clinic Medical Center experience. Am Surg 66: 73–79, 2000.
13. Wajchenberg BL, Albergaria Pereira MA, Medonca BB, et al: Adrenocortical carcinoma: Clinical and laboratory observations. Cancer 88:711–736, 2000.
14. Williamson SK, Lew D, Miller GJ, et al: Phase II evaluation of cisplatin and etoposide followed by mitotane at disease progression in patients with locally advanced or metastatic adrenocortical carcinoma: A southwest oncology group study. Cancer 88:1159–65, 2000.

31. ADRENAL INSUFFICIENCY

Robert E. Jones, M.D.

1. How is adrenal insufficiency classified?

The clinical classification of adrenal insufficiency follows the functional organization of the hypothalamic-pituitary-adrenal axis. Primary adrenal insufficiency is defined as the loss of adrenocortical hormones due to destruction or impairment of the adrenal cortex. Secondary adrenal insufficiency is due to reduced secretion by the pituitary gland of adrenocorticotropin hormone (ACTH), whereas tertiary adrenal insufficiency is caused by failure of the hypothalamus to produce corticotropin-releasing hormone (CRH).

2. What are the causes of primary adrenal insufficiency?

The most common cause of primary adrenal insufficiency is **autoimmune adrenalitis**, which may be either confined to the adrenal gland or part of a polyglandular autoimmune syndrome. **Infectious adrenalitis** due to tuberculosis or disseminated fungal infections also may result in adrenal insufficiency. In patients infected with the human immunodeficiency virus (HIV), adrenalitis due to cytomegalovirus or HIV itself occasionaly results in adrenal failure. Acute, fulminant adrenal insufficiency due to **bilateral adrenal hemorrhage** may occur in the setting of sepsis or anticoagulant therapy. **Adrenomyeloneuropathy**, an X-linked recessive disorder, has become more frequently recognized as a cause of adrenal insufficiency in younger men. Although **bilateral metastatic disease** from lung, breast, or enteric carcinomas is common, the metastases rarely result in adrenal insufficiency, because greater than 90% of the glandular tissue must be replaced by tumor before clinical insufficiency is seen. Lastly, several different medications may reduce circulating levels of adrenal steroids, either by inhibiting one or more steroidogenic enzymes or by enhancing the metabolic clearance rate of steroids. Ketoconazole and aminoglutethimide are examples of the former, whereas rifampin is an example of the latter. Typically, however, adrenal insufficiency does not result unless the medications are given in high doses or the patient has an underlying adrenal condition that limits adrenal secretory reserve.

3. What are the causes of secondary or tertiary adrenal insufficiency?

Secondary adrenal insufficiency typically results from either a loss of anterior pituitary corticotrophs or disruption of the pituitary stalk. Secondary adrenal insufficiency usually occurs in association with panhypopituitarism, but selective ACTH deficiency, either inherited or due to autoimmunity, also has been reported. Most commonly, panhypopituitarism results from space-occupying lesions of the sella turcica. Primary pituitary tumors, craniopharyngiomas, or, on rare occasions, metastatic lesions from breast, prostate, or lung carcinomas may infiltrate and destroy corticotrophs. Aneurysms of the internal carotid artery may erode into the sella, and infiltrative diseases such as histiocytosis X or sarcoidosis have been associated with secondary adrenal insufficiency. Infections due to tuberculosis and histoplasmosis have resulted in a loss of anterior pituitary function. Severe head trauma that disrupts the pituitary stalk and either excessive blood loss that causes shock during deilvery (Sheehan's syndrome) or hemorrhage into a pituitary adenoma (pituitary apoplexy) may result in panhypopituitarism. Lymphocytic hypophysitis, another autoimmune disorder, also causes secondary adrenal insufficiency. Loss of corticotrophs also may occur after pituitary surgery or 5–10 yr after the delivery of 4,800–5,200 R to the pituitary fossa as radiation therapy for a pituitary tumor.

The most common cause of **tertiary adrenal insufficiency** is the long-term use of suppressive doses of glucocorticoids; for example, the use of prednisone in the treatment of rheumatic disease or inflammatory disease. Suppression of CRH with resultant adrenal insufficiency is a paradoxical concomitant of successful therapy for Cushing's syndrome. Loss of hypothalamic function also may result from various tumors, infiltrative diseases, and cranial radiotherapy.

4. Which symptoms are frequenty encountered in adrenal insufficiency?
Most of the symptoms of adrenal insufficiency are relatively nonspecific. Weakness, fatigue, and anorexia are almost universal complaints. Most patients also report minor gastrointestinal symptoms, such as nausea, vomiting, ill-defined abdominal pain, or constipation. On occasion, the gastrointestinal symptoms may be the predominant complaint and, as a result, may divert the physician into a long and fruitless evaluation. Symptoms of orthostatic hypotension, arthralgias, myalgias, and salt-craving are also encountered. Psychiatric symptoms may range from mild memory impairment to overt psychosis.

5. Describe the signs of adrenal insufficiency.
Weight loss occurs in all patients with adrenal insufficiency. Hyperpigmentation, presumably caused by elevated levels of ACTH or related peptide fragments, is noted in over 90% of patients with primary adrenal insufficiency. Hyperpigmentation may be generalized or localized to regions subjected to repeated trauma, such as elbows, knees, knuckles, and buccal mucosa. New scars are also frequently hyperpigmented, and preexisting freckles may increase in number. Vitiligo, areas of cutaneous pigment loss, may coexist in 10–20% of patients with autoimmune adrenalitis. Hypotension is also common in both primary and secondary adrenal insufficiency. Loss of axillary and pubic hair is more pronounced in women because of the loss of adrenal androgen secretion. A peculiar finding—auricular cartilage calcification—may be seen in long-standing adrenal insufficiency from any cause.

6. What laboratory abnormalities are encountered in adrenal insufficiency?
Hyponatremia and hyperkalemia are the most common abnormalities. Patients also may have a mild normocytic, normochromic anemia and may demonstrate eosinophilia and lymphocytosis on a peripheral blood smear. Prerenal azotemia secondary to volume depletion is more common in secondary insufficiency. Modest hypercalcemia is present in less than 10% of patients. Moderate elevations of thyroid-stimulating hormone (TSH) (usually <15 μU/mL) are also common. Whether the elevation is due to underlying autoimmune thyroid disease, to loss of TSH suppression by endogenous steroids, or to the euthyroid sick syndrome is unclear.

7. How do the presentations of primary and secondary adrenal insufficiency differ?
The features of primary and secondary adrenal insufficiency have many similarities and two major differences: hyperpigmentation and hyperkalemia are not seen in secondary adrenal insufficiency. Due to the loss of ACTH secretion, hyperpigmentation does not occur in secondary adrenal insufficiency. Similarly, the adrenal zona glomerulosa remains responsive to the renin angiotensin system in secondary adrenal insufficiency, and secretion of aldosterone is not compromised. Consequently, severe volume depletion is uncommon, and hyperkalemia is not encountered with the loss of ACTH. Cortisol is important in clearance of free water; thus, deficiency of cortisol from any cause may result in hyponatremia.

8. What other autoimmune disease may be associated with autoimmune adrenalitis?
Both type I and type II polyglandular autoimmune syndromes are associated with primary adrenal insufficiency. In type II, the more common syndrome, adrenal insufficiency is universally present Both syndromes are discussed in greater detail in Chapter 55. On rare

occasions, patients with other autoimmune endocrinopathies, such as chronic lymphocytic thyroiditis or insulin-dependent diabetes mellitus, may develop adrenal insufficiency.

9. How is the diagnosis of adrenal insufficiency confirmed?

A low plasma cortisol level (<5 μg/dL) in the face of severe physiologic stress provides reasonably solid evidence for adrenal insufficiency. Conversely, a random plasma cortisol level >20 μg/dL virtually excludes the diagnosis. In the basal or nonstressed state, a morning cortisol level >10 μg/dL generally correlates well with an intact hypothalamic-pituitary-adrenal axis, but cortisol values in this range also may be seen in patients with limited functional reserve of the axis. Screening patients with an ACTH (Cosyntropin) stimulation test may provide misleading information. A plasma cortisol level >20 μg/dL during a short ACTH stimulation test excludes the diagnosis of primary adrenal insufficiency, but it does not rule out a subtle ACTH deficiency, and additional testing is frequently required (see below).

10. Which tests are useful in distinguishing primary from secondary (or tertiary) adrenal insufficiency, and which tests are helpful in differentiating a partial ACTH deficiency from normal adrenal function?

Measuring simultaneous ACTH and cortisol levels will clearly differentiate primary adrenal failure from a central cause. In primary adrenal failure, ACTH levels are elevated, while they are low normal to frankly low in secondary or tertiary hypoadrenalism. The more challenging problem is differentiating a partial deficiency of ACTH from normal adrenal function. A short ACTH (Cortrosyn) stimulation test is always abnormal in primary adrenal insufficiency and may be blunted in central adrenal insufficiency. In order for the short ACTH stimulation test to be abnormal in central adrenal insufficiency, the deficiency of ACTH must be both profound and protracted, resulting in adrenal atrophy due to the loss of the trophic effect of ACTH. Some investigators have advocated using smaller doses of ACTH (1 μg) as opposed to the standard or high dose (250 μg) test to ferret out milder cases of central adrenal insufficiency. However, there may be some overlap in the cortisol responses between normals and those with a partial deficiency of ACTH. Other tests incude insulin induced hypoglycemia (the gold standard) and the metyrapone test. On occasion, the patient may be overlooked during the diagnostic evaluation. Do not forget to give replacement glucocorticoids during metabolic testing, and do not forget that ACTH may be suppressed by exogenous steroids, thereby invalidating the metyrapone test. Dexamethasone is the recommended supplement because it can be used in low doses and does not interfere with the measurement of cortisol.

11. Explain how adrenal crisis is managed.

The five S's of management are salt, sugar, steroids, support, and search for a precipitating illness. Volume should be restored with several liters of 0.9% saline with 5% dextrose. After a sample of blood has been obtained for measurement of cortisol and ACTH, 100 mg of hydrocortisone (cortisol) should be immediately administered intravenously. When hydrocortisone is given in the recommended dose of 100 mg every 8 hr, additional mineralocorticoid is unnecessary. Some authors also advocate the administration of a single dose of dexamethasone (4 mg) during the initial resuscitation of the patient. If the precipitating event or complicating illness has been controlled, the glucocorticoids should be tapered to maintenance levels after 1–3 days.

12. How urgently should a patient with suspected adrenal crisis be treated?

Left untreated, adrenal crisis is fatal. If adrenal crisis is suspected, it must be aggressively treated; stress doses of glucocorticoids carry virtually no morbidity when used in the short term. A formal diagnostic evaluation can be performed at a later time, after the patient has been stabilized.

13. How is chronic adrenal insufficiency best managed?

Maintenance therapy of adrenal insufficiency involves replacement of both glucocorticoid and, if necessary, mineralocorticoid. Hydrocortisone and cortisone acetate are the most frequently used replacement glucocorticoids; however, prednisone also may be used. The usual dose of hydrocortisone is 15–20 mg given in the morning and 5–10 mg in the afternoon, whereas the dose for cortisone acetate is usually 25 mg in the morning and 12.5 mg in the afternoon. The total daily dose for prednisone generally ranges from 2.5–7.5 mg and may be given either as a single dose in the evening or divided into morning and afternoon doses with the morning dose the larger of the two. Fludrocortisone (Florinef), given as a daily dose of 0.05–0.2 mg, is used as a replacement for aldosterone and is generally required to manage the electrolyte abnormalities encountered in primary adrenal insufficiency. The response to replacement therapy may be monitored simply and inexpensively by careful attention to serial weights, blood pressure, electrolytes, and a directed history to assess general health status and well-being. Some authors suggest serial measurements of urinary cortisol excretion to assess the adequacy of cortisol replacement. Care should be taken to avoid excessive doses of glucocorticoids, which may result in osteoporosis or excessive weight gain. The intent of long-term management of adrenal insufficiency is to use the smallest dose of glucocorticoids that provides the maximal benefit in the relief of symptoms.

14. Do patients with adrenal insufficiency require additional hormone supplementation during times of stress?

Any stress, including febrile illnesses, trauma, or diagnostic/surgical procedures, may precipitate an acute adrenal crisis. Therefore, the judicious use of supplemental steroids prevents possible tragedy. Doubling or tripling the glucocorticoid dose is sufficient for mild-to-moderate infections. If vomiting is a feature of the illness or if symptoms consistent with acute adrenal crisis supervene, the patient should be hospitalized for therapy. More severe infections or surgical procedures involving general anesthesia usually require the intravenous administration of hydrocortisone or an equivalent glucocorticoid. Stress doses of hydrocortisone should be tailored to the degree of stress. The dosage for moderate surgical stress should be 50–75 mg of hydrocortisone per day for 1–2 days, whereas major surgical stress should be managed with 100–150 mg of hydrocortisone per day for 2–3 days. The total dose should be divided into thirds and given every 8 hr. If hypotension ensues, the dose of hydrocortisone may be increased to 100 mg every 8 hr. The stress dose of glucocorticoids may be tapered over 1–2 days, and the previous dose of glucocorticoid may be resumed after resolution of the underlying stress. Additional steroid coverage should also be given in the presence of moderate-to-severe trauma.

15. Describe the nonpharmacologic interventions necessary for effective management of patients with adrenal isufficiency.

Education of the patient is paramount. The patient must know what to do during an intercurrent illness. An injectable glucocorticoid, such as dexamethasone, should always be readily available for emergency use. Likewise, a warning tag may prove to be providential in alerting a health care team to the presence of adrenal isufficiency if the patient is incapable of providing an appropriate history.

16. What are the relative potencies of available steroids?

The biologic potency of steroids depends on various factors, including absorption, affinity to corticosteroid-binding globulin (CBG), hepatic metabolism, and affinity to intracellular glucocorticoid receptor. As a general rule, synthetic steroids are poorly bound to CBG and more slowly metabolized; they also have a greater affinity for the glucocorticoid receptor than cortisol. The following table gives the approximate potencies of available preparations.

Relative Potencies of Steroid Hormones

COMPOUND	GLUCOCORTICOID ACTIVITY	MINERALOCORTICOID ACTIVITY	DURATION
Hydrocortisone	1.0	1.0	Short
Cortisone	0.7	0.7	Short
Prednisone	4.0	0.7	Short
Methylprednisolne	5.0	0.5	Short
Dexamethasone	30.0	0.0	Long
Fludrocortisone	10.0	400.0	Long

17. When is diagnostic imaging helpful in the evaluation of adrenal insufficiency?

Pituitary and hypothalamic imaging is absolutely essential to assess the regional anatomy in all patients with newly diagnosed secondary or tertiary adrenal insufficiency. By contrast, adrenal imaging in patients with primary adrenal insufficiency is rarely helpful. The only exception is when the diagnosis of bilateral adrenal hemorrhage is entertained. In this circumstance, an adrenal computed tomographic (CT) scan is virtually diagnostic.

18. What is the prognosis for patients with adrenal insufficiency?

Before isolation of glucocorticoids, the life expectancy of patients with adrenal insufficiency was less than 6 months. With prompt diagnosis and appropriate replacement therapy, patients with autoimmune adrenalitis now enjoy a normal life span. The prognosis of adrenal insufficiency due to other causes depends on the underlying disorder.

19. When patients are given pharmacologic doses of corticosteroids for nonadrenal diseases, how should tapering from steroids be handled?

There are as many suggested regimens of steroid tapering as there are authors who write on the subject. However, certain universal concepts are common to all approaches. The initial tapering of glucocorticoids from pharmacologic to physiologic doses is limited by the behavior of the treated illness. If the illness flares, the higher dose of steroids should be reinstituted and continued until the symptoms stabilize. Later, a more gradual tapering should be reinitiated. When near-physiologic doses of glucocorticoids are reached, the patient may be switched either to hydrocortisone or to alternate-day therapy, with tapering continued. Reestablishment of a normal hypothalamic-pituitary-adrenal axis is heralded by the return of the plasma cortisol to >10 µg/dL 24 hr after the last dose of steroid and normal adrenal responsiveness to exogenous ACTH (short ACTH stimulation). Full recovery of the complete axis may take 6–9 months; the adrenal responsiveness to ACTH is the last limb of the axis to recover. Some patients may develop steroid withdrawal syndrome during rapid tapering or after steroids have been discontinued. This syndrome is characterized by the typical features of adrenal insufficiency; however, arthralgias, myalgias, and, on rare occasions, desquamation may be the predominating symptoms.

20. When should a patient on exogenous glucocorticoids be considered functionally suppressed?

Any patient who has received more than 20 mg of daily prednisone (or glucocorticoid equivalent) for more than 1 month in the preceding year or greater-than-replacement doses of glucocorticoids for more than 1 yr should be considered to have a potentially suppressed axis and therefore should be given stress doses of glucocorticoids during intercurrent illness.

21. What role do adrenal androgens play in the replacement therapy of adrenal insufficiency?

Dehydroepiandrosterone (DHEA) and its sulfated form, DHEA-S, are the major adrenal androgens. Both are weak androgens at best, but in women, they are converted in peripheral tissues to the more potent androgens testosterone and 5α-dihydrotestosterone. This peripheral conversion is a very significant source of circulating testosterone levels in females, and women who have adrenal insufficiency have very low circulating levels of DHEA. This has prompted several groups to investigate the effects of DHEA replacement in women with adrenal insufficiency. Oral DHEA (50 mg/day) essentially normalized circulating levels of androgens in these women and dramatically improved feelings of well-being as well as mental and physical aspects of sexuality.

BIBLIOGRAPHY

1. Arlt W, Callies F, van Vlijmen JC, et al.: Dehydroepiandrosterone replacement in women with adrenal insufficiency. N Engl J Med 341:1013–1020, 1999.
2. Dahlberg PJ, Goellner MH, Pehling GB: Adrenal insufficiency secondary to adrenal hemorrhage: Two case reports and a review of cases confirmed by computed tomography Arch Intern Med 150:905–909, 1990.
3. Grinspoon SK, Bilezikian JP: Current concepts: HIV disease and the endocrine system. N Engl J Med 327:1360–1365, 1992.
4. Huang TS, Jiang YD: Repetitive graded ACTH stimulation test for adrenal insufficiency. J Endocrinol Invest 23:163–169, 2000.
5. Kamilaris TC, Chrousos GP. Adrenal diseases. In Moore WT, Eastman RC (eds): Diagnostic Endocrinology. Philadelphia, B.C. Dekker, 1990, pp. 79–109.
6. Khosa S, Wolfson JS, Demerjian Z, Godine JE: Adrenal crisis in the setting of high-dose ketoconazole therapy. Arch Intern Med 149:802–804, 1989.
7. Merenich JA, McDermott MT, Asp AA, et al.: Evidence of endocrine involvement early in the course of human immunodeficiency virus infection. J Clin Endocrinol Metab 70:572–577, 1990.
8. Nerup J: Addison's disease—clinical studies: A report of 108 cases. Acta Endocrinol 76:572–577, 1990.
9. Oelkers W: Adrenal insufficiency. N Engl J Med 335:1206–1212, 1996.
10. Oelkers W, Diedrich S, Bähr V: Diagnosis and therapy surveillance in Addison's disease: Rapid adrenocortcotropin (ACTH) test and measurement of plasma ACTH, renin activity and aldosterone. J Clin Endocrinol Metab 75:259–264, 1992.
11. Peacey SR, Guo C-Y, Robinson AM, et al: Glucocorticoid replacement therapy: Are patients overtreated and does it matter? Clin Endocrinol 46:255–261, 1997.
12. Salem M, Tainsh RE Jr, Bromberg J, et al.: Preoperative glucocorticoid coverage—a reassessment 42 years after emergence of a problem Ann Surg 219:416–425, 1994.
13. Seidenwurm DJ, Elmer EB, Kaplan LM, et al.: Metastases to the adrenal glands and the development of Addison's disease. Cancer 54:522–527, 1984.
14. Webel SS, Ober KP: Acute adrenal insufficiency. Endocrinol Metab Clin North Am 22:303–328, 1993.

32. CONGENITAL ADRENAL HYPERPLASIA

Jeannie A. Baquero, M.D., and Robert A. Vigersky, M.D.

1. Define congenital adrenal hyperplasia.

Congenital adrenal hyperplasia (CAH) is a family of inherited disorders that result from a decrease in the activity of one of the various enzymes required for the biosynthesis of cortisol. These defects are inherited as autosomal recessive traits and are manifested during both prenatal and postnatal life.

2. What enzyme defects can lead to CAH?

Defects in any of the enzymes required for the synthesis of cortisol from cholesterol can lead to CAH, including steroidogenic acute regulatory protein (StAR), essential in transporting cholesterol to the mitochondria; 3-beta-ol isomerase dehydrogenase, which is responsible for cholesterol side chain cleavage; and three hydroxylases, 17-hydroxylase, essential in converting progesterone to 17-hydroxyprogesterone (17-OHP) and pregnenolone to 17-hydroxypregnenolone; 21-hydroxylase, which converts progesterone to deoxycorticosterone (DOC) and 17-OHP to 11 deoxycortisol; and 11B-hydroxylase, which converts DOC to corticosterone (which then goes on to aldosterone) and 11 deoxycortisol to cortisol. (See figure on page 263.)

3. Discuss the genetics of CAH.

All of the enzyme defects leading to CAH are autosomal recessive disorders; that is, both copies of the involved gene must be abnormal for the condition to occur. There are two 21-hydroxylase genes, *CYP21P* (pseudogene) and *CYP21*, which are located on chromosome 6. Both of these genes are located downstream of the gene coding for complement factor 4 (C4A and C4B). *CYP21P* and *CYP21* genes are about 98% similar, but the pseudogene contains a number of deleterious sequences that ultimately result in a truncated protein. CYP21P is thus an inactive pseudogene while the *CYP21* gene codes for the active 21-hydroxylase enzyme. Modern techniques of molecular biology have determined that the defective enzyme activity may reflect a wide variety of different genetic defects in different families, including gene deletions, point mutations and gene conversions. Most mutations causing 21-hydroxylase deficiency are the result of recombinations between *CYP21* and the *CYP21P* pseudogene (unequal crossing over during meiosis), which inactivate the gene. A relatively new method for rapid simultaneous detection of the 10 mutations found in approximately 95% of 21-hydroxylase deficiency patients uses a polymerase chain reaction (PCR) amplification technique. This technique has been used for prenatal testing around the 9th week of gestation by sampling the chorionic villi; if negative, this procedure prevents the potential long-term complications of glucocorticoid exposure to the fetus and mother. Deficiency of the 11 B-hyroxylase enzyme (CYP11) is also an autosomal recessive defect caused by a mutation on the long arm of chromosome 8.

4. How common is CAH?

CAH is one of the most common inherited diseases. The most common form of CAH (90–95%) is 21-hydroxylase deficiency, which occurs in about 1/10,000 to 1/15,000 births in most populations. The prevalence of this disorder varies greatly among different ethnic groups, being highest among the Jewish population of Eastern Europe (Ashkenazi). The non-classic 21-hydroxlase deficiency may be as common as 1/100 to 1/1000 in persons of European Jewish heritage; the prevalence is similarly high in Yugoslavians and in Hispanics. Less than 2% of the population at large are heterozygote carriers of the 21-hydroxylase defect; that is, one of the two copies of the 21-hydroxylase gene is abnormal. Such heterozygote carriers appear normal in all respects but may have elevated 17-OHP with adrenocorticotropic hormone (ACTH) stimulation testing. The 11-hydroxylase deficiency is the second most frequent form of CAH, occurring in 1/100,000 births in the general population but in 1/5000 births in Jews of Moroccan descent (Sephardic). CAH due to defects of the other enzymes listed here is extremely rare.

5. Explain why adrenal hyperplasia develops.

The process of adrenal hyperplasia begins *in utero*. Reduced production of cortisol in the fetus, due to decreased activity of one of the enzymes needed for cortisol synthesis, results in lowered levels of serum cortisol. Cortisol normally acts through a negative feedback loop to inhibit the secretion of ACTH by the pituitary gland and corticotropin-releasing hormone (CRH) by the hypothalamus. Thus, the low serum cortisol levels that occur in a person with CAH increase the secretion of ACTH and CRH in an attempt to stimulate the adrenal glands to overcome the enzyme block and to return the serum cortisol level to normal. As this process continues over time, the elevated levels of serum ACTH stimulate growth of the adrenal glands, leading to hyperplasia.

6. What is the most serious clinical consequence of CAH?

As a result of a congenital enzyme defect, cortisol production is impaired. In some cases, depending on the precise nature of the enzyme defect, production of aldosterone may also be impaired (see figure). Deficient production of cortisol and/or aldosterone may lead to salt loss, hypovolemia, and a potentially fatal adrenal crisis in the newborn period; this usually occurs after one week of life. Overall, about 2/3 of patients with 21-hydroxylase deficiency have the salt-wasting form. The degree of residual activity of the defective enzyme, which affects the ability to produce glucocorticoids and mineralocorticoids and consequently determines the corresponding clinical manifestations, varies greatly from one affected family to another, depending on the specific genetic alteration. Adrenal crisis in the newborn period usually occurs with genetic defects that result in severe reductions in enzyme activity and steroid biosynthesis, a condition often termed salt-wasting CAH.

7. What are other clinical consequences of CAH in females?

Another important clinical consequence of CAH relates to the cortisol precursors (and their metabolites) that build up behind the blocked enzyme. Many of these precursors and metabolites are androgens; thus, overproduction during fetal development in CAH due to defects in 21-hydroxylase, 11-hydroxylase or 3-beta-hydroxysteroid dehydrogenase may masculinize the external genitalia of a female fetus, leading to ambiguous genitalia at birth (female pseudohermaphroditism). Girls with CAH are more "tomboyish" and have a higher incidence of homosexuality and gender identity disorders. By contrast, in CAH due to deficient activity of 17-hydroxylase or cholesterol side-chain cleavage enzyme, the enzyme defect also blocks synthesis of androgens (see figure); thus masculinization of the external genitalia does not occur, and ambiguous genitalia are not seen in females. Instead, they present with hypogonadism, hypertension and hypokalemia (because of increased mineralocorticoid production) at puberty. In non-classic CAH (alternatively called late-onset CAH), females usually are asymptomatic and have normal external genitalia. They present with premature pubarche, or at the time of normal puberty they may develop severe cystic acne, hirsutism, and/or oligomenorrhea. Adrenal "incidentalomas" are more common in patients

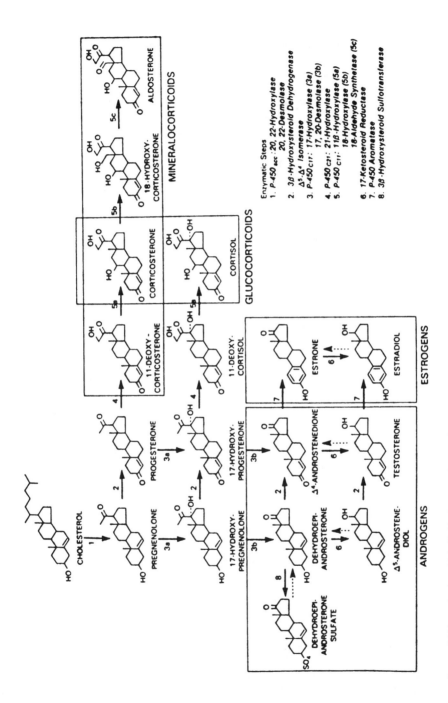

The pathway for steroid biosynthesis, with individual enzymatic steps indicated by number. Deficiencies in enzymes numbered 1, 2, 3a, 4, or 5a can lead to congenital adrenal hyperplasia. (From Becker KL (ed): Principles and Practice of Endocrinology and Metabolism. Philadelphia, J.B. Lippincott, 1990, with permission.)

with CAH and in heterozygotes. Conversely, 60% of patients with "incidentalomas" have exaggerated 17-OH progesterone responses to ACTH.

8. How do the manifestations of CAH in males differ from those in females?
   Like newborn females with CAH, newborn males with CAH also may develop an adrenal crisis related to salt loss and deficient production of glucocorticoid and mineralocorticoid. However, newborn males with CAH due to deficiency of 21-hydroxylase or 11-hydroxylase, the most common forms of CAH, do not manifest ambiguous genitalia (making it more difficult to detect CAH in males). Overproduction of androgens in male fetuses seems to have minimal effect on development of normal male external genitalia. Males with CAH due to deficient activity of 3-beta-hydroxysteroid dehydrogenase, 17-hydroxylase or cholesterol side-chain cleavage enzymes, all of which are rare, are unable to produce androgens such as testosterone in a normal fashion because of the enzyme block (see figure). Because adequate production of androgens during fetal development is necessary for the formation of male external genitalia, the external genitalia at birth are only partially masculinized or, in severe cases, may have a normal female appearance (male pseudohermaphroditism). Males with CAH can present with acne, testicular enlargement due to adrenal rests (rare), and infertility (also rare), but most are asymptomatic. Boys with non-classic CAH are generally asymptomatic.

9. Describe the clinical features that suggest the possibility of CAH.
   Adrenal crisis or severe salt-wasting in the newborn period suggests the possibility of CAH. CAH also must be considered prominently in the differential diagnosis of any newborn with ambiguous genitalia. Because adrenal crisis and salt loss in CAH may be fatal if not treated, the finding of ambiguous genitalia in a newborn should trigger a rapid attempt to confirm or exclude CAH. Most males with CAH do not have ambiguous genitalia; consequently, many cases go unrecognized at birth, unless there is a documented family history of the disorder.

10. What clinical clues help to support or refute the diagnosis of CAH in a newborn with ambiguous genitalia?
The overwhelming majority of genetic males with CAH have unambiguous external genitalia at birth; conversely, CAH is an uncommon cause of ambiguous genitalia in a genetic male. Thus, determination that the infant with ambiguous genitalia is a genetic male makes CAH unlikely and decreases the diagnostic urgency because the disorders giving rise to ambiguous genitalia in genetic males are rarely associated with a fatal outcome. For example, the finding of palpable gonads in the scrotal or inguinal area suggests that the infant is a genetic male, because such palpable gonads are almost always testes. Conversely, the detection of a uterus in an infant with ambiguous genitalia, either by physical examination or by ultrasound, strongly suggests that the infant is a genetic female, thus heightening the possibility of CAH. Modern molecular biology techniques can rapidly confirm the genetic sex of a newborn without the prolonged wait for a traditional chromosome analysis. Because of the potentially severe consequences of CAH, it is probably prudent to assume that any genetic female with ambiguous genitalia has CAH until proved otherwise. Furthermore, it would probably be best to wait to assign gender until molecular testing is done, as gender misassignment may cause long-term psychological problems for the families of such children. Early diagnosis and appropriate therapy also allow one to avoid the progressive effects of excess adrenal androgens, which will cause short stature, gender confusion in girls and psychosexual disturbances in both boys and girls.

11. How is the diagnosis of CAH confirmed?
   The most reliable way to confirm the diagnosis of CAH is to measure blood levels of

the cortisol precursor immediately proximal to the deficient enzyme. For example, in 21-hydroxylase deficiency, one measures the serum level of 17-OHP. In infants with classic 21-hydroxylase deficiency, serum 17-OHP levels are several orders of magnitude above normal. Blood levels of compounds that follow the blocked enzyme in the synthetic pathway, such as cortisol and aldosterone, may be low normal or frankly reduced. In practice, because one does not know a priori which enzyme is deficient in a newborn with suspected CAH (unless there is a documented family history of a particular enzyme defect), serum levels of all steroids that may be in the affected biosynthetic pathway can be measured before and after the administration of 250 μg of ACTH (Cortrosyn). Plasma renin activity and aldosterone levels should also be measured to assess the adequacy of aldosterone synthesis. Determination of which steroid levels are supranormal and which are low facilitates localization of the exact enzyme block. Specific genetic defects may be confirmed with molecular genetic testing. A new method uses PCR amplification for the rapid simultaneous detection of the 10 mutations that are found in approximately 95% of 21-hydroxylase deficiency alleles.

Newborn screening programs for CAH focus on the rapid detection of classic 21-hydroxylase deficiency. In the United States, there are 17 regional programs performing CAH newborn screening based on the measurement of 17-OHP levels in the filter paper blood spot. If CAH is suspected and newborn filter paper screening is not available, ACTH stimulation with steroid precursor measurements should be done after the first 24 hr of life. When non-classic CAH is suspected in the preteenage, teenage or adult patient, ACTH stimulation testing with should be done with 250 μg (not 1 μg) of ACTH; measurement of 17-OHP, 17-OH pregnenolone, and cortisol should be done before and 60 minutes after ACTH injection. Hyperandrogenism can be assessed in women by measuring serum levels of testosterone, androstenedione or 3-alpha androstanediol glucuronide.

12. Describe how CAH is treated.

The most important goal of treatment is to prevent salt loss and adrenal crisis in the newborn period. This requires the prompt administration of glucocorticoids and, in many cases, mineralocorticoids, as well as careful monitoring of salt intake. This treatment not only replaces the deficient hormones but also suppresses elevated serum ACTH levels, thereby reducing adrenal production of androgenic cortisol precursors and metabolites. Such treatment may be given presumptively while awaiting the results of definitive laboratory tests and then discontinued if the tests are not confirmatory. Surgical correction of ambiguous genitalia, such as repair of labioscrotal fusion, usually is carried out at a later time.

In children, the preferred glucocorticoid for chronic replacement is hydrocortisone because of its short half-life, which therefore minimizes growth suppression. Older adolescents and adults can alternatively be placed on prednisone or dexamethasone once growth has been completed. It is sometimes extremely difficult or impossible to find a dosage of glucocorticoid that normalizes production of androgen without impairing growth. In such situations, mineralocorticoids (fludrocortisone) and/or antiandrogens (spironolactone or flutamide) in combination with the aromatase inhibitor testolactone, may be useful adjunctive therapy in combination with nonsuppressive replacement doses of glucocorticoids. Like all patients with deficient adrenal reserve, patients with CAH need increased glucocorticoid doses during times of stress (tripling the maintenance dose of glucocorticoid). If the patient is unable to take oral medication, hydrocortisone (SoluCortef) should be given intramuscularly or intravenously. Those patients with salt-wasting CAH also require mineralocorticoid replacement with fludrocortisone acetate (Florinef). Infant doses are 70 μg/m^2/day and in adults the dose is 0.05–0.3 mg/day. Infants may also need sodium chloride, 1–3 grams/day, to achieve salt and water balance.

13. How is treatment monitored?

The goals of treatment are to prevent symptoms of adrenal insufficiency and to suppress ACTH and adrenal androgen production. For the second goal, it is most appropriate to monitor the levels of the key precursor immediately behind the blocked enzyme (e.g., 17-OHP in the case of 21-hydroxylase deficiency), with the ultimate aim of normalizing its level by adjusting the dosage of glucocorticoid. However, such suppression of 17-OHP and adrenal androgen production often can be achieved only with hydrocortisone doses of 10–20 mg/m^2/day, which are significantly higher than the average replacement doses (6–7 mg/m^2/day). If glucocorticoid dosages are too high, growth and development may be irreversibly impaired. Measurement of 24-hr urinary pregnanetriol (a metabolite of 17-OHP) excretion may also be a useful monitoring tool because of its ability to assess the integrated exposure to increased androgen precursors over a 24-hr period. Androgen levels that should also be monitored include testosterone, androstenedione and 3-alpha-androstanediol glucuronide. In addition, plasma renin activity should be monitored in patients with salt-wasting CAH. Children must have annual bone age determinations and their height should be carefully monitored.

14. What happens to children with untreated CAH?

As noted previously, the degree of cortisol and aldosterone deficiency may vary greatly from one affected family to another, depending on the precise nature of the genetic enzyme alteration. In untreated children with CAH—especially boys, who do not have ambiguous genitalia as a clue to the disorder—severe enzyme defects may lead to a fatal adrenal crisis. If the enzyme defect is milder, death from adrenal crisis in the perinatal period is unusual, but overproduction of androgens continues unabated during childhood, leading to early masculinization and an enhanced initial growth rate. However, production of excessive androgens ultimately leads to premature closure of the epiphyseal growth plates with resultant short stature in adulthood. People with CAH due to enzyme deficiencies that impair production of gonadal steroids, such as 17-hydroxylase deficiency, may present in early adolescence with impaired sexual maturation. Patients with CAH due to deficiency of 11-hydroxylase or 17-hydroxylase also overproduce deoxycorticosterone, a potent mineralocorticoid that is proximal to the enzyme block (see figure on page 263) and thus may have hypertension and hypokalemia. Adult women with untreated CAH often have menstrual irregularity and infertility. Adult men with untreated CAH are often short but otherwise normal; most are fertile although treatment may increase sperm counts in those in whom they are low.

15. What genetic counseling is appropriate for a couple who previously had a child with CAH?

Because all forms of CAH are autosomal recessive disorders, both parents of a child with CAH are obligate heterozygote carriers of the gene defect. Consequently, the chance that another child of the same couple will have CAH is one in four; 50% of the children will be heterozygote carriers. Modern genetic techniques and chorionic villus sampling of fetal DNA at 9 weeks of gestations allow the diagnosis of CAH during the first trimester of pregnancy. The other use for genotypic identification includes the prediction of the phenotype (i.e., severity of the disease). There appears to be good relationship between genotype and phenotype in classic but not in non-classic CAH. Preliminary evidence suggests that prenatal treatment of female fetuses with 21-hydroxylase deficiency in the 5th–7th week of gestation by giving relatively high doses of dexamethasone (0.5–2.0 mg/day) to the mother, may ameliorate the masculinization of genitalia. By contrast, male fetuses with 21-hydroxylase deficiency do not develop ambiguous genitalia and do not require steroid treatment until after birth.

BIBLIOGRAPHY

1. Cassorla FG, Chrousos GP: Congenital adrenal hyperplasia. In Becker KL(ed): Principles and Practice of Endocrinology and Metabolism. Philadelphia, J.B. Lippincott, 1990, p. 604.
2. Chrousos GP, Loriaux DL, Mann DL, et al: Late-onset 21-hydroxylase deficiency mimicking idiopathic hirsutism or polycystic ovarian disease: An allelic variant of congenital virilizing adrenal hyperplasia with a milder enzymatic defect. Ann Intern Med 96:1–43, 1982.
3. Deneux C, Veronique T, Dib A, et al: Phenotype-genotype correlation in 56 women with nonclassical congenital adrenal hyperplasia due to 21-hydroxylase deficiency. J Clin Endocrinol Metab 86:207–213, 2001.
4. Forest MG, Betuel H, David M: Prenatal treatment in congenital adrenal hyperplasia due to 21-hydroxylase deficiency: Update 88 of the French multicenter study. Endocr Res 15:277, 1989.
5. Levine LS: Congenital adrenal hyperplasia. Pediatric Rev 21:159–171, 2000.
6. Linder B, Esteban NV, Yergey AL, et al: Cortisol production rate in childhood and adolescence. J Pediatr 117:892, 1991.
7. Merke DP, Keil MF, Jones JV, et al: Flutamide, testolactone, and reduced hydrocortisone dose maintain normal growth velocity and bone maturation despite elevated androgen levels in children with congenital adrenal hyperplasia. J Clin Endocrinol Metab 85:1114–1120, 2000.
8. Miller WL: Congenital adrenal hyperplasia. Endocrinol Metab Clin North Am 20:721, 1991.
9. Miller WL, Levine LS: Molecular and clinical advances in congenital adrenal hyperplasia. J Pediatr 111:1, 1987.
10. Morel Y, Miller WL: Clinical and molecular genetics of congenital adrenal hyperplasia due to 21-hydroxylase deficiency. Adv Hum Genet 20:1, 1991.
11. Mulaikal RM, Migeon CJ, Rock JA: Fertility rates in female patients with congenital adrenal hyperplasia due to 21-hydroxylase deficiency. N Engl J Med 316:178, 1987.
13. Pang S, Pollack MS, Marshall RN, et al: Prenatal treatment of congenital adrenal hyperplasia due to 21-hydroxylase deficiency. N Engl J Med 322:111, 1990.
12. Pang S: Congenital Adrenal Hyperplasia. Endocrinol Metab Clin North Am 26:853–891, 1997.
14. Sherman SL, Aston CE, Morton NE, et al: A segregation and linkage study of classical and nonclassical 21-hydroxylase deficiency. Am J Hum Genet 42:830, 1988.
15. Speiser PW, White PC: Congenital adrenal hyperplasia due to steroid 21-hydroxylase deficiency. Clin Endocrinol 49:411–417, 1998.
16. Urban MD, Lee PA, Migeon CJ: Adult height and fertility in men with congenital virilizing adrenal hyperplasia. N Engl J Med 299:1392, 1978.
17. Wedell A: Molecular genetics of congenital adrenal hyperplasia (21-hydroxylase deficiency): implications for diagnosis, prognosis and treatment. Acta Paediatr 87:159–164, 1998.
20. White PC, New MI, Dupont B: Structure of the human 21-hydroxylase gene. Proc Natl Acad Sci USA 83:5111, 1986.
18. White PC, New MI, Dupont B: Congenital adrenal hyperplasia (Part 1). N Engl J Med 316:1519, 1987.
19. White PC, New MI, Dupont B: Congenital adrenal hyperplasia (Part 2). N Engl J Med 316:1580, 1987.
21. White PC, Spieser PW: Congenital adrenal hyperplasia due to 21-hydroxylase deficiency. Endocr Rev 21(3):245–291, 2000.
22. Winter JSD, Couch RM: Modern medical therapy of congenital adrenal hyperplasia. Ann N Y Acad Sci 458:165, 1985.

V. Thyroid Disorders

33. THYROID TESTING

Michael T. McDermott, M.D.

1. What is the single best test to screen for abnormal function of the thyroid gland?

The serum thyroid-stimulating hormone (TSH) level, using a highly sensitive TSH assay, is the single best test for assessing thyroid function. This is based on the presumption that one is dealing with primary thyroid disease, as is true in the vast majority of cases. The TSH measurement is misleading, however, when thyroid dysfunction is secondary to hypothalamic or pituitary disease that results in abnormal TSH secretion.

2. How do you interpret the serum TSH measurement in the evaluation of a patient with suspected thyroid disease?

When the TSH level is above the normal range, the patient has primary hypothyroidism. When TSH is below the normal range or undetectable, the patient has primary hyperthyroidism. Exceptions to these rules are rare. The serum TSH value can detect mild hypothyroidism or mild hyperthyroidism long before serum thyroid hormone levels are outside their normal ranges. Measurement of circulating free or total thyroxine (T_4), and sometimes triiodothyronine (T_3), should be performed in all patients with abnormal TSH values.

3. Explain how the serum TSH is used to manage patients on thyroid hormone therapy.

Thyroid hormone therapy is generally given to patients for one of two purposes: replacement therapy for hypothyroidism or suppression therapy for benign nodules or thyroid malignancy. When thyroid hormone is given for replacement, the dosage should be adjusted to maintain the serum TSH level within the normal range. When it is given for suppression, the dosage should be adjusted to maintain the serum TSH level in the low-normal or slightly below the normal range for patients with benign nodular thyroid disease and in the subnormal or undetectable range for patients with thyroid cancer.

4. Discuss the advantages of free thyroid hormone assays.

Free T_4 and free T_3 assays directly determine the amounts of unbound, bioactive thyroid hormones circulating in the bloodstream. Free thyroid hormone tests fall into 2 general categories: equilibrium dialysis assays and analogue assays. Equilibrium dialysis methods are not affected by abnormalities of serum thyroid hormone–binding proteins. Analog methods can be variably affected by protein binding but still give a far more accurate assessment of biologically active thyroid hormone concentrations than do total T_4 and T_3 assays. Analogue assays are used by most commercial laboratories.

5. What do total T_4 and T_3 assays measure?

These assays measure the total T_4 and T_3 concentrations in the circulation. Over 99% of circulating T_4 and approximately 98% of T_3 are bound to proteins such as thyroxine-binding globulin (TBG), thyroxine-binding prealbumin (TBPA), and albumin. Consequently, serum total T_4 and T_3 levels can be altered by disorders of the binding proteins just as they can by disorders of thyroid function.

6. Name the major disorders of thyroid hormone–binding proteins.

The major conditions that increase protein binding of thyroid hormones are pregnancy, estrogen use, congenital TBG excess, and familial dysalbuminemic hyperthyroxinemia. The latter condition is an inherited disorder in which albumin has enhanced affinity for T4, causing an increase in serum levels of total T4 but not T3. Protein binding of thyroid hormones is reduced by androgens and congenital TBG deficiency.

The measurement of T_3 resin uptake (T_3RU) is designed to help clinicians distinguish these disorders of protein binding from true thyroid diseases. The T_3RU is inversely proportional to the percent of T_4 that is protein-bound; accordingly, the T_3RU is low when protein binding of T_4 is increased and high when protein binding is reduced. The T_3RU must be obtained to interpret T_4 and T_3 levels properly. The following table indicates how these values are used to make the correct diagnosis.

	Total T_4	Total T_3	T_3RU
Hyperthyroidism	↑	↑	↑
Increased protein-binding state	↑	↑	↓
Hypothyroidism	↓	↓	↓
Decreased protein-binding state	↓	↓	↑

7. What antithyroid antibody measurements are clinically useful?

Anti-thyroid peroxidase (anti-TPO) antibodies and anti-thyroglobulin (anti-TG) antibodies are present in the serum of most patients with Hashimoto's thyroiditis. Thus either test is useful in establishing a diagnosis of Hashimoto's disease, although the anti-TPO antibodies are more sensitive. Thyroid-stimulating immunoglobulins (TSIs) and TSH receptor antibodies (TRAbs) are positive in the serum of most patients with Graves' disease; their measurement is not necessary in patients with obvious Graves' disease but may be helpful when the diagnosis is in question.

8. How useful are thyroglobulin measurements?

Thyroglobulin is the major iodoprotein constituent of thyroid follicles. Serum thyroglobulin levels are mildly increased in a variety of thyroid diseases. Marked elevations, however, suggest the presence of some type of relatively aggressive or disruptive thyroiditis (subacute, postpartum, or silent thyroiditis), in which large amounts of thyroglobulin leak from the damaged thyroid gland into the circulation. Thyroglobulin measurements are also useful in monitoring patients with thyroid cancer. When a patient has been thyroidectomized and is cancer-free, the serum thyroglobulin level should be undetectable. Normal or elevated serum thyroglobulin levels in such patients, therefore, suggest the presence of residual, recurrent, or metastatic thyroid cancer. One must be aware that most assays for serum thyroglobulin are not reliable in patients who have positive anti-TG antibodies. Methods are available in special labs, however, to circumvent this problem when it arises.

9. Under what circumstances should a serum calcitonin level be measured?

Calcitonin is made by thyroid parafollicular C-cells rather than by thyroid follicular cells. Serum calcitonin is elevated in medullary carcinoma of the thyroid (MCT) and in its familial precursor lesion, C-cell hyperplasia. Since MCT is an uncommon thyroid neoplasm, serum calcitonin measurements should not be used in the routine evaluation of most thyroid nodules; they are indicated, however, if a patient exhibits a feature, such as familial occurrence or associated diarrhea, that is characteristic of MCT.

10. Discuss the utility and interpretation of the radioactive iodine uptake (RAIU) test.

Thyroid follicular cell membranes have iodine symporters or pumps that bring iodine into the cells for subsequent thyroid hormone synthesis. The activity of these iodine pumps can be assessed by measuring the amount of radioactive iodine that is taken up by the thyroid gland over a defined period. The RAIU is thus an index of thyroid gland function; it is not a thyroid imaging test. The normal 24-hour RAIU is approximately 10–25% in the United States, but this value varies somewhat according to location because of geographic differences in dietary iodine intake.

The RAIU is most useful in the differential diagnosis of thyrotoxicosis. According to the results of this test, most cases can be divided into two pathophysiologically distinct categories:

High-RAIU Hyperthyroidism	Low-RAIU Thyrotoxicosis
Graves' disease	Factitious thyrotoxicosis
Toxic multinodular goiter	Iodine-induced thyrotoxicosis
Solitary toxic adenoma	Disruptive thyroiditis
	Subacute thyroiditis
	Postpartum thyroiditis
	Silent thyroiditis

11. When and why should a thyroid scan be ordered?

The thyroid scan is performed by administering a radioactive isotope (iodine or technetium) that localizes in the thyroid gland and then imaging the thyroid by recording the pattern of emitted radioactivity over the gland.

The thyroid scan can be used to distinguish among the three major types of high-RAIU hyperthyroidism (see question 10). Graves' disease (also known as diffuse toxic goiter) is characterized by diffuse tracer uptake; toxic multinodular goiter, by multiple discreet areas of increased uptake; and the solitary toxic adenoma, by a single area of intense uptake. The scan is not helpful in low-RAIU types of thyrotoxicosis because no tracer is absorbed by the thyroid gland.

The thyroid scan is also sometimes used in the evaluation of thyroid nodules, although its cost efficiency in this work-up is doubtful. According to the scan, thyroid nodules may be divided into those that are hot (hyperfunctioning), warm (eufunctioning), and cold (nonfunctioning). Cold nodules have a 20% risk of being a carcinoma; hot nodules, in contrast, are rarely malignant but must be followed because eventually they may cause thyrotoxicosis.

12. What is Thyrogen, and how is it used?

Thyrogen is recombinant human TSH. Thyrogen can be used to stimulate neoplastic thyroid tissue to take up radioactive iodine during an imaging procedure. Thyroid cancer tissue ordinarily traps iodine poorly and can be imaged only if the serum TSH is elevated to a level sufficient to enhance iodine uptake. This can be accomplished either by discontinuing levothyroxine treatment for 6 weeks or by giving injections of Thyrogen. Once the serum TSH level has been increased by either method, serum thyroglobulin is measured and radioiodine (I-131 or I-123) is administered for subsequent whole body scanning. A positive scan or detectable thyroglobulin indicates the presence of residual, recurrent or metastatic thyroid cancer. A Thyrogen scan performed with thyroglobulin measurement has the same accuracy as a levothyroxine withdrawal scan and has the advantage of not causing symptoms of hypothyroidism.

13. Explain the Cytomel and L-thyroxine suppression tests.

The administration of moderately supraphysiologic doses of Cytomel (T_3) for 1 week or L-thyroxine (T_4) for 4–6 weeks completely suppresses pituitary secretion of TSH. In patients with normal thyroid glands, this reduces the RAIU to zero and abolishes the thyroid scan image. However, in patients with autonomy of the thyroid gland (defined as thyroid function that is independent of TSH influence), the RAIU and scan remain unchanged after TSH suppression. The Cytomel and L-thyroxine suppression tests are thus tests of thyroid autonomy. The major causes of autonomy are Graves' disease, toxic multinodular goiters, and toxic adenomas. Patients with thyroid autonomy should not be treated with thyroid hormone suppression because they cannot be suppressed. Many eventually require treatment with antithyroid drugs, radioiodine ablation, or surgical resection for hyperthyroidism.

14. What is the role of the TRH test in the evaluation of thyroid disease?

The intravenous administration of a bolus of thyrotropin-releasing hormone (TRH) normally elicits a brisk increase in the serum TSH and prolactin levels that may last for up to 2 hours. This rise in TSH is exaggerated in patients with primary hypothyroidism and absent in patients with hyperthyroidism. It may exhibit a sluggish or delayed increment in patients with hypothalamic or pituitary disease. Because of the development of highly sensitive serum TSH assays and free thyroid hormone measurements, this test is rarely needed for the diagnosis of primary thyroid disease and is insufficiently accurate for the diagnosis of secondary thyroid disease. Nevertheless, it is occasionally of supportive value when other tests fail to yield a definitive diagnosis.

BIBLIOGRAPHY

 1. Cavaleri R: Thyroid radioiodine uptake: Indications and interpretation. Endocrinologist 2:341, 1992.
 2. Gorman CA: Thyroid function testing: A new era. Mayo Clin Proc 63:1026–1027, 1988.
 3. Haugen BR, Pacini F, Reiners C, et al: A comparison of recombinant human thyrotropin and thyroid hormone withdrawal for the detection of thyroid remnant or cancer. J Clin Endocrinol Metab 84:3877–3885, 1999.
 4. Hay ID, Klee GG: Thyroid dysfunction. Endocrinol Metab Clin North Am 17:473–509, 1988.
 5. Helfand M, Crapo LM: Screening for thyroid disease. Ann Intern Med 112:840–849, 1990.
 6. Klee GG, Hay ID: Biochemical thyroid function testing. Mayo Clin Proc 69:469–470, 1994.
 7. Ladenson PW, Braverman LE, Mazzaferri EL, et al: Comparison of administration of recombinant human thyrotropin with withdrawal of thyroid hormone for radioactive iodine scanning in patients with thyroid carcinoma. N Engl J Med 337:888–896, 1997.
 8. McKenzie JM, Zakarija M: The clinical use of thyrotropin receptor antibody measurements. J Clin Endocrinol Metab 69:1093–1096, 1989.
 9. Nicoloff JT, Spencer CA: The use and misuse of the sensitive thyrotropin assays. J Clin Endocrinol Metab 71:553–558, 1990.
10. Smith SA: Commonly asked questions about thyroid function. Mayo Clin Proc 70:573–577, 1995.
11. Spencer CA, Schwarzbein D, Gutler RB, et al: Thyrotropin (TSH) releasing hormone stimulation test responses employing third and fourth generation TSH assays. J Clin Endocrinol Metab 76:494–498, 1993.
12. Surks MI, Sievert R: Drugs and thyroid function. N Engl J Med 333:1688–1694, 1995.
13. Wang R, Nelson JC, Weiss RM, Wilcox RB: Accuracy of free thyroxine measurements across natural ranges of thyroxine binding to serum proteins. Thyroid 10:31–39, 2000.

34. HYPERTHYROIDISM

Susan T. Wingo, M.D., and Henry B. Burch, M.D.

1. What is the difference between thyrotoxicosis and hyperthyroidism? Define the term *autonomy* as it applies to thyroid hyperfunction.

Thyrotoxicosis is the general term for the presence of increased levels of triiodothyronine (T_3) and/or thyroxine (T_4) due to any cause. It does not imply that a patient is markedly symptomatic or "toxic." **Hyperthyroidism** refers to causes of thyrotoxicosis in which the thyroid overproduces thyroid hormone. Thyroid **autonomy** refers to the spontaneous synthesis and release of thyroid hormone independently of thyroid-stimulating hormone (TSH).

2. What is subclinical thyrotoxicosis?

Subclinical thyrotoxicosis refers to elevation of T_3 and/or T_4 within the normal range, leading to suppression of pituitary TSH secretion into the subnormal range. Clinical symptoms and signs are frequently absent or nonspecific.

3. What are the long-term consequences of subclinical thyrotoxicosis?

Some studies have linked subclinical thyrotoxicosis to accelerated bone loss in postmenopausal women and a higher incidence of atrial dysrhythmia, including atrial fibrillation.

4. List the three most common causes of hyperthyroidism.

1. **Graves' disease** is an autoimmune disorder in which antibodies directed against the TSH receptor result in continuous stimulation of the thyroid gland to produce and secrete thyroid hormone. Extrathyroidal manifestations of Graves' disease include ophthalmopathy, pretibial myxedema, and thyroid acropathy.

2. **Toxic multinodular goiter (TMNG)** generally arises in the setting of a longstanding multinodular goiter in which certain individual nodules have developed autonomous function. Patients with mild or overt TMNG are also at risk for developing iodine-induced thyrotoxicosis (the jodbasedow effect) after exposure to intravenous contrast or treatment with the iodine-containing drug amiodarone.

3. **Toxic adenomas or autonomously functioning thyroid nodules (AFTNs)** are benign tumors that have excessive constitutive activation of the TSH receptor or its signal-transduction apparatus. These tumors frequently produce subclinical thyrotoxicosis and have a predilection for spontaneous hemorrhage. AFTNs generally must be larger than 3 cm in diameter before attaining sufficient secretory capacity to produce overt hyperthyroidism.

5. What are some rarer causes of hyperthyroidism?

Rarer causes of hyperthyroidism include TSH-secreting pituitary adenomas; stimulation of the TSH receptor by extremely high levels of human chorionic gonadotropin (hCG), such as those found in choriocarcinomas in women or germ cell tumors in men; struma ovarii (ectopic thyroid hormone production in thyroid tissue–containing teratomas); and pituitary-specific thyroid hormone resistance. Thyroiditis and ingestion of excessive exogenous thyroid hormone (iatrogenic, inadvertent, or surreptitious) are causes of thyrotoxicosis but not hyperthyroidism (see question 1).

6. How do thyrotoxic patients present clinically?

Common symptoms include palpitations, shakiness, insomnia, difficulty with concentrating, irritability or emotional lability, weight loss, heat intolerance, exertional dyspnea, fatigue, hyperdefecation, menses with lighter flow or shorter duration, and brittle hair. Occasionally patients may experience weight gain rather than loss during thyrotoxicosis, presumably owing to polyphagia beyond that needed to support their increased metabolism.

7. What is apathetic hyperthyroidism?

Older patients with hyperthyroidism may lack typical adrenergic features and present instead with depression or apathy, weight loss, atrial fibrillation, worsening angina pectoris, or congestive heart failure.

8. Describe the physical signs of thyrotoxicosis.

Tremors, tachycardia, flow murmurs, warm moist skin, hyperreflexia with rapid relaxation phases, and a goiter (with a bruit in patients with Graves' disease) may be found in hyperthyroid patients. Eye findings in thyrotoxicosis are discussed in question 9.

9. How does hyperthyroidism cause eye disease?

Lid retraction and stare can be seen with any cause of thyrotoxicosis and are due to increased adrenergic tone. True ophthalmopathy is unique to Graves' disease and is thought to be caused by thyroid autoantibodies that are cross-reactive with antigens in fibroblasts, adipocytes, and myocytes behind the eyes. Common manifestations of ophthalmopathy include proptosis, diplopia, and inflammatory changes such as conjunctival injection and periorbital edema.

10. What laboratory testing should be performed to confirm thyrotoxicosis?

Measurement of TSH with a second- or third-generation assay is the most sensitive test for detecting thyrotoxicosis. Because a low TSH also may be seen in central hypothyroidism, a free T_4 level should be measured to confirm thyrotoxicosis. If the free T_4 level is normal, a T_3 level should be determined to rule out T_3 toxicosis. Other associated laboratory findings may include mild leukopenia, normocytic anemia, elevations of hepatic transaminases and bone alkaline phosphatase, mild hypercalcemia, and low levels of albumin and cholesterol.

11. When is thyroid antibody testing needed for the diagnosis of hyperthyroidism?

The cause of hyperthyroidism usually can be determined with history, physical examination, and radionuclide studies. Testing for TSH receptor antibodies is useful in pregnant women with Graves' disease to determine the risk of neonatal thyroid dysfunction due to transplacental passage of stimulating or blocking antibodies. It is also useful in euthyroid patients suspected of having euthyroid Graves' ophthalmopathy and in patients with alternating periods of hyper- and hypothyroidism as a result of fluctuations in blocking and stimulating TSH receptor antibodies.

12. What is the difference between a thyroid scan and an uptake?

A radioactive iodine uptake (RAIU) uses I^{131} or I^{123} to assess quantitatively the functional status of the thyroid gland. A small dose of radioactive iodine is given orally followed by measurement of radioactivity in the area of the thyroid in 6–24 hours. A high uptake confirms hyperthyroidism. A scan provides a two-dimensional image depicting the distribution of iodine trapping within the thyroid gland. Uniform distribution in a hyperthyroid patient suggests Graves' disease, patchy distribution suggests TMNG, and unifocal activity corresponding to a nodule suggests a toxic adenoma.

13. How should hyperthyroidism be treated?

The three main treatment options are antithyroid drugs (ATDs), including methimazole (MMI) and propylthiouracil (PTU); radioiodine (I^{131}) ablation; and surgery. Unless contraindicated, most patients should receive beta blockers for heart rate control and symptomatic relief. Most thyroidologists in the United States prefer I^{131} over surgery or prolonged courses of ATDs. Patients scheduled to receive I^{131} should be advised to avoid pregnancy and should be cautioned that oral contraceptives may not be fully protective in the hyperthyroid state because of increased levels of sex hormone–binding globulin and increased clearance of the contraceptive.

14. When is surgery indicated for hyperthyroidism?

Surgery is rarely the treatment of choice for hyperthyroidism. It is most often used when a cold nodule is present in a patient with Graves' disease, when I^{131} is contraindicated as in pregnancy, or in patients with extremely large goiters who are less likely to respond to ATDs or I^{131}. Surgery may also be the preferred modality when patients have other serious medical problems that make the rapid attainment of normal thyroid levels crucial. Patients should be euthyroid before surgery to decrease the risk of arrhythmias during induction of anesthesia and the risk of postoperative thyroid storm.

15. Are other treatments available to lower thyroid hormone levels?

Yes. Inorganic iodine acutely reduces the synthesis and release of T_4 and T_3. The inhibition of thyroid hormone synthesis by iodine is known as the Wolff-Chaikoff effect. However, because escape from this effect generally occurs after 10–14 days, iodine is used only to prepare a patient rapidly for surgery or as an adjunctive measure in patients with thyroid storm. Typical doses are Lugol's solution, 3–5 drops 3 times/day, or saturated solution of potassium iodide (SSKI), one drop 3 times/day. Ipodate, an oral radiographic contrast agent, has been shown to cause dramatic reductions in serum T_3 and T_4 levels through inhibition of T_4-5'-deiodinase activity and the effect of the iodine contained in the drug. A typical dose of ipodate is 1 g/day. Recently, the sole manufacturer of ipodate ceased production of this agent. Less experience is available with the use of a related oral contrast agent, iopanoic acid. Other agents occasionally used to treat hyperthyroidism include lithium, which decreases thyroid hormone release, and potassium perchlorate, which inhibits thyroid uptake of iodine.

16. Which medications block conversion of T_4 to T_3?

PTU, propranolol, glucocorticoids, ipodate, and amiodarone inhibit the peripheral conversion of T_4 to T_3.

17. How effective are ATDs?

Ninety percent of patients taking ATDs become euthyroid without significant side effects. Approximately one half of patients attain a remission from Graves' disease after completing a treatment course of 12–18 months. However, only 30% maintain long-term remission; the remainder experience recurrence within 1–2 years after the drugs are withdrawn. The usual starting doses are methimazole, 30 mg/day, or PTU, 100 mg 3 times/day.

18. What side effects are associated with ATDs?

1. Agranulocytosis is a rare but life-threatening complication of ATD therapy, occurring in approximately 1 in every 200–500 patients treated with ATDs. Patients should be instructed to report promptly fever, sore throat, or minor infections that do not resolve quickly.

2. Hepatotoxicity can progress to fulminant hepatitis with necrosis with PTU, and cholestatic jaundice has been reported with MMI. Patients should report right upper quadrant pain, anorexia, nausea, and new pruritus.

3. Rashes can range from limited erythema to an exfoliative dermatitis. Reaction to one ATD does not preclude the use of another, although cross-sensitivity occurs in approximately 50% of cases.

19. What lab tests should be monitored in patients taking ATDs?

Thyroid hormone levels should be monitored to determine when ATD doses can be reduced from the initial high doses to maintenance doses (usually 25–50% of initial doses). TSH may remain suppressed for several months; in this situation, free T_4 levels are more reliable for assessing thyroid hormone status. Hepatic enzymes and complete blood count with differential should be checked every 1–3 months. Because transaminase elevation and mild granulocytopenia can be seen in untreated Graves' disease, it is important to check these parameters before initiating ATD therapy. Many cases of agranulocytosis appear to arise without preceding granulocytopenia; thus, a high index of suspicion is required even if recent testing is normal.

20. How does radioactive iodine work?

Thyroid cells trap and concentrate iodine and use it to make thyroid hormone. I^{131} is organified in the same manner as natural iodine. Because I^{131} emits locally destructive beta particles, cellular damage and death occur over a period of several months after treatment. Doses of I^{131} should be high enough to result in permanent hypothyroidism in order to decrease the recurrence rate. Typical doses for Graves' disease are 8–15 mCi; for TMNG, higher doses of 25–30 mCi are given. These doses are effective in 90–95% of patients.

21. When is pretreatment with ATDs indicated before I^{131} ablation?

Elderly patients and patients with underlying systemic illnesses are often pretreated with ATDs in an effort to deplete the thyroid of preformed hormones and thereby theoretically reduce the risk of I^{131}-induced thyroid storm. When pretreatment with ATDS is used, the drugs are generally stopped 4–7 days before I^{131} is given. However, pretreatment with antithyroid drugs is associated with a rapid increase in thyroid hormone levels upon ATD discontinuation. Most non-pretreated patients experience a rapid decrease in thyroid hormone levels after radioiodine (see figure). Therefore most patients do not require or benefit from ATD pretreatment. Pretreatment also has the disadvantage of lowering the success rate of radioiodine through residual inhibition of organification of the I^{131}.

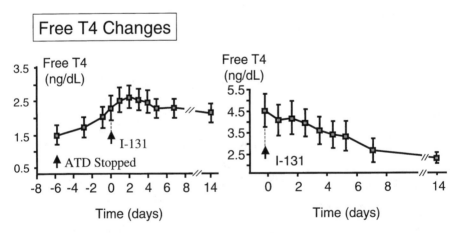

The effect of pretreatment with antithyroid drugs on serum free T4 levels before and after radioiodine therapy for Graves' disease. On the left is shown the mean thyroid hormone level changes following discontinuation of antithyroid drugs and subsequent radioiodine therapy. The right panel shows changes in serum free T4 values after radioiodine therapy in a smaller group of non-pretreated patients. Adapted from Burch HB, Solomon BL, Wartofsky L, Burman KD: Discontinuing antithyroid drug therapy before ablation with radioiodine in Graves' disease. Ann Intern Med 121:553–559, 1994.

22. How long after I^{131} treatment should women wait before becoming pregnant or resuming breast feeding?

Pregnancy should be deferred for at least 6 months after I^{131} ablation. In addition, patients should be on a stable dose of replacement thyroid hormone and free of active ophthalmopathy. Breast milk radioactivity, measured in one study after an 8.3-mCi therapeutic dose of I^{131}, remained unacceptably high for 45 days. If ^{99m}technetium is used for diagnostic studies, breast feeding may be resumed in 2–3 days.

23. Does I^{131} cause or worsen ophthalmopathy in Graves' disease?

This is an area of ongoing controversy. The natural history of Graves' disease is such that 15–20% of patients develop significant ophthalmopathy. The majority of cases arise in the period from 18 months before to 18 months after the onset of thyrotoxicosis. Thus, a fair number of new cases can be expected to coincide with the timing of I^{131} ablation. Two prospective randomized trials have shown that I^{131} is more likely to worsen ophthalmopathy than other treatment modalities. Patients with pre-existing eye disease and those who smoke cigarettes are more likely to experience worsening. As a result, it may be prudent to avoid I^{131} in patients with active moderate-to-severe Graves' ophthalmopathy, or to treat these patients with a course of oral corticosteroids immediately after the dose of I^{131}.

24. How is thyrotoxicosis managed in pregnancy?

Caution must be used in interpreting thyroid laboratory results during pregnancy, because low TSH values are not uncommon in the first trimester and total T_4 levels are elevated by increased thyroxine-binding globulin (TBG) levels. Free T_4 levels are the best indicator of thyroid function during pregnancy. Nuclear medicine testing with RAIU or thyroid scanning is contraindicated in pregnancy because of concerns about fetal exposure to isotopes. Because I^{131} therapy is also contraindicated during pregnancy, treatment options are limited to ATDs or surgery in the second trimester. PTU is generally the preferred ATD during pregnancy because it crosses the placenta to a lesser extent than methimazole. Pregnant patients with Graves' disease require close follow-up to ensure adequate control and to prevent hypothyroidism because the disorder frequently remits during the course of pregnancy. TSH receptor antibodies, which are able to cross the placenta after 26 weeks, should be measured in the third trimester to assess the risk of neonatal thyroid dysfunction.

BIBLIOGRAPHY

1. Bartalena L, Marcocci C, Bogazzi F, et al.: Relation between therapy for hyperthyroidism and the course of Graves' ophthalmopathy. N Engl J Med 338:73–78, 1998.
2. Biondi B, Fazio S, Carella C, et al: Cardiac effects of long term thyrotropin-suppressive therapy with levothyroxine. J Clin Endocrinol Metab 77:334–338, 1993.
3. Burch HB, Wartofsky L: Graves' ophthalmopathy: Current concepts regarding pathogenesis and management. Endocr Rev 14:747–793, 1993.
4. Burch HB, Shakir F, Fitzsimmons TR, et al: Diagnosis and management of the autonomously functioning thyroid nodule: The Walter Reed Army Medical Center experience, 1975-1996. Thyroid 8:871–880, 1998.
5. Burch HB, Solomon BL, Wartofsky L, Burman KD: Discontinuing antithyroid drug therapy before ablation with radioiodine in Graves' disease. Ann Intern Med 121:553–559, 1994.
6. Burrow GN: Thyroid function and hyperfunction during gestation. Endocr Rev 14:194–202, 1993.
7. Cooper DS: Antithyroid drugs for the treatment of hyperthyroidism caused by Graves' disease. Endocrinol Metab Clin North Am 27:225–247, 1998.
8. Faber J, Galloe AM: Changes in bone mass during prolonged subclinical hyperthyroidism due to L-thyroxine treatment: A meta-analysis. Eur J Endocrinol 130:350–356, 1994.
9. Kahaly GJ, Nieswandt J, Mohr-Kahaly S: Cardiac risks of hyperthyroidism in the elderly. Thyroid. 8:1165–1169, 1998.

10. Ladenson PW: Diagnosis of thyrotoxicosis. In Braverman LE, Utiger RD (eds): Werner & Ingbar's The Thyroid, 8th ed. Philadelphia, Lippincott Williams & Wilkins, 2000, pp 685–690.

11. McDermott MT, Ridgway EC: Thyroid hormone resistance syndromes. Am J Med 94:424–432, 1993.

12. McDermott MT, Ridgway EC: Central hyperthyroidism. Endocrinol Metab Clin North Am 27: 187–203, 1998.

13. Sawin CT, Geller A, Wolf PA, et al: Low serum thyrotropin concentration as a risk factor for atrial fibrillation in older persons. N Engl J Med 331:1249–1252, 1994.

14. Singer PA, Cooper DS, Levy EG, et al: Treatment guidelines for patients with hyperthyroidism and hypothyroidism. Standards of Care Committee, American Thyroid Association. JAMA 273: 808–812, 1995.

15. Solomon B, Glinoer D, Lagasse R, Wartofsky L: Current trends in the management of Graves' disease. J Clin Endocrinol Metab 70:1518–1524, 1990.

35. HYPOTHYROIDISM

Bryan R. Haugen, M.D.

1. How common is hypothyroidism?

Hypothyroidism is relatively common with a prevalence of 2–3% in the general population. The mean age at diagnosis is the mid-50s. Hypothyroidism is much more common in women, with a female-to-male ratio of 10:1. Postpartum hypothyroidism, a transient hypothyroid phase after pregnancy, is found in 5–10% of women.

2. What is subclinical hypothyroidism?

Subclinical hypothyroidism (now called mild thyroid failure) is a mild and much more common form of hypothyroidism, often with few or no symptoms. As many as 10–20% of women older than 50 yr have mild thyroid failure. Hypercholesterolemia and subtle cardiac abnormalities have been associated. Biochemically, the levels of thyroxine (T_4) or free T_4 are normal, whereas the level of thyroid-stimulating hormone (TSH) is mildly elevated. When patients are treated with thyroxine, they have an improved sense of well-being (compared with placebo) and the cardiac and lipid abnormalities resolve. Therefore, treatment is generally recommended. Thyroid antibodies, an indicator of autoimmune thyroid disease, may help to predict which patients will progress to clinical hypothyroidism; testing is recommended for patients with a minimally elevated TSH level.

3. Discuss the causes of hypothyroidism.

Many disorders can cause hypothyroidism. The two most common causes are chronic lymphocytic thyroiditis (Hashimoto's disease), an autoimmune form of thyroid destruction, and radioiodine-induced hypothyroidism after treatment of Graves' disease (autoimmune hyperthyroidism). Postpartum thyroiditis occurs in approximately 10% of women, two thirds of whom experience a transient hypothyroid phase (6–12 months) requiring treatment.

Other less common causes of hypothyroidism include subacute thyroiditis, external irradiation to the neck, medications (antithyroid drugs, amiodarone, lithium, interferon), infiltrative diseases, central (pituitary/hypothalamic) hypothyroidism, congenital defects, and endemic (iodine-deficient) goiter, which is fairly common outside the United States.

4. Name the symptoms associated with hypothyroidism.

Hypothyroidism commonly presents with nonspecific symptoms such as fatigue, cold intolerance, depression, weight gain, weakness, joint aches, constipation, dry skin, hair loss, and menstrual irregularities.

5. What findings on physical examination are consistent with hypothyroidism?

Physical examination may be normal with mild thyroid failure and should not deter further work-up if clinical suspicions are high. Common signs of moderate-to-severe hypothyroidism include hypertension (diastolic hypertension is a clue), bradycardia, coarse hair, periorbital swelling, yellow skin (due to elevated levels of beta carotene), carpal tunnel syndrome, and delayed relaxation of the deep tendon reflexes. The thyroid may be enlarged, normal, or small, but thyroid consistency is usually firm.

Unusual presentations of hypothyroidism include megacolon, cardiomegaly, and congestive heart failure (CHF). Severe CHF in one reported patient scheduled for cardiac transplant resolved with thyroid hormone replacement alone.

6. Describe the laboratory tests that may show abnormal results during hypothyroidism.

Laboratory clues to hypothyroidism include normochromic, normocytic anemia (menstruating women may also have iron deficiency anemia due to excessive bleeding from irregular menses), hyponatremia, hypercholesterolemia, and elevated levels of creatine phosphokinase.

7. What tests best confirm the diagnosis of hypothyroidism in the outpatient setting?

Many thyroid function tests are available to the clinician, including assessments of TSH, T_4, triiodothyronine (T_3), resin uptake, free T_4, free T_3, and reverse T_3. In the outpatient setting only one test is usually necessary: assessment of TSH. TSH, which is synthesized and secreted from the anterior pituitary gland, is the most sensitive indicator of thyroid function in the nonstressed state. Basically, if the TSH is normal (range = 0.5–5 mIU/ml), the patient is euthyroid; if the TSH is elevated (>5 mIU/mL), the patient has primary gland failure.

Care must be taken in interpreting total T_4 levels (occasionally done on health-screening panels). Many conditions unrelated to thyroid disease cause low or elevated levels of total T_4, because more than 99% of T_4 is protein-bound and total T_4 levels depend on the amount of thyroid-binding proteins, which may vary greatly. Total T_4 levels must always be compared with the T_3 resin uptake (T3RU), which reflects the amount of thyroid hormone-binding protein.

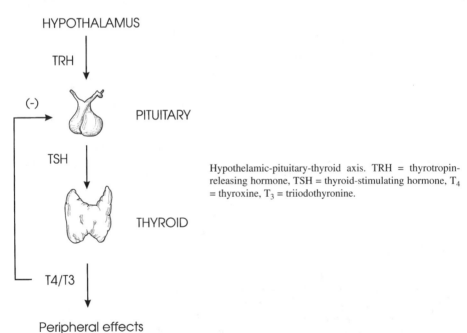

Hypothelamic-pituitary-thyroid axis. TRH = thyrotropin-releasing hormone, TSH = thyroid-stimulating hormone, T_4 = thyroxine, T_3 = triiodothyronine.

8. Name the tests that best confirm hypothyroidism in the inpatient setting.

Interpretation of thyroid function tests in the acutely ill inpatient is more difficult when hypothyroidism is suspected. Acute nonthyroidal illness may cause suppression of the T_4 and T_3 levels, and TSH may be elevated in the recovery phase. (See chapter 40.) Medications such as dopamine and glucocorticoids may suppress the TSH. Severe illness may even cause low levels of free T_4. When hypothyroidism is suspected in the stressed, hospitalized patient, a combination of clinical signs (inappropriate bradycardia, puffy facies, dry skin, delayed relaxation of deep tendon reflexes) and laboratory tests (TSH and free T_4 levels) are necessary to exclude or confirm the diagnosis of hypothyroidism. If these tests are equivocal, a reverse T_3 level, which is normal or elevated in nonthyroidal illness and low in hypothyroidism, may prove helpful. Inpatient TSH testing also may be confounded by normal diurnal variations in TSH. TSH levels in euthyroid people may exceed the normal range at night, when patients are frequently admitted. A morning test may help to clarify the significance of a mildly elevated TSH.

9. Which thyroid hormone preparation should I use?

Since 1891 when sheep thyroid extract was first used to treat myxedema, many preparations have been developed and are still available. Currently the best replacement regimen is levothyroxine (LT_4). Brand-name LT_4 (Synthroid, Levothroid, Levoxyl) is preferred over the generic preparations, because cost is a minor issue (generic LT_4 costs $6/month, whereas brand names cost about $10/month) and because generic LT_4 may vary 15–20% in bioavailability. Other thyroid hormone preparations include L-triiodothyronine (LT_3), which is reserved for special cases because of its potency and short half-life, and desiccated thyroid and thyroglobulin, which give unpredictable concentrations of serum thyroid hormone because of varied content and bioavailability.

10. What is the recommended dose of LT_4 for replacement therapy in a hypothyroid patient?

Otherwise healthy, young patients may be started on full replacement doses of LT_4 (1.6 µg/kg/day). Elderly patients and patients with known or suspected cardiac disease should be started on low doses of LT_4 (25 µg/day), which are increased by 25 µg/day every 2–3 months until the TSH is normal.

11. My patients are asking me about combination T4/T3 therapy. What should I tell them?

The medical and lay literature have taken a renewed interest in combination therapy. A recent placebo-controlled study has suggested that patients taking combination therapy had improved cognitive function and mood scores compared with when they took LT_4 alone. Studies in thyroidectomized animals have shown that T_4 therapy alone does not restore tissue levels of T_4 and T_3 to euthyroid levels, even when the TSH is normalized. While these studies are provocative and intriguing, most experts agree that more information is needed before we can recommend combination T_4/T_3 therapy in most patients. My current approach is to openly discuss this information with inquiring patients. I suggest a trial of LT_4 alone to normalize TSH within the low normal range (0.5–2.0 mU/L) for a period of 2 to 4 months. Many patients do extremely well with this approach, and T_3 is not needed. Patients who have low-normal TSH on LT_4 and still feel "hypothyroid" need further evaluation prior to considering T_3 therapy. I generally exclude anemia and vitamin B12 deficiency (associated with Hashimoto's thyroiditis) and inquire about sleep apnea. If this assessment is negative, I decrease the LT_4 by 12–25 µg and add 5 µg of Cytomel (T_3) in the morning. The goal is to see if the patient's symptoms improve without persistent suppression of the serum TSH (measured in the morning prior to taking medication). There are no data to clearly support or refute this position; I believe it is a position of "good" medical judgment in the absence of "good" medical data.

12. How should the clinician approach surgery in the hypothyroid patient?

There are two broad categories to consider: emergent/cardiac surgery and elective surgery. Hypothyroidism is associated with minor postoperative complications—gastrointestinal (prolonged constipation, ileus) as well as neuropsychiatric (confusion, psychosis); in addition, the incidence of fever with infections is lower. However, rates of mortality and major complications (blood loss, arrhythmias, impaired wound healing) are similar to the rates in euthyroid patients.

Current recommendations are to proceed with emergent surgery in the hypothyroid patient and to monitor for potential postoperative complications while giving replacement therapy with LT_4. Patients with ischemic coronary artery disease requiring surgery should proceed without LT_4 replacement, because T_4 increases myocardial oxygen demands and may precipitate worsening cardiac symptoms if given before surgery. Postoperatively the patient should receive replacement therapy with LT_4 at a slow rate and be followed for CHF (increased in hypothyroid patients undergoing cardiac surgery).

Patients scheduled for elective surgery should wait until TSH is normalized because of the postoperative complications associated with hypothyroidism.

13. How does myxedema differ from hypothyroidism?

Myxedema is a severe, uncompensated form of prolonged hypothyroidism. Complications include hypoventilation, cardiac failure, fluid and electrolyte abnormalities, and coma. (See chapter 39.) Myxedema coma is frequently precipitated by an intercurrent systemic illness, surgery, or narcotic/hypnotic drugs. Patients with myxedema coma should receive replacement therapy with 300–500 mg of intravenous LT_4 followed by 50–100 mg each day. Because conversion of T_4 to T_3 (active hormone) is decreased with severe illness, patients with profound cardiac failure that requires pressors or patients unresponsive to 1–2 days of LT_4 therapy should be given LT_3 at 12.5 mg intravenously every 6 hr.

BIBLIOGRAPHY

 1. Arem R, Patsch W: Lipoprotein and apolipoprotein levels in subclinical hypothyroidism. Arch Intern Med 150:2097–2100, 1990.
 2. Bunevicius R, Kazanavicius G, Zalinkevicius R, Prange AJ: Effects of thyroxine as compared with thyroxine plus triiodothyronine in patients with hypothyroidism. N Engl J Med 340:424-9, 1998.
 3. Cooper DS, Halpern R, Wood LC, et al.: L-thyroxine therapy in subclinical hypothyroidism. Ann Intern Med 101:18–24, 1984.
 4. Elder J, McLelland A, O'Reilly SJ, et al: The relationship between serum cholesterol and serum thyrotropin, thyroxine, and tri-iodothyronine concentrations in suspected hypothyroidism. Ann Clin Biochem 27:110–113, 1990.
 5. Hay ID, Duick DS, Vliestra RE, et al: Thyroxine therapy in hypothyroid patients undergoing coronary revascularization: A retrospective analysis. Ann Intern Med 95:456–457, 1981.
 6. Ladenson PW: Recognition and management of cardiovascular disease related to thyroid dysfunction. Am J Med 88:638–641, 1990.
 7. Ladenson PW, Levin AA, Ridgway EC, Daniels GH: Complications of surgery in hypothyroid patients. Am J Med 77:262–266, 1984.
 8. Mandel SJ, Brent GA, Larsen PR: Levothyroxine therapy in patients with thyroid disease. Ann Intern Med 119:492–502, 1993.
 9. Oppehemer JN, Braverman LE, Toft A, et al.: Thyroid hormone treatment: When and what? J Clin Endocrinol Metab 80:2873–2882, 1995.
10. Patel R, Hughes RW: An unusual case of myxedema megacolon with features of ischemic and pseudomembranous colitis. Mayo Clin Proc 67:369–372, 1992.
11. Rosenthal MJ, Hunt WC, Garry PJ, Goodwin JS: Thyroid failure in the elderly: Microsomal antibodies as discriminant for therapy. JAMA 258:209–213, 1987.
12. Roti E, Minelli R, Gardini E, Braverman LE: The use and misuse of thyroid hormone. Endocr Rev 14:401–423, 1993.

36. THYROIDITIS

Robert C. Smallridge, M.D.

1. Give the differential diagnosis for thyroiditis.
1. Infectious
   a. Acute (suppurative)
   b. Subacute (granulomatous; deQuervain's)
2. Autoimmune
   a. Chronic lymphocytic (Hashimoto's disease)
   b. Atrophic (primary myxedema)
   c. Juvenile
   d. Postpartum
3. Painless (non-postpartum)
4. Drug-induced
5. Riedel's struma
6. Radiation-induced
7. Traumatic

2. What causes acute thyroiditis?
This rare disease is infectious and usually bacterial; at times, however, fungal, tuberculous, parasitic, or syphilitic infections have been reported. *Pneumocystis carinii* has been observed in patients with acquired immunodeficiency syndrome (AIDS). Treatment involves incision/drainage of abscess and antibiotics.

3. Describe the four stages of subacute thyroiditis (see figure).
Stage I   Patients have a painful (uni- or bilateral) tender thyroid and may have systemic symptoms (fatigue, malaise, fever). Inflammatory destruction of thyroid follicles allows release of excess thyroxine (T_4) and triiodothyronine (T_3) into the blood, and thyrotoxicosis may ensue.

Stage II   A transitory period (several weeks) of euthyroidism occurs after the T_4 is cleared from the body.

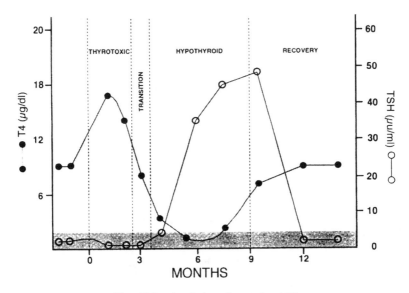

Thyroid function during subacute thyroiditis.

Stage III   With severe disease, patients may become hypothyroid until the thyroid
gland repairs itself.

Stage IV   A euthyroid state returns.

4. What is the natural history of subacute thyroiditis?

Subacute thyroiditis is probably viral in origin. Histologically, the inflammation is granulomatous. Although patients almost always recover clinically, serum thyroglobulin levels remain elevated and intrathyroidal iodine content is low for many months. Patients are also more susceptible to iodine-induced hypothyroidism at a later time. Such findings suggest persistent subclinical abnormalities after an episode of subacute thyroiditis. About 2% of patients have a second episode many years later.

5. What is the most common cause of thyroiditis?

Autoimmune thyroid disease is most common. It is recognized by the presence of thyroid peroxidase (TPO) antibodies and, less frequently, thyroglobulin antibodies in serum.

6. Give the clinical characteristics of autoimmune thyroid disease.

Chronic lymphocytic thyroiditis (Hashimoto's disease) usually presents as a euthyroid goiter that progresses to hypothyroidism in middle-aged and older persons, especially women. Atrophic thyroiditis is characterized by a very small thyroid gland in a hypothyroid patient. Some evidence suggests that thyroid growth inhibitory antibodies may account for the lack of a goiter. Two thirds of adolescents with goiter have autoimmune (juvenile) thyroiditis.

7. Does postpartum thyroiditis follow a different clinical course from that of other types of autoimmune thyroiditis?

Yes. Postpartum disease develops in women between the third and ninth month after delivery. It typically follows the stages seen in patients with subacute thyroiditis, although histologically patients have lymphocytic infiltration.

8. How common is postpartum thyroiditis?

After delivery, 5–10% of women develop biochemical evidence of thyroid dysfunction. About one third of affected women develop symptoms (usually hypothyroidism) and benefit from 6–12 months of therapy with L-thyroxine.

9. What are the differences between subacute and postpartum thyroiditis?

Patients with subacute thyroiditis have thyroid pain, an elevated sedimentation rate, and a transient rise in thyroid antibodies. Most are positive for the HLA-B35 antigen, and histologic examination shows giant cells and granulomas in the thyroid. In postpartum disease, there is no pain, the sedimentation rate is normal, and thyroid antibodies are positive both before and after the episode. The prevalence of HLA-DR3 and HLA-DR5 antigens is increased, and histologic examination shows lymphocytic infiltration of the thyroid gland.

10. Why do women develop postpartum thyroiditis?

Women who develop postpartum thyroiditis have underlying asymptomatic autoimmune thyroiditis. During pregnancy, the maternal immune system is partially suppressed, with a dramatic rebound rise in thyroid antibodies after delivery. Although TPO antibodies are not believed to be cytotoxic, they are currently the most reliable marker of susceptibility to postpartum disease.

11. Does thyroid function in patients with postpartum thyroiditis return to normal, as it does in subacute thyroiditis?

Not always. Approximately 20% of women become permanently hypothyroid, and a similar number have persistent mild abnormalities.

12. Do any factors identify women at increased risk of developing postpartum thyroiditis?

Women with a higher TPO antibody titer are more likely to develop thyroiditis. Approximately 25% of women with type 1 diabetes mellitus develop thyroiditis after delivery. For high-risk patients, screening for thyroid antibodies and careful monitoring of thyroid function are indicated.

13. What is painless thyroiditis?

Both men and non-postpartum women may present with transient thyrotoxic symptoms. As with subacute thyroiditis, they often experience subsequent hypothyroidism. Unlike subacute disease, this disorder is painless. It has been given a variety of names, including hyperthyroiditis, silent thyroiditis, transient painless thyroiditis with hyperthyroidism, and lymphocytic thyroiditis with spontaneously resolving hyperthyroidism. This disease was first described in the 1970s and reached its peak incidence in the early 1980s. It seems to occur less often now.

14. What is the etiology of painless thyroiditis?

Some investigators believe that it is a variant of subacute thyroiditis, because a small percentage of patients with biopsy-proved subacute disease have had no pain (they may have fever and weight loss and may be mistaken for having systemic disease or malignancy). Others believe that painless thyroiditis is a variant of Hashimoto's disease, because the histology of the two is similar. Painless thyroiditis can rarely present with thyroid pain.

15. What is destruction-induced thyroiditis?

Destruction-induced thyroiditis refers to the three disorders (subacute, postpartum, and painless thyroiditis) in which an inflammatory infiltrate destroys thyroid follicles and excessive amounts of T_4 and T_3 are released into the circulation.

16. When a patient presents with hyperthyroid symptoms, an elevated level of T_4, and a suppressed level of TSH, what is the next test that should be ordered?

A 24-hour radioactive iodine uptake (RAIU) should be performed. When the thyroid is overactive (as in Graves' or toxic nodular disease), the RAIU is elevated. In destruction-induced thyroiditis, the RAIU is low, as a result of both suppression of TSH by the acutely increased level of serum T_4 and the diminished ability of damaged thyroid follicles to trap and organify iodine.

17. What is the appropriate therapy for patients with any of the destructive thyroiditides?

In the thyrotoxic stage, beta blockers relieve adrenergic symptoms. All forms of antithyroid therapy (drugs, radioactive iodine ablation, and surgery) are absolutely contraindicated. Analgesics (salicylates or prednisone) provide prompt relief of thyroid pain. Thyroid hormone relieves hypothyroid symptoms and should be continued for 6–12 months, depending on the severity of disease. Many patients need no therapy.

18. Can thyroiditis be drug-induced?

Yes. Amiodarone, an iodine-containing antiarrhythmic drug, may cause thyroid damage and thyrotoxicosis. It may be associated with very high serum interleukin-6 levels and is treated with prednisone. Interferon alpha (less commonly, interferon beta) and interleukin-2 can cause thyroiditis, and both hyper- and hypothyroidism have occurred during therapy.

19. What is Riedel's struma?

Riedel's struma is a rare disorder in which the thyroid becomes densely fibrotic and hard. Local fibrosis of adjacent tissues may produce obstructive symptoms that require surgery. In some cases, fibrosis of other tissues (fibrosing retroperitonitis, orbital fibrosis, or sclerosing cholangitis) may occur.

20. Are there any other causes of thyroiditis?

Yes. External beam radiotherapy can cause painless thyrotoxic thyroiditis. Various forms of neck trauma (neck surgery, cyst aspiration, seat belt injury) have also been reported.

BIBLIOGRAPHY

1. Aizawa T, Watanabe T, Suzuki N, et al: Radiation-induced painless thyrotoxic thyroiditis followed by hypothyroidism: A case report and literature review. Thyroid 8:273–275, 1998.
2. Bartalena L, Brogioni S, Grasso L, et al: Treatment of amiodarone-induced thyrotoxiccosis, a difficult challenge: Results of a prospective study. J Clin Endocrinol Metab 81:2930–2933, 1996.
3. Berger SA, Zonszein J, Villamena P, et al: Infectious diseases of the thyroid gland. Rev Infect Dis 5:108–122, 1983.
4. de Lange WE, Freling NJ, Molenaar WM, et al: Invasive fibrous thyroiditis (Riedel's struma): A manifestation of multifocal fibrosclerosis? A case report with review of the literature. Q J Med 72:709–717, 1989.
5. Gerstein HC: Incidence of postpartum thyroid dysfunction in patients with type I diabetes mellitus. Ann Intern Med 118:419–423, 1993.
6. Guttler R, Singer PA, Axline SG, et al: *Pneumocystis carinii* thyroiditis. Report of three cases and review of the literature. Arch Intern Med 153:393–396, 1993.
7. Iitake M, Momotani N, Ishii J, et al: Incidence of subacute thyroiditis recurrences after a prolonged latency: 24-year survey. J Clin Endocrinol Metab 81:466–469, 1996.
8. Koh LK, Greenspan FS, Yeo PP: Interferon-alpha induced thyroid dysfunction: Three clinical presentations and a review of the literature. Thyroid 7: 891–896, 1997.
9. Ross DS: Syndromes of thyrotoxicosis with low radioactive iodine uptake. Endocrinol Metab Clin North Am 27:169–185, 1998.
10. Rotenberg Z, Weinberger I, Fuchs J, et al: Euthyroid atypical subacute thyroiditis simulating systemic or malignant disease. Arch Intern Med 146:105–107, 1986.
11. Roti E, Minelli R, Gardini E, et al: Iodine-induced hypothyroidism in euthyroid subjects with a previous episode of subacute thyroiditis. J Clin Endocrinol Metab 70:1581–1585, 1990.
12. Seminra SB, Daniels GH: Amiodarone and the thyroid. Endocr Pract 4:48–57, 1998.
13. Shigemasa C, Ueta Y, Mitani Y, et al: Chronic thyroiditis with painful tender thyroid enlargement and transient thyrotoxicosis. J Clin Endocrinol Metab 70:385–390, 1990.
14. Smallridge RC: Postpartum thyroid disease: A model of immunologic dysfunction. Clin Appl Immunol Rev. 1:89–103, 2000.
15. Smallridge RC: Postpartum thyroid dysfunction: A frequently undiagnosed endocrine disorder. Endocrinologist 6:44–50, 1996.
16. Smallridge RC, De Keyser FM, Van Herle AJ, et al: Thyroid iodine content and serum thyroglobulin: Cues to the natural history of destruction-induced thyroiditis. J Clin Endocrinol Metab 62: 1213–1219, 1986.
17. Volpé R: The management of subacute (DeQuervain's) thyroiditis. Thyroid 3:253–255, 1993.
18. Woolf PD: Transient painless thyroiditis with hyperthyroidism: A variant of lymphocytic thyroiditis? Endocr Rev 1:411–420, 1980.

37. THYROID NODULES AND GOITER

William J. Georgitis, M.D., FACP

1. What is the definition of goiter?

Goiter is defined as an enlargement of the thyroid gland visible as a swelling of the front of the neck. Dictionary-listed roots include French *goitre*, Middle French *goitron* or throat, the assumed Vulgar Latin term *guttrion*, and Latin terms *guttrio* and *guttur* for throat, dated 1625.

2. Describe how nontoxic goiter develops.

The pathogenesis for euthyroid goiter is still being studied. TSH-dependent enlargement of the thyroid to compensate for diminished thyroid hormone production resulting from environmental goitrogens, iodine deficiency, or inherited biosynthetic defects may be important. Regression of goiter after iodine supplementation or thyroxine suppression of TSH supports this mechanism. However, TSH levels are not elevated in endemic goiter. Genetic factors may be important and can possibly involve thyroglobulin, thyroperoxidase, intracellular signaling pathways affecting cell life cycles, and the Na^+/I^- symporter.

3. What is the natural history of diffuse nontoxic goiter?

Simple goiter over time tends to become multinodular and heterogenous in morphology and function. Autonomous function, defined as TSH-independent production and secretion of thyroid hormone, may evolve. Iodine supplementation treatment programs introduced to decrease the incidence of cretinism and goiter in populations with iodine deficient goiter have led to hyperthyroidism (jodbasedow hyperthyroidism) in some individuals with underlying thyroid autonomy. This form of hyperthyroidism, which may be transient, also appears following iodine exposure to radiographic contrast agents or medications rich in iodine.

4. How does lithium cause goiter?

Lithium has many diverse effects on the thyroid. It inhibits iodine uptake, dampens iodotyrosine coupling, alters thyroglobulin structure, blocks thyroid hormone secretion, and has mitogenic actions. The blocking effect on thyroid hormone release is most important for the development of goiter and hypothyroidism. During lithium therapy in patients free of thyroid disease, TSH secretion increases and compensatory thyroid enlargement occurs but hypothyroidism generally does not appear.

However, in euthyroid patients with compromised thyroid function, the addition of lithium may result in symptomatic hypothyroidism. Hypothyroid symptoms are easily overlooked during lithium treatment for depression or bipolar disorder. Thyroid tests before and during lithium treatment are especially appropriate for patients with underlying chronic lymphocytic thyroiditis, partial thyroidectomy, or past history of injury to the thyroid from radiation or viral thyroiditis.

5. What diagnosis should be suspected when a thyroid nodule suddenly is painful and increases in size?

Hemorrhagic degeneration of a benign adenoma with cyst formation should be suspected. Expansion of the nodule stretches visceral pain fibers in the thyroid capsule. The resulting deep aching pain may be referred to the jaw or ear. Needle aspiration yields hemorrhagic fluid.

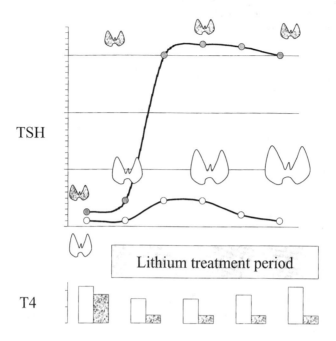

6. How can patients with low radioactive uptake forms of hyperthyroidism including viral subacute thyroiditis, lymphocytic thyroiditis with spontaneously resolving hyperthyroidism (also called silent or painless thyroiditis), and factitious thyroid hormone ingestion be differentiated?

Patients with any of these disorders might have an abnormal thyroid gland by palpation. This is true even of the patient surreptitiously taking thyroid hormone, since he/she may have originally had a goiter that gave them access to a prescription for thyroid hormone. As shown in the table below, each disorder has some features that help distinguish it from the others. Subacute thyroiditis has symptoms, signs, and laboratory findings suggestive of a systemic viral illness, whereas painless thyroiditis and factitious thyroid hormone use do not. Elevated serum thyroid hormone levels in both types of thyroiditis result from the release of thyroid hormone from an inflamed thyroid gland, and therefore serum thyroglobulin levels are usually normal or high. In contrast, thyroglobulin release should be suppressed by surreptitious thyroid hormone ingestion. Finally, the course over time may help to define the correct diagnosis because thyroiditis eventually resolves to euthyroidism or evolves to hypothyroidism.

	Subacute Thyroiditis	Painless thyroiditis	Factitious hyperthyroidism
Thyrotoxicosis	+	+	+
Fever	+	–	–
Constitutional symptoms	+	–	–
Neck and jaw pain	+	–	–
Goiter	+	+	±
Sedimentation rate	↑↑	N	N
Serum thyroglobulin	↑	↑	N
Anti-TPO antibodies	–	+	–

N = normal, TPO = thyroid peroxidase.

7. How are most thyroid cancers discovered?

Most thyroid cancers are discovered just by chance in asymptomatic patients. A lump in the neck may be noted first by the patient, by an examining physician, or during imaging studies to investigate structures adjacent to the thyroid. Neck pain, hoarseness, or symptoms of tracheal compression are unusual and when present suggest rapid growth from aggressive forms of thyroid malignancy like lymphoma or anaplastic thyroid cancer that fortunately are rare. Thyroid nodules are common, with a lifetime occurrence approaching 6% and an autopsy prevalence of 50%. The vast majority are benign. The frequency of thyroid cancer in surgical series before the widespread use of fine-needle aspiration averaged about 10%.

8. List a differential diagnosis for nodules of the thyroid.

Adenoma	Thyroiditis	Metastatic cancer
Carcinoma	Thyroid hemiagenesis	Parathyroid cyst
Thyroid cyst	Lymphoma/sarcoma	

9. Can the nature of a thyroid nodule be suspected on the basis of history or physical examination?

Most patients with thyroid nodules, both benign and malignant, have no symptoms and have normal thyroid function. Certain clinical features are worth noting, however. Symptoms attributable to a neck mass, such as hoarseness, dysphagia, dyspnea, or hemoptysis from tracheal invasion, suggest malignancy. Recent painless growth typifies thyroid cancer, whereas the sudden appearance of thyroid pain and enlargement most often results from hemorrhagic degeneration of a benign nodule. Family history is usually not helpful except in medullary thyroid cancers associated with the multiple endocrine neoplasia syndromes; inheritance of these tumors is autosomal dominant with almost complete penetrance for the abnormal gene. Nodules greater than 3 cm in size and those fixed to adjacent neck structures or accompanied by enlarged cervical lymph nodes are more likely to be cancerous.

10. If a nodule is cancer, what kind is it likely to be?

A papillary thyroid cancer or variant of papillary is the most common by far.

Thyroid Cancer Classified in Descending Order of Frequency

Papillary	50–70%
Follicular	10–15%
Medullary	1–2%
Anaplastic	Rare
Primary thyroid lymphoma	Rare
Metastatic to thyroid	Rarely detected in vivo

11. Is examination of thyroid cyst fluid helpful in making a diagnosis?

First, the amount and gross appearance of aspirated cyst fluid are worth recording. After aspiration, about one third of cysts reaccumulate fluid. If the volume on sequential aspirations does not decline, surgical removal of the cyst should be considered. Simple thyroid cysts have yellow, burgundy, or chocolate-colored fluid and are generally benign. Complex thyroid nodules with both cystic and solid components contain brown or hemorrhagic fluid and have a higher risk of being malignant. Cytology of cyst fluid is almost always nonspecific, showing histiocytes and crenated erythrocytes. Fine-needle biopsy directed at any solid component palpable after the fluid has been drained may help to define nature of the lesion. Crystal-clear watery fluid is indicative of a parathyroid cyst. Because hyperparathyroidism in association with parathyroid cysts occurs about half the time, a serum calcium level should be checked.

12. What is the risk of cancer in patients with multinodular goiter and Hashimoto's disease?

Although autopsy series indicate that up to 75% of thyroid nodules are multiple and that malignancy is rare, any thyroid nodule can be cancerous. Contrary to old axioms, a nodule in the presence of multinodular goiter or lymphocytic thyroiditis has the same risk of cancer as a solitary nodule.

13. What is the role of fine-needle aspiration biopsy in the evaluation of a thyroid nodule?

Fine-needle aspiration (FNA) is a safe, outpatient procedure with an accuracy of 90–95% in adequate specimens interpreted by experienced cytopathologists. Most FNAs return with benign diagnoses, including adenomatous hyperplasia (benign multinodular goiter), colloid adenoma, and autoimmune thyroiditis. Surgery is thus avoided. A reading of papillary thyroid cancer helps the surgeon to plan the operation of choice. Follicular neoplasms are more vexing because FNA cannot reliably differentiate adenoma from carcinoma. Finally, FNA may yield a specimen that is inadequate for interpretation in about 15% of patients; this circumstance deserves further investigation. In summary, the information obtained from FNA of a thyroid nodule helps to direct proper management. FNA should be performed on all readily palpable solitary thyroid nodules and on dominant nodules in a multinodular goiter. In addition to a serum TSH level, many clinicians consider FNA to be the first test to be performed in the evaluation of a thyroid nodule.

14. What is the difference between a "cold," "warm," and "hot"nodule on thyroid scan?

The cold nodule displays diminished radiolabeling compared with surrounding normal thyroid tissue. Most cold nodules are benign, but virtually all thyroid cancers are cold nodules. The hot nodule avidly absorbs tracer, whereas uptake by the remainder of the thyroid is suppressed. Solitary toxic nodules (STNs) are usually larger than 3 cm in diameter and most often occur in patients older than 40. Toxic adenomas are never cancerous. The majority have gain of function mutations in the thyrotropin receptor. In contrast, a warm nodule may be malignant. Some warm nodules are really cold nodules that appear warm because they are invested by normal thyroid tissue. Others are autonomous but, unlike a STN, fail to secrete sufficient thyroid hormone to suppress TSH secretion and dampen tracer uptake by surrounding normal thyroid tissue. Repeat thyroid scanning with the patient taking a dose of thyroid hormone that suppresses the serum TSH level may help by demonstating automous function in a nodule that initially appeared warm on scan. Autonomous nodules may be observed, whereas all others deserve FNA to exclude thyroid cancer.

15. Who invented the incision used for thyroidectomy?

Theodor Kocher (1841–1917), a Swedish surgeon, devised the incision. He was an innovator. So be cautiou, when you ask for a "Kocher" in the operating room. Kocher's name is also associated with a surgical forcep, a wrist operation, and a right subcostal incision for cholecystectomy.

16. Which treatment was used first for diffuse toxic goiter (Graves' disease), radioactive iodine or antithyroid medications?

Both were developed in the early 1940s. Thiourea, the first goitrogenic substance to be used, had undesirable toxicities and soon was replaced by methimazole and propylthiouracil. Of the fission products developed during World War II, [130]I was used before [131]I. Radioiodine became widely available in about 1946.

17. What thyroid conditions are treated with radioactive iodine?

Radioiodine treatment is effective for diffuse toxic goiter, toxic nodular goiter, and solitary toxic nodules. Compressive symptoms from benign multinodular goiters in patients judged to be poor surgical risks can also be relieved by radioactive iodine. Although the goiter shrinks only about 30% or less, relief of symptoms is common. Finally, radioactive iodine is used as an adjunctive therapy for differentiated forms of thyroid cancer and has been shown to decrease cancer recurrence.

18. When is suppression therapy with thyroxine useful?

Although thyroxine suppression therapy was widely used in the past in the belief that it reduced the size of thyroid nodules, this issue is not so clear now that objective measurements with thyroid ultrasound are being used in randomized studies. For euthyroid patients, thyroid hormone administration to induce regression of thyroid nodules has not proven to be very effective except under special circumstances, such as in iodine deficient subjects or in preventing new nodules after lobectomy in radiation-exposed patients. For solitary nodules, the apparent reduction in size with thyroid hormone administration may represent regression of surrounding thyroid tissue rather than the nodule itself. Routine administration to all patients may be associated with more iatrogenic side effects than benefit but may still be valuable in certain cases. For example, in a patient with goiter and evidence of recent thyroid enlargement and an elevated serum TSH, thyroid hormone replacement may cause regresson of the goiter. Less clear is the question of whether TSH should be suppressed to low-normal levels or below the normal range.

BIBLIOGRAPHY

1. Bennedbæk FN, Nielsen LK, Hegedüs L: Effect of percutaneous ethanol injection therapy vs. suppressive doses of L-thyroxine on benign solitary solid cold thyroid nodules: A randomized trial. J Clin Endocrinol Metab 83:830–835,1998.
2. Bennedbæk FN, Perrild H, Hegedüs L: Diagnosis and treatment of the solitary thyroid nodule. Results of a European survey. Clin Endocrinol 50:357–363, 1999.
3. Cheung PSY, Lee JMH, Boey JH: Thyroxine suppressive therapy of benign solitary thyroid nodules: a prospective randomized study. World J Surg 13:818–822, 1989.
4. Dremier S, Coppee F, Delange F, et al: Thyroid autonomy: Mechanism and clinical effects. J Clin Endocrinol Metab 81:4187–4193, 1996.
5. Hegedus L, Nygaard B, Hansen JM: Is routine thyroxine treatment to hinder postoperative recurrence of nontoxic goiter justified? J Clin Endocrinol Metab 84:756–760, 1999.
6. Lazarus JH: The effects of lithium therapy on thyroid and thyrotropin-releasing hormone. Thyroid 8:909–913, 1998.
7. Mazzaferri EL: Management of a solitary thyroid nodule. N Engl J Med 328:553–559, 1993.
8. Mortensen JD: Gross and microscopic findings in clinically normal thyroid glands. J Clin Endocrinol Metab 15:1270–1280, 1955.
9. Ridgway EC: Medical treatment of benign thyroid nodules: Have we defined a benefit? Ann Intern Med 128:403–405, 1998.
10. Rojeski MT: Nodular thyroid disease. N Engl J Med 313:428–436, 1985.
11. Ross DS: Evaluation of the thyroid nodule. J Nucl Med 32:2181–2192, 1991.

38. THYROID CANCER

Arnold A. Asp, M.D.

1. What are the most common types of thyroid cancer?

The thyroid consists predominantly of follicular epithelial cells, which incorporate iodine into thyroid hormone to be stored in follicles, and of smaller numbers of parafollicular cells, which produce calcitonin. Malignant transformation of either type of cell may occur, but the parafollicular malignancy (medullary carcinoma of the thyroid) is much less common than cancers derived from follicular epithelial cells. Malignancies originating from follicular epithelial cells are designated according to their microscopic appearance and include papillary, follicular, and anaplastic carcinomas.

Papillary carcinoma and its variants comprise approximately 60–80% of thyroid cancers, whereas follicular carcinoma makes up approximately 15–30% of primary thyroid malignancies. These two forms are frequently referred to as the differentiated thyroid carcinomas. Medullary carcinoma of the thyroid (MCT) comprises 2–10% of thyroid carcinomas, whereas anaplastic forms of thyroid carcinoma make up 1–10%.

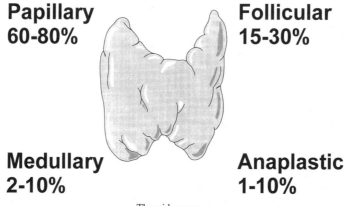

**Papillary
60-80%**

**Follicular
15-30%**

**Medullary
2-10%**

**Anaplastic
1-10%**

Thyroid cancer.

2. Describe the differentiated forms of thyroid carcinoma.

Malignant transformation of the iodine-concentrating cells of the thyroid follicle results in two main forms of differentiated thyroid carcinoma: papillary and follicular carcinoma. The two malignancies are histologically distinct. Papillary carcinoma is generally an unencapsulated tumor marked by enlarged cells with dense cytoplasm and overlapping nuclei that have granular, powdery chromatin, nucleoli, and pseudonuclear inclusion bodies (often called "Orphan Annie eyes"), all arranged in papillary fronds. Follicular carcinoma is generally characterized by atypical-appearing thyroid cells with dense, uniform, overlapping nuclei, and a disorganized microfollicular architecture. Follicular carcinoma cannot be differentiated reliably from benign follicular adenomas on cytomorphologic criteria alone; follicular cancer must demonstrate invasion of the tumor capsule or blood vessels. Tumors that contain histologic elements of both types of carcinoma are classified as mixed papillary-follicular cancer and are considered to be variants of papillary carcinoma. Two additional pathologic variants of papillary carcinoma, tall cell and insular cell, may be slightly more aggressive than other papillary forms.

Papillary and follicular carcinoma also behave as clinically distinct entities. Most endocrinologists consider follicular carcinoma to be the more aggressive of the differentiated cancers, with a higher rate of metastases, more frequent recurrence after therapy, and an exaggerated mortality rate compared with the relatively indolent papillary carcinoma. This view is not universal. Some authors believe that the sharp dichotomy between the clinical courses of papillary and follicular carcinoma is artificial and attribute the apparent aggressiveness of follicular carcinoma to its occurrence in an older population; they argue that when cases are controlled for age, outcomes of patients with either form of differentiated carcinoma are comparable.

3. What is the clinical course of papillary carcinoma?

Papillary carcinoma usually presents as a painless nodule within the thyroid gland or cervical lymphatics. The disease may occur at any age but has a peak incidence during the fourth decade. Women are more commonly affected than men and comprise 62–81% of patients in most series. The primary tumor is rarely encapsulated (4–22% in most series) but is less aggressive if a capsule is present. Papillary carcinoma is more commonly multifocal within the thyroid than is follicular carcinoma; 20–80% of glands have multiple lesions at resection. Extrathyroidal invasion through the capsule of the thyroid occurs in 5–16% of cases.

Papillary carcinoma frequently metastasizes to regional cervical and high mediastinal lymphatics. At the time of surgery, 35–43% of patients have enlarged regional lymph nodes that harbor cancer. If lymph nodes are systematically "picked" and examined for microscopic foci, the prevalence of cervical metastases increases to 90%. Unlike other neoplasms, the presence of papillary carcinoma in regional lymph nodes does not increase mortality; it does, however, increase the likelihood of recurrence after therapy. Up to 20% of recurrent lesions cannot subsequently be eradicated. Although lymphatic metastases are common, only 3–7% of patients with papillary carcinoma manifest distant metastatic lesions during initial therapy. Distant metastases involve the lung (76% of distant foci), bone (23% of distant foci), and brain (15% of distant foci).

Compared with other malignancies, papillary carcinoma is relatively indolent. Cancer-related death occurs in only 4–12% of patients during 20-year follow-up. Prognostic factors at the time of diagnosis that augur a poor outcome include male sex, age > 40 years, extrathyroidal invasion, distant metastases, and large primary tumor (> 1.5 cm diameter).

4. What is the clinical course of follicular carcinoma?

Follicular carcinoma usually presents as an asymptomatic nodule within the thyroid, but unlike papillary carcinoma, it may present as an isolated metastatic pulmonary or osseous focus without a palpable thyroid lesion. Very rarely metastatic foci of follicular carcinoma retain hormonal synthetic capability and overproduce thyroid hormones, causing thyrotoxicosis. Follicular carcinoma may occur at any age, but has a later peak incidence (fifth decade) than papillary carcinoma. Women outnumber men, comprising approximately 60% of cases. Follicular carcinoma occurs more commonly in areas of iodine deficiency; the incidence of this malignancy has decreased as iodine supplementation has increased. The tumor is nearly always encapsulated, and the degree of vascular or capsular invasiveness (minimal to extensive) is indicative of malignant potential. Follicular carcinoma is usually unifocal (< 10% multifocal).

Hematogenous metastases occur in follicular carcinomas; for this reason, cervical and mediastinal lymphatic involvement is less common than in papillary carcinoma (only 6–13% of patients during initial surgery). In contrast to cases of papillary carcinoma, the presence of cervical metastases indicates advanced disease. Distant metastases to the lung, bone, and central nervous system (in descending order of occurrence) are discovered more commonly in follicular than in papillary carcinoma, occurring in 12–33% of cases. Death due to follicular carcinoma occurs in 13–59% of patients followed for 20 years. Prognostic factors at the time of initial therapy that portend a poor outcome include age greater than 50 years, male sex (in some settings), marked degree of vascular invasion, and distant metastases.

5. Do any other factors predict the course of differentiated carcinoma?

Differentiated carcinoma is discovered in 5–10% of the surgical resections performed for the treatment of Graves' disease. In some series of patients with Graves' disease, up to 45% of palpable nodules contain papillary carcinoma. Such data have led to the speculation that the thyroid-stimulating immunoglobulins responsible for thyrotoxicosis may potentiate the growth of neoplastic cells and predispose to aggressive forms of differentiated carcinoma.

Chronic lymphocytic thyroiditis is found concomitantly with papillary carcinoma in 5–10% of cases. Local recurrence and metastatic disease are less common in such cases and may indicate a favorable effect of Hashimoto's disease.

Distant metastatic disease, as mentioned above, occurs more commonly in follicular carcinoma than in papillary cancer. Regardless of the primary type of cancer, the prognosis associated with distant metastases is dismal. Overall, 50–66% of patients with pulmonary, osseous, or central nervous system lesions die within 5 years. On rare occasions, pulmonary metastases may be compatible with 10–20 year survival in younger patients. Metastases to bone are associated with brief survival, despite aggressive therapy.

6. How are the differentiated carcinomas treated?

No other subject in endocrinology inflames passions or sparks controversy more than the therapy of differentiated thyroid carcinoma. Meetings of specialists are all too often subjected to the sad spectacle of fisticuffs between members as the merits of therapy are debated; balding bespectacled men in bowties circle one another, fists and arms gamely pumping the air, while female counterparts shriek biostatistics peppered with vernacular epithets and common finger gestures seldom encountered outside the confines of the roller-derby rink. Simply stated, therapy of differentiated thyroid carcinoma is based on the surgical removal of the primary tumor and eradication of all metastatic disease with radioactive iodine (^{131}I). Lifelong suppression of thyroid-stimulating hormone (TSH) with exogenous thyroid hormone subsequently reduces the risk of recurrence.

7. What type of surgery is preferred?

Opinions about the extent of initial surgical resection have been tempered by the possible complications of thyroid surgery; recurrent laryngeal nerve damage with resultant hoarseness and/or iatrogenic hypoparathyroidism occur, in 1–5% of thyroid resections. Fear of complications, coupled with the relatively low mortality rate associated with differentiated thyroid carcinoma, has prompted some surgeons to remove only the thyroid lobe in which cancer is apparent at the time of exploration.

Most surgeons, however, are cognizant of the frequency of clinically inapparent multicentric lesions, the increased recurrence rates in patients treated with simple lobectomy, and the low rate of postsurgical complications; thus they have rejected simple lobectomy and instead prefer near-total thyroidectomy, which entails the removal of the thyroid lobe containing the tumor, the isthmus, and the majority of the contralateral thyroid lobe. The posterior capsule of the contralateral lobe is left undisturbed in an attempt to preserve the underlying parathyroid glands and the recurrent laryngeal nerve. With this procedure, the surgeon is able to remove the primary tumor and the bulk of normal thyroid tissue that may harbor microscopic malignancy.

Cervical and high mediastinal lymph nodes that appear to harbor metastatic disease are harvested at the time of surgery. Radical neck dissections do not reduce mortality or rate of recurrence and should be avoided, unless there are direct extensions of the tumor through-out the neck. In the event that a single, small (< 1.5 cm) papillary or minimally invasive fol-licular carcinoma is discovered, lobectomy and isthmusectomy may be curative.

8. How does ^{131}I therapy benefit the patient?

Most (but not all) differentiated thyroid malignancies retain the ability to trap inorganic iodine when stimulated by TSH. When ^{131}I is concentrated within normal or malignant thy-roid tissue, beta-irradiation results in cellular damage or death. If a metastatic lesion is capa-ble of concentrating ^{131}I, it becomes visible with a gamma camera; if it absorbs enough ^{131}I to impart 8000 cGy of irradiation, the tumor focus may be eradicated. This is the basis of postsurgical radioiodine scans (^{131}I or ^{123}I) for whole-body surveillance and the therapeu-tic use of ^{131}I to treat residual, recurrent, and metastatic disease. Patients with one thyroid lobe intact (after lobectomy and isthmusectomy) concentrate the entire scanning dose of radioiodine within the remaining lobe. Metastatic foci outside the thyroid cannot be detected in these patients, and surveillance scans are therefore uninformative and should be avoided. To optimize the efficacy of whole-body scans and to maximize the concentration of thera-peutic radioiodine in metastatic lesions, serum levels of TSH must be elevated. Withdrawal of exogenous L-thyroxine for 6 weeks before the scan allows the protein-bound fraction of the hormone to be exhausted. To alleviate symptoms of hypothyroidism, liothyronine (Cytomel, 25 mg twice daily) is administered for the first 4 weeks of the withdrawal period but discontinued during the 2 weeks before the scan. Liothyronine, with a shorter half-life than thyroxine, is rapidly depleted after withdrawal. During the 2-week period in which no exogenous thyroid hormone is available, a rapid rise in serum TSH (> 30 mU/ml) ensues. Normal remnant thyroid tissue (on the posterior capsule of the thyroid bed) and malignant tissue are maximally stimulated by elevated levels of TSH and usually concentrate any available radioiodine.

During the whole-body scan, 3–5 mCi of ^{131}I or 1.5 mCi of ^{123}I is administered orally to the patient, who is subsequently positioned under a gamma camera after the radioiodine is allowed to equilibrate (48–72 hours for ^{131}I; 5 hours for ^{123}I). The resultant image indi-cates the amount of thyroid tissue remaining in the thyroid bed and the extent of local and distant metastatic disease. Therapeutic ^{131}I is then administered.

9. How much ^{131}I is administered to the postsurgical patient?

A discussion of the studies supporting the various doses of therapeutic radioiodine exceeds the scope of this chapter. Generally, in the patient with a single, small papillary tumor (< 1.5 cm) free of extrathyroidal metastases at the time of surgery and on subsequent whole-body scan, many endocrinologists consider the resection curative and do not admin-ister radioiodine. In such cases, the use of adjunctive radioiodine does not alter the course of the disease. The author prefers, however, to administer a small dose of ^{131}I (30 mCi) in an attempt to ablate the thyroid bed and thereby to improve the accuracy of future surveil-lance scans. This "small" dose ablates up to 80% of thyroid remnants. Other endocrinolo-gists believe that this dose is insufficient to ablate all residual normal and malignant tissue and prefer a dose of 70–150 mCi of radioiodine.

Patients with large or aggressive tumors, metastatic disease evident during surgery, or extrathyroidal lesions visible on postsurgical whole-body scans usually receive 100–200 mCi of ^{131}I in an attempt to eradicate the malignancy. These "large" doses of radioiodine have tra-ditionally been administered only in an approved inpatient facility under the auspices of the Nuclear Regulatory Commission (NRC). Patients remain isolated until ambient levels of radioactivity fall to acceptable levels. Radionuclide is excreted renally, but significant amounts are also present in saliva and sweat; such wastes must be disposed of appropriately. More recently the NRC has lifted the absolute requirement for inpatient administration of high dose ^{131}I, and this procedure is now being performed in some centers on an outpatient basis.

10. Are there complications of ^{131}I therapy?

Radioiodine is absorbed by the salivary glands, gastric mucosa, and thyroid tissue. Within 72 hours of oral administration of ^{131}I, patients may experience radiation sialadenitis and transient nausea. Such symptoms are self-limited. Thyroid tissue may become edematous and tender but rarely requires corticosteroid therapy. Radioiodine, borne in the blood, causes transient, clinically insignificant suppression of the bone marrow.

Late complications of high-dose radioiodine therapy may include gonadal dysfunction and predisposition to nonthyroidal malignancies. Some studies have demonstrated reduced sperm counts in male patients proportional to the administered dose of ^{131}I. Older women may experience temporary amenorrhea and reduced fertility. Two deaths from bladder cancer and three deaths from leukemia have been reported among patients treated with lifetime cumulative doses of radioiodine exceeding 1000 mCi. Most studies suggest that cumulative doses of ^{131}I less than 700–800 mCi, given in increments of 100–200 mCi separated by 6–12 months, are not leukemogenic.

11. How are bony and pulmonary metastases treated?

Radioiodine (^{131}I) is often used to treat bony and pulmonary metastases. Multifocal skeletal metastases from differentiated thyroid cancer are generally treated with 200 mCi of ^{131}I. However, isolated bony lesions are often treated instead with surgical resection or curettage or with external beam radiation therapy. Pulmonary metastases present a therapeutic dilemma, because radiation absorbed by the malignant cells often causes fibrosis of the underlying lung parenchyma. For this reason, pulmonary metastases that absorb more than 50% of the scanning dose of radioiodine are usually treated with no more than 75–80 mCi of ^{131}I.

12. How are patients monitored for recurrent disease?

Following surgery and radioiodine therapy, all patients are placed on a large enough dose of exogenous thyroid hormone to render serum levels of TSH undetectable. A whole-body scan should be repeated, after proper preparation, approximately 6–12 months after the initial surgery and ^{131}I therapy. After two serial scans, separated by at least 6–12 months, are free of evident disease, semiannual scans may be discontinued. Some centers subsequently repeat surveillance scans every 5 years, but because the procedure is distinctly uncomfortable for the patient, many centers do not adhere to this schedule.

Another means of detecting recurrent disease in the asymptomatic patient is annual measurement of serum thyroglobulin. This protein, manufactured only by normal or malignant thyroid cells, should be undetectable in the serum of a patient who has undergone complete surgical and radioiodine ablation. Evidence of recurrent tumor (rising levels of thyroglobulin or palpable neck mass) warrants the repetition of a whole-body scan. Although the measurement of serum thyroglobulin levels while the patient is on levothyroxine suppression therapy with a low or undetectable serum TSH level has some value, the diagnostic accuracy of thyroglobulin determinations is greatly enhanced by measuring serum thyroglobulin when the patient's serum TSH level is elevated, following levothyroxine withdrawal.

13. Isn't there an alternative to withdrawal of thyroid hormone prior to a whole body scan?

Recombinant human TSH (rhTSH; Thyrogen) has been approved for use in scanning patients with differentiated thyroid carcinoma. The rhTSH acts just as native TSH produced by the pituitary, stimulating iodine uptake and thyroglobulin secretion from remnant thyroid tissue and metastatic foci of cancer. The rhTSH (0.9 mg) is administered intramuscularly once daily for two consecutive days, followed by a scanning dose of ^{131}I (3-5 cGy) given orally on the third day. The patient is then imaged under a gamma camera on the fifth day. Serum thyroglobulin levels are drawn before administration of rhTSH and compared with those obtained on the fifth day. The rhTSH stimulated scans, when coupled with concomitant serum thyroglobulin measurements, are generally as accurate as standard whole-body scans, and do not cause the significant hypothyroid symptoms that patients experience with levothyroxine withdrawal scans. Unfortunately, rhTSH has not yet been approved for use in raising serum TSH levels prior to therapeutic I administration. Therefore rhTSH scans should be avoided if recurrent or metastatic thyroid cancer requiring ^{131}I treatment is anticipated.

14. Which malignancy is associated with prior radiation exposure?

From 1940 through the early 1970s, external irradiation of the head and neck was used in the treatment of acne, enlarged thymus, enlarged tonsils and adenoids, tinea capitis, and asthma. It was recognized belatedly that such radiation exposure caused neoplastic transformation of thyroid cells; after a 10–20 year latency period, 33–40% of exposed individuals developed benign thyroid nodules, and 5–11% developed carcinoma. The carcinomas in irradiated glands mirror those found within the non-irradiated population, with papillary cancer predominating. The tumors are no more aggressive but are more often multicentric (55%) than in non-irradiated individuals (22%).

15. What is a Hurthle cell?

Hurthle, or Askanazy, cells are large polygonal cells with abundant cytoplasm and compact nuclei; they are found in benign nodules, Hashimoto's disease, and either form of differentiated thyroid carcinoma. Hurthle-cell carcinoma, composed solely of these cells, is believed to be a particularly aggressive variant of follicular cancer that is characterized by frequent pulmonary metastases.

16. What is anaplastic thyroid carcinoma? How is it treated?

Anaplastic thyroid carcinoma is one of the most aggressive and resistant forms of human cancer. This malignancy comprises only 1–10% of all thyroid carcinomas in the Western hemisphere but accounts for up to 50% of thyroid carcinomas in some areas of eastern Europe. Like follicular carcinoma, it is more prevalent in areas of iodine deficiency; the incidence is currently declining throughout North America.

Four histologic variants of anaplastic carcinoma are currently recognized: giant cell, spindle cell, mixed spindle-giant cell, and small cell carcinoma. True small cell carcinoma is extremely rare, and most "small cell" tumors are actually a malignant form of lymphoma that is more amenable to therapy. Microscopic examination of the anaplastic malignancies reveals bizarre fibrous whorls, primitive follicles, and cartilage and osteoid reminiscent of chondrosarcoma.

Anaplastic carcinoma occurs more commonly in the elderly (peak age: 65–70 years) and affects equal numbers of males and females. These cancers may arise in preexisting differentiated thyroid carcinomas (dedifferentiation), in benign nodules, or, most commonly, de novo. The miniscule number of anaplastic malignancies within large series of patients followed for decades with differentiated carcinoma may discredit the theory of dedifferentiation of established cancers. Anaplastic carcinoma expands rapidly; most patients present with steric symptoms, such as dyspnea, dysphagia, hoarseness, and pain. Nearly one-half of all patients require tracheostomy as a result of explosive tumor growth.

The type of histologic variant does not appear to affect outcome; prognosis is dismal in most cases. Surgical extirpation has been combined with external beam irradiation

(4500–6000 cGy) or chemotherapy (usually doxorubicin or paclitaxel) in an attempt to eradicate the malignancy. Despite vigorous therapy, average survival is approximately 6–8 months.

17. What is medullary carcinoma of the thyroid (MCT)?

MCT is a neoplasm that arises from the parafollicular cells (or C-cells) of the thyroid. Embryologically, these cells originate in the neural crest and migrate to the thyroid, where despite close proximity, there is no apparent physical or hormonal interaction with the follicular cells. The parafollicular cells elaborate calcitonin (CT), which acts on osteoclasts to modulate release of calcium from skeletal stores. The DNA that contains the genetic code for CT also contains the code for another peptide, calcitonin gene-related peptide (CGRP). Tissue-specific alternative splicing allows parafollicular cells to secrete CT, whereas neural cells produce only CGRP. Neoplastic transformation of parafollicular cells results in unbridled expression of normal cell products (CT) and abnormal products (CGRP, chromogranin A, carcinoembryonic antigen [CEA], adrenocorticotropin [ACTH]). CT serves as an excellent tumor marker for the malignancy, and the abnormal products mediate the clinical syndromes associated with MCT. Accumulation of massive amounts of procalcitonin within the thyroid is detectable histologically as amyloid (AE type).

18. How common is MCT?

MCT comprises approximately 2–10% of all thyroid malignancies and occurs in sporadic and hereditary forms. Sporadic MCT is the more common form. Most patients present in the fourth or fifth decade, with most series reporting nearly equal numbers of men and women. Sporadic MCT is usually unifocal within the thyroid and may originate in any portion of the gland. One half of all patients manifest metastatic disease at the time of presentation; metastatic sites include (in descending order) local lymphatics, lung, liver, and bone.

The hereditary form of MCT occurs within kindreds as an isolated condition (familial MCT), as a component of multiple endocrine neoplasia (MEN) 2A (MCT, hyperparathyroidism, pheochromocytoma), as a component of the MEN 2B syndrome (MCT, pheochromocytoma, mucosal neuromas), or in conjunction with pheochromocytoma and cutaneous lichen amyloidosis. All forms are transmitted as an autosomal dominant trait. Hereditary tumors are bilateral and arise in the junction of the upper one third and lower two thirds of the thyroid lobes, where the concentration of C-cells is highest. Biochemical screening for MCT to detect early disease within affected kindreds enhances the survival of individuals with hereditary MCT compared with those with the sporadic form. An erudite discussion of the MEN syndromes is included in Chapter 54, the belletristic presentation of which will undoubtedly move the reader to tears.

19. Are extrathyroidal manifestations associated with MCT?

The wide array of peptides and prostaglandin products secreted by MCT tumors results in multiple extrathyroidal symptoms. The most common is diarrhea, which occurs in up to 30% of patients with MCT. Although CT, CGRP, prostaglandins, 5-hydroxytryptamine, and vasoactive intestinal peptide have been proposed as the causative secretagogue, none has been convincingly implicated.

On rare occasions, Cushing's syndrome may occur in MCT and is attributable to the secretion of either ACTH, corticotropin-releasing hormone (CRH), or both. Successful therapy of the underlying malignancy ameliorates the cushingoid features.

There are no reported cases of hypocalcemia due to the chronic production of CT by MCT.

20. How can CT be used as a clinically useful tumor marker?

CT is secreted by normal parafollicular cells and cells undergoing neoplastic transformation. Most certainly in the hereditary form, and probably in the sporadic form of MCT, malignant degeneration of the C-cells is preceded by a period of "benign" hyperplasia, during which curative resection is theoretically feasible. The serum level of CT is proportional to the mass of hyperplastic or malignant parafollicular cells. Unfortunately, the Kulchitsky cells of the lung as well as cells of the thymus, pituitary, adrenal glands, and prostate also secrete small amounts of CT, as do certain malignancies, such as small cell lung cancer and breast cancer.

A clinically relevant test is required to allow the discrimination of the CT of non-MCT sources from the CT produced by hyperplastic and malignant C-cells. The pentagastrin stimulation test satisfies this requirement. The test involves the intravenous administration of pentagastrin (0.5 μg/kg body weight) with the collection of CT at baseline, 1.5, 2, 5, and 10 minutes after injection. Normal subjects demonstrate little or no response to the infusion, whereas subjects with C-cell hyperplasia or MCT manifest an exaggerated response. Absolute values depend on the assay used for determining CT. When pentagastrin is unavailable, a calcium infusion (2 mg/kg over 5 minutes) can similarly be used to stimulate CT secretion. As assays for the MEN 2 gene on chromosome 10 become clinically available (see Chapter 54), screening of kindreds for the hereditary form of MCT with stimulation tests may be unnecessary. The test, however, will remain valuable in elucidating residual disease after therapy.

21. How is MCT treated?

The therapy of MCT remains frustrating. When MCT is discovered on biopsy or suspected as a result of the screening of kindred members, the entire thyroid should be surgically removed, with care to preserve the parathyroids and laryngeal nerves. A dissection of the lymphatics of the central neck also should be undertaken, because 50–70% of these nodes contain metastases. Because parafollicular cells do not accumulate radioiodine, postsurgical radioablation is not warranted. External beam radiotherapy and chemotherapy do not appear to improve survival, although they are sometimes used in desperation against recurrent disease. Residual disease grows slowly, causing obstructive symptoms and the symptoms listed in question 18. Rates of 10- and 20-year survival in one large series were 63% and 44%, respectively.

22. Now that we know all about the thyroid malignancies, what is the correct approach to a patient with a thyroid nodule?

The prevalence of nodular thyroid disease increases with age and is approximately 4 times higher in women than in men. By the sixth decade of life, 5–10% of the general population in developed nations have one or more palpable thyroid nodules. Detection by palpation is relatively insensitive, however; ultrasonographic or pathologic (autopsy) examination of the population reveals a much higher prevalence of thyroid nodules (20% by 40 years of age, 50% by 70 years of age). Only 8–17% of surgically resected nodules are cancerous; the remainder are nonmalignant and mandate excision only for obstructive symptoms or cosmesis. The responsibility of the internist is to steer patients with nodules of malignant potential to resection, but to stay the hand of the surgeon when excision of a benign nodule is proposed.

Fine-needle aspiration (FNA) of a palpable nodule is the first test performed by most endocrinologists. Collection of the sample is relatively simple for most sighted individuals; cytologic interpretation of the sample is the limiting factor in this procedure. The diagnostic accuracy of FNA is reported to range between 70–97%. Interpretation of the aspiration sample may indicate that the nodule is malignant, benign, or "suspicious for malignancy." The sample also may be judged to have inadequate material for interpretation, requiring reaspiration. Papillary carcinoma may be diagnosed with some certainty from FNA samples, but the diagnosis of follicular carcinoma requires the demonstration of vascular invasion. Some large centers boast cytopathologists who can reliably differentiate follicular carcinoma from follicular adenoma; these uncommon, grizzled old demigods of pathology have forsaken the company of mortals for the solace of their microscopes. Most cytopathologists designate such samples as "follicular neoplasm" or "suspicious for malignancy."

Some endocrinologists advocate the performance of a radionuclide scan to determine the metabolic activity of the nodule and to discern the existence of other unsuspected nodules. Such data are potentially valuable; autonomous or "hot" nodules rarely harbor malignancy but may yield cytopathologic specimens that mimic malignancy. Detractors of radionuclide scanning, however, criticize the cost and delay in performance of FNA and tout the rare cancer found in autonomous nodules. Ultrasound of thyroid nodules provides little significant value as a diagnostic tool for an individual nodule but may help detect other nodules that are difficult to palpate because of their posterior or substernal location. Furthermore, ultrasound-guided FNA can be very useful for obtaining tissue from these difficult-to-palpate nodules and from nodules that are discovered incidentally during imaging procedures that were ordered to evaluate other conditions.

Nodules designated as malignant on FNA should be resected. Those designated as "suspicious for malignancy" or "follicular neoplasm" also should be referred for excision, because up to 20% are malignant. Benign nodules should be observed for change in size or obstructive symptoms; the administration of suppressive amounts of exogenous thyroid hormone is controversial because of the attendant risk for osteoporosis and the lack of data demonstrating unequivocal efficacy of this intervention.

The internist occasionally encounters a patient who chooses surgical resection of a nodule despite benign results with FNA. This prompts a final word of advice: "Never stand between a ready surgeon and a willing patient who has been thoroughly apprised of the risks of thyroid surgery." False-negative results of FNA range between 1–6%, and up to 35% of thyroids in autopsy series contain clinically insignificant papillary carcinomas, either of which, if discovered at a later date, will engender distrust on the part of the patient.

23. Has a molecular defect been associated with thyroid carcinoma?

Mutation of a single protooncogene or tumor suppressor gene has not been associated with thyroid carcinogenesis. Several mutations have been described in thyroid neoplasms; however, none appears to be able to induce malignant changes without concomitant cooperating mutations. Although the practical relevance of these defects is limited at this time, further research may identify these or others as clinical indicators of the malignant potential of individual tumors.

The *ras* protooncogenes code for a family of receptor-associated proteins, named p21, that serve as signal transducers between membrane receptors and intracellular effectors. When the receptors are stimulated, p21 becomes complexed with guanosine triphosphate (GTP) and activates MAP kinase. Because excessive kinase activity would be detrimental, native p21 possesses intrinsic GTP-ase activity, which eventually inactivates the complex and terminates the activity of MAP kinase. Mutation of the *ras* protooncogene results in p21 that lacks GTP-ase activity, causing uncontrolled accumulation of kinase activity and prompting disordered cellular growth. *Ras* oncogene has been described in 10–50% of follicular carcinomas in iodine-deficient areas.

Closely related to *ras*-coded p21 are the G-stimulatory (Gs) proteins, which also link transmembrane receptors to intracellular effectors, such as adenyl cyclase. Gs proteins consist of α, β, and γ subunits, noncovalently bound together, that become active when GTP complexes to the α subunit. Native Gsα possesses intrinsic GTP-ase activity that functions as a timer, stopping the reaction at an appropriate point. Mutations of the Gsα gene that code for proteins lacking intrinsic GTP-ase activity have been discerned. These constitutively activated Gs proteins promote both cell growth and function; they have been detected primarily in functioning benign thyroid nodules and rarely in differentiated thyroid carcinomas.

Another mutation that has been described in differentiated thyroid carcinomas is the *ret/ptc* oncogene. The *ret* protooncogene is found on chromosome 10 and normally codes a receptor (*ret*) with intrinsic tyrosine kinase activity. The ligand for *ret* is a glial cell derived neurotrophic factor; *ret* is not normally expressed on thyroid follicular cells. The *ret/ptc* mutation results in constitutively activated tyrosine kinase, which causes disordered cellular development and is found in 2-70% of papillary thyroid carcinomas, depending on the ethnic group. Although tumors expressing this mutation are no larger than other papillary cancers, they may be more likely to metastasize.

A final mutation associated with up to 25% of anaplastic thyroid carcinomas codes for abnormal protein p53. Normal p53 is found in the cytoplasm, where it forms a complex with heat shock protein-70 (hsp70) and crosses the nuclear membrane to interact with nuclear transcription factors. Mutation of the gene coding for p53 results in translation of a protein that cannot interact with these nuclear proteins. Loss of this tumor suppressor causes unrestricted cell growth and, along with other coexisting mutations, malignant degeneration.

BIBLIOGRAPHY

1. Brennan MD, Bergstralh EJ, van Heerden JA, McConahey WM: Follicular thyroid cancer treated at the Mayo Clinic, 1946 through 1970: Initial manifestations, pathologic findings, therapy, and outcome. Mayo Clin Proc 66:11–22, 1991.
2. Chua EL, Wu WM, Tran KT, et al: Prevalence and distribution of ret/ptc 1, 2, and 3 in papillary thyroid carcinoma in New Caledonia and Australia. J Clin Endocrinol Metab 85:2733–2739, 2000.
3. DeGroot LJ, Kaplan EL, McCormick M, Straus FJ: Natural history, treatment, and course of papillary thyroid carcinoma. J Clin Endocrinol Metab 71:414–424, 1990.
4. Demeter JG, DeJong SA, Lawrence AM, Paloyan E: Anaplastic thyroid carcinoma: Risk factors and outcome. Surgery 110:956–963, 1991.
5. Dulgeroff AJ, Herschman JM: Medical therapy for differentiated thyroid carcinoma. Endocr Rev 15:500–515, 1994.
6. Farid NR, Shi Y, Zou M: Molecular basis of thyroid cancer. Endocr Rev 15:202–232, 1994.
7. Fogelfeld L, Wiviott MBT, Shore-Freedman E, et al: Recurrence of thyroid nodules after surgical removal in patients irradiated in childhood for benign conditions. N Engl J Med 320:835–840, 1989.
8. Gagel RF, Robinson MF, Donovan DT, Alford BB: Medullary thyroid carcinoma: Recent progress. J Clin Endocrinol Metab 76:809–814, 1993.
9. Gharib H, McConahey WM, Tiegs RD, et al: Medullary thyroid carcinoma: Clinicopathologic features and long-term follow-up of 65 patients treated during 1946 through 1970. Mayo Clin Proc 67:934– 940, 1992.
10. Gharib, H: The use of recombinant thyrotropin in patients with thyroid cancer. Endocrinologist 10: 255–263, 2000.
11. Grauer A, Raue F, Gagel RF: Changing concepts in the management of hereditary and sporadic medullary thyroid carcinoma. Endocrinol Metab Clin North Am 19:613–635, 1990.
12. Kebebew E, Clark OH: Differentiated thyroid cancer: "Complete" rational approach. World J Surg 24:942–951, 2000.
13. Mazzaferi EL: Controversies in the management of differentiated thyroid cancer. Endocrine Post-Graduate Syllabus 167–189, 1990.
14. Mazzaferi EL: Management of a solitary thyroid nodule. N Engl J Med 328:553–559, 1993.
15. McConahey WM, Hay ID, Woolner L, et al: Papillary thyroid cancer treated at the Mayo Clinic, 1946 through 1970: Initial manifestations, pathologic findings, therapy, and outcome. Mayo Clin Proc 61:978–996, 1986.
16. Nel CJC, van Heerden JA, Goellner JR, et al: Anaplastic carcinoma of the thyroid: A clinicopathologic study of 82 cases. Mayo Clin Proc 60:51–58, 1985.
17. Robbins J (moderator): Thyroid cancer: A lethal endocrine neoplasm. Ann Intern Med 115: 133–147, 1991.

39. THYROID EMERGENCIES

Michael T. McDermott, M.D.

1. What is thyroid storm?
Thyroid storm or crisis is a life-threatening condition characterized by an exaggeration of the manifestations of thyrotoxicosis.

2. How do patients develop thyroid storm?
Thyroid storm generally occurs in patients who have unrecognized or inadequately treated thyrotoxicosis and a superimposed precipitating event, such as thyroid surgery, non-thyroid surgery, infection, or trauma.

3. What are the clinical manifestations of thyroid storm?
Fever (> 102° F) is the cardinal manifestation. Tachycardia is usually present, and tachypnea is common, but the blood pressure is variable. Cardiac arrhythmias, congestive heart failure, and ischemic heart symptoms may develop. Nausea, vomiting, diarrhea, and abdominal pain are frequent features. Central nervous system manifestations include hyperkinesis, psychosis, and coma. A goiter is a helpful finding but is not always present.

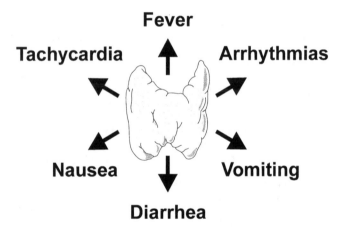

Thyroid storm.

4. What laboratory abnormalities are seen in thyroid storm?
Serum thyroxine (T_4), triiodothyronine (T_3), T_3 resin uptake (T3RU), free T_4 and free T_3 are usually all elevated, and serum thyrotropin (TSH) is undetectable. Other common laboratory abnormalities include anemia, leukocytosis, hyperglycemia, azotemia, hypercalcemia, and elevated liver-associated enzymes.

5. How is the diagnosis of thyroid storm made?
The diagnosis must be made on the basis of suspicious but nonspecific clinical findings. Serum thyroid hormone levels are elevated but, if the diagnosis is strongly suspected, waiting for the results of tests may cause a critical delay in the initiation of effective life-saving therapy. Furthermore, thyroid hormone levels do not reliably distinguish patients with thy-

roid storm from those who have uncomplicated thyrotoxicosis as a coincident disorder. Clinical features are therefore the key.

6. What other conditions may mimic thyroid storm?
Similar presentations may be seen with sepsis, pheochromocytoma, and malignant hyperthermia.

7. How should patients with thyroid storm be treated?
As soon as the diagnosis is made, measures should be taken to decrease thyroid hormone synthesis, to inhibit thyroid hormone release, to reduce the heart rate, to support the circulation and to treat the precipitating condition. Specific medications that can be used for these purposes are listed below.

Decrease Thyroid Hormone Synthesis
Propylthiouracil (PTU)	200 mg q4h (orally, rectally, or NG tube)
Methimazole (Tapazole)	20 mg q4h (orally, rectally, or NG tube)

Inhibit Thyroid Hormone Release
Sodium iodide (NaI)	1 g over 24 hours IV
Potassium iodide (SSKI)	5 drops q8h orally
Lugol's solution	10 drops q8h orally

Reduce the Heart Rate
Propranolol	40–80 mg q4–6h orally, or
	1–2 mg at 1 mg/min q4-6 hours IV
Esmolol	.25–.50 mg/kg over 1 min. IV, then
	.05–.10 mg/kg/min infusion
Diltiazem	60–90 mg q6–8h orally, or
	.25 mg/kg over 2 min. IV, then 10 mg/min infusion

Support the Circulation
Dexamethasone	2 mg q6h IV, or
Hydrocortisone	100 mg q8h IV
Intravenous fluids	

Treat the Precipitating Condition

8. What is the prognosis for patients with thyroid storm?
When thyroid storm was first described, the acute mortality rate was nearly 100%. Today, the prognosis is significantly improved when aggressive therapy, as described above, is initiated early; however, the mortality rate continues to be approximately 20%.

9. What is myxedema coma?
Myxedema coma is a life-threatening condition characterized by an exaggeration of the manifestations of hypothyroidism.

10. What are the clinical manifestations of myxedema coma?
Hypothermia, bradycardia, and hypoventilation are common; blood pressure, while generally reduced, is more variable. Pericardial, pleural, and peritoneal effusions are often found. An ileus is present in about two thirds of patients, and acute urinary retention also may be seen. Central nervous system manifestations include seizures, stupor, and coma; deep tendon reflexes are either absent or exhibit a delayed relaxation phase. Typical hypothyroid changes of the skin and hair may be apparent. A goiter, although frequently absent, is a helpful finding; a thyroidectomy scar also may be an important clue.

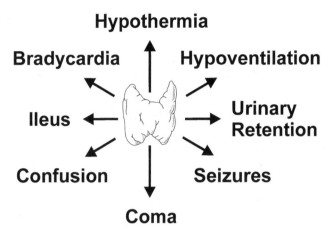

Hypothermia

Bradycardia ↑ **Hypoventilation**

Ileus ← → **Urinary Retention**

Confusion ↓ **Seizures**

Coma

Myxedema coma.

11. How do patients develop myxedema coma?

Myxedema coma usually occurs in elderly patients who have inadequately treated or untreated hypothyroidism and a superimposed precipitating event. Important events include prolonged cold exposure, infection, trauma, surgery, myocardial infarction, congestive heart failure, pulmonary embolism, stroke, respiratory failure, gastrointestinal bleeding, and administration of various drugs, particularly those that have a depressive effect on the central nervous system.

12. What laboratory abnormalities are seen in myxedema coma?

Serum T_4, T_3, T3RU, free T_4 and free T_3 are usually low, and the TSH is significantly elevated. Other frequent abnormalities include anemia, hyponatremia, hypoglycemia, and elevated serum levels of cholesterol and creatine kinase (CK). Arterial blood gases usually reveal retention of carbon dioxide and hypoxemia. The electrocardiogram often shows sinus bradycardia, various types and degrees of heart block, low voltage, and T-wave flattening.

13. How is the diagnosis of myxedema coma made?

The diagnosis must be made on clinical grounds based on the findings described above. Serum levels of thyroid hormones are reduced and the TSH level is elevated, but the delay involved in waiting for test results may unnecessarily postpone the initiation of effective therapy.

14. How should patients with myxedema coma be treated?

As soon as the diagnosis is made, steps should be taken to rapidly replete circulating thyroid hormone levels, to replace glucocorticoids, to support vital functions and to treat the precipitating conditions. The issue of whether to use levothyroxine (LT4), liothyronine (LT3), or a combination of the LT4 and LT3 remains controversial and has not been settled by an adequate prospective investigation. Specific measures that can be used are listed below.

Rapid Repletion of Circulating Thyroid Hormones

Levothyroxine (LT4)	300–500 µg over 5 min IV, then 50–100 µg qd orally or IV.
Liothyronine (LT3)	50–100 µg over 5 min IV, then LT4 50–100 µg qd orally or IV

LT4 plus LT3	LT4 150–300 μg over 5 min IV, plus
	LT3 10 μg over 5 min IV, then
	LT4 50–100 μg qd orally or IV

Glucocorticoid Replacement
  Hydrocortisone   100 mg q8h IV

Support Vital Functions
  Oxygen
  Intravenous fluids
  Rewarming (blankets or central rewarming)
  Mechanical ventilation (if needed)

Treat the Precipitating Condition

15. What is the prognosis for patients with myxedema coma?

Myxedema coma originally had a mortality rate of 100%. Today, the outlook is much improved for appropriately treated patients, although the mortality rate in recent studies has varied from 0–45%.

BIBLIOGRAPHY

1. Brooks MH, Waldstein SS: Free thyroxine concentrations in thyroid storm. Ann Intern Med 93:694, 1980.
2. Burch HD, Wartofsky L: Life threatening thyrotoxicosis: Thyroid storm. Endocrinol Metab Clin North Am 22:263–278, 1993.
3. Dillmann WH: Thyroid storm. Curr Ther Endocrinol Metab 6:81–85, 1997.
4. Jordan RM: Myxedema coma. Pathophysiology, therapy, and factors affecting prognosis. Med Clin North Am 79 (1):185–194, 1995.
5. Nicoloff JT: Myxedema coma: A form of decompensated hypothyroidism. Endocrinol Metab Clin North Am 22:279–290, 1993.
6. Olsen CG: Myxedema coma in the elderly. J Am Board Fam Pract 8:376–383, 1995.
7. Pittman CS, Zayed AA: Myxedema coma. Curr Ther Endocrinol Metab 6:98–101, 1997.
8. Tietgens ST, Leinung MC: Thyroid storm. Med Clin North Am 79 (1):169–184, 1995.
9. Tsitouras PD: Myxedema coma. Clin Geriatr Med 11:251–258, 1995.
10. Yamamoto T, Fukuyama J, Fujiyoshi A: Factors associated with mortality of myxedema coma: Report of eight cases and literature survey. Thyroid 9:1167–1174, 1999.
11. Yeung S-CJ, Go R, Balasubramanyam A: Rectal administration of iodide and propylthiouracil in the treatment of thyroid storm. Thyroid 5:403–405, 1995.

40. EUTHYROID SICK SYNDROME

Michael T. McDermott, M.D.

1. What is the euthyroid sick syndrome?

The euthyroid sick syndrome refers to a group of changes in serum thyroid hormone and TSH levels that occur in patients with a variety of non-thyroidal illnesses including infections, trauma, surgery, myocardial infarction, malignancies, inflammatory conditions and starvation. This condition is also called the non-thyroidal illness syndrome. It is not a primary thyroid disorder but instead results from changes in the peripheral metabolism and transport of thyroid hormones induced by the non-thyroidal illness.

2. What hormone changes characterize the euthyroid sick syndrome?

Patients with mild to moderate non-thyroidal illnesses often develop low serum total T_3 and free T_3 levels. This results from decreased conversion of T_4 to T_3 by peripheral tissues, predominantly the liver. Serum TSH levels generally remain in the normal range.

With more severe non-thyroidal illnesses, serum T3 levels may become very low; in addition, the total T_4 concentrations become depressed while the T3RU increases. The latter changes result from reduced binding of thyroid hormones to their transport proteins owing both to impaired hepatic protein synthesis and to the presence of circulating inhibitors of thyroid hormone protein binding. Free T_4 levels are more variable, however, having been observed in numerous studies to be either normal, increased, or decreased. Serum TSH levels remain normal or become slightly decreased at this stage.

When non-thyroidal illnesses resolve, thyroid hormone levels also return to normal. However, as hepatic protein synthesis improves and circulating inhibitors of thyroid hormone binding disappear, there may be a transient drop in serum free T_4 values with a resultant increase in serum TSH levels before complete normalization occurs.

3. How can the euthyroid sick syndrome be distinguished from hypothyroidism?

In the euthyroid sick syndrome, serum T_3 is decreased proportionately more than T_4, the T3RU tends to be high, and the TSH is normal or mildly decreased. In primary hypothyroidism, serum T_4 is reduced proportionately more than T_3, the T3RU tends to be low, and the TSH is increased. Other tests also may be helpful. In the euthyroid sick syndrome, free T_4 is usually normal and reverse T_3 (RT_3) is increased; in hypothyroidism, both free T_4 and RT_3 are decreased.

4. What causes the euthyroid sick syndrome?

The euthyroid sick syndrome is believed to be caused by increased circulating levels of cytokines and other mediators of inflammation that result from the underlying non-thyroidal illness. These mediators can alter multiple aspects of thyroid economy at the level of the hypothalamus, the pituitary, the thyroid, serum transport proteins, and peripheral tissues.

5. Is the euthyroid sick syndrome an adaptive mechanism, or is it harmful?

Many experts consider the euthyroid sick syndrome to be an adaptive mechanism that may reduce peripheral tissue energy expenditure during the non-thyroidal illness. Conversely, others argue that the alterations in circulating thyroid hormone levels may themselves be harmful and may accentuate the effects of the non-thyroidal illness. This issue is likely to remain controversial for years to come.

6. Should patients with the euthyroid sick syndrome be treated with thyroid hormones?

Management of the euthyroid sick syndrome is also highly controversial. Currently, there are no consistent or convincing data demonstrating a recovery or survival benefit from treating euthyroid sick syndrome patients with either levothyroxine (LT4) or liothyronine (LT3). Experts continue to debate this issue, however, and agree that large, prospective studies are needed to answer this question. In the absence of more definitive data, thyroid hormone therapy cannot be recommended at this time.

7. Does the euthyroid sick syndrome have any prognostic significance?

Current evidence indicates that the prognosis for recovery from critical nonthyroidal illnesses may be fairly well predicted from the severity of the reduction in serum levels of T_3 and T_4. Patients with extremely low serum T_3 levels have a very high mortality rate.

8. Are levels of thyroid hormone ever elevated in patients with non-thyroid diseases?

The serum T_4 may be transiently elevated in patients with acute psychiatric illnesses and in patients with various acute medical illnesses. The mechanisms underlying such elevations of T_4 are not well understood, but may be mediated by alterations in neurotransmitters or cytokines. This condition must be distinguished from true thyrotoxicosis.

BIBLIOGRAPHY

1. Brennan MD, Bahn RS: Thyroid hormones and illness. Endocr Pract 4:396–403, 1998.
2. Brent GA, Hershman JM: Thyroxine therapy in patients with severe nonthyroidal illness and low serum thyroxine concentration. J Clin Endocrinol Metab 63:1–8, 1986.
3. Camacho PM, Dwarkanathan A: Sick euthyroid syndrome. What to do when thyroid function tests are abnormal in critically ill patients. Postgrad Med 105:215–219, 1999.
4. Chopra I: Euthyroid sick syndrome: Is it a misnomer? J Clin Endocrinol Metab 82:329–334, 1997.
5. DeGroot LJ: Dangerous dogmas in medicine: The nonthyroidal illness syndrome. J Clin Endocrinol Metab 84:151–164, 1999.
6. Kimura T, Kanda T, Kotajima N, et al: Involvement of circulating interleukin-6 and its receptor in the development of euthyroid sick syndrome in patients with acute myocardial infarction. Eur J Endocrinol 143:179–184, 2000.
7. McIver B, Gorman CA: Euthyroid sick syndrome: An overview. Thyroid 7:125–132, 1997.
8. Morley JE, Slag MF, Elson MK, Shafer RB: The interpretation of thyroid function tests in hospitalized patients. JAMA 249:2377–2379, 1983.
9. Nagaya T, Fujieda M, Otsuka G, et al: A potential role of activated NF-kappaB in the pathogenesis of euthyroid sick syndrome. J Clin Invest 106:393-402, 2000.
10 Simons RJ, Simon JM, Demers LM, Santen RJ: Thyroid dysfunction in elderly hospitalized patients: Effect of age and severity of illness. Arch Intern Med 150:1249–1253, 1990.

41. THYROID DISEASE IN PREGNANCY

Linda A. Barbour, M.D., M.S.P.H.

1. What are the physiologic changes in thyroid function seen in normal pregnancy?

Pregnancy results in a number of hormonal changes and increased metabolic demands that significantly alter thyroid function (see table). The influence of estrogen and human chorionic gonadotropin (hCG) on circulating thyroid hormone levels requires that thyroid function tests in pregnancy be interpreted cautiously. Estrogen increases thyroid binding globulin (TBG) 2–3 fold beginning a few weeks after conception. This results in a 30–100% increase in serum total T_4 and total T_3 levels since circulating thyroid hormones are highly protein bound. Measurement of the T_3 resin uptake (T3RU), which is inversely related to serum thyroid binding capacity, is correspondingly low, so that the free T_4 index (FT4I; calculated by multiplying the total T_4 by the T3RU) is usually normal. The free T_4, free T_3, and TSH levels, in contrast, are usually normal during all three trimesters, although slight variation in their values can be seen in a number of circumstances at different periods of gestation.

During the first trimester, high levels of hCG may stimulate thyroid T4 secretion sufficiently to suppress the serum TSH into the 0.1–0.5 μU/ml range in up to15% of pregnant women. This is because the beta-subunit of hCG has 85% sequence homology in the first 114 amino acids with TSH and can bind to and stimulate the TSH receptor. It has been estimated that a 10,000 IU/L increase in circulating hCG corresponds to a mean free T_4 increment of 0.6 ng/ml. Levels of hCG above 50,000 IU/L, which may be seen when hCG peaks at the end of the first trimester, can therefore increase the free T_4 level enough to suppress the serum TSH. However, the TSH remains in the low-normal range and the free T_4 is in the upper-normal range in the majority of cases. A TSH in the high-normal range during the first trimester is therefore suspicious for subclinical hypothyroidism and should be rechecked in 4–6 weeks.

The mother must increase her hormonal output of thyroid hormone during pregnancy for a number of reasons. First, there appears to be some thyroid hormone loss as a result of limited transplacental passage of thyroid hormone. Second, thyroid hormone may undergo enhanced metabolism owing to high activity of a placental Type III monodeiodinase, which converts T_4 to reverse T_3 (rT3) and T3 to T2. Finally, iodine requirements increase in pregnancy as a result of a marked increase in the maternal glomerular filtration of iodine (~50%) and owing to increasing fetal iodine requirements for the synthesis of fetal thyroid hormone. Women in iodine-replete areas often show a slight increase in TSH and a slight decrease in free T_4 in the third trimester, probably owing to both a 2–3 fold increase in TBG and the increasing thyroid hormone requirements during pregnancy. However, TSH and free T_4 in the third trimester are usually maintained in the normal range as long as the functional capacity of the maternal thyroid is normal.

Thyroid Function Tests During Normal Pregnancy

	First Trimester	Second Trimester	Third Trimester
Total T4	↑	↑	↑
T3RU	↓	↓	↓
Free Thyroxine Index	Normal	Normal	Normal
Total T3 (RIA)	↑	↑	↑
Free T4	Normal	Normal	Normal
TSH	Normal or ↓	Normal	Normal

2. What is the "goiter of pregnancy," and is it necessary to evaluate an enlarged thyroid gland in pregnancy?

The "goiter of pregnancy" has been well described in iodine-deficient areas of the world but does not generally occur in geographic regions that are iodine-replete. In fact, one of the first pregnancy tests to be developed in these iodine-deficient areas was a tightly fitting loosely braided necklace that broke when a woman developed such a goiter. Iodine requirements increase markedly during pregnancy as a result of increased urinary iodine losses, diversion of iodine to the fetus for thyroid hormone synthesis, and increased maternal thyroid hormone requirements. The World Health Organization (WHO) recommendations for iodine intake are 200 μg/day during pregnancy and 150 μg/day in the non-pregnant state. If iodine intake is insufficient, thyroid hormone production drops, resulting in increased secretion of TSH, which then stimulates thyroid gland growth. Thyroid volume commonly increases by 30% or more during pregnancy in these iodine-deficient regions and often does not completely regress following delivery. Many European and Third World countries with endemic iodine deficiency do not supplement with iodine and therefore women are at risk of iodine deficiency goiters during pregnancy. When iodine intake is severely deficient, overt hypothyroidism results. Endemic cretinism occurs if severe hypothyroidism due to iodine deficiency goes unrecognized and untreated at birth.

In iodine-replete areas such as the U.S., the thyroid gland volume may increase by 10–15% as a result of pregnancy-induced vascular swelling of the gland; although this enlargement can be recognized by ultrasound, it cannot usually be appreciated by palpation. Therefore, any goiter found during pregnancy in an iodine-replete area should be evaluated in the same manner as one occurring outside of pregnancy.

3. Which thyroid hormones and thyroid-related medications cross the placenta?

Thyroid hormone crosses the placenta poorly owing in part to the high placental activity of the Type III monodeiodinase that converts T_4 to rT_3 and T_3 to T_2. However, it is now clear that some T_4 does cross, since fetuses with complete thyroid agenesis have about 30% of the normal amount of thyroid hormone at birth. Significant amounts of thyroid hormone also appear to cross in the first trimester before the fetal thyroid begins functioning. In contrast, iodine easily crosses the placenta for use by the fetal thyroid, which, after 12 weeks' gestation, takes up iodine even more avidly than the maternal thyroid. PTU, methimazole, and beta blockers also cross the placenta well. Thyrotopin-releasing hormone (TRH), but not TSH, also crosses and has been used in experimental protocols to attempt to accelerate fetal lung maturity. Immunoglobulin (IgG) antibodies, such as thyroid stimulating immunoglobulins (TSI), cross the placenta especially in the late second and third trimesters and can occasionally cause fetal or neonatal hyperthyroidism in infants of women with Graves' disease. Although thyroid peroxidase antibodies (TPO antibodies) and anti-thyroglobulin antibodies (TG antibodies) can also cross, this is usually of no clinical significance. However, very rarely they may be associated with thyrotropin receptor–blocking antibodies that can cause transient neonatal hypothyroidism.

4. When does the fetus begin making thyroid hormone, and is fetal thyroid hormone production independent of maternal thyroid status?

At about 10–12 weeks, the fetal thyroid gland develops and the hypothalamic-pituitary-thyroid axis begins to function. Prior to this, the fetus is dependent on maternal thyroid hormone. Inadvertent exposure to I-123 prior to 8 weeks is worrisome but unlikely to cause fetal hypothyroidism because the half-life of this isotope is short and fetal uptake is negligible until 10 weeks. Ablative doses of I-131, however, can cause fetal hypothyroidism even in the first trimester because it has a longer half-life. A pregnancy test should therefore always be done before administering I-123 or I-131 to a woman of child-bearing age.

After the first trimester, the fetal hypothalamic-pituitary-thyroid axis is fairly independent of the mother with the exception of its dependence on adequate maternal iodine stores. Anti-thyroid drugs or high levels of TSI may, however, affect fetal thyroid function or cause goiter development at this stage. Thyroid hormone and TBG levels increase in the fetus and plateau at about 35–37 weeks' gestation. High levels of rT3 and low levels of T_3 are maintained throughout the pregnancy as a result of the high placental activity of Type III monodeiodinase. The axis is relatively immature, however, considering the increased fetal TSH levels relative to the low level of T_4 production at birth. At the time of labor and in the early neonatal period, there is a dramatic increase in the capacity of the liver to convert T_4 to T_3.

5. What is gestational thyrotoxicosis or hyperthyroidism related to hyperemesis gravidarum? How can it be differentiated from other types of hyperthyroidism in pregnancy?

Gestational thyrotoxicosis refers to hyperthyroidism caused by elevated levels of hCG. This molecule has significant sequence homology with TSH, enabling it to bind and weakly activate the TSH receptor. At levels exceeding 50,000 IU/ml, which are commonly seen during the first trimester, hCG has sufficient thyrotropic effects to raise serum thyroid hormone levels enough to suppress the serum TSH level. Higher levels of hCG are seen in women with twin pregnancies and especially in molar pregnancies, during which hyperthyroidism is commonly seen. In fact, a woman who presents with hyperthyroidism and a positive pregnancy test should have an ultrasound to exclude a molar pregnancy.

Women with hyperemesis gravidarum (persistent nausea and vomiting accompanied by electrolyte derangements and weight loss) commonly have abnormal thyroid function tests. In one of the largest series yet published, half of the 57 women with hyperemesis gravidarum had elevated free T_4 measurements. It may be difficult to differentiate this disorder from other causes of hyperthyroidism, since autoimmune hyperthyroidism also commonly presents during the first trimester of pregnancy and the biochemical profile of the two conditions is similar. However, it is extremely important to determine whether the thyrotoxicosis is due to Graves' disease or to hyperemesis gravidarum because the latter usually resolves without anti-thyroid treatment by ~18 weeks when hCG levels decline and the hyperemesis usually resolves. Clues pointing to the diagnosis of hCG-induced hyperthyroidism include the absence of a goiter, ophthalmopathy, or pre-existing hyperthyroid symptoms antedating the pregnancy. In addition, TSI levels are usually negative and T_3 levels are generally not as high as those in Graves' disease because the compromised nutritional state of these women results in decreased conversion of T4 to T3 in peripheral tissues. It is rarely necessary to treat with beta-blocker therapy or anti-thyroid drugs, since the hyperthyroid state is usually self-limited. Hyperthyroidism is probably not the cause of the nausea. Instead, it appears that hCG is mediating both the hyperthyroidism and nausea by different mechanisms.

6. What are the most common causes of hyperthyroidism in pregnancy, and during what period of gestation is it most likely to present?

Hyperthyroidism complicates pregnancy in about 0.2% of women. Graves' disease is the most common cause of hyperthyroidism in pregnancy, accounting for nearly 85% of the cases. Autoimmune thyroid disease is most likely to present in the first trimester or the postpartum period, because the immune suppression of pregnancy has been shown to significantly decrease thyroid antibody levels during the second and third trimesters. Other causes include toxic multinodular goiters, solitary toxic adenomas, iodine-induced hyperthyroidism, and subacute thyroiditis. As noted above, hCG-induced hyperthyroidism is common in women with hyperemesis gravidarum or hydatidiform moles.

7. What is the diagnostic evaluation of women with hyperthyroidism?

Normal pregnancy can produce clinical features that mimic hyperthyroidism; these include heat intolerance, mild tachycardia, increase in cardiac output, a systolic flow murmur, peripheral vasodilation, and a widened pulse pressure. Weight loss may be obscured by the weight gain of pregnancy. As in the nonpregnant state, hyperthyroidism in pregnancy is usually characterized by low serum TSH levels and increased serum levels of free T_4. However, when interpreting thyroid tests in pregnant women, it is important to realize that serum TSH levels are also frequently low in normal women during the first trimester of pregnancy.

Radioisotope scans are contraindicated during pregnancy, and therefore the differential diagnosis of hyperthyroidism in pregnant women must be based on the history, physical exam, and laboratory testing. An obstetric ultrasound may be indicated to exclude a hydatidiform mole or to look for twin pregnancies. Although a diffusely enlarged thyroid gland with a bruit in a woman with ophthalmopathy and pre-pregnancy symptoms is strongly suggestive of Graves' disease, the diagnosis is often less clear, since these findings may be absent. If a woman is actively vomiting, the distinction between early Graves' disease and hyperemesis gravidarum may be particularly difficult. It is unusual, however, for women to develop hCG-induced hyperthyroidism at hCG levels less than 50,000 IU/ml. The presence of onycholysis, pretibial myxedema, and high serum levels of T_3 or TSI also supports a diagnosis of Graves' disease. Women who have goiters from endemic areas of iodine deficiency and who move to the U.S. may develop iodine-induced hyperthyroidism when they suddenly become iodine-replete.

8. What are the risks of Graves' disease to the mother?

Inadequately treated hyperthyroidism in the mother can result in pre-eclampsia, weight loss, proximal muscle weakness, anxiety, and atrial fibrillation. Left ventricular dysfunction can occur and is usually reversible but may persist for several weeks after biochemical hyperthyroidism has been corrected. This may place the pregnant woman at risk for the development of congestive heart failure, especially in the presence of superimposed pre-eclampsia, infection, anemia, or at the time of delivery. Thyroid storm can also occur in these women.

9. What are the risks to the fetus of maternal Graves' disease?

Inadequately treated maternal hyperthyroidism can result in fetal tachycardia, severe growth restriction, premature births, and a 9-fold increased incidence of low birth weight in the infants. Congenital malformations are probably not increased in babies born to mothers with either treated or untreated hyperthyroidism.

In about 2–5% of cases, fetal or neonatal hyperthyroidism can develop as a result of very high levels of maternal TSI. Transplacental passage of IgG is limited, and therefore this is an unusual occurrence unless the TSI levels are at least 5-fold elevated. Treatment consists of administering higher doses of PTU to the mother in order to deliver a sufficient amount of medication into the fetal circulation. Occasionally mothers are rendered hypothyroid with these high PTU doses, and T_4 supplementation is required. Neonatal hyperthyroidism is more common than fetal hyperthyroidism because of the high activity of placental type III monodeiodinase, relatively low serum T_3 levels in utero, and the effects of maternal anti-thyroid drugs on the fetus. Neonatal hyperthyroidism may manifest as irritability, failure to thrive, hyperkinesis, diarrhea, poor feeding, jaundice, tachycardia, poor weight gain, thrombocytopenia, goiter, and, less commonly, exophthalmos, cardiac failure, hepatosplenomegaly, hyperviscosity syndrome, or craniosynostosis. Neonatal mortality may be as high as 30% if the condition is unrecognized. These infants may need to be placed on anti-thyroid medications until the antibody levels wane, which usually occurs by 20 weeks.

If the mother has been receiving anti-thyroid drugs during pregnancy, it may take 5–10 days for the neonate to manifest symptoms because of the residual effects of these medications. Rarely, women who are euthyroid from previous ablative therapy still have high enough levels of TSI to cause their infants to develop fetal or neonatal hyperthyroidism.

10. How can pregnant women with Graves' disease be safely treated in pregnancy?

Treatment of clinical hyperthyroidism is definitely indicated to decrease morbidity in both the mother and fetus. Thionamide therapy with the judicious use of beta blockers until thyroid hormone levels are reduced is the preferred treatment because radioiodine readily crosses the placenta and will be concentrated by the fetal thyroid after 10–12 weeks of gestation.

Propylthiouricil (PTU) remains the preferred anti-thyroid medication in the U.S. because of previous reports that it crosses the placenta less well than methimazole (MMI) and that MMI may be associated with a scalp deformity in the baby (aplasia cutis). Both of these concerns about MMI have been recently challenged, however, and it is currently believed that MMI can be used safely if necessary. Because PTU is more highly protein bound and crosses less well into breast milk than MMI, it is also considered preferable to use PTU in women who breast feed their infants.

Since PTU and MMI both cross the placenta, the lowest possible doses should be given with a goal of maintaining the mother's serum free T_4 or T_3 (if the mother is predominantly T_3 thyrotoxic) in the high-normal range. The serum TSH level often remains persistently suppressed in women with free T_4 and T_3 levels in this range, and therefore it cannot be used to accurately titrate the dose of anti-thyroid drugs during pregnancy. Approximately 1–3% of newborns exposed to PTU in utero develop transient neonatal hypothyroidism or a small goiter. However, this is rare if PTU doses can be decreased to < 400 mg/day at term. Fortunately, anti-thyroid drugs can usually be markedly decreased by the third trimester because of the decreasing levels of TSI that accompany the natural immunosuppression of pregnancy. In fact, many women require minimal or no drug at term, especially if they have a small goiter but it is important to ensure that they are not hyperthyroid at delivery in order to reduce the risk of thyroid storm. The majority of women will have a rebound in their hyperthyroidism postpartum, and thionamide therapy will need to be increased.

Beta-blockers are indicated to treat symptomatic hyperadrenergic signs and symptoms until anti-thyroid drug therapy has rendered the patient euthyroid. However, they should be discontinued when the patient becomes euthyroid because long-term treatment with beta-blockers has been associated with intrauterine growth restriction. There are no compelling data that one beta-blocker is safer than another.

Radioactive iodine is contraindicated in pregnancy because after 12 weeks' gestation the fetal thyroid gland has an avidity for iodine that is 20–50 times that of the maternal thyroid. Accordingly, any dose of radioiodine will be more highly concentrated in fetal thyroid tissue and can easily ablate the fetal gland. Cold iodine (e.g., Lugol's solution or SSKI) should also be avoided in pregnancy except in women with thyroid storm. If it must be given after 10–12 weeks, the baby should be monitored for the development of a goiter. Surgery is rarely indicated during pregnancy but may be necessary in women who are unable to take anti-thyroid drugs (i.e. because of agranulocytosis) or who are refractory to high doses of anti-thyroid medications. If done, it is best to perform surgery in the second trimester before fetal viability. The rationale for this is that there is a significant increase in the risk of miscarriage in the first trimester and of preterm labor when surgery is done after 24 weeks.

11. What should be done if a woman inadvertently receives an I-123 scan or an ablative dose of I-131 and is subsequently found to be pregnant?

A woman who receives I-123 for a thyroid scan early in pregnancy can be reassured for the most part because the fetus has not developed the ability to concentrate iodine before 10 weeks and the radiation exposure from this test is very low. An ablative dose of I-131 given early in pregnancy, however, is cause for greater concern because the half-life of I-131is 8 days and the radiation is more destructive to the thyroid gland. Generally, if the dose is given very early, when the fetal thyroid gland is not yet trapping iodine, the relatively low thyroid and total body irradiation dose is probably not sufficient to justify termination of the pregnancy. Nonetheless, it may be useful in these situations to give PTU to block the recycling of I-131 in the fetal thyroid gland if it can be given within 1 week of I-131 treatment. Fetal hypothyroidism can be diagnosed in utero by percutaneous umbilical sampling, and T4 treatment may be given via amniotic fluid injections, although such treatment is still experimental. Certainly, all women of childbearing age regardless of contraceptive measures should have a pregnancy test before receiving any dose of I-123 or I-131.

12. How should women with Graves' disease be counseled in regards to treatment alternatives before becoming pregnant?

Many experts would recommend definitive treatment with I-131 (after a negative pregnancy test) in a woman of childbearing age who wishes to become pregnant. In a series of nearly 300 women given radioiodine for cancer therapy, no significant difference in stillbirths, preterm births, low birth weight infants, or congenital malformations were reported in subsequent pregnancies. Effective birth control needs to be established, and then women should optimally wait for at least 3–6 months after regaining a stable euthyroid status before trying to conceive. Women who are stable on low doses of thionamides should not have a problematic pregnancy, but it is highly likely that thionamide doses will need to be adjusted during pregnancy and the postpartum period. Furthermore, thionamides are known to pass across the placenta as well as into breast milk. Rarely, women who have been definitively treated for Graves' disease still have high levels of circulating TSI, which can place the fetus at increased risk for developing fetal or neonatal hyperthyroidism despite the mother's euthyroid state. For this reason, TSI levels should be checked during pregnancy in women with active or previous Graves' disease.

13. What is the natural history of Graves' disease in the postpartum period, and what treatment options can be recommended for women who wish to breast feed?

The majority of women (~70%) will have a postpartum relapse of their Graves' disease, usually within the first 3 months after delivery, as the natural immunosuppression of pregnancy disappears. Anti-thyroid therapy must almost always be increased during this time. For the nursing mother, PTU is the preferred anti-thyroid drug because it is highly protein bound and crosses less well into breast milk than MMI. The infant will need to have thyroid function tests monitored while the mother is taking PTU. If the etiology of the hyperthyroidism is in question, a diagnostic I-123 scan can be done provided the woman is willing to interrupt breast feeding for 2–3 days. Both I-123 and 99-Tc pertechnetate are excreted into breast milk with an effective half-life of 5–8 hours and 2–8 hours, respectively. Ablative therapy with I-131 cannot be offered unless the women is willing to give up nursing altogether because even a 5-mCi dose requires discontinuation of breast feeding for at least 56 days. Beta-blockers can be used if necessary in the breastfeeding mother. However, atenolol may produce higher breast milk concentrations than other beta-blockers, and there are rare reports of neonatal bradycardia in mothers who nursed while taking this drug.

14. What are the risks to the mother of hypothyroidism in pregnancy, and how do thyroid hormone requirements change during pregnancy?

Hypothyroidism in pregnancy can cause maternal anemia, myopathy, congestive heart failure, and an increased risk of pre-eclampsia, placental abruption, low birth weight infants and postpartum hemorrhage. Thyroid hormone requirements rise during pregnancy with up to 75% of pregnant women requiring an increase in thyroxine dosage of up to 50 μg over their pre-pregnancy dose. The mean levothyroxine dose required by pregnant women is reported to be ~146 μg/day compared with the usual dose in nonpregnant women of 110–115 μg/day. Women who are athyreotic may need to increase their thyroid hormone dose by 25% as soon as pregnancy is confirmed. The rapid increase in thyroid hormone requirements that occurs in the first trimester may be due to the sudden increase in the TBG pool associated with pregnancy. The serum TSH level should be checked as soon as pregnancy is confirmed, and, if it is even minimally elevated, an appropriate increase in thyroid hormone should be given. As discussed above, the TSH may be mildly suppressed in normal women during the first trimester as a result of the thyrotropic influence of hCG. Therefore, unless a woman is symptomatically hyperthyroid or has frankly elevated serum free T_4 levels, the thyroxine dosage should not be reduced in response to the finding of a low first trimester TSH level. The TSH should be checked again every 6–8 weeks and titrated to maintain a normal serum TSH concentration. In women who have had a thyroidectomy for thyroid cancer, the goal of maintaining a suppressed serum TSH without rendering the woman thyrotoxic should be adhered to during pregnancy. It is extremely important to advise the pregnant woman to take her thyroid hormone at a different time than her prenatal vitamins or iron supplements since ferrous sulfate can bind to thyroxine and decrease its bioavailability. Thyroid hormone will need to be reduced almost immediately after delivery to pre-pregnancy doses to avoid hyperthyroidism postpartum.

15. What is the risk of abnormal fetal and neonatal intellectual development in infants born to mothers who are hypothyroid during the first trimester of pregnancy?

All newborns in the U.S. are screened for hypothyroidism, since it is well established that infants who have severe congenital hypothyroidism but receive thyroid hormone replacement at birth appear to have fairly normal intellectual growth and development. However, the fetal effects of maternal hypothyroidism during the first trimester, when the fetal brain is dependent on maternal thyroid hormone, is a subject of ongoing debate. There have been several recent publications suggesting that psychomotor and intellectual development might be impaired in infants born to mothers who were hypothyroid during the first trimester of pregnancy, although the differences from controls in these studies were small and often became insignificant when the infants were tested later in childhood.

Nonetheless, considering the current level of evidence, it seems prudent to attempt to identify and appropriately treat hypothyroidism in women of childbearing age who wish to become pregnant (preconception) as well as in pregnant women in the first trimester. It must be remembered, however, that serum TSH levels often decline in the first trimester as a result of the influence of hCG. Thus a TSH level of 4–5 μU/ml in the first trimester may be inappropriately high while a TSH level of 0.1 μU/ml may be appropriately low because of the thyroid-stimulating activity of high levels of hCG.

16. How should a thyroid nodule be evaluated during pregnancy?

There are data to suggest that thyroid nodules discovered during pregnancy may have a higher risk of being malignant. However, this is likely due in part to selection or sampling bias, since many young women do not have systematic health examinations until they become pregnant. Depending on the patient population, the incidence of biopsied nodules being benign is > 60%, whereas differentiated thyroid cancer has been found in 5–40% of cases. The majority of malignant nodules are papillary thyroid carcinoma. Fine-needle aspiration (FNA) cytology is highly accurate in diagnosing papillary carcinoma whereas cytology showing a follicular or Hurthle cell neoplasm predicts only a 5–15% risk of malignancy. When the serum TSH is normal, < 20% of FNA specimens will be non-diagnostic. In one series of 61 patients with differentiated thyroid cancer (87% papillary), there were no differences in the rates of recurrence, distant spread, or outcomes related to whether neck surgery was performed during or after pregnancy.

There is no absolute consensus about the management of nodular thyroid disease in pregnancy, but the following generalizations can be made:

1. The evaluation of a solitary or dominant nodule in a pregnant woman is similar to that in nonpregnant women. FNA should be offered when nodules are > 1–2 cm, especially if they are detected before 20 weeks or if there are other risk factors for malignancy such as lymphadenopathy or rapid growth.

2. FNA specimens should be evaluated using the same criteria as established for nonpregnant patients.

3. If the cytology is suspicious or confirms papillary thyroid cancer, the best time to offer a thyroidectomy is probably in the second trimester, to avoid the risk of miscarriage in the first trimester and preterm labor in the third trimester. If the nodule is < 2 cm, has not rapidly increased in size, and the patient has no lymphadenopathy, it may be reasonable to postpone thyroidectomy until after pregnancy and place the woman on thyroid suppression therapy in the meantime.

17. What is postpartum thyroiditis, and who is at risk?

Postpartum thyroid dysfunction occurs in approximately 5–10% of women, with a much higher incidence in certain populations. In one series, 25% of women with type 1 diabetes mellitus developed postpartum thyroid dysfunction; it is therefore recommended that this population should be screened in the postpartum period on a routine basis. The disorder is highly associated with circulating TPO antibodies, while the histology is identical to that of Hashimoto's thyroiditis with profuse mononuclear cell infiltration and destruction of thyroid follicles. In one series of 152 women with TPO antibodies detected at 16 weeks' gestation, postpartum thyroiditis occurred in 50%; of these, 19% had hyperthyroidism alone, 49% had hypothyroidism alone, and the remaining 32% had hyperthyroidism followed by hypothyroidism. Women with a family history of thyroid disease are also at increased risk and may be candidates for screening with TPO antibodies during pregnancy or with thyroid function tests in the postpartum period.

Classically, the clinical course consists of three phases but not all women manifest each phase. At 1–3 months, affected women often develop hyperthyroidism as a result of immunologically mediated destruction of thyroid follicles resulting in the release of stored thyroid hormone into the circulation. These women may experience anxiety, irritability, palpitations, fatigue, and insomnia, but commonly this phase does not come to the attention of the clinician. Symptomatic patients are best treated with beta blockers, which must soon be tapered and discontinued as the thyrotoxic phase spontaneously resolves. Occasionally, there is a question as to the etiology of the hyperthyroidism, since Graves' disease commonly appears or exacerbates in the first several months postpartum. Distinguishing between the two conditions is facilitated by measurement of a serum thyroglobulin level and TPO antibodies (both are high in postpartum thyroiditis) and, if the mother is willing to interrupt nursing for 2–3 days, an I-123 uptake (low in postpartum thyroiditis and high in Graves' disease).

More commonly, women present with hypothyroidism alone at ~4–8 months postpartum. Non-specific symptoms include fatigue, depression, impaired concentration, poor memory, aches and pains, dry skin, and weight gain, all of which may be overlooked by the clinician. Symptoms may predate the onset of thyroid function abnormalities in women with positive TPO antibodies and may persist for some time after an euthyroid state is achieved. Women with abnormal thyroid function tests and symptoms consistent with hypothyroidism should be treated with thyroxine replacement for approximately 6–12 months or at least until 1 year postpartum. At that time, discontinuation of thyroxine therapy can be attempted to identify the 80% of women who will return to the euthyroid state by 12 months after delivery. Thyroid function testing should then be followed at least every 6 months in those women who become euthyroid, since permanent hypothyroidism may later develop. In one series of 43 patients with postpartum thyroiditis, 23% of the women were hypothyroid at 2–4 years, and, in a longer series, 48% of women were hypothyroid 7–9 years later. Women with the highest TPO antibody titers and most the severe hypothyroidism appear to be at the highest risk of developing permanent hypothyroidism. If a woman becomes euthyroid within a year postpartum, she has a very high likelihood (70%) of developing postpartum thyroiditis after a subsequent pregnancy.

REFERENCES

1. Fisher DA: Fetal thyroid function: Diagnosis and management of fetal thyroid disorders. Clin Obstet Gynecol 40(1):16–31, 1997.
2 Gerstein HC: Incidence of postpartum thyroid dysfunction in patients with type I diabetes mellitus. Ann Intern Med 118:419–423, 1993.
3. Glinoer D: What happens to the normal thyroid during pregnancy? Thyroid 9(7):631–635, 1999.
4. Goodwin TM, Hershman JM: Hyperthyroidism due to inappropriate production of human chorionic gonadotropin. Clin Obstet Gynecol 40:32–44, 1997.
5. Hay ID: Nodular thyroid disease diagnosed during pregnancy: How and when to treat. Thyroid 9(7):667–670, 1999.
6. Lazarus JH: Clinical manifestations of postpartum thyroid disease. Thyroid 9(7):685–690, 1999.
7. Masiukiewicz US, Burrow GN: Hyperthyroidism in pregnancy: Diagnosis and treatment. Thyroid 9(7):647–652, 1999.
8. Mestman JH, Goodwin TM, Montoro MM: Thyroid disorders of pregnancy. Endocrin Metab Clin North Am 24(1):41–71, 1995.
9. Moosa M, Mazzaferri EL: Outcome of differentiated thyroid cancer diagnosed in pregnant women. J Clin Endocrinol Metab 82:2862–2866, 1997.
10. Othman S, Phillips DIW, Parkes AB, et al: A long-term follow-up of postpartum thyroiditis. Clin Endocrinol 32:559–564, 1990.
11. Terry AJ , Hague WM: Postpartum thyroiditis. Sem Perinatol 22(6):497–502, 1998.

42. PSYCHIATRIC DISORDERS AND THYROID DISEASE

James V. Hennessey, M. D.

1. How well established is the relationship between thyroid disease and psychiatric symptoms?

For over a century, since the publication of the Clinical Society of London's "Report on Myxoedema" in 1888, it has been recognized that thyroid disease may give rise to psychiatric disorders that can be corrected by re-establishment of normal thyroid function. Later, Asher re-emphasized the fact that patients with profound hypothyroidism may present with depressive psychosis. As outlined in the table below, the symptoms of hypothyroidism often mimic those of depression, while those of hyperthyroidism include anxiety, dysphoria, emotional lability, and intellectual dysfunction, as well as mania or depression, the latter being especially characteristic among the elderly presenting with (so called) apathetic thyrotoxicosis.

Clinical Features Common to Both Thyroid Diseases and Mood Disorders

	HYPOTHYROIDISM	MOOD DISORDERS	HYPERTHYROIDISM
Depression	Yes	Yes	Yes
Diminished interest	Yes	Yes	Yes
Diminished pleasure	Yes	Yes	No
Decreased libido	Yes	Yes	Sometimes
Weight loss	No	Yes	Yes
Weight gain	Yes	Sometimes	Occasionally
Appetite loss	Yes	Yes	Sometimes
Increased appetite	No	Yes	Yes
Insomnia	No	Yes	Yes
Hypersomnia	Yes	Yes	No
Agitation/anxiety	No	Yes	Yes
Fatigue	Yes	Yes	Yes
Poor memory	Yes	Yes	Occasionally
Cognitive dysfunction	Yes	Yes	Yes
Impaired concentration	Yes	Yes	Yes
Constipation	Yes	Sometimes	No

Adapted from Hennessy JV, Jackson IMD: The interface between thyroid hormones and psychiatry. Endocrinologist 6:214–223, 1996.

2. What abnormalities of thyroid function are found in psychiatric disorders?

Since patients with thyroid disease may manifest frank psychiatric disorders that are reversible with endocrine therapy, the thyroid axis has been extensively studied in patients presenting with a wide variety of behavioral disturbances. Various abnormalities of thyroid function have been identified, particularly in depression (see below). In most depressed subjects the basal serum TSH, thyroxine (T_4) and triiodothyronine (T_3) are within the normal range, though in one report a third of such patients were observed to have suppressed TSH levels.

3. What abnormalities of TRH Stimulation may be observed in the depressed patient?

Following the introduction of TRH for clinical testing in the early 1970s, the TRH stimulation test was evaluated in a wide variety of psychiatric conditions. It was soon recognized that patients with depression as well as those with alcohol withdrawal frequently had a "blunted" TSH response to TRH administration. Data from over 40 studies in 917 depressed patients have shown a blunted TSH response(as defined by a TSH rise $< 5\mu U/mL$)in approximately 25% of such subjects. Although a blunted TSH response may be more likely in unipolar than in bipolar depression, attempts to differentiate these disorders on the basis of the TRH stimulation test have been disappointing.

In most instances, the blunted TSH response is a "state" marker that normalizes on recovery from the depression. The mechanism responsible for the blunted TSH response in affective disorders is not known for sure. However, glucocorticoids, which are known to inhibit the hypothalamic-pituitary-thyroid axis, are elevated in depression and could be responsible.

However, the suppressed TSH response to TRH is not specific to depression, and may be observed in other conditions such as alcohol withdrawal, starvation, normal aging males, renal failure, acromegaly, Cushing's syndrome, and hypopituitarism. The blunting may also be induced by medications such as thyroxine, glucocorticoids, growth hormone, somatostatin, dopamine and phenytoin, all of which have been reported to diminish this response.

4. Can abnormalities in the TSH circadian rhythm be identified in depression?

In normal subjects, the TSH begins to rise in the evening before the onset of sleep, reaching a peak between 11:00 p.m. and 4 a.m. In depression, the nocturnal surge of TSH is frequently absent, resulting in an overall reduction in thyroid hormone secretion; this supports the view that a degree of functional central hypothyroidism might occur in some depressed subjects. Sleep deprivation, which has an antidepressant effect, brings about a return of the normal TSH circadian rhythm. The mechanism responsible for the impaired nocturnal rise of TSH is unknown.

5. Is autoimmune thyroid disease frequently present in the depressed patient?

Although the blunted TSH response is well recognized in depression, it is less clearly appreciated that an enhanced response may occur in up to 15% of depressed subjects with normal baseline thyroid function tests. The majority of such patients have anti-thyroid antibodies, suggesting that the TSH hyper-response may indicate latent hypothyroidism caused by autoimmune thyroiditis. When autoimmunity is tested utilizing the antithyroid peroxidase antibody (anti-TPO) rather than the less specific antimicrosomal antibody, the prevalence of autoimmune thyroid disease is even higher. Not all studies, however, have found an increased prevalence of antithyroid antibodies in depressed subjects when compared with matched control groups.

6. What is the frequency with which an elevated thyroxine value is encountered in the psychiatric patient?

Approximately 20% of patients admitted to the hospital with acute psychiatric presentations, including schizophrenia and major affective disorders, but rarely dementia or alcoholism, may demonstrate mild elevations in their serum T_4 levels, and less often their T_3 levels. The basal TSH is usually normal but may demonstrate blunted TRH responsiveness in up to 90% of such patients. These findings do not appear to represent thyrotoxicosis, and the abnormalities spontaneously resolve within 2 weeks without specific therapy. Such phenomena may be due to central activation of the hypothalamic-pituitary-thyroid axis resulting in enhanced TSH secretion with consequent elevation in circulating thyroxine levels.

In depressed patients, the most consistent abnormality of the thyroid axis appears to be an increase in serum T_4 and/or free T_4 levels, though usually within the conventional normal range. This generally regresses following successful treatment of the depression.

7. What is the prevalence of hypothyroid dysfunction seen in psychiatric populations?

Thyroid function test abnormalities are common in older individuals. In otherwise normal female subjects over 60 years of age, the prevalence of elevated TSH values and/or positive antithyroid antibodies is 10% or more. Subjecting apparently asymptomatic individuals with slight elevations of serum TSH but normal T_4 and T_3 levels to a battery of psychologic tests has revealed significant differences from control subjects on scales measuring memory, anxiety, somatic complaints and depression. It is becoming increasingly recognized that depression is much more common in elderly individuals. Whether borderline hypothyroidism plays a role in these behavioral disturbances requires further investigation. Among alcoholics and those suffering from anorexia nervosa, suppressed T_3 levels with elevations in reverse T_3 and normal TSH values are consistent with the "sick thyroid state." These findings likely result from caloric deprivation.

8. Which medications affect thyroid function and thyroid function tests?

A number of medications commonly used to treat psychiatric illness have been shown to affect thyroid function tests.

Impact of Psychotropic Medications on Thyroid Function Tests

MEDICATION	MECHANISM	TEST FINDINGS
Lithium carbonate	↓ thyroglobulin hydrolysis ↓ T_4 and T_3 release	TSH ↑ (transiently) Hypothyroidism, goiter
ANTIPSYCHOTICS Perphenazine	↑ TBG concentration	↑ (T_4, nl free T_4

ANTICONVULSANTS
  Phenytoin
  Carbamazepine
  Phenobarbital
  Valproic acid
	↑ Hepatic clearance of T_4
	↓ T_4 binding, ↑ hepatic clearance
	↑ hepatic clearance
	↓ T_4 binding (?),
	↑ hepatic clearance (?)
		↓ T_4, ± ↓ free T_4, nl TSH
		↓ T_4, ± ↓ free T_4, nl TSH
		↓ T_4, ± ↓ free T_4, nl TSH
		
		↓ T_4, ± ↓ free T_4, nl TSH

NARCOTICS
  Heroin
  Methadone
	↑ TBG concentration
	↑ TBG concentration
		↑ T_4, nl free T_4
		↑ T_4, nl free T_4

MISCELLANEOUS Amphetamines	↑ TSH secretion (?)	↑ T_4, nl free T_4

Adapted from Hennessy JV, Jackson IMD: The interface between thyroid hormones and psychiatry. Endocrinologist 6:214–223, 1996.

9. How does lithium effect the pituitary-thyroidal axis?

Lithium carbonate, used to treat bipolar disorders, interferes with both the release and organification of thyroid hormone. Therapeutic lithium levels diminish both T_3 and T_4 release from the thyroid gland, while at higher (probably toxic) levels iodine uptake and organification may also be inhibited. Following a 3-week therapeutic course of lithium carbonate, suppression of serum T_4 and T_3 levels and associated elevations of basal serum TSH values and exaggerated TSH responses to TRH administration may be noted; these abnormalities generally return to normal within 3–12 months, even if the medication is continued.

Goiter is the most common thyroid disorder occurring in lithium-treated patients. Hypothyroidism can also occasionally develop, particularly in patients who have thyroid glands that have been compromised by disorders such as Hashimoto's thyroiditis and Graves' disease previously treated with I-131 therapy. However, it is uncommon for hypothyroidism to occur if pre-treatment thyroid function is completely normal and patients are thyroid antibody–negative. If considered clinically necessary, lithium may be continued and thyroxine added to treat patients who develop goiter or hypothyroidism.

10. How does phenytoin effect the interpretation of laboratory tests and the function of the thyroid?

The effects of phenytoin (Dilantin®), occasionally used in the treatment of bipolar disorder, on thyroid function are quite complex. Suppressed values of total and, occasionally, free thyroxine are observed in a significant minority of patients who are chronically treated with phenytoin alone and in upwards of 75% of those in whom the drug is combined with carbamazepine (Tegretol®). The lower total T_4 levels are likely due to displacement of T_4 from thyroxine-binding globulin (TBG), while the reduced free T_4 levels result from enhanced clearance of T4 through phenytoin-induced hepatic microsomal oxidative enzyme activity. Generally, the suppressed T_4 levels are accompanied by normal T_3 and free T_3 levels and normal TSH concentrations. Normal basal TSH values with diminished TSH responses to TRH have been attributed to potential phenytoin agonism at the T_3 receptor, due to possible structure homology with thyroid hormone. However, other studies have suggested that this may be an assay artifact because free T_4 values have been found to be normal or mildly elevated in analyses using undiluted serum.

11. What are the effects of other psychotropic medications in determining thyroid function?

Carbamazepine (Tegretol®) is used increasingly in the management of bipolar disorder. Chronic use with maintenance of therapeutic serum levels may lead to suppressed serum T_4 values in more than 50% of patients. This is thought to be due to enhanced hepatic microsomal enzyme metabolism of thyroxine. TRH stimulation testing before and after initiation of Tegretol therapy reveals that TSH responsiveness is reduced by the addition of this drug; this has led to speculation that carbamazepine may inhibit thyroid function through effects on the pituitary gland. Displacement of T_4 from TBG, similar to that seen with phenytoin, has additionally been cited as a potential effect.

Both phenobarbital and valproic acid have also been reported to lower serum levels of T_4 in chronically treated patients, the former via enhanced hepatic T_4 clearance and the latter likely due to protein binding changes. Heroin, methadone, and perphenazine commonly increase serum TBG levels and therefore may elevate serum total T_4 levels, although TSH and free thyroxine values remain normal. Amphetamines induce hyperthyroxinemia through enhanced secretion of TSH, an effect that appears to be centrally mediated.

12. How do antidepressant therapies effect thyroid function?

Antidepressants do not generally cause abnormal peripheral thyroid hormone levels but may affect thyroid hormone metabolism in the CNS. However, circulating total T_4 and free T_4, but not T_3, levels often show a modest decline, though still within the normal range, after treatment with various pharmacologic classes of antidepressants, as well as with electroconvulsive therapy (ECT).

13. Are there caveats of antidepressant usage in individuals with thyroid disease?

The use of tricyclic antidepressants (TCA) in thyrotoxic patients should be pursued with caution, as cardiac dysrhythmias may be exacerbated or precipitated. Further, the MAO inhibitors have been noted to cause hypertension in thyrotoxic patients, although they generally do not affect thyroid function or serum thyroid hormone levels.

THYROID HORMONE IN THE TREATMENT OF PSYCHIATRIC ILLNESS (DEPRESSION)

14. Has thyroxine been used as sole treatment for depression?

Asher's report on "myxoedema madness" demonstrating that thyroid hormone deficiency could result in depression that was reversible with thyroid hormone administration led to studies of the role of thyroid hormone therapy alone in the treatment of depression and other psychiatric diseases. Although initial reports of T_3 as single therapy were promising, these studies were methodologically flawed, so that the role of thyroid hormone by itself in the treatment of depression in the absence of abnormalities of thyroid function has not been established.

15. Are neuropsychiatric abnormalities demonstrable and reversible among patients with mild thyroid failure?

Recent studies have shown that symptomatic patients with subclinical hypothyroidism (slightly elevated serum TSH but normal T_4 and T_3 levels) can have significant impairment of memory-related abilities, and significant differences in anxiety, somatic complaints and depressive features when compared with euthyroid controls. Normalization of the serum TSH with L-thyroxine therapy may completely reverse these neuropsychiatric features. Further, when thyroid hormone is withdrawn from subjects with underlying hypothyroidism, gradually increasing sadness and anxiety symptoms are observed over the ensuing few weeks. These findings indicate that the patient presenting with depression must be assessed for thyroid dysfunction, since the presence of even subclinical hypothyroidism may provide an opportunity for resolution of the depression with thyroid hormone treatment.

16. Can a combination of thyroid hormone and antidepressant therapy enhance an individuals' response to depression treatment?

Utilization of adjuvant therapy is logical when depression fails to resolve after 6 weeks of adequate anti-depressant medication. Such resistance occurs in about 30–45% of cases. The role of adjuvant thyroid hormone therapy along with antidepressant medication, especially tricyclic antidepressants (TCAs), has been investigated in euthyroid patients with depression over the past 25 years. T_3 doses of 25–50 µg daily will generally increase serum T_3 levels significantly and cause suppression of serum TSH and T_4 values. Two separate therapeutic effects of T_3 therapy have been studied: first, its ability to accelerate the onset of the antidepressant response; second, its ability to augment antidepressant responses among those considered pharmacologically resistant.

17. How effective is the addition of thyroid hormone for the acceleration of the antidepressant response?

Because the antidepressant effect of TCAs is known to be delayed, the role of T_3 in accelerating the therapeutic onset of these drugs has been investigated. Several reports detailing the clinical outcomes of starting T_3 along with varying doses of TCAs at the outset of therapy have appeared in the literature. In these studies, doses of T_3 ranged anywhere from 5–40 µg daily. The study populations were also inhomogeneous, consisting of patients with various different types of depression. Furthermore, there were important methodologic limitations, including small sample sizes, inadequate medication doses, lack of serum medication level monitoring, and variable outcomes measures. As a result, it still has not been clearly established that T_3 accelerates the antidepressant effect of TCAs. These early studies have therefore had relatively little impact on the current clinical approach to the depressed patient, and T_3 is not generally used by most workers in the field to accelerate antidepressant responses.

18. Can triiodothyronine augment the clinical antidepressant response?

An additional hypothesis is that adding small doses of T_3 to the antidepressant therapy of patients who have little or no or initial response will enhance the clinical effectiveness of the antidepressant. Resistance to antidepressants is defined as inadequate remission after 2 successive trials of monotherapy with different anti-depressants in adequate doses, each for 4–6 weeks before changing to alternative therapies. However, 8–12 weeks of ineffective antidepressant therapy is commonly deemed unacceptable and strategies designed to augment the response are being sought.

Early studies assessing T_3 effectiveness in augmenting the antidepressant response were neither placebo controlled nor focused on patient populations that could be directly compared. The first placebo-controlled, double-blind, randomized study reported results in 16 unipolar depressed outpatients who had experienced no improvement in their clinical outcomes with TCAs alone. The intervention consisted of adding 25 µg of T_3 or placebo daily for 2 weeks before the patients were crossed over to the opposite treatment for an additional 2 weeks. No beneficial effect of T_3 was apparent. The only other placebo-controlled, randomized double blind trial investigating this question involved 33 patients with unipolar depression treated with either desipramine or imipramine for 5 weeks prior to random assignment to placebo or 37.5 µg of T_3 daily. After 2 weeks of observation on T_3, during which TCA levels were monitored, significantly more patients treated with T_3 (10 of 17; 59%) had a positive response than did placebo treated patients (3 of 16; 19%). A subsequent open clinical trial of imipramine-resistant depression, using a prolonged period of TCA treatment preceding the addition of T_3, showed no demonstrable T_3 effect.

Although it is clear that a large multicenter double-blind, placebo-controlled study to determine the role of T_3 as augmentation therapy is needed, many antidepressant-resistant patients currently receive T_3 in an attempt to augment the response of therapy.

19. What evidence is there that the effect of selective serotonin re-uptake inhibitors (SSRIs) and electro convulsive therapy (ECT) may be enhanced by the addition of T_3?

The SSRI group of substances (including fluoxetine and sertraline), is the preferred antidepressant medication in the United States today. Only two case reports are available addressing the role of thyroid hormone as adjuvant therapy for SSRIs, and the limited information to date suggests that SSRIs behave similarly to TCAs in this regard. Of interest, T_3 has been reported to augment the antidepressant effect of ECT.

20. Are any psychiatric conditions recognized to respond to pharmacologic doses of thyroxine?

For the 10–15% of bipolar disorder patients with 4 or more episodes of manic-depressive psychosis yearly (rapid cyclers), the prevalence of autoimmune thyroid disease may reach 50% or higher. Therapeutic intervention with standard therapy such as lithium is frequently disappointing. Treating such patients with levothyroxine in pharmacologic doses sufficient to suppress serum TSH and elevate T_4 levels to approximately 150% of normal may decrease the manic and depressive phases in both amplitude and frequency and has led to remission in some of the patients. Given these encouraging results, controlled studies on the efficacy of levothyroxine or triiodothyronine seem warranted.

21. Are mechanisms of thyroid hormone action on the brain known?

Thyroid hormones play a critical role in the development and function of the central nervous system. Triiodothyronine receptors are widely distributed throughout the brain, and there is much evidence that thyroid hormone regulates brain function through interaction with the catecholaminergic system. Thyroid hormone action in brain tissue is accomplished through the binding of T_3 to its nuclear receptor. The T_3 is derived from T_4 by the action of (type II) 5'-deiodinase, which is located throughout the CNS.

22. Should T_4 or T_3 be used in treating the depressed patient?

Most studies using thyroid hormone as adjuvant therapy have utilized T_3 rather than T_4 and in those reports where the advantages of one over the other were assessed, T_3 was considered superior. In a randomized trial combining T_4 or T_3 with antidepressants, only 4 of 21 patients (19%) treated with 150 μg/day of T_4 for 3 weeks responded, whereas 9 of 17 (53%) responded with 37.5 μg/day of T_3. Further studies of open T_4 treatment in anti-depressant-resistant patients have appeared, but the lack of control makes outcome interpretation difficult. One of these indicated that responders to levothyroxine had significantly lower pre-treatment serum T_4 and reverse T_3 levels, leading the authors to believe that the responders might have been subclinically hypothyroid. Combination therapy with T_4 rather than T_3 may be indicated when subclinical hypothyroidism or rapid cycling bipolar disease is present. Since T_4 equilibrates in tissues more slowly than T_3, treatment with T_4 for at least 6–8 weeks, and preferably longer, would be necessary to determine its efficacy in this situation.

23. What are proposed mechanisms linking thyroid function and depression?

It has been postulated that type II 5'-deiodinase activity in the CNS is deficient in depression giving rise to a state of brain hypothyroidism co-existing with systemic euthyroidism. If this is so, it would account for the apparent efficacy of thyroid hormone treatment in depression and the observation that T_3 is more effective than T_4.

24. Do antidepressant medications have a mechanistic connection to the action of thyroid hormone in the brain?

It has been shown that desipramine, a TCA, and fluoxetine, a SSRI, both enhance type II 5'-deiodinase activity in the CNS, thus presumably increasing the availability of T_3 in the brain. This could conceivably account for the clinical efficacy of these classes of drugs.

25. Can management recommendations in regards to thyroid evaluation in the psychiatric patient be made?

It would seem prudent to check thyroid function tests in those psychiatric patients who are at increased risk for developing thyroid disease. Women over 45 years of age, patients with known autoimmune diseases, individuals with a family history of thyroid disease, and those receiving lithium or suffering from dementia should be screened for underlying thyroid abnormalities. Patients receiving medications known to influence the interpretation of thyroid function tests should have these effects considered when interpreting the results of testing.

26. Who should be treated with thyroid hormone with the intent of relieving psychiatric symptoms?

It is recommended that thyroxine therapy be offered to any depressed patient with an elevated serum TSH, especially if accompanied by increased anti-thyroid antibody titers. Thyroid hormone replacement by itself may be sufficient to alleviate the depression in these individuals without the need for antidepressant medication. On the other hand, antidepressant therapy, if required, may be ineffective prior to normalization of thyroid axis parameters. In patients with refractory depression but normal systemic thyroid function, adjuvant T_3 therapy is possibly worth considering.

BIBLIOGRAPHY

1. Asher R: Myxoedematous madness. Br Med J 22:555–562, 1949.
2. Chopra IJ, Solomon DH, Huang T-S: Serum thyrotropin in hospitalized psychiatric patients: Evidence for hyperthyrotropinemia as measured by ultrasensative thyrotropin assay. Metabolism 93:538–543, 1990.

3. 1888 Report on myxoedema. Transact Clin Soc Lon 21 (Suppl).

4. Fava M: New approaches to the treatment of refractory depression. J Clin Psychiatr 61(suppl 1): 26–32, 2000.

5. Fava M, Labbate LA, Abraham ME, Rosenbaum JF: Hypothyroidism and hyperthyroidism in major depression revisited. J Clin Psychiatr 56:186–92, 1995.

6. Hein MD, Jackson IMD: Thyroid function in psychiatric illness. Gen Hosp Psych 12:232–44, 1990.

7. Hennessey JV, Jackson IMD: The interface between thyroid hormones and psychiatry. Endocrinologist 6:214–223, 1996.

8. Jackson IMD, Whybrow PC: The relationship between psychiatric disorders and thyroid dysfunction. Thyroid Update 9:1–7, 1995.

9. Manzoni F, DelGerra P, Caraccion N, et al: Subclinical hypothyroidism: Neuro-behavioral features and beneficial effect of L-thyroxine treatment. Clin Invest 71:367–371, 1993.

10. Nelson JC: Augmentation strategies in depression 2000. J Clin Psychiatr 61(suppl 2):13–19, 2000.

11. Stockigt JR: Hyperthyroxinemia secondary to drugs and acute illness. Endocrinologist 3:67–73, 1993.

12. Surks MI, Sievert R: Drugs and thyroid function. N Engl J Med 333:1688–94, 1995.

13. Whybrow PC: The therapeutic use of triiodothyronine and high dose thyroxine in psychiatric disorders. Acta Med Austr 21:47–52, 1994.

VI. Reproductive Endocrinology

43. DISORDERS OF SEXUAL DIFFERENTIATION

Sharon Zemel, M.D., and Robert H. Slover, M.D.

1. Describe the levels of sexual differentiation and their relationship to sex assignment.

We are used to thinking of chromosomal sex as the determinant of sex assignment, and in the vast majority of children this is the case. For some individuals, however, chromosomal sex and phenotypic sex are clearly discordant.

Chromosomal sex, or more specifically genetic sex, is the first level of differentiation. The great majority of infants are 46 XX females or 46 XY males. Genetic sex determines gonadal sex. Gonadal sex is determined by the presence or absence of the testis-determining factor called SRY (sex-determining region of the Y). Coded by a gene on the short arm of the Y chromosome, SRY stimulates the undifferentiated gonad to become a testis. If a 46 XY individual has a defective or absent SRY gene on the Y chromosome, testes will fail to develop. If a 46 XX individual has had a translocation of the SRY gene onto an X chromosome, testes will develop.

The next level of sex determination involves the genital duct structures. In the normal male, testicular Leydig cells produce testosterone, which is necessary to maintain ipsilateral Wolffian duct structures (e.g., vas deferens, epididymis, seminal vesicles). Normal testes also produce müllerian-inhibiting factor (MIF), which acts ipsilaterally to cause regression of müllerian duct structures (fallopian tubes, uterus, upper third of the vagina). In the absence of testosterone and MIF—as in normal females and some abnormal males—müllerian duct structures are preserved and wolffian duct structures regress.

At this time, the external genitalia also begin to develop. Male and female external genitalia arise from the same embryologic structures. In the absence of androgen stimulation, these structures remain in the female pattern, whereas the presence of androgens causes male differentiation (virilization). For complete virilization, testosterone must be converted to dihydrotestosterone (DHT) by the enzyme 5-alpha-reductase, and androgen receptors must be functional. Excessive androgens virilize a female, whereas inadequate production of androgen, inability to convert testosterone to DHT, or androgen receptor defects result in undervirilization of a male.

Finally, many external factors join to create gender identity. Exogenous and endogenous hormones are clearly important, as is the appearance of the genitalia. In utero influences are being increasingly recognized. In ambiguous infants, confusion about sex of rearing may result in gender confusion and psychological trauma. Each level of sex determination must be considered in diagnosing the infant with ambiguity and suggesting a sex of rearing.

2. What is testis-determining factor?

The testis-determining factor (TDF) promotes differentiation of the gonad into a testis. Originally considered the H-Y antigen, then ZFY (zinc finger on Y), SRY was eventually characterized as the TDF. SRY belongs to a family of DNA binding proteins. Specific manipulations have shown that the introduction of SRY will sex reverse XX mice, and site-directed mutagenesis of the SRY gene in XY mice will yield XY females. Other genes on the sex chromosomes and autosomal chromosomes are involved in the regulation of SRY.

3. Describe the Lyon hypothesis. In which cells are two X chromosomes needed for normal development?

Dr. Mary Lyon addressed the question of the extra X chromosomal material in females. Simply put, if two X chromosomes are needed in each cell, how can males be developmentally normal? Lyon suggested that in each cell, one of the two X chromosomes is inactive and that in any given cell line, *which* X is active is determined randomly. In fact, the inactive X may be identified in many cells as a clump of chromatin at the nuclear membrane (Barr body). However, two functional X chromosomes are needed for normal sustained ovarian development. Without two X chromosomes per cell (as in 45 XO Turner syndrome), the ovary involutes and leaves only fibrous tissue.

4. Discuss normal male sexual differentiation.

The figure below shows schematically how male development is accomplished.

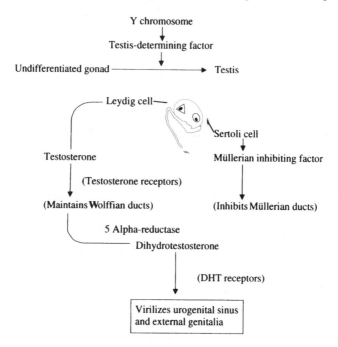

The fetus is sexually bipotential. The undifferentiated gonad is derived from coelomic epithelium, mesenchyme, and germ cells, which, in the presence of SRY, give rise to Leydig cells, Sertoli cells, seminiferous tubules and spermatogonia. Testes are formed at seven weeks. Testicular production of testosterone (Leydig cells) and MIF (Sertoli cells) then leads to wolffian duct development and müllerian duct regression, respectively. Conversion of testosterone to DHT by 5-alpha-reductase and subsequent binding of DHT to androgen receptors cause masculinization of the external genitalia.

5. Describe normal female sexual differentiation.

In the absence of SRY, the undifferentiated gonad gives rise to follicles, granulosa cells, theca cells, and ova. Ovarian development occurs in the thirteenth to sixteenth week of gestation. Lack of testosterone and MIF allows regression of the Wolffian ducts and maintenance of the Müllerian ducts, respectively. Lack of DHT results in the maintenance of female external genitalia.

6. How is external genital development determined?

The external genitalia arise from the urogenital tubercle, urogenital swelling, and urogenital folds. In females these become the clitoris, labia majora, and labia minora, respectively. In males, under the influence of DHT, the genital tubercle becomes the glans of the penis, the urogenital folds elongate and fuse to form the shaft of the penis, and the genital swellings fuse to form the scrotum. Fusion is completed by 70 days of gestation and penile growth continues to term.

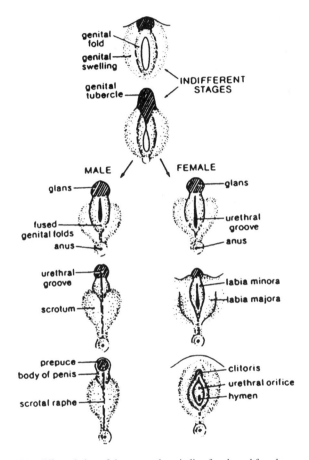

The differentiation of the external genitalia of male and female.

Female differentiation does not require ovaries or hormonal influence, whereas normal development of male genitalia requires normal testosterone synthesis, conversion to DHT by 5-alpha reductase, and normal androgen receptors.

7. The differential diagnosis of sexual differentiation disorders is complex but may be simplified by an approach based on a understanding of the process of sexual differentiation. Can you devise such a classification?

There are four large categories of ambiguity:
1. Virilized 46 XX females
2. Undervirilized 46 XY males

3. Disorders of gonadal differentiation
4. Unclassified forms, including cryptorchidism, hypospadias, and developmental anomalies

---

Differential Diagnosis of Sexual Ambiguity

Virilized 46 XX females (female pseudohermaphroditism)
  Congenital adrenal hyperplasia
    21-hydroxylase deficiency
    11-beta-hydroxylase deficiency
    3-beta-hydroxysteroid dehydrogenase deficiency
  Maternally derived androgens and synthetic progesterones
Undervirilized 46 XY males (male pseudohermaphroditism)
  Testicular unresponsiveness to human chorionic gonadotropin (hCG) and luteinizing hormone (LH) (Leydig cell agenesis or hypoplasia)
  Testosterone biosynthesis defects
    Congenital lipoid adrenal hyperplasia (cholesterol side-chain cleavage defect)
    3-beta-hydroxysteroid dehydrogenase deficiency
    17-alpha-hydroxylase deficiency
    17,20-lyase (desmolase) deficiency
    17-beta-hydroxysteroid dehydrogenase deficiency
  Peripheral unresponsiveness to androgen
    Androgen insensitivity syndromes (receptor defects)
    5-alpha-reductase deficiency
  Defects in synthesis, secretion or response to MIF
  Maternal estrogen or progesterone ingestion
Disorders of gonadal differentiation
  46 XY partial gonadal dysgenesis
  45 X/46 XY gonadal dysgenesis
  "Vanishing testes" (embryonic testicular regression; 46 XY agonadism; anorchia)
  True hermaphroditism
Unclassified
  In males
    Hypospadias
    Cryptorchidism
    Ambiguity secondary to congenital anomalies
  In females
    Absence or anomalous development of vagina, uterus and tubes (Rokitansky syndrome)

---

8. What is a virilized female?

A virilized female (previously called female pseudohermaphroditism) is characterized by a 46 XX karyotype, ovaries, normal müllerian duct structures, absent wolffian duct structures, and virilized genitalia due to exposure to androgens during the first trimester.

The most common cause of female pseudohermaphroditism is congenital adrenal hyperplasia due to 21-hydroxylase deficiency. In fact, this disorder is the single most common cause of sexual ambiguity across the board. The gene responsible for encoding the 21-hydroxylase enzyme is inactive. To produce adequate amounts of cortisol, the fetus makes large amounts of adrenocorticotropic hormone (ACTH), which stimulates increased production of the precursor, 17-hydroxyprogesterone, and of adrenal androgens.

Of importance, affected infants may present with a wide spectrum of ambiguity, ranging from clitoromegaly alone to complete fusion of the labial swellings to form a scrotum and large phallus. Even in the most virilized girls, however, a penile urethra is rare.

Virilization may also may be caused by maternal ingestion of androgens or synthetic progesterones during the first trimester of pregnancy.

9. What is an undervirilized male?

An undervirilized male (previously called male pseudohermaphroditism) refers to a 46 XY male who has ambiguous or female external genitalia. The abnormality may range from hypospadias to a completely female phenotype. Such disorders result from deficient androgen stimulation of genital development and most often are due to Leydig cell agenesis, testosterone biosynthetic defects and partial or total androgen resistance (androgen receptor defects).

10. Which boys with hypospadias should be evaluated for sexual ambiguity?

First-degree (coronal or glandular) hypospadias as the sole presenting genital abnormality has no apparent endocrine basis and need not be evaluated. The incidence of this anomaly is between 1 and 8 of 1,000 births. On the other hand, perineoscrotal hypospadias is a feature of many etiologies of sexual ambiguity, and a child with this finding should be fully evaluated as ambiguous.

11. What is gonadal dysgenesis?

Patients with Y-related chromosomal or genetic disorders that cause maldevelopment of one or both testes are said to have gonadal dysgenesis. They present with ambiguous genitalia and may have hypoplasia of wolffian duct structures and inadequate virilization. MIF may be absent, allowing müllerian duct structures to persist. Duct asymmetry is therefore common. The Y-containing dysgenetic testes are at risk for developing gonadoblastomas and need to be removed at diagnosis.

12. An infant is born with ambiguous genitalia, and the sex of the infant is uncertain. How do you approach the parents?

Honesty and diplomacy are essential. You need to explain that the genitalia are not yet fully developed and that further testing is needed to determine the infant's sex. Reference to more commonly understood birth defects may be useful. Explain that 2–3 days may be necessary to complete the testing and that a team will participate to make an accurate diagnosis and a considered recommendation. Completion of the birth certificate should be postponed, and the infant should be admitted to the nursery without a sex assignment. You should encourage the family to delay naming the baby and not to give a name applicable to either sex.

13. What history do you need to evaluate the infant?

Maternal history is particularly important and should include illnesses, drug ingestion, alcohol intake and ingestion of hormones during pregnancy. Was progestational therapy used for threatened abortion or androgens for endometriosis? Does the mother have signs of excessive androgen? Explore family history for occurrence of ambiguity, neonatal deaths, consanguinity or infertility.

14. How should you direct the physical examination?

The diagnosis of the etiology of sexual ambiguity can rarely be made by examination alone, but physical findings can help to direct further evaluation. Look for the following:

1. Are gonads present? Are they normal in size, texture, and position?
2. What is the phallic length? Measure along the dorsum of the phallus from the pubic ramus to the tip of the glans. At term, a stretched phallic length of 2.5 cm is 2.5 SD below the mean. Assess phallic width and development.
3. Note the position of the urethral meatus, and look for evidence of hypospadias and chordee (ventral curvature secondary to shortened urethra).
4. What is the degree of fusion of the labioscrotal folds? The folds may range from normal labia majora to a fully fused scrotum. In subtle cases, the ratio of the distance from the posterior fourchette to the anus is compared with the total distance from the urethral meatus.

5. Is there an apparent vaginal orifice?
6. Evaluate other areas. Certain forms of congenital adrenal hyperplasia may cause areolar or genital hyperpigmentation, dehydration or hypertension. Turner's stigmata may be present, including webbed neck, low hairline and edema of hands and feet. Other associated congenital anomalies may indicate a complex that includes ambiguity.

15. Explain which radiographic and laboratory studies are needed.

1. Structural studies are needed to address the presence of gonads and müllerian structures. Pelvic ultrasound by qualified personnel should be done as soon as possible to look for a uterus. The presence of gonads, fallopian tubes, and a vaginal vault may also be determined. If necessary, a genitogram may be performed by inserting contrast material into the urogenital orifice (or vaginal orifice) to define vaginal size, presence of a cervix and any fistulae.
2. A karyotype is essential and must be obtained expeditiously. Buccal smears are absolutely contraindicated because they are inaccurate. In many laboratories, a karyotype can be completed within 48–72 hr. Some labs can also do FISH analysis for the presence of the SRY gene.
3. Because 21-hydroxylase deficiency is a relatively common cause of sexual ambiguity, we assess the level of 17-hydroxyprogesterone in all such infants who do not have palpable gonads.

Further evaluation must be directed by information provided through the history, examination and initial studies. Determining presence or absence of palpable gonads (presumably testes), presence or absence of a uterus and karyotype allows classification of the infant as virilized female, undervirilized male, a disorder of gonadal differentiation or one of the unclassified forms.

16. The infant has no palpable gonadsand has fused labioscrotal folds and a prominent phallus. The ultrasound reveals a uterus and tubes with possible ovaries. The karyotype is 46 XX. How do you proceed now?

The infant is a virilized female. If there is no history of maternal androgen ingestion or virilization, the infant has one of three forms of congenital adrenal hyperplasia (CAH). Of these, 21-hydroxylase deficiency is most common and is confirmed by finding an elevated serum level of 17-hydroxyprogesterone. In 11-beta-hydroxylase deficiency, 11-deoxycortisol is elevated, whereas 17-hydroxypregnenolone and dehydroepiandrosterone (DHEA) are elevated in 3-beta-hydroxysteroid dehydrogenase deficiency. The baseline levels are usually diagnostic but can be confirmed by an ACTH stimulation test. The electrolyte disturbances seen, with such disorders do not usually occur until 8–14 days of life. Many states now screen for CAH.

17. An undervirilized male represents a more complex diagnostic dilemma. In an infant with palpable gonads, no müllerian structures and a 46 XY karyotype, how do you proceed?

Defects in testosterone synthesis include three enzyme blocks common to the adrenal and testicular pathways (cholesterol side-chain cleavage defect, 3-beta-hydroxysteroid dehydrogenase deficiency and 17-alpha-hydroxylase deficiency). Enzyme blocks are diagnosed with ACTH stimulation testing and measurement of precursors. Cholesterol side-chain cleavage defects have no measurable precursors but show high levels of ACTH and a low cortisol response. Patients with 17-alpha-hydroxylase deficiency have elevated levels of progesterone, desoxycorticosterone and corticosterone, with associated hypertension. Infants with 3-beta hydroxysteroid dehydrogenase deficiency have elevated levels of 17-hydroxypregnenolone and DHEA.

The two remaining defects in testosterone synthesis involve deficiencies of testicular rather than adrenal enzymes: 17,20-lyase and 17-beta-hydroxysteroid dehydrogenase. Thus, they are not associated with elevations of ACTH or electrolyte disturbances. Both deficiencies are diagnosed by measuring the precursor response to administration of hCG. Infants with 17,20-lyase deficiency have elevated levels of 17-hydroxypregnenolone and 17-hydroxyprogesterone, whereas infants with 17-beta-hydroxysteroid dehydrogenase deficiency have elevated levels of DHEA and androstenedione.

Infants with Leydig cell hypoplasia have low levels of testosterone after hCG stimulation but normal adrenal function. Testicular biopsy reveals normal seminiferous tubules but absent or few Leydig cells.

Stimulation with hCG also allows measurement of the testosterone-to-dihydrotestosterone ratio. If the ratio is elevated, 5-alpha-reductase deficiency should be suspected and may be confirmed by cultures of genital skin fibroblasts.

Finally, normal testosterone levels with no abnormalities in ACTH and hCG testing lead to the diagnosis of partial androgen insensitivity (androgen receptor defects). The diagnosis is made by demonstrating abnormal androgen binding in cultures of genital skin fibroblasts in a research laboratory or molecular analysis.

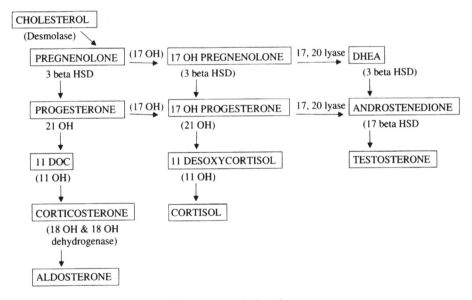

Testosterone synthesis pathway.

18. What is complete androgen insensitivity?

Strictly speaking, complete androgen insensitivity (testicular feminization) rarely presents as ambiguity in the newborn period or early childhood. Unless the testes have descended and are palpable in the labia majora, affected infants appear as phenotypically normal females.

The androgen receptor, encoded on the X chromosome, binds testosterone and, more avidly, dihydrotestosterone. Androgen insensitivity results from abnormalities of the androgen receptor. Complete androgen resistance occurs with a frequency of 1 in 20,000 to 1 in 64,000 XY individuals. Affected children grow as normal females until puberty. They feminize with normal breast development, because high levels of testosterone are aromatized to estrogen, but they have no pubic or axillary hair and no menses. Because they produce

MIF, they lack müllerian duct structures. Wolffian duct structures are also rudimentary or absent because they lack normal testosterone receptors. Gender identity is usually female. Patients come to medical attention because of primary amenorrhea. The diagnosis is therefore frequently missed until patients are in their mid- to late teens.

The intra-abdominal testes are at risk for malignancy, particularly after the onset of puberty. Timing of gonadectomy is debated. Because the risk of malignancy is low until puberty, some prefer to leave the gonads intact until spontaneous pubertal development; on the other hand, because carcinoma in situ has been found in prepubertal patients, others recommend early removal. If the testes are removed before puberty, estrogen therapy is necessary for normal pubertal progression. Because the upper section of the vagina is müllerian in origin, affected individuals may have shortened vaginas and need plastic surgical repair.

19. Describe the clinical picture in children with 5-alpha-reductase deficiency.

Deficiency of 5-alpha-reductase impairs the conversion of testosterone to DHT, leading to incomplete virilization and differentiation of the external genitalia. The disorder is particularly well documented in large kindreds in the Dominican Republic and Gaza, in whom it is inherited as an autosomal recessive condition.

Male infants with 5-alpha-reductase deficiency are born with sexual ambiguity. External genitalia range from a penis with simple hypospadias to a blind vaginal pouch and clitoris-like phallus. The most common presentation is a urogenital sinus with a blind vaginal pouch. During puberty, affected boys undergo virilization; affected females are normal. Traditionally, infants with 5-alpha-reductase deficiency were raised as females until puberty, then continued life as males and, in some cases, achieved fertility. Recently, however, the condition has been recognized early in life, and affected males are now raised from infancy as boys.

20. What is a "true hermaphrodite"?

"True hermaphroditism," a disorder of gonadal differentiation, refers to individuals with both ovarian and testicular elements. Affected children may have bilateral ovotestes, an ovary or testis on one side with an ovotestis on the other, or an ovary on one side and testis on the other. Because the effects of MIF and testosterone on duct structures are ipsilateral and localized, internal duct development is often asymmetrical. Thus, a fallopian tube and unicornuate uterus, with absent or vestigial male duct structures, may develop on the side without testicular elements, whereas epididymis, vas deferens and seminal vesicles without müllerian structures may develop on the side with testicular elements. The genitalia may be male, female or ambiguous, depending on the amount of functioning testicular tissue.

21. Why is a multidisciplinary team needed in approaching an infant with sexual ambiguity?

Sexual ambiguity is a complex issue in numerous ways. Accurate diagnosis is essential and may take a fair amount of time. Sex of assignment must be based not only on underlying diagnosis and karyotype but also on potential for adult sexual function, fertility and psychological health. For these reasons, input from several specialties, including endocrinology, genetics, neonatology, psychology, and urology, is important. All members of the team must communicate adequately with each other, and parents must receive a single message.

22. Once the etiology of sexual ambiguity has been determined in an infant, what factors should be considered in assigning a sex of rearing?

Arriving at a precise diagnosis provides the treating team an understanding of potential risks and benefits of either sex assignment. For example, in a poorly virilized male, the difference in outcome among children with defects in testosterone synthesis, complete androgen insensitivity, and 5-alpha-reductase deficiency is enormous. A child with defective synthesis of testosterone may be raised male or female, depending on other factors; a child with complete androgen insensitivity should be raised female; and a boy with 5-alpha-reductase deficiency usually is raised male. Yet children affected by any of the three conditions have 46 XY karyotypes.

Several factors must be considered: What is the potential for unambiguous genital appearance? What is the potential for normal sexual function? Is there a potential for fertility? What was the in utero hormone exposure What are the factors likely to affect gender identity and pyschological health? Phallic size, urethral position, vaginal anatomy and presence or absence of müllerian or wolffian duct structures, as well as gonadal characteristics and karyotype, must be considered.

Virilized females are usually assigned a female sex. They have normal ovaries as well as müllerian structures and, with surgical correction and steroid replacement, can have normal sexual function and achieve fertility.

Undervirilized males are often infertile, and sex assignment has usually been based on phallic size. Because a stretched penile length of 2.5 cm is 2.5 SD below the mean, an infant with a phallus smaller than 2.5 cm usually is assigned a female sex of rearing. Deficiency of 5-alpha-reductase is an obvious exception. If male sex assignment is contemplated, a trial of depot testosterone (50 mg every 3–4 weeks) for 1–3 months indicates whether phallic growth is possible.

In patients with gonadal dysgenesis and Y chromosomal material, gonadectomy is necessary and fertility is not possible. Internal duct structure is also frequently deranged. Small phallic size usually leads to a female sex assignment.

True hermaphrodites who have a unilateral ovary and müllerian structures may have spontaneous puberty and normal fertility and are raised as females. External genital size and structure may allow male assignment, but more commonly, external genitalia are poorly virilized and affected infants are assigned a female sex.

We need to learn much more about gender identity and consider which decisions might be made later than previously thought. Some surgical interventions are cosmetic, and some affected patients have expressed the wish that they should make the decisions in adolescence or adulthood. This field challenges many of our perceptions of sex and gender and our role as physicians.

BIBLIOGRAPHY

1. Goodall J: Helping a child to understand her own testicular feminization. Lancet 337:33, 1991.
2. Jasso N, Boussin L, Knebelmann B, et al.: Anti-müllerian hormone and intersex states. Trends Endocrinol Metab 2:227, 1991.
3. Kaplan S: Clinical Pediatric Endocrinology. Philadelphia, W.B. Saunders, 1990.
4. McGillivray BC: The newborn with ambiguous genitalia. Semin Perinatol 16:365, 1992.
5. Meyers-Seifer CH, Charest NJ: Diagnosis and management of patients with ambiguous genitalia. Semin Perinatol 16:332, 1992.
6. Mulaikal RM, Migeon CJ, Rock JA, et al.: Fertility rates in female patients with congenital adrenal hyperplasia due to 21-hydroxylase deficiency. N Engl J Med 316:178, 1987.
7. Pagona R: Diagnostic approach to the newborn with ambiguous genitalia. Pediatr Clin North Am 34:1019, 1987.
8. Penny R: Ambiguous genitalia. Am J Dis Child 144:753, 1990.
9. Thigpen AE, Davis DL, Gautier T, et al.: Brief report: The molecular basis of steroid 5 alpha-reductase deficiency in a large Dominican kindred. N Engl J Med 327:1216, 1992.
10. Zucker KJ, et al.: Psychosexual development of women with congenital adrenal hyperplasia. Hormone Behav 30:300, 1996.

44. DISORDERS OF PUBERTY

Sharon H. Travers, M.D., and Robert H. Slover, M.D.

1. What physiologic events initiate puberty?

Maturation of the hypothalamic-pituitary axis initiates puberty. The hypothalamus begins to secrete gonadotropin-releasing hormone (GnRH) in pulses during sleep and eventually during waking hours as well. GnRH pulses stimulate the pituitary gland to secrete pulses of gonadotropins, of which there is luteinizing hormone (LH) predominance. In response to the increased secretion of gonadotropins, there is increased secretion of gonadal hormones that lead to the progressive development of secondary sexual characteristics.

2. What is adrenarche?

Adrenarche refers to the time during puberty when the adrenal glands increase their production and secretion of adrenal androgens. Plasma concentrations of DHEA and DHEA-S, the most important adrenal androgens, begin to increase in children by about 6–8 years. However, the signs of adrenarche, such as pubic and axillary hair development, acne, and body odor, do not typically occur until early to mid-puberty. The control of adrenal androgen secretion is not clearly understood, but it does appear to be separate from GnRH and the gonadotropins.

3. What is the normal pattern of puberty in males?

The mean age of onset of puberty in boys is 11.5 years with a range of 9–14 years. In both sexes, puberty requires maturation of gonadal function and increased secretion of adrenal androgens (adrenarche). The first evidence of puberty in the majority of boys is enlargement of the testes to greater than 4 ml in volume or greater than 2.5 cm in length. It is not until midpuberty, when testosterone levels are rapidly rising, that boys experience voice change, axillary and facial hair, and the peak growth spurt. Spermatogenesis is mature at a mean age of 13.3 years.

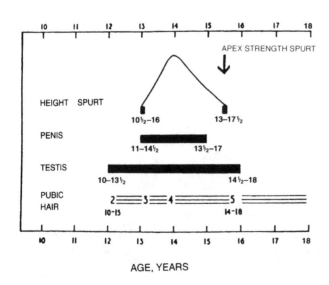

Sequence of events at puberty in males. (From Marshall WE, Tanner JM: Variations in the pattern of pubertal changes in boys. Arch Dis Child 45:13–23, 1970.)

4. Describe the normal pattern of female pubertal development.

Girls normally begin puberty between ages 8 and 13 years (mean age: 10.6 years for white girls and 9.5 years for black girls). The initial pubertal event is typically the appearance of breast buds, although in a small percentage of girls, pubic hair development may appear first. Initial breast development often occurs asymmetrically and should not be of concern. Breast development is primarily under the control of estrogens secreted by the ovaries, whereas pubic and axillary hair growth result mainly from adrenal androgens. Unlike boys, the pubertal growth spurt in girls occurs at the onset of puberty. Menarche usually occurs 18–24 months after the onset of breast development (mean age: 12.8 years). Although most girls have reached about 97.5% of their maximum height potential at menarche, this can vary considerably. Consequently, age of menarche is not necessarily a good predictor of adult height.

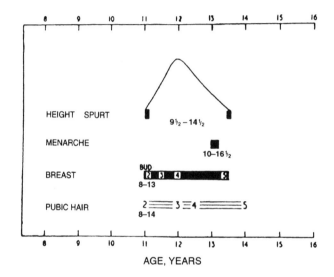

The sequence of events at puberty in females. An average is represented in relation to the scale of ages. (From Marshall WE, Tanner JM: Variations in the pattern of pubertal changes in girls. Arch Dis Child 44: 291–303, 1969, with permission.)

5. What controls the pubertal growth spurt?

In both boys and girls, the pubertal growth spurt is primarily controlled by gonadal steroids. Gonadal steroids augment growth hormone secretion and also have direct stimulatory effects on bone and cartilage. At the end of puberty, linear growth is near complete as a result of the effects of gonadal steroids on skeletal maturation and epiphyseal fusion.

6. How is pubertal development measured?

Sexual maturity is determined by examination and is described by a scale devised by John Tanner in 1969. Because of the distinct actions of adrenal androgens and gonadal steroids, it is important to distinguish between breast and pubic hair development in girls and between genital and pubic hair development in boys. In all cases, Tanner stage I is prepubertal and Tanner stage V is complete maturation. In addition to the physical examination, the tools to assess pubertal development may include determination of bone age, growth velocity and pattern, and specific endocrine studies.

Tanner Stages of Pubertal Development

STAGE	CHARACTERISTICS	STAGE	CHARACTERISTICS
Girls	**Breast Development**		**Pubic Hair Development**
I	Prepubertal; elevation of papilla only	I	Prepubertal; no pubic hair
II	Breast buds are noted or palpable; enlargement of areola	II	Sparse growth of long, straight, or slightly curly, minimally pigmented hair, mainly of labia
III	Further enlargement of breast and areola, with no separation of their contours	III	Considerably darker and coarser hair spreading over mons pubis
IV	Projection of areola and papilla to form secondary mound above level of breast	IV	Thick, adult-type hair that does not yet spread to medial surface of thighs
V	Adult contour breast with projection of papilla only	V	Hair adult in type and distributed in classic inverse triangle
Boys	**Genital Development**		**Pubic Hair Development**
I	Prepubertal; testicular length < 2.5 cm	I	Prepubertal; no pubic hair
II	Testes > 2.5 cm in longest diameter andscrotum thinning and reddening	II	Sparse growth of slightly pigmented, slightly curly pubic hair, mainly at base of penis
III	Growth of penis in width and length and further growth of testes	III	Thicker, curlier hair, spread to mons pubis
IV	Penis further enlarged; testes larger, withdarker scrotal skin color	IV	Adult-type hair that does not yet spread to medial surface of thighs
V	Genitalia adult in size and shape	V	Adult-type hair spread to medial thighs

Data from Marshall WE, Tanner JM: Variations in the pattern of pubertal changes in girls. Arch Dis Child 44:291–303, 1969; and Variations in the pattern of pubertal changes in boys. Arch Dis Child 45:13–23, 1970.

7. What constitutes sexual precocity in boys and girls?

Precocious puberty is defined as pubertal development occurring below the limits of age set for normal onset of puberty. In girls, this is puberty before 8 years of age and for boys, before 9 years of age. Recently, it has been noted that breast development can occur normally as early as 7 years in white girls, and 6 years in black girls. Consequently, evaluation and treatment of girls who start puberty between 6 and 8 years should depend on factors such as family history, rapidity of development, presence of CNS symptoms, and family concern. Girls who are short and start puberty between 6 and 8 years may also benefit from evaluation. In children who present with early pubertal signs, precocious puberty must be distinguished from normal variants of puberty such as benign premature thelarche and benign premature adrenarche.

Precocious puberty, regardless of the cause, is associated with increased linear growth and skeletal maturation secondary to elevated sex steroid levels. Children with precocious puberty are often tall for their age during childhood. However, skeletal maturation may become more advanced than stature, leading to premature fusion of the epiphyseal growth plates and a compromised adult height. In addition to the physical consequences of early puberty, there are social and psychological aspects that the practitioner needs to consider.

8. In which sex is precocity more prevalent? Why?

Precocious puberty predominantly affects girls. The disparity in overall prevalence of precocity is explained by the large numbers of precocious girls with central idiopathic precocity, a condition that is unusual in boys. At least 80% of all precocious puberty in girls is central idiopathic in nature. The prevalence of organic etiologies of precocious puberty (central nervous system lesions, gonadal tumors, and specific underlying diseases) is similar in both sexes.

9. Two common benign conditions in girls are often confused with precocious puberty. The first is premature thelarche. How is it diagnosed and treated?

Premature thelarche refers to isolated breast development in girls without accompanying signs of adrenarche such as pubic/axillary hair, body odor, and acne. There are several characteristics of premature thelarche that distinguish it from the breast development that occurs in precocious puberty. First of all, premature thelarche is most common in girls who are either under 2 years or between 6 and 8 years of age. Breast development can occur secondary to increased sensitivity of breast tissue to low levels of estrogen being produced, or secondary to a transient increase in ovarian estrogen secretion, perhaps from a cyst. Girls with premature thelarche may have a history of slowly progressing breast development or waxing and waning of breast size. Growth rate and bone age are not accelerated and on physical examination, the breast tissue rarely develops beyond Tanner stage 2–3. GnRH stimulation may provoke a FSH-predominant response as opposed to the typical LH-predominant response seen in true central precocity. The natural course of benign thelarche is for the breast tissue to regress or fail to progress. Because of its benign nature, treatment is not necessary except for reassurance and follow-up. Follow-up is critical because premature thelarche occasionally is the first sign of what later becomes apparent as central precocious puberty.

10. The second benign condition is premature adrenarche. How is it diagnosed and treated?

Premature adrenarche occurs in both genders and is the early development of pubic hair with or without axillary hair, body odor, and acne. There are no signs of gonadarche in this condition, so girls have no breast development and boys show no testicular enlargement. Premature adrenarche is caused by early secretion of the adrenal androgens, primarily DHEA and DHEA-S. A child who has premature adrenarche and Tanner stage 2 pubic hair development will have adrenal androgen values similar to those normally found in a pubertal child at the same stage of development. The natural course of premature adrenarche is for the signs to slowly progress without having an effect on the timing of true puberty. Since pubic hair development may be the first sign of puberty, especially in girls, follow-up is necessary to evaluate for evidence of gonadarche (i.e. breast development). As in premature thelarche, growth rate and bone age are not accelerated. If signs of puberty are rapidly progressing or if there is evidence of increased linear growth and advanced bone age, measurement of androgens (DHEA-S, androstenedione, and testosterone) is performed to evaluate for a serious virilizing disorder such as congenital adrenal hyperplasia (CAH) or an adrenal tumor.

11. How is the diagnosis of precocious puberty made?

The diagnosis of precocious puberty requires the appearance of the physical signs of puberty before the age of 8 years in girls or 9 years in boys. The disorders that cause precocity are either GnRH-dependent (central) or GnRH-independent (peripheral). Central precocious puberty involves activation of the GnRH pulse generator, an increase in gonadotropin secretion, and a resultant increase in the production of sex steroids. Consequently, the sequence of hormonal and physical events in central precocious puberty is identical to the progression of normal puberty. In evaluating a child with early pubertal development, the presence of any of the following warrants further investigation or referral to a specialist:

1. Growth velocity and/or bone age are increased.
2. Levels of sex steroids are elevated (levels may be difficult to interpret, however, early in the course of pubertal development).
3. Girls show evidence of both estrogen and androgen events (such as breast development and pubic hair) or menses.
4. Boys show virilization with testicular enlargement.
5. Girls with isolated breast development or boys with virilization and no testicular enlargement may also require evaluation depending on their age, and the degree and tempo of their development.

In both boys and girls, a complete history should be taken, with careful consideration of any exposure to exogenous steroids, onset of pubertal signs and rate of progression, presence or history of CNS abnormalities, and pubertal history of other family members. Height measurements should be plotted on a growth chart to determine growth velocity. A physical examination is performed with focus on Tanner staging, presence of café-au-lait spots, and neurologic signs. One of the first steps in evaluating a child with early pubertal development is obtaining a radiograph of the left hand and wrist to determine skeletal maturity (bone age). If the bone age is advanced, further evaluation is typically warranted.

12. After making the general diagnosis of precocity, how do I proceed to a specific diagnosis?
It is usually difficult to distinguish GnRH-dependent (central) from GnRH-independent (peripheral) precocity on physical examination. Although the possible causes of peripheral precocious puberty are more numerous (see below), central precocity accounts for the overwhelming majority of cases.

Sex steroid levels, especially in boys, should be measured; testosterone levels above the prepubertal range (>10 ng/dl) confirm pubertal status but do not indicate the cause. Estrogen values in girls are not as helpful because slightly elevated levels may indicate either early puberty or benign thelarche. Consequently, the single most important test is a GnRH stimulation test to determine whether gonadotropin responses are consistent with central or peripheral precocious puberty. The diagnosis of central precocious puberty is made by demonstrating a LH response to GnRH greater than 7–10 IU/L. Measurement of random gonadotropins is not helpful because of overlap between prepubertal and pubertal values. In all boys and in girls less than 6 years of age who are diagnosed with central precocious puberty, a MRI study of the brain should be done to evaluate for CNS lesions. It is unlikely that an abnormality will be found in girls between 6 and 8 years, so the need for a MRI in this age group should be individually assessed.

A suppressed or prepubertal LH response to GnRH suggests that there are high sex steroid levels (causing negative feedback) being produced independent of gonadotropin stimulation, a pattern consistent with peripheral precocious puberty. In girls, pelvic ultrasound and serum estradiol levels are obtained in this scenario to evaluate for an ovarian cyst, tumor, or McCune-Albright Syndrome. In boys with suspected peripheral precocious puberty, additional laboratory studies should include serum hCG, DHEA-S, and androstenedione levels. Elevated adrenal androgens suggest congenital adrenal hyperplasia (CAH) or an adrenal tumor. Asymmetric or unilateral enlargement of the testes suggests a Leydig cell tumor.

Causes of isosexual precocious puberty
Central (GnRH-dependent)
    Idiopathic true precocious puberty*
    Central nervous system tumors (hamartomas*, hypothalamic tumors)
    Central nervous system disorders (meningitis, encephalitis, hydrocephalus, trauma, abscesses, cysts, granulomas, radiation therapy)

Peripheral (GnRH-independent)
    Males
        Human chorionic gonadotropin (hCG)–secreting tumors (CNS, liver)
        Congenital adrenal hyperplasia (21-hydroxylase or 11-hydroxylase deficiency)
        Adrenal tumors
        Leydig cell testicular tumors
        Familial gonadotropin-independent Leydig cell maturation (testotoxicosis)
        McCune-Albright syndrome (polyostotic fibrous dysplasia)
    Females
        Follicular cysts*
        Ovarian tumors
        Adrenal tumors
        Exogenous estrogen
        McCune-Albright syndrome (polyostotic fibrous dysplasia)

Causes of contrasexual precocious puberty (rare)
    Feminization in males
        Adrenal tumors (feminizing)
        Increased peripheral steroid-to-estrogen conversion
    Virilization in females
        Congenital adrenal hyperplasia (21-hydroxylase deficiency*, 11-hydroxylase
            deficiency, 3-beta-hydroxysteroid dehydrogenase deficiency)
        Adrenal tumors (virilizing)
        Ovarian tumors (virilizing)
*More common.

13. How is central idiopathic precocious puberty treated?

Children with central precocious puberty can be treated with GnRH analogues such as leuprolide. GnRH analogues down-regulate pituitary GnRH receptors and thus decrease gonadotropin secretion. With treatment, physical changes of puberty regress or cease to progress, and linear growth slows to a prepubertal rate. Projected final heights often increase as a result of slowing of skeletal maturation. Usually, GnRH analogues are given as a monthly depot intramuscular injection, and side effects are rare. After discontinuation of therapy, pubertal progression resumes and in girls, ovulation and pregnancy have been documented. Therapy is considered for both psychosocial and final height considerations. For example, in a girl who is near the normal age of puberty and who has slowly progressing development, treatment would not necessarily be indicated. However, the same age girl who has already progressed to menarche may benefit psychosocially from treatment.

14. What is the association of hypothyroidism with precocity?

Precocious puberty, specifically breast development, has been described in girls with severe acquired hypothyroidism. Although affected children exhibit secondary sex characteristics of precocity, growth is delayed—and perhaps bone ages—because of the hypothyroidism. The mechanism for this association is not known, but elevated levels of TSH may cross-react with ovarian gonadotropin receptors to stimulate ovarian enlargement and secretion of estrogen. Patients are easily diagnosed with studies of thyroid function and treated with L-thyroxine. Once the hypothyroidism is adequately treated, breast development regresses.

15. What is McCune-Albright syndrome? How is it treated?

McCune-Albright syndrome is a triad consisting of irregular (coast-of-Maine) café-au-lait lesions, polyostotic fibrous dysplasia, and GnRH-independent precocious puberty. It affects both sexes but is seen infrequently in boys. In girls, breast development and vaginal bleeding occur with sporadic increases in estradiol. Serum gonadotropin levels are low, and GnRH testing elicits a prepubertal response. With time, however, increased estradiol may mature the hypothalamus, thus leading to true central GnRH-dependent precocity. The syndrome is often associated with other endocrine dysfunction, including hyperthyroidism, hyperparathyroidism, adrenal hyperplasia, Cushing's syndrome and gigantism. In affected tissues, there is an activating mutation in the gene that encodes the α subunit of G_s, the G protein that stimulates adenylate cylase. Endocrine cells with this mutation have autonomous hyperfunction and secrete excess amounts of their respective hormones.

Girls with McCune-Albright syndrome are generally treated with testolactone, a medication that inhibits the aromatization of testosterone to estrogen. Testolactone, however, is not effective in many girls, and recently there have been trials using tamoxifen, an estrogen receptor antagonist. In boys, treatment consists of either inhibiting androgen production with ketoconazole or a combination of inhibiting estrogen production with testolactone and blocking androgen action with spironolactone.

16. Describe testotoxicosis. How is it treated?

Familial testotoxicosis is an autosomal dominant, gonadotropin-independent form of male precocity. Boys with this condition begin to develop true precocity with testicular and phallic enlargement and growth acceleration by the age of 4 years. Serum testosterone levels are high, but serum gonadotropins are low and GnRH testing shows a prepubertal response. By mid-adolescence to adulthood, GnRH stimulation demonstrates a more typical LH-predominant pubertal response. The cause, in some families, has been found to be an activating mutation in the gene encoding the LH receptor. The mutant LH receptors in the testes are constitutively overactive and do not require LH binding for their activity but produce testosterone autonomously. Treatment options are the same as for boys with McCune-Albright syndrome.

17. How does non–salt-wasting congenital adrenal hyperplasia present in boys?

The most common adrenogenital syndrome is 21-hydroxylase deficiency. Girls develop virilization in utero, resulting in a degree of sexual ambiguity. They are discovered at birth and should be diagnosed within the first few days of life by the finding of greatly elevated serum 17-hydroxyprogesterone levels. In the more common salt-losing form of this disease, boys present with vomiting, shock, and electrolyte disturbances at 7–10 days of age. A small subset of affected boys, however, do not waste salt; they present in early or late childhood with precocity consisting of pubic hair, acne, body odor, deepening of the voice, penile but not testicular enlargement, acceleration of linear growth, and skeletal maturation. A similar presentation occurs in boys with the much less common 11-hydroxylase deficiency, which, in contrast to 21-hyroxylase deficiency, may cause hypertension. Treatment is directed at reducing serum androgen levels by replacing glucocorticoids to reduce pituitary secretion of corticotropin (ACTH).

18. What is adolescent gynecomastia? When and how should it be treated?

Normal boys can have either unilateral or bilateral breast enlargement during puberty. Breast development generally starts during early puberty and resolves within 2 years. The cause of gynecomastia is not clearly understood but may be related to an elevated ratio of estradiol to testosterone levels. Treatment primarily consists of reassurance and support; however, if resolution does not occur or if the breast enlargement is excessive, surgery may be warranted. Pathologic conditions associated with gynecomastia include Klinefelter's syndrome and various other testosterone-deficient states.

19. At what age does failure to enter puberty necessitate investigation?

Delayed puberty should be evaluated if there are no pubertal signs by 13 years of age in girls and by 14 years of age in boys. An abnormality in the pubertal axis may also present as lack of normal pubertal progression, which is defined as more than 4 years between the first signs of puberty and menarche in girls, or more than 5 years for completion of genital growth in boys.

20. What is constitutional growth delay, and how does it affect puberty?

Constitutional growth delay is the most common cause of delayed puberty. Children with this growth pattern have a fall off in their linear growth within the first 2 years of life; after this, growth returns to normal, albeit at a lower growth channel than would be expected for parental heights. Skeletal maturation is also delayed, and the onset of puberty is commensurate with bone age rather than chronological age. For example, a 14-year-old boy with a bone age of 11 years will appropriately start puberty when his bone age is closer to 11.5–12 years. The delay in puberty postpones the pubertal growth spurt and closure of growth plates, so that the child continues to grow after his/her peers have reached their final height. A key feature of this growth pattern is normal linear growth after 2 years of age. There is often a family history of "late bloomers."

It is often challenging to differentiate between constitutional delay and hormonal disorders of pubertal development, such as gonadotropin deficiency, in the prepubertal period. Time and careful observation are important tools.

21. When is hypogonadism diagnosed?

Functional or permanent hypogonadism should be considered when there are no signs of puberty and bone age has advanced to beyond the normal ages for puberty to start. An eunuchoid body habitus is often evident in children with abnormally delayed puberty; a decreased upper to lower body ratio and long arm span characterize this habitus. As a rule, serum gonadotropin levels are measured first to determine whether there is hypogonadotropic hypogonadism (gonadotropin deficiency) or hypergonadotropic hypogonadism (primary gonadal failure). If a child's bone age is below the normal age for puberty to start, gonadotropin levels are not a reliable means of making an accurate diagnosis.

Causes of Delayed Adolescence in the Phenotypic Male and Female

---

Hypergonadotropic conditions
    Variants of ovarian and testicular dysgenesis
    Gonadal toxins (antimetabolite and/or radiation treatment)
    Enzyme defects (17-alpha-hydroxylase deficiency in the genetic male or female; 17-keto-
        steroid reductase deficiency in the genetic male)
    Androgen insensitivity (testicular feminization)
    Other miscellaneous disorders
Hypogonadotropic conditions
    Multiple pituitary hormone deficiencies
    Isolated growth hormone deficiency
    Isolated gonadotropin deficiency
    Miscellaneous syndrome complexes (e.g., Prader-Willi syndrome)
    Systemic conditions, nutritional and psychogenic disorders, increased energy expenditure
    Other endocrine causes: hypothyroidism, glucocorticoid excess, hyperprolactinemia
    Constitutional delay in growth and development
Eugonadotropic conditions: delayed menarche
    Gonadal dysgenesis variants with residual functioning ovarian tissue
    Polycystic ovarian disease
    Hyperprolactinemia

From Rosenfeld R: Diagnosis and management of delayed puberty. J Clin Endocrinol Metab 70:559, 1990, with permission.

22. What causes hypogonadotropic hypogonadism?

Chronic illnesses, malnutrition, exercise, and anorexia can all cause a functional deficiency of gonadotropins that reverses when the underlying condition improves. Hyperprolactinemia can also present as delayed puberty and only 50% of the time will there be a history of galactorrhea. Permanent gonadotropin deficiency is suspected if these conditions are ruled out and gonadotropin levels are low. Gonadotropin deficiency may be associated with other pituitary deficiencies from conditions such as septo-optic dysplasia, craniopharyngioma, or cranial irradiation. Various syndromes, such as Prader-Willi, are also associated with gonadotropin deficiency. Isolated gonadotropin deficiency (i.e., occurring without another pituitary deficiency) is often difficult to diagnose, as hormonal tests do not absolutely distinguish whether a child can produce enough gonadotropins or whether he/she simply has very delayed puberty. If gonadotropin deficiency cannot be clearly distinguished from delayed puberty, a short course of sex steroids can be given for 4–6 months. Individuals with constitutional delay will often enter puberty after such an intervention. If spontaneous puberty does not occur after this treatment or after a second course, the diagnosis of gonadotropin deficiency may be made.

23. What is Kallmann's syndrome?

Kallmann's syndrome is one of a class of disorders referred to as idiopathic hypogonadotropic hypogonadism or idiopathic hypothalamic hypogonadism (IHH). It occurs as frequently as 1:10,000 boys and 1:50,000 girls. The classic form is characterized by hypogonadotropic hypogonadism with hyposmia or anosmia and is associated with hypoplasia or aplasia of other structures of the rhinencephalon (e.g., cleft lip/cleft palate, congenital deafness, and color blindness). Undescended testes and gynecomastia are common.

24. What causes hypergonadotropic hypogonadism?

Elevated gonadotropin levels indicate that there is a failure of the gonads to produce enough sex steroids to suppress the hypothalamic-pituitary axis. These levels are diagnostic for gonadal failure at two periods of time: before 3 years of age, and once the bone age is at or beyond the normal age for puberty to start. Surgery, radiation, and chemotherapy are all potential causes of gonadal failure in both sexes.

In girls with gonadal failure and no apparent cause, a karyotype evaluation should be performed; Turner syndrome (45,XO) will be the most likely explanation. 46,XX gonadal dysgenesis can also occur and may be inherited as an autosomal recessive trait. A karyotype will also identify 46,XY gonadal dysgenesis in a phenotypic female who is actually a genetic male. In this condition, there is complete lack of testicular development and consequently, except for the absence of gonads, normal female genital differentiation occurs. Boys may have gonadal failure secondary to testicular torsion, radiation, chemotherapy, or the vanishing testis syndrome. Noonan and Klinefelter's syndrome (47,XXY) are other potential causes of primary testicular insufficiency. Consequently, in a boy with unexplained gonadotropin elevations, a karyotype should be done.

25. What is Turner syndrome? How is it treated?

Any consideration of pubertal delay in girls must include the possibility of Turner syndrome. An absent or structurally abnormal second X chromosome characterizes Turner syndrome (45,XO). The incidence of Turner syndrome is approximately 1:2000 live female births. However, the chromosomal abnormality is actually more common than this, as 99% of XO fetuses do not survive beyond 28 weeks gestation, and the XO karyotype occurs in 1 out of 15 miscarriages. In the absence of a second functional X chromosome, oocyte degeneration is accelerated, leaving fibrotic streaks in place of normal ovaries. Because of primary gonadal failure, serum gonadotropin levels rise and are elevated at birth and again at the normal time of puberty.

In approximately 10–20% of Turner girls, there will be some ovarian function at puberty that allows for slight breast development. A small percentage of this group will also have normal periods, and an even smaller percentage (<1% of all girls with Turner syndrome) will actually be fertile. Treatment is with unopposed estradiol or conjugated estrogen for a year, followed by cycling with estrogen and progestins. The short stature of girls with Turner syndrome is treated with growth hormone. Final height in girls with Turner syndrome is related to when growth hormone is initiated, with better outcomes in girls who are started at a young age. Consequently, early diagnosis of Turner syndrome is essential.

Clinical Findings Commonly Described in Patients with Turner Syndrome

PRIMARY DEFECTS	SECONDARY FEATURES	INCIDENCE (%)
Physical features		
Skeletal growth disturbances	Short stature	100
	Short neck	40
	Abnormal upper to lower segment ratio	97
	Cubitus valgus	47
	Short metacarpals	37
	Madelung deformity	7.5
	Scoliosis	12.5
	Genu valgum	35
	Characteristic facies with micrognathia	60
	High arched palate	36
Lymphatic obstruction	Webbed neck	25
	Low posterior hairline	42
	Rotated ears	Common
	Edema of hands/feet	22
	Severe nail dysplasia	13
	Characteristic dermatoglyphics	35
Unknown factors	Strabismus	17.5
	Ptosis	11
	Multiple pigmented nevi	26
Physiologic features		
Skeletal growth disturbances	Growth failure	100
	Otitis media	73
Germ cell chromosomal defects	Gonadal failure	96
	Infertility	99.9
	Gonadoblastoma	4.0
Unknown factors—embryogenic	Cardiovascular anomalies	55
	Hypertension	7
	Renal and renovascular anomalies	39
Unknown factors—metabolic	Hashimoto's thyroiditis	34
	Hypothyroidism	10
	Alopecia	2
	Vitiligo	2
	Gastrointestinal disorders	2.5
	Carbohydrate intolerance	40

From Hall J, Gilchrist D: Turner syndrome and its variants. Pediatr Clin North Am 37:1421, 1990, with permission.

26. Why do boys with Klinefelter's syndrome have pubertal delay?

Klinefelter's syndrome, or seminiferous tubular dysgenesis, is the most common cause of testicular failure. It results from at least one extra X chromosome; thus the most common karyotype is 47, XXY. The incidence is 1:1000 male births.

Eunuchoid proportions are present from early childhood. Other features include gynecomastia, tall stature, small testes, and elevated serum gonadotropins. Learning disabilities and behavioral problems may also be present. Seminiferous tubular dysgenesis is universal in patients with Klinefelter's syndrome, but Leydig cell function (testosterone production) is variable; thus they may have either delay in pubertal onset or failure to progress normally through puberty. In most patients, testosterone replacement is necessary.

Features That May Be of Value in the Clinical Detection of Klinefelter's Syndrome

FEATURES	CHILD	ADULT
Psychosocial	Delay in language development; placid; poorly organized motor function	Increased psychopathology; disturbed body image
Testes	May be small in size (decreased germ cell mass)	Small size with hyalinization; incomplete virilization or fibrosis; gynecomastia
Phallus	May be small in size; may have hypo-spadias	Small size secondary to inadequate testosterone production
Body habitus	Long legs with decreased upper to lowersegment ratio; slim build with decreasedweight for height; hypoplasia of middle phalanges of fifth fingers; limitation of pronation and supination of forearms	Eunuchoid habitus; increased truncal adiposity and decreased muscle mass

From Rosenfeld R: Diagnosis and management of delayed puberty. J Clin Endocrinol Metab 70:559, 1990, with permission.

27. Describe the history and physical examination for an adolescent with pubertal delay.

The history should include questions regarding the presence of chronic illnesses, nutritional disorders, exercise history, galactorrhea, family history of infertility, and timing of puberty in parents and siblings. Weight gain or loss should also be noted. Physical examination should include measurement of arm span and upper-to-lower segment ratio. Eunuchoid proportions occur early in patients with Klinefelter's syndrome and late in those with other forms of hypogonadism. Signs of any chronic illness, malnutrition, anorexia, and features of Turner syndrome (girls) and Klinefelter's syndrome (boys) should be noted. A careful search should be made for any signs of puberty, such as pubic hair and axillary hair, acne, testicular size and penile length (boys), and breast development (girls). Pubic hair may represent only adrenal androgen production. Testicular length of greater than 2.5 cm indicates gonadotropin stimulation. Estrogen effect is evaluated by breast development and vaginal maturity. In addition, visual field and olfaction should be evaluated (80% of boys with Kallmann's syndrome have reduced or absent sense of smell). Signs of hypothyroidism and Cushing's syndrome must also be evaluated. In addition, the growth chart should be analyzed to determine if there is short stature and if linear growth has been normal.

28. What laboratory tests help in the diagnosis of pubertal delay?

Assessment of bone age is critical in determining biologic age and the time of expected pubertal development. If linear growth is normal and the bone age is less than the normal age for pubertal onset, the diagnosis is likely to be constitutional growth delay. If linear growth is subnormal with bone age delay, it may be necessary to investigate the poor growth with evaluation of growth hormone or thyroid status. If bone age has advanced to beyond the age for normal puberty, gonadotropin levels are very helpful in distinguishing between gonadotropin deficiency and primary gonadal failure. Additional laboratory studies may include chemistry panels, electrolytes, thyroid function tests, estradiol (girls), testosterone (boys), and prolactin levels. If gonadotropins are elevated, chromosome analysis is indicated for both genders to evaluate for Turner syndrome in girls and Klinefelter's syndrome in boys. In the case of low serum gonadotropins, olfactory testing and cranial MRI are recommended.

The GnRH test is difficult to interpret in prepubertal or peripubertal children. Although GnRH testing may suggest the diagnosis of constitutional delay if there is a clear rise in LH levels, the overlap in response among prepubertal, hypogonadotropic, and early pubertal children is significant.

29. How is delayed puberty managed?

The treatment of delayed puberty depends on the underlying cause. If the delayed pubertal development is secondary to anorexia, hypothyroidism, or illness, treatment of these underlying conditions will result in spontaneous onset of puberty. Puberty will also begin spontaneously, albeit late, in constitutional growth delay so that reassurance alone to the patient and family may be sufficient. However, treatment may be offered for psychological reasons. Both boys and girls may be distressed because of their small size and sexually immature appearance. They are often treated as if they were younger, teased by peers, and denied participation in certain athletic activities. In boys, a 4–6 month course of low-dose depot testosterone (50–100 mg intramuscularly every 4 weeks) can be offered if the bone age is at least 11–11½ years. This treatment results in some early virilization without adversely affecting final height. Spontaneous puberty usually begins, as evident by testicular enlargement, 3–6 months after the end of the testosterone course. Treatment of delayed puberty in girls with constitutional growth delay is more controversial and less frequent. After a thorough initial evaluation, however, some endocrinologists use low doses of conjugated estrogen (Premarin, 0.3 mg) or ethinyl estradiol (5–10 μg) daily for 3–4 months. Therapy is then stopped, and physical changes are evaluated. Withdrawal bleeding is unusual after one course of estrogen therapy but may occur with subsequent courses.

30. How are boys with hypogonadism treated?

In boys with hypogonadotropic hypogonadism for whom fertility is not an immediate issue and in all boys with primary hypogonadism, long-term testosterone therapy is required. While the patient is growing, careful attention must be paid to growth velocity and bone age. Most commonly, depot testosterone esters (enanthate or cypionate) are used in 25–50 mg doses every 3–4 weeks for the first 1–2 years of therapy. By the second or third year, the dose is raised to 50–100 mg intramuscularly every 3–4 weeks. The adult maintenance level is 200–300 mg intramuscularly every 3–4 weeks. Alternatively, the cutaneous testosterone patch or gel may be used.

31. How is estrogen treatment given for girls with hypogonadism?

Replacement therapy in hypogonadal girls is begun with estrogen treatment alone, either as ethinyl estradiol (5–10 μg) or as Premarin (0.15–0.3 mg) for 12 to 18 months. Following this, progesterone is added for 10 days of each month or a birth control pill may be prescribed. Progesterone therapy is needed to counteract the effects of estrogen on the uterus; unopposed estrogen can cause endometrial hyperplasia and carcinoma. Replacement of gonadal steroids in both sexes is also necessary for normal bone mineralization and to prevent osteoporosis.

32. Do body habitus and lifestyle influence the timing of puberty and final height?

In the early 1980s, a number of reports suggested that extremely active and thin girls had a high incidence of primary amenorrhea and delay of puberty. Gymnasts, runners, and ballet dancers, among others, were evaluated. A high incidence of primary amenorrhea, secondary amenorrhea, and dysmenorrhea was found among this group of athletes and appears to have been related to their low fat-lean ratios as well as to the exercise itself. Indeed, when forced by injury to discontinue activity, such athletes gained weight and quickly progressed to menarche.

A recent study evaluated the effect of intensive physical training during puberty on final height in girls. Predicted height decreased significantly with time in gymnasts but not in swimmers. The author concluded that heavy training in gymnastics, starting before and lasting through puberty, may reduce final adult height.

33. What is the definition of amenorrhea?

A girl who has not had menarche by 16 years of age or within 4 years after the onset of puberty is considered to have primary amenorrhea. Secondary amenorrhea is diagnosed if more than 6 months has elapsed since the last menstrual period.

34. How do you begin to evaluate a girl with amenorrhea?

In order to sort out the many causes of amenorrhea, it is helpful to distinguish those girls who produce sufficient estrogen from those who do not by performing a progesterone challenge. Girls who are producing estrogen will have a withdrawal bleed after 5–10 days of oral progesterone, whereas those who are estrogen-deficient will have no or very little bleeding. There are two situations in which girls have sufficient estrogen but do not have a withdrawal bleed. In Rokitansky syndrome, maldevelopment of the mullerian structures leads to an absent or hypoplastic uterus and/or cervix. Complete androgen insensitivity syndrome (testicular feminization) in a genetic male results in a phenotypic female who has normal breast development secondary to the aromatization of testosterone to estrogen. However, the production of mullerian-inhibiting factor in these patients leads to regression of the mullerian structures and thus the absence of a uterus. The absence of a cervix is a diagnostic finding in both of these conditions; consequently, a pelvic examination should be considered in all girls who present with amenorrhea, especially primary amenorrhea. The causes of amenorrhea associated with estrogen insufficiency include hypogonadism, and this is described in the previous section of delayed puberty.

35. What causes amenorrhea in girls who are producing estrogen?

Amenorrhea in girls who are producing normal or even elevated amounts of estrogen is a manifestation of anovulatory cycles. Irregular menses may also be a sign of chronic anovulation; estrogen production, unopposed by progesterone, leads to endometrial hyperplasia and intermittent shedding. Since menarche is normally followed be a period of anovulatory cycles and irregular menses, many adolescents with a pathologic etiology may be missed. Consequently, it is important to evaluate all girls who do not have regular menses by 3 years after menarche. The most common cause of chronic anovulation is polycystic ovarian syndrome (PCOS), a disorder characterized by increased ovarian androgen production. The clinical presentation varies and may include amenorrhea, oligomenorrhea, dysfunctional uterine bleeding, hirsutism, acne, and obesity.

BIBLIOGRAPHY

1. Comite F, et al: Cyclical ovarian function resistant to treatment with an analogue of luteinizing hormone releasing hormone in McCune-Albright syndrome. N Engl J Med 311:1032, 1984.
2. Evans SJ: The athletic adolescent with amenorrhea. Pediatr Ann 13:605, 1984.

3. Frisch R, Wyshak G, Vincent L: Delayed menarche and amenorrhea in ballet dancers. N Engl J Med 303: 17, 1980.
4. Ghai K, Cara JF, Rosenfeld RL: Gonadotropin releasing hormone agonist (Nafarelin) test to differentiate gonadotropin deficiency from constitutionally delayed puberty in teen-age boys—a clinical research center study. J Clin Endocrinol Metab 80:2980, 1995.
5. Grumbach MM, Stybe: Puberty: Ontogeny, neuroendocrinology, physiology, and disorders. In Wilson JD, Foster DW, Kronenberg HM, Larsen PR (eds): Williams Textbook of Endocrinology, 9th ed. Philadelphia, WB Saunders, 1998, pp 1509–1625.
6. Hall J, Gilchrist D: Turner syndrome and its variants. Pediatr Clin North Am 37:1421, 1990.
7. Herman-Giddens ME, Slora EJ, Wasserman RC, et al.: Secondary sexual characteristics and menses in young girls seen in office practice: A study from the Pediatric Research in Office Setting network. Pediatrics 99(4):505–512, 1997.
8. Ibanez L, et al: Natural history of premature pubarche and auxological study. J Clin Endocrinol Metab 74:254, 1992.
9. Kaplan S (ed): Clinical Pediatric Endocrinology. Philadelphia, W.B. Saunders, 1990.
10. Kaplan S, Grumbach M: Pathophysiology and treatment of sexual precocity. J Clin Endocrinol Metab 71:785, 1990.
11. Kappy MS, Ganong CS: Advances in the treatment of precocious puberty. Adv Pediatr 41:223, 1994.
12. Kulin H, Rester E: Managing the patient with a delay in pubertal development. Endocrinologist 2:231, 1992.
13. Levine M: The McCune-Albright syndrome: The whys and wherefores of abnormal signal transduction. N Engl J Med 325:1738, 1991.
14. Pescovitz O: Precocious puberty. Pediatr Res 11:229, 1990.
15. Root AW: Precocious puberty. Pediatr Rev 21(1):10–19, 2000.
16. Rosenfeld R: Diagnosis and management of delayed puberty. J Clin Endocrinol Metab 70:559, 1990.
17. Rosenfield RL: The ovary and female sexual maturation. In Sperling MA (ed): Pediatric Endocrinology. Philadelphia, WB Saunders, 1996, pp 75–86.
18. Styne DM: The testes: Disorders of sexual differentiation and puberty. In Sperling MA (ed): Pediatric Endocrinology. Philadelphia, WB Saunders, 1996, pp 423–476.
19. Theinz G, et al: Evidence for a reduction of growth potential in adolescent female gymnasts. J Pediatr 122:306, 1993.
20. Wheeler M, Styne D: Diagnosis and management of precocious puberty. Pediatr Clin North Am 37:1255, 1990.
21. Zachman M: Therapeutic indications for delayed puberty and hypogonadism in adolescent boys. Horm Res 35:141, 1991.

45. MALE HYPOGONADISM

Derek J. Stocker, M.D., and Robert A. Vigersky, M.D.

1. What is male hypogonadism?

Male hypogonadism refers to the clinical and/or laboratory syndrome that results from a failure of the testis to work properly. The normal testis has two functions: synthesis and secretion of testosterone (from the Leydig cells) and production of sperm (from the seminiferous tubules). Deficiency of one or both functions is termed male hypogonadism. Depending on the stage of development, hypogonadism may have varied manifestations (see Table 1). For instance, in utero androgen deficiency leads to a female phenotype or ambiguous genitalia (male pseudohermaphroditism). This may be caused by a block in the production of testosterone due to congenital testosterone biosynthetic enzyme defects or, in rare instances, to the inability of peripheral tissues to respond normally to testosterone. These complete and incomplete androgen insensitivity syndromes (testicular feminization and Reifenstein's syndrome, respectively) fall under the general category of male hypogonadism. Childhood androgen deficiency results in delayed or absent pubertal development. In adulthood, a decrease in sperm output without deficient production of testosterone is common and results in male infertility; thus, infertility is a form of male hypogonadism. A decrease in production of testosterone in adulthood is usually accompanied by a decline in production of sperm. When it is not, the term *fertile eunuch* (eunuchoid proportions [see below]), low levels of luteinizing hormone (LH), low levels of testosterone, normal levels of follicle-stimulating hormone (FSH) and spermatogenesis) is appropriately applied. The most frequent circumstance in which adult hypogonadism is seen is in the middle age or senescent man complaining of decreased libido or potency without concerns of fertility and consequently, semen analysis is not performed.

Forms of Hypogonadism

STAGE OF DEVELOPMENT	CLINICAL MANIFESTATION
In Utero	Female or ambiguous genitalia (male pseudohermaphroditism)
Peripubertal	Delayed or absent puberty Eunuchoid proportions Reduced peak bone mass
Early adulthood	Infertility with normal androgen levels (azoospermia/oligospermia) Fertility with low androgen levels (fertile eunuch) Diminished libido and/or potency
Mid-to-late adulthood	Osteoporosis Decreased libido and/or potency Diminished androgen production

2. How is production of testosterone normally regulated?

LH is episodically secreted from the anterior pituitary in response to pulses of gonadotropin-releasing hormone (GnRH) thus stimulating production of testosterone by Leydig cells. Once testosterone is secreted into the bloodstream, it is bound by sex hormone–binding globulin (SHBG). The non–SHBG-bound (or "free") testosterone provides negative feedback to the hypothalamic-pituitary unit and thus inhibits output of LH. This classic endocrine feedback loop serves to maintain serum testosterone at a predetermined level; if serum testosterone falls below the set point, the pituitary is stimulated to secrete LH, which in turn stimulates testicular output of testosterone until serum levels return to the set point. Conversely, if serum testosterone rises above the set point, decreased output of LH results in decreased testicular output of testosterone until serum levels have declined to the set point.

3. Describe how production of sperm is normally regulated.

The regulation of sperm production is complex and less clearly understood than regulation of testosterone production. There are both hormonal and non-hormonal factors that are important. The Sertoli cells within the seminiferous tubules seem to play an important coordinating role. They maintain a blood-testis barrier, similar to the blood-brain barrier, that establishes the ideal environment for spermatogenesis by allowing penetration of glucose and testosterone but preventing some larger molecules and proteins from entering the seminiferous tubule. Sertoli cells respond to FSH by producing inhibin (secreted into the blood) and androgen-binding protein, transferrin and other proteins (secreted into the seminiferous tubular lumen). Inhibin appears to inhibit the output of FSH from the pituitary gland, thus completing a feedback loop. In theory, if spermatogenesis declines, production of inhibin also should decline; thus the negative feedback effect on the pituitary would be reduced, leading to an increased output of FSH, which then presumably stimulates spermatogenesis. However, not all aspects of this feedback loop (FSH-inhibin-spermatogenesis) have been verified experimentally. Moreover, spermatogenesis depends on intratesticular production of testosterone mediated by androgen receptors within Sertoli cells. Initiation of spermatogenesis during puberty requires both LH and FSH. However, reinitiation of the process if it is disrupted by exogenous factors (see below), requires only LH (or HCG), although FSH may be needed to produce a normal number of sperm.

4. Define primary hypogonadism and secondary hypogonadism.

Failure of testicular function may result from a defect either in the testis or at the hypothalamic-pituitary level. Testicular disorders leading to hypogonadism are termed primary hypogonadism, whereas disorders of hypothalamic-pituitary function leading to hypogonadism are termed secondary hypogonadism (see figure).

5. What are the causes of primary hypogonadism?

Primary hypogonadism may be either congenital or acquired. The most common cause of congenital primary hypogonadism is Klinefelter's syndrome, caused by an abnormal chromosomal complement (47XXY). It is often associated with the clinical triad of gynecomastia, small firm testes and azoospermia (sperm count of zero). The production of testosterone is usually reduced by about 50%. Other congenital causes of primary hypogonadism include cryptorchidism, myotonic dystrophy and rarely, congenital adrenal hyperplasia due to deficiency of 3 beta-hydroxysteroid dehydrogenase, 17 alpha-hydroxylase or 17 beta-hydroxysteroid dehydrogenase. Mutations of the androgen receptor gene resulting in mild quantitative or qualitative abnormalities of the androgen receptor have been associated with a normal male phenotype exhibiting only oligospermia or azoospermia, whereas more severe mutations may result in ambiguous genitalia or a normal-appearing female phenotype (testicular feminization). Rare mutations of the LH receptor on the Leydig cell have been reported and can result in a male phenotype (if mild) or a female phenotype (if severe).

Currently, the most common acquired cause of primary hypogonadism results from cancer chemotherapy. Particularly potent are the alkylating agents: their effects are usually much more devastating on production of sperm than on production of testosterone. Cisplatin and carboplatin also cause oligospermia but only temporarily, as does radioactive iodine treatment for thyroid cancer. Another pharmaceutical agent that causes primary hypogo-

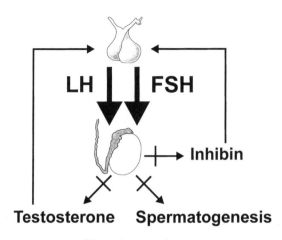

Primary hypogonadism.

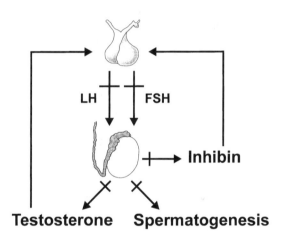

Secondary hypogonadism.

nadism is ketoconazole, which directly inhibits androgen synthesis. Testicular trauma, exposure to diagnostic or therapeutic radiation, hemochromatosis and infections, such as postpubertal mumps orchitis, also may lead to primary hypogonadism. Certain acquired systemic disorders such as AIDS, uremia, and hepatic cirrhosis, are also associated with primary hypogonadism. However, the mechanism in these cases may be multifactorial and include effects on the hypothalamic-pituitary unit. A considerable number of cases of primary hypogonadism are idiopathic.

6. Is normal aging associated with primary hypogonadism?

A number of cross-sectional studies have noted that older men seem to have mildly reduced levels of total serum testosterone but significantly reduced levels of free testosterone (due to a rise in SHBG with age) compared with younger men. This decline is associated with a rise in LH and FSH and probably reflects an intrinsic part of the aging process on which are superimposed the various chronic diseases that develop as one ages.

7. Discuss the causes of secondary hypogonadism.

Any disease that affects the hypothalamic-pituitary axis can cause secondary hypogonadism. Involvement of the hypothalamus or pituitary stalk will interfere with the secretion
of GnRH or the ability of GnRH to communicate with the pituitary. A number of anatomic
lesions of the pituitary will cause secondary hypogonadism by interfering with the release of
LH and FSH. Such lesions include benign tumors and cysts, malignant tumors (both primary
central nervous system tumors and metastatic tumors from distant sources), vascular
aneurysms, infiltrative diseases, pituitary hemorrhage and pituitary trauma. The most
common pituitary tumor found in the adult patient is a prolactin-secreting adenoma. These
tumors primarily cause hypogonadism as a result of local destruction and compression,
inhibiting the production and release of LH and FSH. Elevated prolactin levels can also interrupt secretion of GnRH, although this is usually of much less significance in men than the
mass effect. Pituitary adenomas that produce growth hormone (acromegaly) or adrenocorticotropic hormone (Cushing's disease) and nonfunctioning pituitary tumors may similarly
cause secondary hypogonadism by their mass effects. Hypothalamic-pituitary dysfunction
from surgery, trauma, hemorrhage or infiltrative diseases, such as hemochromatosis, may
also cause hypogonadism. Congenital disorders in which output of LH and FSH is impaired,
such as Kallmann's syndrome (associated with anosmia or hyposmia and other midline
defects like cleft palate, short third or fourth metacarpals and/or metatarsals), also lead to secondary hypogonadism. Some cases of Kallmann's syndrome have been shown to be due to a
deletion of the *KAL* gene (located on the short arm of the X chromosome [Xp22.3]), which
encodes an extracellular matrix glycoprotein called anosmin-1, one of a class of neural adhesion molecules that allows GnRH-secreting neurons to enter the olfactory bulb and migrate
to the hypothalamus during embryogenesis. Iatrogenic causes, such as the use of anabolic
steroids by athletes, represent another possible cause of hypogonadism.

8. What clinical symptoms are seen in male hypogonadism?

Loss of the sperm-producing function of the testis leads to infertility, usually defined as
failure of a normal female partner to conceive after 12 months of unprotected intercourse.
Loss of the testosterone-producing function of the testis may lead to loss of libido and erectile dysfunction as well as diminution of secondary sexual characteristics, such as facial and
pubic hair. Decreased production of testosterone also may cause more generalized symptoms,
such as decreased muscle mass and strength, malaise and fatigue. Osteoporosis is now a well-
recognized result of both primary and secondary hypogonadism. Hypogonadism is found in
up to 30% of men with vertebral fractures. Estradiol that is aromatized from testosterone may
be the most important factor in preserving bone density in both men and women. However,
androgen receptors are also found in bone and may explain the sexual dimorphism of bone
density. In boys who develop hypogonadism before sexual maturation, delay or absence of
the onset of puberty is typical. Tender gynecomastia is frequently seen in hypogonadism.

9. Describe the physical findings observed in male hypogonadism.

Reduction in testis size to < 20 mL (approximately 4.5 x 3.0 cm) is seen in virtually all
cases of male hypogonadism, except those of recent onset. Because most of the testis
volume is composed of seminiferous tubules, the decline in testis size usually correlates
roughly with the decline in sperm production. Decreased testosterone production may lead
to reduction in body hair, arrest of temporal balding, and small prostate size. Gynecomastia,
which usually reflects a decrease in the androgen/estrogen ratio, is also common, particularly in primary hypogonadism, because the elevated LH levels stimulate aromatization of
testosterone to estradiol. Onset of hypogonadism before the epiphyses of the long bones fuse
may lead to a delayed epiphyseal closure. This delay prolongs the longitudinal growth phase
of the extremities, resulting in the development of eunuchoid proportions, in which the ratio

of the upper body segment (pubis to vertex) to the lower body segment (pubis to floor) is less than 0.9 and the arm span is more than 5 cm. greater than the height. Impaired production of testosterone during fetal development may lead to ambiguous external genitalia, hypospadias, micropenis and cryptorchidism.

10. What laboratory tests help to confirm a suspected diagnosis of male hypogonadism?

The main functions of the testis, production of sperm and production of testosterone, are readily assessed by semen analysis and measurement of serum testosterone, respectively. Normal semen analysis values in men following two to three days of abstinence are: 20 million sperm per milliliter and > 60% motility of the sperm. Because sperm density is highly variable from day to day in all men, accurate assessment usually involves several semen analyses done with the same abstinence period each time. The best initial test for testosterone production is measurement of the nonfasting morning serum total testosterone level. Serum testosterone also varies considerably from moment to moment and from morning to night in response to LH secretion; again, several samples may be needed to establish an accurate measurement. In addition, most testosterone in serum is bound to plasma proteins, particularly SHBG; thus, in elderly or obese patients who have increased and decreased SHBG levels, respectively, and in those men in whom plasma protein levels may be disrupted, measurement of the physiologically active "free" testosterone may prove informative. Bone density measurement using a DEXA scan may provide helpful baseline information and assist in deciding whether to provide androgen replacement therapy.

11. Can laboratory tests help to distinguish primary from secondary hypogonadism?

As noted previously, the testis is normally regulated by a series of negative feedback loops. LH from the pituitary stimulates production of testosterone by the testis, and serum testosterone then inhibits output of LH. FSH from the pituitary stimulates spermatogenesis, which then inhibits FSH via inhibin. Thus, primary hypogonadism resulting from a testicular disorder leads to a decline in production of testosterone and sperm, a consequent decrease in the negative feedback effects on the pituitary and a corresponding increase in serum levels of LH and FSH. Conversely, in secondary hypogonadism due to a hypothalamic-pituitary disorder, serum LH and FSH may be subnormal or "inappropriately" normal (explainable, in part, by decreased bioactivity). A subnormal sperm count and normal testosterone level with a normal LH and elevated FSH suggests primary hypogonadism with a dysfunction of the seminiferous tubules and sperm production but intact Leydig cell function.

12. What other diagnostic tests are useful in defining the cause of male hypogonadism?

Additional diagnostic testing should be based on clinical suspicion and the results of preliminary testing. For example, in cases of secondary hypogonadism, measurement of serum prolactin and pituitary radiography, preferably magnetic resonance imaging with gadolinium, should be done. Computed tomography directed at the sella is also acceptable, but skull films are not considered adequate. Visual field testing and measurement of other pituitary hormones also may be appropriate to assess either possible tumoral hypersecretion (e.g., Cushing's disease, acromegaly) or tumor-related hypopituitarism. Likewise, the initial findings in primary hypogonadism may suggest additional tests. For example, small firm testes, gynecomastia, azoospermia, modestly reduced serum testosterone, and high levels of serum LH and FSH in a young man may lead to chromosome analysis to confirm a presumptive diagnosis of Klinefelter's syndrome. Measurement of serum estradiol levels may be helpful when feminization is prominent clinically, as with secondary hypogonadism related to production of estrogen by testicular or adrenal tumors. Determination of bone age in a young male may be of benefit in the evaluation of delayed maturity. Testis biopsy rarely provides information that is useful in establishing a specific diagnosis, prognosis or treatment.

13. How is hypogonadism treated?

Deficiency of testosterone is easily treated with testosterone replacement therapy. Current testosterone preparations include injected testosterone esters, transdermal patches (scrotal and nonscrotal) and testosterone gel. Oral alkylated androgens such as fluoxymesterone, oxandrolone and danazol are not recommended because of potential hepatotoxicity and dyslipidemia. Furthermore, their inability to be aromatized may lead to loss of bone density. Intramuscular injections of testosterone esters, such as testosterone enanthate or cypionate, have been used for decades to treat hypogonadism. Generally, these medications are given in a dosage of 200 mg every 2 weeks or 100 mg every week. However, lower doses are often used in teenagers when initiating therapy and in older men. Less frequent injections may lead to a period of inadequate testosterone replacement between injections. Due to the discomfort and complications of regular intramuscular injections, these formulations are losing favor now that alternatives exist. Nevertheless, they remain an effective and inexpensive option. The transdermal patches have gained favor over the past few years owing to their ease of use and the stable serum testosterone concentrations they provide, but they cost several times more than injectable forms of testosterone. These patches deliver approximately 5 mg of testosterone over a 24-hr period and are changed daily. Even more recently, a testosterone gel has become available in the United States as well. The gel is also applied daily and is generally dosed to deliver 25–100 mg per application. All of these transdermal preparations can be complicated by local skin irritation, but this usually does not necessitate the cessation of therapy. Sublingual and implantable preparations are not approved in the United States. The treatment goal for all of these preparations is a normalization of the serum LH in primary hypogonadism and a serum total testosterone level in the normal range for secondary hypogonadism. Some older men with testosterone deficiency are unconcerned about sexual function and may not desire testosterone replacement. However, in testosterone-deficient men of any age, low bone density and/or reduced hematopoiesis may be indications for testosterone replacement therapy even in the absence of decreased libido or erectile dysfunction. Because of its potential abuse by athletes and others, testosterone is presently designated a schedule III drug.

14. Is testosterone treatment dangerous?

Testosterone administration is generally quite safe; as with any drug, however, there is always the potential for adverse effects. Gynecomastia and acne may occur in the first few months after initiating testosterone treatment; these may resolve with continued treatment, although temporary dose reduction may be helpful. Abnormalities in liver function are uncommon with currently used injectable and transdermal preparations. In older men, effects of testosterone on the prostate must be considered, including the possibility of precipitating urinary retention due to testosterone-induced enlargement of the prostate. While there is no evidence that testosterone treatment causes prostate carcinoma, the potential for testosterone stimulation of occult prostate carcinoma exists. Therefore, it is advisable to perform a digital rectal exam of the prostate and monitor prostate-specific antigen in middle-age and older men before and annually while they are receiving testosterone replacement. A testosterone-induced increase in hematocrit is common, although clinically significant polycythemia is quite rare unless the drug is being abused. Testosterone treatment may also precipitate sleep apnea; marked increases in hematocrit may be a clue to this side effect. In boys who have not yet gone through puberty, the rapid increase in serum testosterone after initial treatment may lead to considerable psychological difficulties and physically aggressive behavior; initiating treatment with smaller doses may be helpful. Testosterone replacement therapy has no adverse effect on lipid profiles compared with eugonadal men, but overtreatment can lead to several lipid abnormalities, including decreases in the high-density lipoprotein cholesterol level.

15. How does one treat the deficiency of sperm production?

In men with primary hypogonadism, as manifested by elevated levels of serum FSH, there seems to be no effective pharmacologic treatment for increasing the sperm count. Anatomic lesions, such as varicoceles and ejaculatory duct obstructions, can be corrected surgically, but improvement in spermatogenesis may not result. If one plans to use a medication that is known to cause hypogonadism (e.g., cancer chemotherapeutic agents), it may be desirable to cryopreserve semen specimens before treatment, provided that treatment is not unduly delayed. The outlook is much less pessimistic with secondary hypogonadism, particularly if the condition developed after puberty. Treatment with gonadotropins (human chorionic gonadotropin with or without added FSH) may be successful in restoring production of sperm as well as testosterone. The pretreatment size of the testis is often a clue to prognosis; larger testis size is associated with a better outcome. Production of testosterone and sperm in men with secondary hypogonadism also may be enhanced with pulsatile administration of GnRH via a portable infusion pump, provided that the pituitary retains the capability to make gonadotropins. Treatment with gonadotropins or GnRH tends to be both costly and prolonged.

In men with primary or secondary hypogonadism who have not responded to specific therapy when appropriate and who have preservation of some germ cells in either ejaculate or testis, the newer methods of assisted reproductive technology, particularly intracytoplasmic sperm injection, may offer some hope, although at a high financial cost.

16. Does prolactin-related hypogonadism require a special approach?

Yes. The mechanism by which hyperprolactinemia, usually from a pituitary adenoma, causes hypogonadism is not clearly defined. However, prolactin seems to have an inhibitory effect on the action of testosterone in addition to other effects on its production. Thus, patients with high levels of serum prolactin and low levels of serum testosterone often do not respond clinically to testosterone replacement therapy unless serum concentrations of prolactin are lowered. The most effective way to lower serum concentrations of prolactin in such circumstances is usually treatment with dopamine agonists, such as bromocriptine or cabergoline. The latter is more potent and has fewer side effects.

BIBLIOGRAPHY

1. Adamopoulos DA, Lawrence DM, Vassilopoulos P, et al: Pituitary-testicular relationships in mumps orchitis and other viral infections. BMJ 1:1177, 1978.
2. Bagatell CJ, Bremner WJ: Androgens in men—uses and abuses. N Engl J Med 334:707–14, 1996.
3. Baker HWG, Burger HF, DeKretser DM, et al: Changes in the pituitary-testicular system with age. Clin Endocrinol 5:349, 1976.
4. Bannister P, Handley T, Chapman C, Losowsky MS: Hypogonadism in chronic liver disease: Impaired release of luteinising hormone. BMJ 293:1191, 1986.
5. Bhasin S: Androgen treatment of hypogonadal men. J Clin Endocrinol Metab 74:1221, 1992.
6. Carter JN, Tyson JE, Tolis G, et al: Prolactin-secreting tumors and hypogonadism in 22 men. N Engl J Med 299:847, 1978.
7. Castro-Magana M, Bronsther B, Angulo MA: Genetic forms of male hypogonadism. Urology 35:195, 1990.
8. Griffin JL, Wilson JD: The syndromes of androgen resistance. N Engl J Med 302:198, 1980.
9. Gromoll J, Eiholzer U, Nieschlag E, Simoni M: Male hypogonadism caused by homozygous deletion of exon 10 of the luteinizing hormone (LH) receptor: Differential action of human chorionic gonadotropin. J Clin Endocrinol Metab 85:2281, 2000.
10. Guo CY, Jones TH, Eastell R: Treatment of isolated hypogonadotropic hypogonadism effect on bone mineral density and bone turnover. J Clin Endocrinol Metab 82:658–665, 1997.
11. Harman SM, Metter EJ, et al: Longitudinal effects of aging on serum total and free testosterone levels in healthy men. Baltimore Longitudinal Study of Aging. J Clin Endocrinol Metab 86:724–731, 2001.

12. Hayes FJ, Seminara SB, et al: Hypogonadotropic hypogonadism. Endocrinol Metab Clin North Am 27(4):739–63, 1998.
13. Holdsworth S, Atkins RC, DeKretser DM: The pituitary-testis axis in men with chronic renal failure. N Engl J Med 296:1245, 1977.
14. Hsueh WA, Hsu TH, Federman DD: Endocrine features of Klinefelter's syndrome. Medicine 57:447, 1978.
15. Lee PA, O'Dea LS: Primary and secondary testicular insufficiency. Pediatr Clin North Am 37:1359, 1990.
16. Lieblich JM, Rogol AD, White BJ, Rosen SW: Syndrome of anosmia with hypogonadotropic hypogonadism (Kallman syndrome): Clinical and laboratory studies in 23 cases. Am J Med 73:506, 1982.
17. Matsumoto AM, Bremner WJ: Endocrinology of the hypothalamic-pituitary-testicular axis with particular reference to the hormonal control of spermatogenesis. Baillieres Clin Endocrinol Metab 1:71, 1987.
18. Schilsky RL, Lewis BJ, Sherins R, Young RC: Gonadal dysfunction in patients receiving chemotherapy for cancer. Ann Intern Med 93:109, 1980.
19. Schwartz ID, Root AW: The Klinefelter syndrome of testicular dysgenesis. Endocrinol Metab Clin North Am 20:153, 1991.
20. Seminara SB, Hayes FJ, Crowley WF Jr: Gonadotropin-releasing hormone deficiency in the human (Idiopathic hypogonadotropic hypogonadism and Kallmann's syndrome): Pathophysiological and genetic considerations. Endocrine Rev 19:521, 1998
21. Snyder PJ, et al: Effects of testosterone replacement in hypogonadal men. J Clin Endocrinol Metab 85:2670, 2000.
22. Swerdloff RS, Wang C, et al: Long-term pharmacokinetics of transdermal testosterone gel in hypogonadal men. J Clin Endocrinol Metab 85:4500–4510, 2000.
23. Szulc P, Munoz F, Claustrat B, et al: Bioavailable estradiol may be an important determinant of osteoporosis in men: The MINOS study. J Clin Endocrinol Metab 86:192, 2001.
24. Tenover JL: Male hormone replacement therapy including "andropause." Endocrinol Metab Clin North Am 27(4):969–87, 1998.
25. Wang C, Baker HWG, Burger HG, et al: Hormonal studies in Klinefelter's syndrome. Clin Endocrinol 4:399, 1975
26. Whitcomb RW, Crowley WF: Male hypogonadotropic hypogonadism. Endocrinol Metab Clin North Am 22:125, 1993.

46. IMPOTENCE

Robert A. Vigersky, M.D.

1. What is impotence?

Classically, impotence has been defined as the inability to attain and maintain an erection of sufficient rigidity for sexual intercourse in 50% or more attempts. A more descriptive term for impotence is *erectile dysfunction.*

2. Do men with impotence have disturbances in other sexual functions?

Most impotent men are able to ejaculate. Premature ejaculation may precede the development of impotence and is sometimes associated with drug therapy. Sexual desire (libido) is also usually preserved; loss of libido is suggestive of hypogonadism or severe systemic or psychiatric illness.

3. Is impotence common?

At least 10 million American men and perhaps as many as 20 million are impotent. Another 10 million may suffer from partial erectile dysfunction. The prevalence of impotence increases with age; about 2% of 40-year-old, 20% of 55-year-old, and 50–75% of 80-year-old men are impotent. Of interest, there is a libido-potency gap in that many elderly men continue to have active libidos, but only 15% of them engage in sexual activity.

4. How does a normal erection occur?

Erection is primarily a vascular event that results from the complex interplay of the hormonal, vascular, peripheral nerve and central nervous systems. Erection is usually initiated by various psychic and/or physiologic stimuli in the cerebral cortex. The stimuli are modulated in the limbic system and other areas of the brain, integrated in the hypothalamus, transmitted down the spinal cord, and carried to the penis via both autonomic and sacral spinal nerves. (For you Latin scholars, these are the nervi erigentes derived from the verb "erigo, erigere, erexi, erectus.") Sensory nerves from the glans of the penis enhance the message and help to maintain erection during sexual activity via a reflex arc. These stimuli may mediate the release of several neurotransmitters that reverse the tonic smooth muscle constriction maintained by norepinephrine, endothelin and other vasoconstrictive factors. Perhaps more importantly, the neural stimuli cause the release of nitric oxide (NO) and prostaglandin E1 (PGE1), which are potent vasodilating substances. NO stimulates guanyl cyclase activity, which increases cyclic guanosine monophosphate (cGMP) and thereby causes a decrease in intracellular calcium, producing dissociation of actin-myosin in vascular smooth muscle cells. Phosphodiesterase 5, by causing a decrease in cGMP, allows for reversal of the process; i.e., detumescence. Sildenafil citrate (Viagra) inhibits phosphodiesterase 5 (see below).

5. Describe the vascular changes in the penis that result in erection.

Within the two spongy corpora cavernosa of the penis are millions of tiny spaces called lacunae, each lined by a wall of trabecular smooth muscle. As neurotransmitters dilate cavernosal and helicine arteries to the penis and relax the trabecular smooth muscle, the lacunar spaces in the penis become engorged with blood. This results in entrapment of outflow vessels between the expanding trabecular walls and the rigid tunica albuginea that surrounds the corpora cavernosa, thereby greatly reducing venous outflow from the penis. This veno-occlusive mechanism accounts for tumescence and rigidity. Failure of venous occlusion (venous leak) is one of the intractable causes of impotence.

6. What types of nerves and neurotransmitters play a role in penile erection?

At least three neuroeffector systems play a role in penile erection. Adrenergic nerves generally inhibit erection; cholinergic nerves and nonadrenergic, noncholinergic (NANC) substances enhance erection as follows:

- Sympathetic nerves (via alpha-adrenergic receptors)
    Constrict cavernosal and helicine arteries
    Contract trabecular smooth muscle
- Parasympathetic nerves (via cholinergic receptors)
    Inhibit adrenergic fibers
    Stimulate NANC fibers
- NANC messengers (nitric oxide, vasoactive intestinal polypeptide, prostaglandins or other endothelium-derived factors)
    Dilate cavernosal and helicine arteries
    Relax trabecular smooth muscle

7. What are the common causes of impotence?

The frequency of the various causes of impotence is difficult to assess because of the large number of patients who do not report the problem, confusion regarding the diagnosis, and variability in the sophistication of the initial evaluation. Primary causes of impotence in men presenting to a medical outpatient clinic are approximated below:

Endocrine factors	30%
Diabetes mellitus	15%
Medications	20%
Systemic disease and alcoholism	10%
Primary vascular causes*	5%
Primary neurologic causes	5%
Psychogenic or unknown causes	15%

*Alterations of blood flow are thought to play a role in many causes of impotence, but specific lesions amenable to therapy are relatively rare.

8. Besides diabetes mellitus, what are the most common causes of endocrinologic impotence?

The three main endocrinologic disorders associated with impotence are the following:
- Primary (hypergonadotropic) hypogonadism (increased luteinizing hormone [LH] and decreased testosterone)
- Secondary (hypogonadotropic) hypogonadism (decrease LH and decreased testosterone)
- Hyperprolactinemia

Less common causes include hyperthyroidism, hypothyroidism, adrenal insufficiency and Cushing's syndrome.

9. Describe the most common drugs known to induce impotence.

Non-prescription drugs such as alcohol (as the porter says to Macduff in Act II, scene 3 of Macbeth, "it provokes the desire but takes away the performance") and illicit drugs such as cocaine, methadone, and heroin can cause impotence. The prescription drugs most commonly associated with impotence include the following:
- Antihypertensive agents, especially methyldopa, clonidine, beta blockers, vasodilators (e.g., hydralazine), thiazide diuretics and spironolactone

- Antipsychotic medications
- Antidepressants and tranquilizers
- Other (especially cimetidine, digoxin, phenytoin, carbamazepine, ketoconazole and metoclopramide)

10. Which antihypertensive agents should be used in patients with impotence?

Virtually every blood pressure medication has been associated with impotence. However, erectile dysfunction is relatively uncommon, even in healthy older men on antihypertensive therapy. There is little overall difference in the rate of erectile problems among the commonly prescribed antihypertensive agents, but angiotensin-converting enzyme inhibitors and calcium channel blockers are the agents least likely to affect erectile ability. When beta blockade is required, selective beta agonists such as atenolol or acebutolol also have minimal impact on sexual function.

11. What is "stuttering" impotence? What is its significance?

Impotence alternating with periods of entirely normal sexual function is termed stuttering impotence. Multiple sclerosis (MS) is the most significant organic cause of stuttering impotence. It may be the initial manifestation of MS and may be present in up to 50% of men with the disease.

12. What historical information helps to separate organic from psychogenic impotence?

True psychogenic impotence is uncommon and should be a diagnosis of exclusion. Questions that may help to separate psychogenic from organic impotence are listed below:

	ORGANIC	PSYCHOGENIC
Was onset abrupt?	No	Yes
Is impotence stress dependent?	No	Yes
Is libido preserved?	Yes	No
Do you have morning erections?	No	Yes
Do you have orgasms?	Yes	No
Can you masturbate?	No	Yes
Does impotence occur with all partners?	Yes	No

13. Name the essential components of a physical exam in a man complaining of impotence.

- Secondary sexual characteristics, such as muscle development, hair pattern and presence of breast tissue
- Vascular examination, especially of the femoral and lower extremity pulses and the presence of bruits
- Focused neurologic examination, including assessing the presence of peripheral neuropathy with vibratory and light touch sensation and of autonomic neuropathy using the cremasteric reflex, anal sphincter tone and/or the bulbocavernosus reflex, evaluation of standing and supine blood pressure and measurement of the heart rate response to deep breathing and valsalva (diabetics rarely have autonomic neuropathy as a cause of impotence in the absence of peripheral neuropathy)
- Examination of the genitalia to determine penile size, shape, presence of plaque or fibrous tissue (Peyronie's disease); size and consistency of the testes; prostate examination
- Thyroid examination

14. What is the appropriate laboratory assessment for men with impotence?

Laboratory assessment should be based on history and physical examination findings but generally includes the following:

- Complete blood count
- Urinalysis
- Fasting glucose and (in diabetics) HbA1C
- Fasting lipid profile
- Serum creatinine
- Thyroid function tests
- Serum testosterone and LH

15. Should prolactin levels be measured in all impotent men?

Whether serum prolactin should be measured in all men with impotence is somewhat controversial. In general, patients with normal levels of testosterone and LH and a normal neurologic examination do not require measurement of prolactin. However, if testosterone is low and associated with low or low normal normal LH or if history or examination suggests a pituitary lesion, prolactin should be measured. Because prolactin interferes with the action of testosterone, prolactin status should be assessed in hypogonadal men unresponsive to testosterone replacement therapy. Hypothyroidism and renal failure also may elevate prolactin.

16. What is a penile brachial index?

Comparison of the penile and brachial systolic blood pressure allows a general assessment of the vascular integrity of the penis. This technique is not highly sensitive, but it is noninvasive and easy to perform and may help to identify men who require more extensive vascular studies. Penile systolic blood pressure obtained with Doppler ultrasound should be the same as brachial systolic pressure (i.e., ratio approximately=1.0). An index <0.7 is highly suggestive of vasculogenic impotence. Diagnostic yield is increased if the penile brachial index is repeated after exercising the lower extremities for several minutes. This maneuver may uncover a pelvic steal syndrome (loss of erection due to pelvic thrusting) that is characterized by a difference of >0.15 between the resting and exercise ratios.

17. What is nocturnal penile tumescence monitoring?

Most men experience three to six erections during the night that are entrained to REM sleep. By monitoring such events, one can assess the frequency, duration, and, with some instruments, even the rigidity of erection. This procedure helps to distinguish organic from psychogenic impotence. This can be done at home either semi-quantitatively (using a Snap-Gauge) or more quantitatively (using the Rigi-Scan).

18. Discuss the therapeutic options in the treatment of impotence.

- Medical treatments
  - Remove offending drugs
  - Treat underlying medical conditions
  - Replace testosterone in hypogonadal men
  - Reduce hyperprolactinemia with bromocriptine
  - Prescribe sildenafil citrate (Viagra)
  - Prescribe adrenergic receptor blockers (e.g., yohimbine)
  - Consider an SSRI for premature ejaculation
- Intracavernosal injection of vasoactive substances, especially prostaglandin E, papaverine and phentolamine individually or in combination for those in whom sildenafil citrate has failed or is contraindicated
- Transurethral delivery of alprostadil (PGE1)
- External mechanical aids and vacuum/suction devices
- Surgical treatments
  - Revascularization procedures

        Obliteration of venous shunts
        Surgical penile implants
    • Psychological therapy, especially for men whose impotence has no obvious organic cause

19. Are medical treatments for impotence safe and effective?

The introduction of sildenafil citrate (Viagra), a selective phosphodiesterase 5 inhibitor, in 1998 has produced a paradigm shift in the approach to the treatment of impotence. Given 1 hour before anticipated sexual activity (and avoiding a fatty meal, which inhibits its absorption by one third), it is successful in up to 80% of men with organic impotence (although only about 50% of diabetic men). The few side effects that it has (headache, flushing, dyspepsia and a blue haze in vision) rarely cause discontinuation of its use. Since it causes vasodilatation similar to that of nitrates, it is contraindicated in those taking any form of nitrates. Sildenafil has been shown to be safe in patients with known coronary artery disease who are not using nitrates. Nevertheless, it should be given with care in men with a recent myocardial infarction or stroke, resting hypotension, class III or IV congestive heart failure, and unstable angina. Because sildenafil citrate is metabolized via CYP3A4, any drugs that block that enzyme (e.g., erythromycin and other macrolide antibiotics, ketoconazole and other antifungal drugs, HIV protease inhibitors such as saquinavir and ritonavir, and cimetidine) will increase its plasma concentrations and, therefore, it should be started at lower (25 mg) doses than usual (50 mg). Androgen replacement therapy for hypogonadal men is relatively safe, provided that liver enzymes, prostate size and prostate-specific antigen are monitored. Androgen therapy can be given intramuscularly in the form of long-acting testosterone enanthate or cypionate, 200–300 mg every 2–3 weeks or transdermally via a non-scrotal or scrotal patch or a gel. These topical forms eliminate the peaks and troughs associated with intramuscular injection but are more expensive than the intramuscular form and may cause transient local skin irritation. Bromocriptine is helpful in men with elevated levels of prolactin, even when levels of testosterone are normal. Many other oral and parenteral treatments for impotence are under investigation. Sublingual apomorphine, working through an unknown mechanism, looks particularly promising. Yohimbine hydrochloride (6.5 mg orally 3 times/day) is rarely effective except in patients with psychogenic impotence.

20. Discuss the role of intracavernosal or intraurethral injection.

Injection of vasodilatory substances directly into the corpora cavernosa of the penis should be reserved for those men in whom sildenafil is either ineffective, contraindicated, or has produced intolerable adverse effects. Such "sildenafil salvage" therapy results in erection satisfactory for intercourse in some men with impotence. PGE1 (Caverject), papaverine and phentolamine may be used alone or in combination (trimix). Side effects, which depend on the type and quantity of substances injected, include hypotension, elevation of liver enzymes and headache. Local complications include hematoma, swelling, inadvertent injection into the urethra and local fibrosis with long-term use. The most serious local complication is priapism (a sustained erection) for more than 4 hr, which may necessitate injection of alpha-adrenergic agonists or corpora cavernosal aspiration. PGE1 is also available as an intraurethral suppository (MUSE) and, since it is less invasive and easier to use, may be a more appropriate second line agent that intracavernosal injection. There are no controlled studies evaluating the success of either approach in sildenafil citrate failures.

21. What other modalities are available to treat impotent men?

Vacuum erection devices provide a noninvasive, mechanical solution for impotence. They are somewhat cumbersome to use and require the placement of an occlusive ring at the base of the penis to prevent venous outflow. They may be particularly effective in those men who have a "venous leak" as the etiology of their impotence. The constrictive ring prevents antegrade ejaculation because of the urethral constriction. Surgical revascularization has a limited place in the treatment of impotent men because of its invasiveness and limited success rate. Similarly, penile prosthesis insertion is rarely done because of the availability of several effective and noninvasive alternatives. In those men in whom premature ejaculation is the major problem, intermittent use of SSRIs have been efficacious in delaying time to ejaculation.

BIBLIOGRAPHY

1. Adams MA, Banting BD, Maurice DH, et al: Vascular control mechanism in penile erection: Phylogeny and the inevitability of multiple overlapping systems. Int J Impotence Res 9:85–95, 1997.
2. Bagatell CJ, Bremner WJ: Androgens in men—Use and abuses. N Engl J Med 334:707–714, 1997.
3. Cookson MS, Nadig PW: Long-term results with vacuum constriction device. J Urol 149:290-294, 1993.
4. Feldman HA, Goldstein I, Hatzichristou DJ, et al: Impotence and its medical and psychosocial correlates: Results of the Massachusetts male aging study. J Urol 151:54-61, 1994
5. Goldstein I, Lue TF, Padma-Nathan H, et al: Oral sildenafil in the treatment of erectile dysfunction. N Engl J Med 338:1397-1404, 1998.
6. Grimm RH, et al, for the TOHMS Research Group: Long-term effects on sexual function of five antihypertensive drugs and nutritional hygienic treatment in hypertensive men and women. Treatment of Mild Hypertension Study (TOHMS). Hypertension 29:8–14, 1997.
7. Hanash KA: Comparative results of goal oriented therapy for erectile dysfunction. J Urol 157: 2135–2139, 1997.
8. Herrmann HC, Chang G, Klugherz BD Mahoney PD: Hemodynamic effects of sildenafil in men with severe coronary artery disease. N Engl J Med 342:1622-1626, 2000.
9. Korenman SG: New insights into erectile dysfunction: A practical approach. Am J Med 105135-144, 1998.
10. Krane RJ, Goldstein I, DeTejada JS: Impotence. N Engl J Med 321:1648–1659, 1989.
11. Lerner SF, Melman A, Christ GJ: A review of erectile dysfunction: New insights and more questions. J Urol 149 (5 pt 2):1246–1252, 1993.
12. Linet OI, Ogring FG, et al: Efficacy and safety of intracavernosal prostaglandin in men with erectile dysfunction. N Engl J Med 334:873–878, 1996.
13. McMahon CG, Touma K: Treatment of premature ejaculation with paroxetine hydrochloride as needed: Two single-blind placebo controlled crossover studies. J Urol 161:1826–1830, 1999.
14. Morley JE, Kaiser FE: Impotence: The internists' approach to diagnosis and treatment. Adv Intern Med 38:151–168, 1993.
15. Neisler AW, Carey NP: A critical reevaluation of nocturnal penile tumescence monitoring in a diagnosis of erectile dysfunction. J Nerv Ment Dis 178:78–79, 1990.
16. NIH Consensus Conference: Impotence. JAMA 270:83–90, 1993.
17. Padma-Nathan H, et al for the Medicated Urethral System for Erection (MUSE) Study Group: Treatment of men with erectile dysfunction with transurethral alprostadil. N Engl J Med 336:1–7, 1997.
18. Rajfer J, Aronson WJ, Bush PA, et al: Nitric oxide as a mediator of relaxation of the corpus cavernosum in response to nonadrenergic, noncholinergic neurotransmission. N Engl J Med 326:90–94, 1992.
19. Rendell MS, Rajfer J, Wicker PA, et al: Sildenafil for treatment of erectile dysfunction in men with diabetes. A randomized controlled trial. JAMA 281:421–426, 1999.
20. Sidi AA: Vasoactive intracavernous pharmacotherapy. Urol Clin North Am 15:95–101, 1988.
21. Witherington R: Mechanical aids for treatment of impotence. Clin Diabetes 7:1–22, 1989.

47. GYNECOMASTIA

Brenda K. Bell, M.D.

1. What is the definition of gynecomastia?
Gynecomastia is defined as the presence of palpable breast tissue in a male.

2. How does gynecomastia present clinically?
Gynecomastia usually presents as a palpable discrete button of firm subareolar breast tissue or as a diffuse collection of fibroadipose tissue. The examiner can differentiate fibroadipose tissue from simple fat by pinching the breast tissue in question and comparing the texture and consistency with the fat tissue in the anterior axillary fold.

3. What is the significance of painful gynecomastia?
Pain or tenderness implies recent, rapid growth of breast tissue.

4. Is gynecomastia always bilateral?
The involvement tends to be bilateral, but asymmetry is common. Unilateral enlargement is present in 5–25% of patients and may be a preliminary stage in the development of bilateral disease.

5. Does gynecomastia have a racial predilection?
No.

6. What is the pathophysiology of gynecomastia?
Estrogens stimulate ductal proliferation. Androgens may inhibit breast development. Gynecomastia results from an increase in the ratio of estrogens to androgens, which may be due to increased production of estrogens, decreased production of testosterone, or increased conversion of androgens to estrogens in peripheral tissue.

7. Where are estrogens produced in the male?
Direct testicular production of estrogens accounts for less than 15%. The majority of estrogens come from the conversion of adrenal and testicular androgens to estrogens in peripheral tissues, particularly adipose tissue and the liver.

8. What is the most common etiology of gynecomastia?
Asymptomatic palpable breast tissue is common in normal males, particularly in the neonate (60–90%), at puberty (60–70% between the ages of 12 and 15 years), and with increasing age (30–85% over age 45 years). Because of this high prevalence, gynecomastia is considered a relatively normal finding during the above periods of life. Gynecomastia at these ages is often called physiologic or idiopathic and accounts for 50% of cases.

9. Why does gynecomastia occur so commonly during these stages of life?
Neonatal gynecomastia is due to placental transfer of estrogens. During early puberty, production of estrogens begins sooner than production of testosterone, causing an imbalance in the ratio of estrogens to androgens. With aging, production of testosterone decreases, and peripheral conversion of androgens to estrogens often increases because of an age-associated increase in adipose tissue.

10. What are the other causes of gynecomastia?

Drugs account for 10–20% of cases; primary hypogonadism for 10%; and adrenal or testicular tumors for less than 3%. Other causes combined, including secondary hypogonadism, androgen-resistant disorders, malnutrition, cirrhosis, alcohol abuse, renal disease, congenital adrenal hyperplasia, extragonadal tumors, and hyperthyroidism, account for less than 10%.

11. What drugs cause gynecomastia?

Many drugs have been implicated, some with known steroid effects, others with no clear mechanism:

Anabolic steroids	Metoclopramide	Nifedipine	Protease inhibitors
Estrogen creams	Reserpine	Verapamil	Finasteride
Spironolactone	Marijuana	Tricyclic antidepressants	Resperidone
Flutamide	Heroin	Phenothiazines	Fluoxetine
Cimettidine	Methadone	Captopril	Minocycline
Ranitidine	Phenytoin	Enalapril	Ethionamide
Isoniazid	Diazepam	Omeprazole	Chemotherapy
Digitoxin	Metronidazole	Amlodipine	Growth hormone
Ketoconazole	Theophylline	Diltiazem	Androgens
Methyldopa	Amiodarone	Cyproterone acetate	Methotrexate
Haloperidol	Amphetamines	Auranofin	Domperidone
Diethylproprion	Etretinate	Penicillamine	Sulindac
Melatonin			

12. How do testicular tumors cause gynecomastia?

Germ cell tumors can produce human chorionic gonadotropin (hCG). Like luteinizing hormone (LH), hCG increases testicular production of estradiol. Leydig cell tumors may directly secrete estradiol.

13. What extragonadal tumors cause gynecomastia?

Pancreatic, gastric, and pulmonary tumors have been associated with production of hCG. Hepatomas may have increased aromatase activity that results in increased conversion of androgens to estrogens.

14. Who should undergo evaluation for gynecomastia?

History and physical examination are indicated in all cases and will determine the cause in 30–40%. Gynecomastia is so common, however, that many experts are cautious about attaching importance to the detection during routine examination of a small amount of breast tissue in an otherwise asymptomatic man.

Acute development of enlargement and tenderness in males greater than age 25 warrants additional evaluation.

15. What information is significant in the history?

Age	Thyroid symptoms
Duration of enlargement	Drugs
Breast symptoms (tenderness, discharge)	Alcohol use
Other illnesses	Congenital abnormalities
Nutritional status and recent changes in weight	Pubertal progression
Impotence and libido	

16. What should be noted on the physical examination?

The most important features include characteristics of the breast tissue (irregular, firm, eccentric; nipple discharge), testes (size, asymmetry), abdomen (liver enlargement, ascites, spider angioma), secondary sexual characteristics, thyroid status (goiter, tremor, reflexes), and any signs of excessive cortisol (buffalo hump, central obesity, hypertension, purple stria, moon facies).

17. Should laboratory tests be ordered?

Some believe that hormonal testing is not cost effective and favor checking testicular ultrasound alone to rule out the 3% incidence of feminizing tumors. Most, however, favor measuring liver enzymes, blood urea nitrogen, creatinine, thyrotropin (TSH), and testosterone. Estradiol, LH, follicle-stimulating hormone (FSH), prolactin, and hCG may follow the initial screen. Many would obtain a chest radiograph. If the hCG or estradiol level is elevated, a testicular ultrasound is indicated. For prepubertal patients, an adrenal computed tomographic (CT) scan should also be considered.

18. What findings raise the suspicion of breast cancer?

Breast cancer is rare in men (0.2%) and does not increase with gynecomastia, except in Klinefelter syndrome (3–6%). Carcinoma is usually unilateral, painless, and nontender. Bloody discharge, ulceration, firmness, fixation to the underlying tissue, eccentric location (not subareolar), and adenopathy are suspicious findings. If doubt remains, biopsy should be considered. The diagnostic accuracy of fine-needle aspiration cytology is greater than 90%. Excisional biopsy or mastectomy would be recommended for malignant or suspicious cytology.

19. Will gynecomastia spontaneously regress?

Neonatal gynecomastia usually resolves within 4 months. Gynecomastia resolves within 18 months in 95% of pubertal boys. Persistent tissue becomes more fibrous with time, however, and is less likely to remit spontaneously. More highly developed breast tissue (Tanner stages III, IV, and V) is also less likely to regress. Gynecomastia in older men does not usually resolve spontaneously.

20. What is the treatment when gynecomastia does not regress?

Hormonal therapy can be attempted. Tamoxifen, clomiphene, danazol, dihydrotestosterone, and testolactone have all been used. Tamoxifen has the fewest side effects and the highest response rate for both improvement in tenderness and decrease in size. Medication is more likely to work if gynecomastia has been present less than 4 months and the size of the tissue is less than 3 cm. Once the medication is stopped, gynecomastia recurs in 25–30%. For recurrent or persistent gynecomastia greater than 3 cm, surgery is the recommended therapy.

BIBLIOGRAPHY

1. Bowers S, Pearlman N, McIntyre R, et al: Cost-effective management of gynecomastia. Am J Surg 176:638–641, 1998.
2. Braunstein G: Gynecomastia: Current concepts. N Engl J Med 328:490–495, 1993.
3. Braunstein G, Glassman H: Gynecomastia: Current Therapy in Endocrinology and Metabolism, 6th ed. Toronto, BC Decker, 1997.
4. Carlson H: Gynecomastia: Pathogenesis and therapy. Endocrinologist 1:337–342, 1991.
5. Glass AR: Gynecomastia. Endocrinol Metab Clin North Am 23:825–837, 1994.
6. Joshi A, Kapila K, Verma K: Fine needle aspiration cytology in the management of male breast masses. Acta Cytol 43:334–338, 1999.
7. Neuman J: Evaluation and treatment of gynecomastia. Am Fam Physician 55:1835–1844, 1997.

8. Niewohner C, Nuttall F: Gynecomastia in a hospitalized male population. Am J Med 77:633–638, 1984.
9. Scully R, Mark E, McNeely W, et al: Case 12-2000. N Engl J Med 342(16):1196–1204, 2000.
10. Ting A, Chow L, Leung Y: Comparison of tamoxifen with danazol in the management of idiopathic gynecomastia. American Surgeon 66:38–40, 2000.
11. Volpe C, Raffetto J, Collure D, et al: Unilateral male breast masses: Cancer risk and their evaluation and management. American Surgeon 65:250–253, 1999.
12. Webster D: Benign disorders of the male breast. World J Surg 13:726–730, 1989.
13. Wilson J, Aiman J, MacDonald P: The Pathogenesis of Gynecomastia. Chicago, Year Book, 1980.

48. AMENORRHEA

Margaret E. Wierman, M.D.

1. What is amenorrhea?

Amenorrhea is the absence of menstrual periods. Oligomenorrhea refers to lighter, irregular menses. Primary amenorrhea is the failure to begin menses, whereas secondary amenorrhea refers to cessation of menstrual periods after cyclic menses have been established.

2. Describe the normal maturation process of the hypothalamic-pituitary-ovarian axis.

In girls, puberty usually begins after age 8 years and is heralded by the initiation of breast development. The average age for girls in the U.S. to begin menses is 12 years. This event generally signals the end of the pubertal process, occurring after the growth spurt and most somatic changes are completed. The process is triggered by gonadotropin-releasing hormone (GnRH)–induced episodic secretion of luteinizing hormone (LH) and follicle-stimulating hormone (FSH) from the pituitary gland. The pulsatile release of gonadotropins activates the ovaries, causing maturation of follicles and production of estrogen and, later, progesterone. These gonadal steroids give feedback at the level of the hypothalamus and pituitary to regulate GnRH and gonadotropin secretion. A final maturation event is the development of positive feedback by estradiol to induce the midcycle LH surge that stimulates ovulation. In many adolescents, menstrual cycles are anovulatory and thus irregular for the first 6–12 months. As the hypothalamic-pituitary-gonadal (HPG) axis matures, ovulatory cycles become more frequent. In normal adult women, all but one or two cycles per year are ovulatory.

3. What are the most common causes of primary amenorrhea?

Primary amenorrhea is defined as lack of menses by age 16 or lack of secondary sexual characteristics by age 14. It usually results from abnormal anatomic development of the female reproductive organs or from a hormonal disorder involving the hypothalamus, pituitary gland, or ovaries. The presence of normal secondary sexual characteristics in such patients suggests an anatomic problem, such as obstruction or failure of development of the uterus or vagina. In contrast, a lack of secondary sexual characteristics indicates a probable hormonal cause. GnRH deficiency due to maturational arrest of GnRH-producing neurons in the olfactory placode during embryonic development is a hypothalamic cause of primary amenorrhea. The pituitary gland itself may be compressed by pituitary tumors, craniopharyngiomas, and Rathke pouch cysts, causing impaired LH and FSH secretion. The ovaries also may be defective because of gonadal dysgenesis due to Turner syndrome (45 XO karyotype) or destruction by chemotherapy. Finally, the presence of ambiguous genitalia or palpable gonads in the labia or inguinal area may indicate a disorder of sexual differentiation such as congenital adrenal hyperplasia (21-hydroxylase deficiency) or an androgen resistance syndrome (testicular feminization).

4. What disorders cause secondary amenorrhea?

Secondary amenorrhea, which is much more common than primary amenorrhea, occurs postpubertally as a result of pregnancy, menopause, hypothalamic amenorrhea, hyperprolactinemia, and hyperandrogenic anovulatory disorders such as polycystic ovarian syndrome (PCOS).

5. How do you evaluate a patient with amenorrhea?

One must determine whether the disorder is anatomic or hormonal, congenital or acquired, and where the defect is located. A complete history and physical examination provide the first essential clues. Measurement of serum gonadotropin levels (LH and FSH) separates patients into one of two categories. Patients with low or normal levels of LH and FSH (hypogonadotropic hypogonadism) have a disorder at the level of the hypothalamus or pituitary gland. However, patients with high LH and FSH levels (hypergonadotropic hypogonadism) may have a defect at the level of either the ovary or hypothalamic-pituitary unit (e.g., gonadotropin-producing pituitary tumors and PCOS, in which the hypothalamic GnRH pulse generator is abnormally accelerated).

6. Discuss the major congenital causes of hypogonadotropic hypogonadism.

Congenital or idiopathic hypogonadotropic hypogonadism is due to GnRH deficiency. Female patients present with primary amenorrhea. When associated with anosmia, the disorder is termed Kallmann's syndrome. GnRH deficiency occurs in 1/10,000 males and 1/80,000 females and may be X-linked, autosomal dominant, autosomal recessive, or sporadic. The X-linked form is associated with a mutation in the annexin gene that encodes a neural cell adhesion protein thought to be important in providing the scaffolding for GnRH neurons in their migration from the olfactory placode to the hypothalamus during embryonic development. Thus, GnRH-secreting neurons fail to reach their target in the hypothalamus but instead remain in the olfactory area. All other hypothalamic-pituitary function is normal. Gonadal steroid administration is used to initiate the development of secondary sexual characteristics, and fertility can be attained using pulsatile GnRH or gonadotropin therapy.

7. What are the acquired forms of amenorrhea due to hypogonadotropic hypogonadism?

- Hyperprolactinemia
- Hypothalamic amenorrhea

8. How does hyperprolactinemia cause amenorrhea?

Elevated prolactin levels may be due to prolactinomas, hypothyroidism, medications (usually psychotropic drugs), and pregnancy. Hyperprolactinemia impairs function of the HPG axis at all levels, but the major site of inhibition is the hypothalamic GnRH pulse generator. As prolactin levels rise, luteal phase defects develop, ovulation ceases, and menstrual cycles become shorter and irregular. Still higher levels of prolactin are associated with amenorrhea. Treatment of the elevated prolactin levels usually normalizes menstrual cycles.

9. What is hypothalamic amenorrhea?

Hypothalamic amenorrhea refers to amenorrhea resulting from acquired disorders of the GnRH pulse generator. Excessive stress, exercise, and weight loss have been shown to act centrally to disrupt the GnRH-induced pulsatile gonadotropin secretory pattern. In men, GnRH-induced LH pulses normally occur every 2 hours. In contrast, the LH pulse pattern in women must change across the menstrual cycle, accelerating from every 90 minutes in the early follicular phase to every 30 minutes at ovulation and then slowing from every hour to every 8 hours across the luteal phase. Disruption of this sensitively timed pattern results in anovulation, irregular menses, and, eventually, amenorrhea.

Hypothalamic amenorrhea may result from several different types of gonadotropin secretory disorders. Some women with anorexia nervosa have absent LH pulsations (prepubertal pattern), some have pulsations only at night (early pubertal pattern), and still others have LH pulses throughout the 24-hour period but they are significantly reduced in amplitude or frequency. The diagnosis relies heavily on a history of weight loss and/or high levels of exercise or stress. Supportive findings on physical examination include evidence of decreased estrogen effects and absence of other major illnesses. Laboratory testing usually reveals low serum estradiol and low or low-normal serum LH and FSH levels; the test for beta-hCG is negative, and the prolactin level is normal. Elevated gonadotropin levels, in contrast, indicate probable premature ovarian failure.

10. What are the consequences of amenorrhea?

Short-term consequences of estrogen deficiency may include painful intercourse and hot flashes. Among the more important long-term consequences are osteoporosis and premature coronary artery disease.

11. What treatment options are available for hypothalamic amenorrhea?

Interventions to increase body weight and to reduce stress and/or exercise should be attempted initially. If these interventions are unsuccessful, estrogen replacement therapy should be instituted. Fertility, if desired, may be achieved by ovulation induction with clomiphene in mild cases or with human menopausal gonadotropins or pulsatile GnRH administration if the disorder is more severe.

12. What disorders cause amenorrhea with hypergonadotropic hypogonadism?

- Premature ovarian failure (high FSH, later high LH)
- Polycystic ovarian syndrome (low FSH, high LH)
- Gonadotropin-secreting pituitary tumors (high FSH and/or LH)

13. How do you make a diagnosis of premature ovarian failure?

Premature ovarian failure, which is defined as menopause before the age of 40, may be due to surgical removal or autoimmune destruction of the ovaries. Autoimmune destruction of the ovaries is characterized by a history of normal puberty and regular menses followed by the early onset of hot flashes, irregular menses, and eventual amenorrhea. Elevated serum FSH levels are the laboratory hallmark of gonadal failure. To avoid misdiagnosis, blood for FSH measurement must be drawn in the early follicular phase, if the woman still has menses, because FSH levels rise along with LH at mid-cycle in normally ovulating women. Turner syndrome mosaics may have several menses before they undergo menopause; therefore, a karyotype may be helpful if ovarian failure occurs in adolescence or the early 20s.

14. What other disorders may coexist with premature ovarian failure?

Both patients and family members are at risk for other autoimmune disorders, including primary adrenal insufficiency (Addison's disease), autoimmune thyroid disorders (Graves' disease, Hashimoto's disease), type 1 diabetes mellitus, pernicious anemia (vitamin B_{12} deficiency), celiac sprue, and rheumatologic disorders.

15. What are the treatment options for women with premature ovarian failure?

Estrogen replacement therapy, usually in combination with progesterone, is critical to decrease postmenopausal bone loss and premature coronary artery disease. New options for fertility in women with premature ovarian failure include donor eggs with the partner's sperm and in vitro fertilization with hormonal preparation of the patient to enable her to carry the fetus.

16. What is hyperandrogenic anovulation?

Hyperandrogenic anovulation refers to the cluster of disorders that present with irregular menses or amenorrhea and signs of androgen excess, such as hirsutism and virilization. The disorders in this group include PCOS, androgen-secreting tumors of the ovaries or adrenal glands, congenital adrenal hyperplasia (CAH; classic or attenuated form), and obesity-induced amenorrhea.

17. How are these hyperandrogenic disorders differentiated clinically?

Tumors are suggested by rapid progression of hirsutism and virilization (temporal hair recession, clitoris enlargement, breast atrophy) and by high serum androgen levels; they may be excluded by a serum testosterone level less than 200 ng/dl or dehydroepiandrosterone sulfate (DHEAS) levels less than 1000 ng/ml. CAH (most commonly due to 21-hydroxylase deficiency) is diagnosed by high basal or adrenocorticotropic hormone (ACTH)–stimulated levels of 17-hydroxyprogesterone. Obesity-induced amenorrhea is suggested by a history of normal puberty and menses until progressive weight gain triggers the development of hirsutism, acne, oligomenorrhea, and, later, amenorrhea. Affected women have low serum levels of FSH and LH in the follicular phase in contrast to women with PCOS (see below).

18. Describe the pathophysiology of obesity-induced amenorrhea.

Fat tissue contains aromatase and 5-alpha-reductase enzymes. Aromatase converts androgens to estrogens; when aromatase is present in increased amounts, as in obesity, constant elevated (rather than normally fluctuating) serum estrogen levels are produced, impairing normal ovulation. Increased activity of 5-alpha-reductase, which converts testosterone to dihydrotestosterone (DHT), results in excessive DHT production, promoting the development of hirsutism and acne. Primary treatment of obesity results in restoration of normal reproductive function.

19. How does the patient with PCOS present clinically?

Most patients with PCOS present in adolescence with a history of early menarche (<12 yr) and persistently irregular menses. Hirsutism and acne beginning in the teenage years are other common features of the disorder. About 60% of patients become overweight in their 20s and 30s. Patients also frequently have signs of insulin resistance, including acanthosis nigricans, a velvety, hyperpigmented cutaneous lesion on the neck and in the axillae. Irregular, anovulatory menses lead to infertility, and the resultant unopposed estrogen exposure increases the risk of endometrial hyperplasia and carcinoma.

20. What is the pathogenesis of PCOS?

Experts disagree as to whether PCOS is a primary disorder of the central nervous system, the adrenal glands, or the ovaries. Existing data most strongly support the presence of an abnormal hypothalamic GnRH pulse generator that, in contrast to hypothalamic amenorrhea, is set too fast. The pituitary gonadotropin response to GnRH is pulse rate–dependent; rapid GnRH pulses stimulate LH secretion but inhibit FSH production. The increased LH/FSH secretory ratio results in inadequate ovarian follicle recruitment and/or development, causing anovulation and the appearance of multiple subcapsular cysts, and triggers constant estrogen and enhanced androgen production by the ovaries. The ovarian androgens—DHEA, androstenedione, and testosterone—may be elevated; for unclear reasons, the adrenal androgens, DHEA and DHEAS, may be increased as well. High levels of circulating androgens decrease hepatic production of sex hormone–binding globulin (SHBG), allowing more free androgen to target the skin and hair follicles, inducing the development of acne and hirsutism. Insulin resistance also plays a role in the ultimate picture because hyperinsulinemia augments ovarian androgen production and further reduces SHBG levels.

21. What are the treatment options for patients with PCOS?

The initial goals are to suppress androgen production and action and to ensure regular shedding of the endometrium to decrease the risk of developing endometrial hyperplasia. Birth control pills are the treatment of choice; an antiandrogen, such as spironolactone, may be added if hirsutism is a major problem. Intermittent cycling with medroxyprogesterone (Provera) is an alternative for endometrial protection but does not suppress the elevated androgens and their ultimate impact on ovarian morphology and function. Fertility may be achieved with clomiphene, human menopausal gonadotropins, or pulsatile GnRH administration, but only with difficulty because of the already overactive hormonal environment. Recently designed regimens using progesterone pretreatment to slow the GnRH pulse generator or a GnRH agonist to inhibit endogenous GnRH, coupled with induction of ovulation by human menopausal gonadotropins, have been more successful. A new approach that has shown some promise is reducing insulin resistance and serum insulin levels with insulin sensitizers such as metformin. Studies using metformin thus far have shown modest decreases in serum androgen levels, some improvement in menstrual regularity, and improved ovulation in response to clomiphene. The thiazolidinedione class of insulin sensitizers has shown promise, but the first-generation agent, troglitazone, was taken off the market. Data on rosiglitazone and pioglitazone are not yet available. Further investigation is necessary before these or similar medications gain popular acceptance.

BIBLIOGRAPHY

1. Berga SL: Functional hypothalamic chronic anovulation. In Adashi WY, Rock JA, Rosenwaks Z (eds): Reproductive Endocrinology, Surgery, and Technology. Philadelphia, Lippincott-Raven, 1996, pp 1061–1075.
2. Cumming DC: Exercise-associated amenorrhea, low bone density, and estrogen replacement therapy. Arch Intern Med 156:2193–2195, 1996.
3. Ehrmann DA: Insulin lowering therapeutic modalities for polycystic ovary syndrome. Endocrine Metabolic Clin North Am 28 (2):423–38, 1999.
4. Kiningham RB, Apgar BS, Schwenk TL: Evaluation of amenorrhea. Am Fam Physician 53:1185–1194, 1996.
5. Pralong FP, Crowley WF Jr: Gonadotropins: Normal physiology. In Wierman ME (ed): Diseases of the Pituitary: Diagnosis and Treatment. Totowa, Humana Press, 1997, pp 203–219.
6. Schlechte JA: Differential diagnosis and management of hyperprolactinemia. In Wierman ME (ed): Diseases of the Pituitary: Diagnosis and Treatment. Totowa, Humana Press, 1997, pp 71–77.
7. Taylor AE, Adams JM, Mulder JE, et al: A randomized, controlled trial of estradiol replacement therapy in women with hypergonadotropic amenorrhea. J Clin Endocrinol Metab 81:3615–3621, 1996.
8. Warren MP: Anorexia, bulimia, and exercise-induced amenorrhea: Medical approach. Curr Ther Endocrinol Metab 6:13–17, 1997.
9. Welt CK, Hall JE: Gonadotropin deficiency: Differential diagnosis and treatment. In Wierman ME (ed): Diseases of the Pituitary: Diagnosis and Treatment. Totowa, Humana Press, 1997, pp 221–246.
10. Wierman ME: Gonadotropin releasing hormone. In Adashi WY, Rock JA, Rosenwaks Z (eds): Reproductive Endocrinology, Surgery, and Technology. Philadelphia, Lippincott-Raven, 1996, pp 665–681.

49. GALACTORRHEA

William J. Georgitis, M.D., FACP

1. What hormones are essential for lactation?

Both estrogen and prolactin are necessary for milk production. Estrogens promote cellular proliferation and ductular development. Prolactin, which rises dramatically during pregnancy, stimulates differentiation of acini in preparation for production of milk protein. Paradoxically, high levels of estrogen inhibit milk production. Shortly after delivery, estrogen levels decline and lactation begins. Growth hormone, insulin, and cortisol are necessary permissive factors for cell growth in cultured breast tissue. Androgens inhibit breast tissue growth and differentiation, and thus galactorrhea rarely occurs in men.

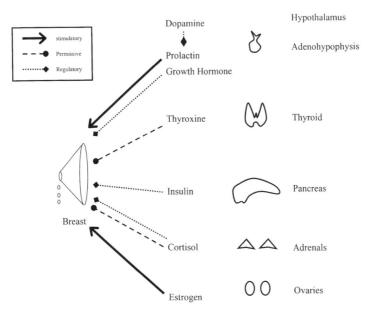

Hormones essential for lactation. Bold arrows indicte major stimulatory hormones, dashed arrows indicate permissive hormones, and dotted arrows indicate hormones that play predominantly regulatory roles.

2. Can failure to lactate and menstruate postpartum indicate a serious disorder?

The inability to lactate and menstruate after delivery are signs of Sheehan's syndrome. Postpartum pituitary necrosis is associated with difficult deliveries complicated by obstetrical hemorrhage and hypotension. In the United States, pituitary insufficiency from Sheehan's syndrome is usually limited to the adenohypophysis. In developing countries, vasopressin deficiency may also occur, indicating more severe necrosis of the pituitary involving the neurohypophysis.

3. How frequent is galactorrhea?

A milklike discharge from the breast of a nongravid woman or milk secretion persisting for 6 months after nursing has ceased is fairly common. The lifelong frequency of galactorrhea has been reported to range from 2–20%. Milk should not be found in normal nulligravidas, postmenopausal women not receiving hormone replacement, or men.

4. Does galactorrhea always look like milk?

No. Breast milk is basically an emulsion of fat and water. It has over 100 known constituents. Because the quantity of fat varies, the gross appearance may range from milky to opalescent or clear. Microscopic examination confirms that a breast secretion is galactorrhea by revealing fat globules. Special stains for fat or chemical analysis for lactate or specific milk proteins are rarely necessary.

5. Is galactorrhea always expressed from both breasts?

Galactorrhea may be unilateral or bilateral. Although many patients report frank leaking or staining of garments, some may not notice the discharge. Small amounts of serous fluid can be expressed from the majority of normal women who have experienced pregnancy.

6. Is the differential diagnosis for galactorrhea simple or complex?

The differential diagnosis for galactorrhea is actually quite lengthy and complex. Causes of nonpuerperal galactorrhea are not easy to arrange in a logical manner. Some lists categorize diagnoses by anatomic location, some by causality, and some by symptoms or signs. Most attempts at a logical approach seem to lose their structure before the differential is complete. A shift in gender often creeps into many of the differential lists. Another attempt appears in the table below but certainly has room for improvement. Examples appear in parentheses.

Causes of Nonpuerperal Galactorrhea

Idiopathic	Endocrinopathies
Pituitary tumors	Primary hypothyroidism
Prolactinoma	Hyperthyroidism
Somatotropinoma	Primary adrenal insufficiency
Hypothalamic disorders	Endogenous estrogens
Tumor (craniopharyngioma)	Adrenocortical carcinoma
Infiltrative disease (sarcoid)	Reflex arc activation
Infundibular disruption (trauma)	Nipple stimulation
Medications	Thoracic nerve irritation (shingles)
Psychotropic (chlorpromazine)	Miscellaneous associations
Antihypertensive (methyldopa)	Stress
Cannabinoid (morphine)	Empty sella syndrome
Estrogens (oral contraceptives)	Renal or hepatic failure
Antiemetics (metoclopramide)	Polycystic ovary syndrome

7. Which medications cause galactorrhea?

Psychotropic medications are the leading culprits. The most common are phenothiazines, tricyclic antidepressants, haloperidol, benzodiazepines, butyrophenones, amphetamines, and monoamine oxidase (MAO) inhibitors. Other commonly prescribed drugs implicated as causes include cimetidine, metoclopramide, verapamil, and estrogens in numerous formulations.

8. Is the presence or absence of amenorrhea significant?

It is very important to obtain a comprehensive menstrual history from any woman complaining of galactorrhea. A common physiologic cause for galactorrhea and amenorrhea is pregnancy. The galactorrheic woman without amenorrhea has a 20% chance of having a pituitary tumor. When amenorrhea accompanies galactorrhea, the percentage increases to 34%. Furthermore, when amenorrhea is present, hyperprolactinemic hypogonadotropic hypogonadism may be present and be accompanied by infertility and osteopenia.

9. What percentage of women with elevated levels of serum prolactin have galactorrhea?

Women with elevated prolactin levels have a prevalence of galactorrhea ranging from 50–80%. The degree of prolactin elevation correlates poorly with the amount of lactation. However, the level of prolactin does crudely correlate with the possible causes.

10. How can the serum level of prolactin be used to help determine the cause of galactorrhea?

Prolactin is a dynamic, not a static, hormone. Blood levels display diurnal fluctuations and respond to various stimuli. Prolactin rises after meals and in response to hypoglycemia, seizures, intercourse, and vigorous nipple stimulation. Normal levels range as high as 20 ng/ml. Drug-induced galactorrhea is accompanied by normal or moderately elevated serum prolactin levels but mild hyperprolactinemia may also result from pituitary, hypothalamic, or parasellar processes. Since many drugs cause galactorrhea by decreasing dopaminergic inhibition of prolactin secretion, it is understandable that mass lesions compressing or disrupting normal hypothalamic-pituitary portal connections might result in prolactin levels that overlap with those associated with drug-induced hyperprolactinemia.

Medications are generally not adequate explanations for prolactin levels above 100 ng/ml. Prolactin values in this range are most often due to pregnancy or prolactinomas. In a non-pregnant individual, the odds of finding a pituitary tumor are proportionate to the degree of hyperprolactinemia. Levels above 300 ng/ml usually indicate the presence of a prolactinoma that can be readily demonstrated with current pituitary imaging methods. Patients with levels ranging from 100–300 ng/ml should also have pituitary imaging studies. If a tumor is not detected, continued surveillance is necessary because the majority probably harbor microprolactinomas below the resolving power of current imaging modalities.

11. Should other lab tests be included in the evaluation?

Yes. A serum TSH level should be measured since primary hypothyroidism can present with the amenorrhea-galactorrhea syndrome. Pituitary hyperplasia develops in these patients and may mimic a pituitary adenoma. Published reports include patients with massive hyperplasia and optic chiasmal compression. Hypothyroidism may easily be overlooked in this situation. Both the pituitary hyperplasia and the amenorrhea-galactorrhea usually resolve with thyroxine therapy. A TSH level should therefore be measured in every patient with a pituitary mass and galactorrhea, especially before pituitary surgery is used to treat a condition that most often responds to thyroid hormone replacement alone.

12. It seems odd that hyperthryoidism is listed. Why is that?

In one report, a high prevalence of galactorrhea was described in hyperthyroid patients. The mechanism is obscure since prolactin levels were normal. The galactorrhea was not spontaneous but was expressible only on examination and was thus of questionable significance. Perhaps, this condition does not truly belong on the list.

13. Has galactorrhea been seen following surgery and chest wall lesions?

Galactorrhea has appeared after various types of major surgery involving both the thorax and the abdomen. In women, prolactin levels may rise while estrogen levels fall postoperatively. There does not seem to be a higher frequency of galactorrhea in patients who have had chest wall surgery compared with other major surgical precedures, and the hyperprolactinemia that develops is not sustained. Galactorrhea also occurs with processes like herpes zoster that involve the chest wall. In this condition, the increased prolactin secretion is thought to result from stimulation of nerves somehow involved in a reflex arc between the breast and pituitary-hypothalamic unit.

14. Galactorrhea in renal failure seems odd. What is the connection?

Hyperprolactinemia in renal failure is modest in degree and results from decreased metabolic clearance of prolactin, although in some cases medications with dopamine inhibitory actions also play a role. Most of these patients with elevated prolactin levels do not have have galactorrhea.

15. Can galactorrhea be present in the absence of excessive prolactin?

Yes. One third of women with acromegaly have galactorrhea. Most of these patients have hyperprolactinemia as a result of secretion of prolactin directly by the tumor or indirectly from pituitary stalk disruption. Some patients, however, have normal serum levels of prolactin. Galactorrhea in these cases appears to result from activation of breast prolactin receptors by growth hormone. This cross-activation at high growth hormone levels stems from structural homology between growth hormone and prolactin.

16. Is galactorrhea associated with an increased risk of breast cancer?

No. When a breast discharge occurs in someone with breast cancer, a palpable mass is usually present. Nonmilky breast discharge is not a common presentation for breast cancer, and even bloody breast secretions more often result from benign conditions like mastitis. Some evidence suggests that the risk of breast cancer is reduced in premenopausal women who have lactated.

17. Are medications used to treat galactorrhea?

Not much any more. Dopamine agonists, such as bromocriptine, pergolide, and cabergoline, are still the drugs of choice for patients with prolactinomas. They are also effective for other types of galactorrhea, but in 1994, the manufacturer of bromocriptine withdrew the treatment indication for postpartum lactation following case reports of vascular side effects including stroke and myocardial ischemia that were attributed to the drug. For women choosing not to breast feed, measures including garments providing firm breast support, analgesics, and ice packs can be helpful.

18. What about galactorrhea in men?

Galactorrhea is a rare complaint in men, although men comprise about 5% of patients evaluated for galactorrhea in some reported series. The rarity of this complaint, even in hyperprolactinemic men, is probably due to the lack of estrogen priming necessary for milk production. Men with galactorrhea need to be examined for feminizing syndromes and pro-lactin-producing pituitary tumors.

19. Does galactorrhea always need treatment?

Not always. Generally, galactorrhea unaccompanied by amenorrhea, infertility, osteopenia, or a pituitary tumor will not have serious long-term consequences if left untreated. Treatment is indicated to restore fertility and may be indicated when a pituitary tumor is present, depending upon the tumor size.

Microadenomas, less than 1 cm in diameter by definition, rarely seem to grow to macroadenomas. Spontaneous improvement with falling prolactin levels and return of menstruation can occur. However, if estrogen deficiency and osteopenia are present, even microprolactinomas may need treatment. Continued observation is necessary in all cases, and especially if oral contraceptives are used, to monitor for the rare case that progresses from a microadenoma to a macroadenoma.

Macroadenomas often require treatment, especially if threat of visual loss is a concern or if cosecretion causes a morbid condition such as acromegaly. The most common functional pituitary tumors with galactorrhea are prolactinomas. Trans-phenoidal surgery for small prolactinomas initially showed postoperative success in about 80% of cases compared with the lower success rate of 50% for macroprolactinomas. Trans-phenoidal surgery as the initial treatment of choice for microprolactinomas fell into disfavor when recurrence rates assessed several years postoperatively ranged from 17-91%. Now medical therapy with dopamine agonists is first-line therapy for all size categories of prolactinomas.

Serum prolactin levels need to be reduced near or into the normal range in order to restore menses and control galactorrhea. Dopamine agonists, including bromocriptine, pergolide, and cabergoline, all lower prolactin levels, shrink tumors, and can restore cyclic menstrual function in premenopausal women. Galactorrhea can decrease within hours of starting treatment with bromocriptine. Some reduction in tumor size occurs in close to 9 out of 10 patients, and a 25% reduction in size occurs in nearly 8 out of 10. Surgery and radiation therapy are effective for tumors failing to respond to medications and occasionally for drug-intolerant patients. Radiotherapy stops tumor growth and results in a gradual decline in prolactin levels over many years. The slow prolactin response is accompanied by a progressive increase in the prevalence of radiation-induced hypopituitarism, ranging from 13-100%. Comparing the treatment responses to medical, surgical, and radiation therapy, it is understandable that surgery and radiation are now viewed as adjuncts to medical treatment for most prolactinoma patients.

20. Did Hippocrates have anything to say relevant to amenorrhea or galactorrhea?
His aphorisms show that he did.

"If a woman who is neither pregnant nor has given birth produces milk, her menstruation has stopped." (Aphorisms, Section V, # 39.) "If the catamenia are suppressed, without being followed by rigor or fever, but by disinclination for food, pregnancy may be suspected." (Aphorisms, Section V, # 61.)

The first patient sounds like the young woman who now comes to you with a negative home pregnancy test, a normal TSH from a health fair screening, and an Internet printout to ensure that you measure a prolactin and possibly order an MRI, while the second reminds us all not to overlook important historical clues and physical signs for the most common disorders like pregnancy.

BIBLIOGRAPHY

1. Bevan JS, Webster J, Burke CW, Scanlon MF: Dopamine agonists and pituitary tumor shrinkage. Endocr Rev 13:220–240, 1992.
2. Biller BM: Diagnostic evaluation of hyperprolactinemia. J Reprod Med 44 (12 Suppl):1095–1099, 1999.
3. Dalkin AC, Marshall JC: Medical therapy of hyperprolactinemia. Endocrinol Metab Clin North Am 18:259–276, 1989.
4. Fiorica JV: Nipple discharge. Obstet Gynecol Clin North Am 21:453–460, 1994.
5. Fradkin JE, Eastman RC, Lesniak MA, et al: Specificity spillover at the hormone receptor— exploring its role in human disease. N Engl J Med 320:640–645, 1989.
6. Kapcala LP: Galactorrhea and thyrotoxicosis. Arch Intern Med 144:2349–2350, 1984.
7. Kleinberg DL, Noel GL, Frantz AA: Galactorrhea: A study of 235 cases, including 48 pituitary tumors. N Engl J Med 296:589–600, 1977.
8. Klibanski A, Biller BMK, Rosenthal DI, et al: Effects of prolactin and estrogen deficiency in amenorrheic bone loss. J Clin Endocrinol Metab 67:124–130, 1988.
9. Koppelman MC, Jaffe MJ, Rieth KG, et al: Hyperprolactinemia, amenorrhea and galactorrhea. Ann Intern Med 100:115–121, 1984.
10. Luciano AA: Clinical presentation of hyperprolactinemia. J Reprod Med 44(12 Suppl): 1085–1090, 1999.
11. Mehta AE, Reyes FI, Faiman C: Primary radiotherapy of prolactinomas: Eight- to 15-year follow-up. Am J Med 83:49–58, 1987.

12. Molitch ME, Elton RL, Blackwell RE, et al: Bromocriptine as primary therapy for prolactin-secreting macroadenomas: Results of a prospective multicenter study. J Clin Endocrinol Metab 60:698–705, 1985.
13. Poretsky L, Garber J, Kleefield J: Primary amenorrhea and pseudoprolactinoma in a patient with primary hypothyroidism: Reversal of clinical, biochemical and radiologic abnormalities with levothyroxine. Am J Med 81:180–182, 1986.
14. Rayburn WF: Clinical commentary: The bromocriptine (Parlodel) controversy and recommendations for lactation suppression. Am J Perinatol 13:69–71, 1996.
15. Reichlin S: Neuroendocrinology. In Wilson JD (ed): Williams Textbook of Endocrinology, 9th ed., Philadelphia, W. B. Saunders, 1998, pp 881–892.
16. Thomson JA, Davies DL, McLaren EH, et al: Ten-year follow-up of microprolactinoma treated by transsphenoidal surgery. BMJ 309:1409–1410, 1994.

50. HIRSUTISM AND VIRILIZATION

Tamis M. Bright, M.D.

1. What is hirsutism?

Hirsutism is the excessive growth of terminal hair in androgen-dependent areas: tip of the nose, upper lip, chin, side burns, ear lobes, back, chest, areolae, axillae, lower abdomen, pubic triangle, and anterior thighs. Hirsutism is frequently associated with irregular menses and acne. Hirsutism should be distinguished from hypertrichosis, which is a non–androgen-dependent diffuse increase in vellus hair.

2. What is virilization?

Virilization consists of hirsutism, acne, and irregular menses along with signs of masculinization: deepening of the voice, increased muscle mass, temporal balding, clitoromegaly, and increased libido. Virilization results from high circulating levels of androgens, close to or in the male range, and is usually due to an androgen-secreting tumor.

3. What is the cause of hirsutism?

Hirsutism is caused by hyperandrogenism. Androgens transform the fine, downy, minimally pigmented vellus hair in androgen-sensitive areas into coarse, pigmented, terminal hair. Twenty-five percent of testosterone comes from the ovaries, 25% from the adrenal glands, and 50% from peripheral conversion of androstenedione, which is produced by both the ovaries and adrenals. Testosterone is converted into dihydrotestosterone (DHT) by the enzyme 5-alpha-reductase, which is present in hair follicles. DHT is responsible for the transformation of vellus into terminal hair. Hair follicles also contain the enzymes that convert dehydroepiandrosterone (DHEA), which is produced by the adrenals, and androstenedione into testosterone. Consequently, an increase in any of the androgenic steroids may cause high levels of DHT in the hair follicle and result in hirsutism.

Low levels of sex hormone–binding globulin (SHBG), which is produced by the liver, may promote hirsutism. Eighty percent of circulating testosterone is bound to SHBG, 19% is bound to albumin, and 1% is free. Decreases in SHBG increase the free fraction of hormone available to androgen-sensitive hair.

Increased activity of 5-alpha-reductase, even with normal circulating androgen levels, also may cause hirsutism by the excessive conversion of testosterone into DHT.

4. List the conditions that result in hirsutism.

- Polycystic ovarian syndrome (PCOS)
- Congenital adrenal hyperplasia (CAH)
- Cushing's syndrome
- Hypothyroidism
- Prolactinoma
- Ovarian hyperthecosis
- Idiopathic/familial hirsutism
- Medications

5. What is the pathophysiology of PCOS?

PCOS affects 5–10% of premenopausal women and is a common cause of hirsutism and oligomenorrhea. The hirsutism is gradually progressive, usually beginning at puberty, and most patients have irregular menses from the onset of menarche. However, in a study of hirsute patients with regular menses, 50% had polycystic ovaries. Thus, PCOS presents as a spectrum: some patients have minimal findings, whereas others have the entire constellation of hirsutism, acne, obesity, infertility, amenorrhea or oligomenorrhea, male pattern alopecia, acanthosis nigricans, hyperinsulinemia, and hyperlipidemia.

The exact cause of PCOS is unknown, but affected patients have been shown to have an accelerated rate of pulsatile gonadotropin-releasing hormone (GnRH) secretion from the hypothalamus. The gonadotropin secretory profile is highly dependent on the rate of GnRH pulsatility. Rapid GnRH pulses stimulate the secretion of luteinizing hormone (LH), but not follicle-stimulating hormone (FSH), from the pituitary gland. The increased LH/FSH secretory ratio results in arrested ovarian follicle development with cyst formation and hypertrophy of theca cells, leading to constant estrogen and increased androgen production with chronic anovulation.

Mild elevations of prolactin, of uncertain etiology, are seen in 5–10% of patients. Some also have mild elevations of dehydroepiandrosterone sulfate (DHEAS), suggesting an intrinsic abnormality of adrenal steroidogenic enzyme activity in this subset of cases.

Patients with PCOS and irregular menses frequently have insulin resistance and hyperinsulinemia. Current research shows decreased adipocyte and muscle sensitivity to insulin without detectable abnormalities of insulin binding, but there is no change in hepatic sensitivity compared with weight-matched controls. A post–insulin-binding defect in insulin receptor-mediated signal transduction has been shown to be caused by defective autophosphorylation of the insulin receptor in some patients. Others have normal phosphorylation, indicating a probable defect further downstream in the signaling pathway. A decrease in the glucose transporter, GLUT4, also has been demonstrated in some patients. DNA studies have not yet uncovered a common etiologic genetic defect to explain these findings. However, because insulin decreases SHBG and increases the ovarian androgen response to LH stimulation, hyperinsulinemia resulting from insulin resistance contributes to the elevated free androgen levels in PCOS.

6. What is the pathophysiology of the hyperandrogenism in CAH?

CAH results from a deficiency of one of the key enzymes in the cortisol biosynthesis pathway; it often presents with precocious puberty and childhood hirsutism. Partial or late-onset CAH, owing to milder deficiencies of the same enzymes, may cause postpubertal hirsutism. Ninety percent of CAH is due to 21-hydroxylase (21-OH) deficiency, which causes a defect in the conversion of 17-hydroxyprogesterone (17-OHP) to 11-deoxycortisol and of progesterone to desoxycorticosterone (DOC). The resulting low cortisol production rate leads to hypersecretion of pituitary adrenocorticotropic hormone (ACTH), which stimulates overproduction of 17-OHP and progesterone as well as adrenal androgens, particularly androstenedione. Hirsutism results from the androgen excess.

Deficiency of 11-beta-hydroxylase decreases the conversion of 11-deoxycortisol to cortisol and of DOC to corticosterone. Again, reduced production of cortisol stimulates hypersecretion of ACTH, with consequent overproduction of 11-deoxycortisol, DOC, and adrenal androgens, mainly androstenedione. In addition to hirsutism, patients frequently develop hypertension from the high levels of DOC, a mineralocorticoid.

Deficiency of 3-beta-hydroxysteroid dehydrogenase decreases the conversion of pregnenolone to progesterone and 17-hydroxypregnenolone to 17-OHP. This defect increases production of pregnenolone, 17-hydroxypregnenolone, and the androgens DHEA, DHEAS, and androstenediol, which promote the development of hirsutism.

Deficiency of 17-ketosteroid reductase causes a defect in the conversion of androstenedione to testosterone, DHEA to androstenediol, and estrone to estradiol. Affected patients have elevated basal levels of androstenedione, DHEA, and estrone.

7. How does Cushing's syndrome cause hirsutism?

All causes of Cushing's syndrome may result in hypertrichosis because of increased vellus hair on the face, forehead, limbs, and trunk owing to cortisol hypersecretion. Cushing's syndrome due to an adrenal tumor also may produce hirsutism and virilization from increased secretion of androgens with cortisol.

8. How do prolactinomas and hypothyroidism cause hyperandrogenism?

Hyperprolactinemia suppresses GnRH activity. which diminishes pulsatile LH secretion from the pituitary gland, resulting in decreased ovarian estrogen production and amenorrhea. Prolactin also increases the adrenal androgens, DHEA and DHEAS. Hypothyroidism decreases SHBG, leading to an increase in free testosterone.

9. What is the pathophysiology of the hyperandrogenism in ovarian hyperthecosis?

Ovarian hyperthecosis is a non-neoplastic condition of the ovaries with proliferating islands of luteinized thecal cells in the ovarian stroma. Hyperthecosis causes overproduction of testosterone, androstenedione, and DHT to an even higher level than is usually seen in PCOS. LH and FSH are either normal or low, and the degree of insulin resistance and hyperinsulinemia is greater than in PCOS.

10. Describe the pathophysiology of idiopathic and familial hirsutism.

Idiopathic hirsutism is believed to be caused by increased cutaneous activity of 5-alpha-reductase or enhanced skin sensitivity to androgens. Familial hirsutism is an ethnic tendency to have a higher density of hair follicles per unit area of skin. Mediterraneans and Hispanics have increased hair density, whereas Asians have lower density. Patients with idiopathic or familial hirsutism usually have the onset of hirsutism shortly after puberty with a slow subsequent progression. They have normal menses and fertility as well as a normal hormonal profile.

11. Which medications can cause hirsutism?

Danazol, testosterone, glucocorticoids, metyrapone, phenothiazines, anabolic steroids, and oral contraceptives containing norgestrel and norethindrone can cause hirsutism. Phenytoin, diazoxide, minoxidil, glucocorticoids, streptomycin, penicillamine, and psoralens can cause hypertrichosis.

12. What conditions cause virilization?

Ovarian tumors	Adrenal disorders
Thecoma	Congenital adrenal hyperplasia
Fibrothecoma	Adenoma
Granulosa and granulosa-theca cell tumors	Carcinoma
Arrhenoblastoma (Sertoli-Leydig cell tumors)	
Hilus cell tumors	
Adrenal rest tumors of the ovary	
Luteoma of pregnancy	

13. When should a patient be evaluated for hirsutism?

Any patient with rapid development of hirsutism or coexistence of amenorrhea, irregular menses, or virilization should be evaluated. A patient with regular menses who shows significant concern about hirsutism also may warrant a work-up.

14. What information is important in the history?
- Age of onset, progression, and extent of hair growth
- Current measures of hair removal and frequency of use
- Age at menarche, regularity of menses, and fertility
- Change in libido or change in voice
- Family history of hirsutism
- Symptoms of Cushing's disease, prolactinoma, or hypothyroidism
- Medications

15. What findings are important on physical examination?

•Distribution and degree of hirsutism
•Increased muscle mass, temporal balding, clitoromegaly, or acne
•Obesity
•Acanthosis nigricans
•Visual field defects
•Moon facies, plethora, buffalo hump, supraclavicular fat pads, striae, or thin skin
•Galactorrhea
•Goiter, loss of lateral eyebrows, periorbital edema, dry skin, or delayed reflexes
•Abdominal or pelvic masses

16. When should laboratory tests be ordered for a patient with hirsutism?

Laboratory testing should be guided by the results of the history and physical examination. Many authors advocate against testing in patients with regular menses and only gradual progression of hirsutism. However, serum levels of total testosterone, DHEAS, 17-OHP, LH, and FSH can be useful tests, depending on the individual patient. Patients with signs or symptoms of hypothyroidism, hyperprolactinemia, or Cushing's syndrome also should be evaluated with serum TSH, prolactin, or 24-hour urine cortisol testing, respectively. Otherwise, these tests need not be obtained for every patient.

For a patient without signs of virilization, it is important to differentiate idiopathic hirsutism, PCOS, and CAH, because each is treated differently. Total testosterone, DHEAS, and 17-OHP help in the differential. Idiopathic hirsutism has normal levels on all three tests. PCOS has mildly increased testosterone, normal or slightly increased DHEAS, and normal 17-OHP. CAH has elevated testosterone and DHEAS and mild-to-marked elevation of 17-OHP. An early morning follicular phase level of 17-OHP > 500 ng/dl (normal = < 200 ng/dl) is diagnostic. A borderline elevated level requires an ACTH stimulation test with assessment of 17-OHP levels at baseline and 60 minutes after stimulation with ACTH. The levels are then plotted on a nomogram to determine normals, heterozygous carriers of the 21-OH gene, and patients with late-onset 21-OH deficiency. Some patients with late-onset 21-OH deficiency have normal baseline 17-OHP levels; however, the ACTH-stimulated levels are usually diagnostic.

In most patients with PCOS, LH is elevated, FSH is normal or low, and the ratio of LH to FSH should be greater than 2. However, not all patients with PCOS have an elevated LH, particularly those with obesity; thus, LH and FSH are helpful in confirming but not excluding the diagnosis of PCOS.

17. What laboratory tests should be ordered in a patient with virilization?

A patient with virilization needs to be evaluated to determine if she has an ovarian tumor, an adrenal tumor, or CAH. As in patients without virilization, tests should include serum total testosterone, DHEAS, and 17-OHP. A markedly increased testosterone level (> 200 ng/dl) with normal values on the other tests points to an ovarian tumor. High levels of DHEAS with or without high testosterone levels suggest an adrenal tumor. Increased levels of 17-OHP with modest elevations of DHEAS and testosterone are more consistent with CAH. Laboratory values suggesting tumors need to be followed with a transvaginal ultrasound of the ovaries or CT of the adrenals or ovaries. If no mass is found, iodocholesterol scanning of the adrenals or venous sampling of the ovaries or adrenals can be performed for localization before surgical removal.

18. How is PCOS treated?

If the patient's primary concern is infertility, clomiphene is the usual drug of choice. If clomiphene fails to induce ovulation, cyclic gonadotropin administration is often useful.

Pulsatile GnRH also has been used with some success. In obese patients, weight reduction alone has been shown to increase the spontaneous ovulation rate. If a component of adrenal androgen (DHEAS) hypersecretion appears to be present, low-dose dexamethasone can be added in doses of 0.125–0.375 mg at night. This regimen may improve the ovulation rate as well as decrease hirsutism.

If fertility is not the issue, oral contraceptives or cyclic progestins are used to induce regular menses and thereby decrease the risk of endometrial cancer. Preparations containing androgenic progestins such as norgestrel and norethindrone should be avoided. As above, dexamethasone may be added in patients with an elevated DHEAS; however, this may increase glucose in an already glucose-intolerant patient. If hirsutism does not improve with these measures, the agents listed in question 20 may be needed.

Patients also should be evaluated with a fasting blood glucose or an oral glucose tolerance test and a lipid profile because of the high prevalence of glucose intolerance, diabetes, and hyperlipidemia in this disorder. These problems need to be addressed separately because they are not resolved by treating the hyperandrogenism alone. Troglitazone and metformin have been used in PCOS patients with and without increased glucose levels. Both agents improved glucose levels in patients with hyperglycemia, and they also seemed to have benefit in treating the other aspects of PCOS. Treatment with metformin resulted in improved regularity of menses, fertility, and hyperandrogenism in some studies. Other studies have not shown an effect beyond that which would be expected with the weight loss that is induced by metformin. Treatment with troglitazone, a thiazolidinedione, decreased androgens and increased SHBG but was withdrawn from the market owing to liver toxicity. Other newer thiazolidinediones are currently under study.

19. What is the treatment for CAH?

Glucocorticoid replacement decreases ACTH secretion and thereby reduces excessive adrenal androgen production. Mineralocorticoid replacement is also required in some causes of CAH. Treatment with the regimens listed in question 20 can hasten improvement of hirsutism.

20. Describe the therapies that are available for the treatment of hirsutism.

No matter what therapy is chosen, the patient must be made aware that results will not be seen for at least 3–6 months. Although many different medications and combinations have been used, only topical eflornithine HCl is currently approved by the Food and Drug Administration for treatment of hirsutism.

1. **Estrogens.** Oral contraceptive pills (OCPs) are the most commonly used therapy. They increase serum estrogens and SHBG, which decreases free testosterone levels. Monophasic and triphasic preparations work equally well. Preparations containing the progestins desogestrel, norgestimate, and gestodene are believed to be the best because they are the least androgenic. Potential side effects include weight gain, bloating, nausea, emotional liability, breast pain, and deep venous thrombosis.

2. **Antiandrogens**

(a) Spironolactone is an androgen receptor blocker and a weak inhibitor of testosterone production. It is often given in combination with OCPs for additive effects. It can be used alone if the patient cannot tolerate OCPs; however, adequate birth control should be used because spironolactone can feminize a male fetus. Other side effects include diuresis for the first few days of treatment, fatigue, and dysfunctional uterine bleeding. Initial doses are 25–100 mg twice daily, tapered to 25–50 mg/day once an effect has been seen.

(b) Flutamide blocks androgen receptors and can be used alone or in combination with OCPs. Combination therapy gives slightly better results than flutamide alone, and recurrence of hirsutism after stopping the medications is decreased. Side effects include feminization of a male fetus, increased liver function tests (LFTs), and fatal hepatotoxicity. One trial comparing flutamide with spironolactone showed more improvement and fewer side effects with flutamide; however, other studies have shown no difference. Dosage is 125–250 mg once or twice daily.

(c) Finasteride, a 5-alpha-reductase inhibitor, also effectively decreases hirsutism. Side effects include feminization of a male fetus, headache, and depression. One study showed no difference in improvement of hirsutism between finasteride and spironolactone (100 mg/day); another showed spironolactone to be better. Some studies comparing flutamide to finasteride have shown equal efficacy, whereas others show flutamide to be superior to finasteride. Dosage is 5–7.5 mg/day.

(d) Cimetidine is a weak antiandrogen but has not proved to be effective in treating hirsutism.

3. **GnRH agonists.** By providing constant rather than pulsatile GnRH levels to the pituitary, GnRH agonists reduce gonadotropin secretion and thereby decrease ovarian production of both estrogen and androgen. Estrogen replacement must be given to avoid hot flashes, vaginal dryness, and bone density loss. Leuprolide (3.75 mg/month IM), buserelin or nafarelin nasal spray (3 times/day), and goserelin subcutaneous implants effectively reduce hirsutism. Some studies demonstrate an increased effect over OCPs alone, whereas others show similar effects. The preparations are expensive and thus are usually reserved for severe PCOS.

4. **Progestational agents.** Cyproterone acetate is a potent progestin and moderate antiandrogen used in Canada and Europe, but it is not available in the U.S. It has been used alone or in combination with estrogen. Side effects include weight gain, fluid retention, mood changes, decreased libido, and increased LFTs. Treatment with cyproterone has shown good results compared with controls, but studies have shown no difference between cyproterone and finasteride, flutamide, or OCPs combined with spironolactone (100 mg/day). Cyproterone also has been combined with GnRH agonists but without clinical improvement compared with cyproterone plus estrogen.

5. **Topical agents.** Eflornithine HCl 13.9% cream is the newest agent for the treatment of facial hirsutism. Eflornithine HCl irreversibly inhibits ornithine decarboxylase, an enzyme necessary for hair follicle cell division. Inhibition of ornithine decarboxylase results in a decreased rate of hair growth. In clinical trials, 32% of patients have had marked improvement or better as compared with 8% of controls after 24 weeks of treatment. Twenty-six percent of both the treatment group and the controls showed some improvement. Forty-two percent of the treatment group showed no improvement as compared with 66% of controls with no improvement. The most common side effects encountered were acne, pseudofolliculitis barbae, burning, tingling, erythema, or rash over the applied area. Generally side effects resolved without treatment and rarely required discontinuation of the medication. The cream is applied to the face twice daily. The patients' hirsutism returned to baseline by 8 weeks following discontinuation of the medication.

6. **Cosmetic measures**

(a) Bleaching, shaving, plucking, waxing, depilating, and electrolysis are effective measures that can be used alone or in combination with the above treatments. They remove terminal hair that is already present while the patient waits for medications to decrease new growth and rate of transformation to terminal hair.

(b) Laser-assisted hair removal is an effective treatment for hirsutism. It is an outpatient procedure that uses either a ruby or YAG laser, both of which cause thermal injury to the hair follicle. The ruby laser is targeted directly at the hair follicle. The YAG laser requires a pretreatment application of a mineral oil lotion containing carbon particles to the target area. Both techniques result in removal of hair, and a period of 2–6 months before the regrowth of hair, which is thinner and lighter. The side effects include minimal discomfort, local edema and erythema lasting 24–48 hours, rare petechiae, and infrequent hyperpigmentation lasting less than 6 months.

(c) Because weight loss effectively decreases androgens and increases SHBG in obese women, a weight reduction diet should be recommended in overweight patients.

In summary, most patients are given a trial of OCPs, with or without spironolactone, and are advised to use cosmetic measures while waiting for the medications to work. The new topical cream, eflornithine HCl, may be used alone or in combination with cosmetic measures. Eflornithine could also be used with OCPs and spironolactone, but there are no trials with these combinations yet. Because of their more serious side effects and high cost, the other medications are reserved for the most severe cases in which OCPs and spironolactone fail. Unfortunately, most patients will have a relapse of hirsutism approximately 12 months after discontinuation of medical therapy.

BIBLIOGRAPHY

1. Conn J, Jacobs H: Managing hirsutism in gynaecological practice. Br J Obstet Gynaecol 105: 687–96, 1998.
2. Dunaif A: Hyperandrogenic anovulation (PCOS): A unique disorder of insulin action associated with an increased risk of non-insulin-dependent diabetes mellitus. Am J Med 98 (1A): 33S–39S, 1995.
3. Erenus M, Yucelten D, Gurbuz O, et al: Comparison of spironolactone–oral contraceptive versus cyproterone acetate–estrogen regimens in the treatment of hirsutism. Fertil Steril 66:216–219, 1996.
4. Fruzzetti F, Bersi C, Parrini D, et al: Treatment of hirsutism: Comparisons between different antiandrogens with central and peripheral effects. Fertil Steril 71:445-451, 1999.
5. Heiner JS, Greendale GA, Kawakami AK, et al: Comparison of gonadotropin-releasing hormone agonist and a low dose oral contraceptive given alone or together in the treatment of hirsutism. J Clin Endocrinol Metab 80:3412–3418, 1995.
6. Schrode K, Huber F, Staszak J, et al: Randomized, double-blind, vehicle-controlled safety and efficacy evaluation of eflornithine 15% cream in the treatment of women with excessive facial hair. Am Acad Derm Annual Meeting, Abstract P291, 2000.
7. Speroff L, Glass R, Kase N: Clinical Gynecologic Endocrinology and Infertility, 6th ed. Baltimore, Lippincott Williams & Wilkins, 1999.
8. Venturoli S, Marescalchi O, Colombo F, et al: A prospective randomized trial comparing low dose flutamide, finasteride, ketoconazole, and cyproterone acetate–estrogen regimens in the treatment of hirsutism. J Clin Endocrinol Metab 84:1304-1310, 1999.
9. Wheeland RG: Laser-assisted hair removal. Derm Clin 15:469–477, 1997.
10. Yen S, Jaffe R: Reproductive Endocrinology, 4th ed. Philadelphia, WB Saunders, 1999.

51. INFERTILITY

Robert E. Jones, M.D.

1. What is the definition of infertility?

Unprotected sexual intercourse without conception for at least 1 year. One half of normally fertile couples conceive by 3 months, three quarters by 6 months, and 90% by 1 year. Thus, the normal fecundity rate (frequency of pregnancy in 1 month) is 20%; in other words, the chance of fertility with each ovulation is at best 20%.

2. How common is infertility?

Approximately 10–15% of married couples are unable to conceive. The contributions of male and female factors are roughly equal. Population studies have documented that 8–9% of women of childbearing age are unable to become pregnant, and a similar percentage of men are unable to father a child. Roughly, one half of the infertile women have primary infertility (no previous delivery), and one half have secondary infertility (previous delivery).

3. Describe the initial evaluation of the infertile couple.

The initial evaluation for the woman should consist of a history, physical examination, and laboratory evaluation, including a blood count, urinalysis, fasting glucose level, and Papanicolaou smear. The man should have several semen analyses. Ovulation may be documented by serial measurement of basal body temperatures or by measurement of serum or urine levels of progesterone 7–8 days after the midcycle (ovulation) temperature rise or 21 days after the beginning of menstrual flow. A postcoital test (PCT) is performed at the expected time of ovulation to look for possible cervical or immunologic causes of infertility. A PCT entails the evaluation of a specimen of cervical mucus obtained from the fornix within 2 hours of sexual intercourse. Any abnormality identified at this point must be pursued before more invasive tests are performed. If the above evaluation is normal, hysterosalpingography should be performed to determine tubal patency and to visualize uterine anatomy. Laparoscopy may be required to evaluate other pelvic causes. Further evaluation of the man is discussed in questions 12–20.

Infertility Tests

TEST	EVALUATES
CBC, UA, FBS, Pap smear	Maternal health
Semen analysis	Male factor
Menstrual history, BBT, LPP	Ovulation
Postcoital test	Cervical factor
Hysterosalpingogram	Tubal patency, anatomy of uterus
Laparoscopy	Pelvic factor

CVC = complete blood count, UA = urinalysis, FBS = fasting blood sugar, BBT = basal body temperature, LPP = luteal phase progesterone level.

4. What are the common causes of infertility?

Common Causes of Infertility

CAUSE OF INFERTILITY	FREQUENCY (%)
Male factor	30–40
Pelvic factor	30–40
Anovulation	10–15
Cervical factor	10–15

5. What is the initial laboratory evaluation for the patient with secondary amenorrhea or oligomenorrhea?

The most common cause of secondary amenorrhea in a woman of reproductive age is pregnancy. A timely serum or urine pregnancy may prevent embarrassment on the physician's part. Hyperprolactinemia and hypothyroidism are relatively common, potentially remediable causes of menstrual dysfunction; therefore, assessment of basal levels of thyroid-stimulating hormone (TSH) and prolactin is essential. Follicle-stimulating hormone (FSH) provides a prognosis for future fertility, because levels greater than 30 mIU/mL indicate probable menopause. If the above laboratory values are normal, it is reasonable to continue the evaluation by obtaining serum levels of testosterone, dehydroepiandrosterine sulfate (DHEAS), luteinizing hormone (LH), and 17-hydroxyprogesterone (drawn during the follicular phase if the patient is not amenorrheic) to evaluate for neoplasm, polycystic ovarian syndrome, or congenital adrenal hyperplasia. Such conditions, of course, may be suspected earlier in the evaluation on the basis of historical facts or evidence of androgenization on physical examination.

6. How does clomiphene stimulate ovulation?

Clomiphene citrate (Clomid) is usually considered an estrogen antagonist, but it also has weak estrogenic activity. By competing with estrogen for receptor sites in the hypothalamus, clomiphene prevents the normal feedback inhibition of estrogen on release of gonadotropin-releasing hormone (GnRH). The resulting increase in GnRH pulses stimulates an increase in LH and FSH pulses, which in turn stimulates recruitment of ovarian follicles and ovulation.

7. Are any other treatments available to a woman with polycystic ovarian syndrome (PCOS) who fails to ovulate on clomiphene?

In more than 80% of women with PCOS, insulin resistance has been implicated in the pathogenesis of their condition. Hyperinsulinemia directly stimulates the ovarian production of testosterone and suppresses the hepatic production of sex hormone binding globulin, thereby increasing circulating levels of bioavailable (or free) testosterone. Elegant short-term studies have shown that either suppression of insulin production or a reduction of tissue resistance to insulin ameliorates many clinical and biochemical features of PCOS including anovulation. Both metformin and thiazolidinediones have been effective in reducing insulin resistance in these women; however, metformin is considered to be the preferred agent if fertility is the clinical goal. Metformin may be used by itself, or it can be used in conjunction with clomiphene to assist in restoring ovulation.

8. How are human menopausal gonadotropin and human chlorionic gonadotropin used to stimulate ovulation?

Human menopausal gonadotropin (hMG) is purified LH and FSH extracted from the urine of postmenopausal women. An individualized injection schedule is given to stimulate follicle development. The dose and frequency are based on close monitoring of either serum or urine levels of estrogen and ovarian ultrasound When a mature follicle is visualized ultrasonically, hMG infections are halted, and human chorionic gonadotropin (hCG) is used to stimulate ovulation. An additional injection of hCG is usually given in approximately 7 days to maintain the corpus luteum.

9. Are twins more common with ovulation stimulation?

The normal frequency of multiple pregnancies is about 1%. Ovulation stimulation with either hMG or clomiphene results in increased frequencies of multiple gestations. The data for multiple gestations in over 2,000 pregnancies with clomiphene are 92% singletons, 7% twins, 0.5% triplets, 0.3% quadruplets, and 0.1% quintplets. The frequency of birth defects, spontaneous abortion, and ectopic pregnancy with clomiphene is the same as in the normal population. The frequency of spontaneous abortion after use of hMG is about 20–30% compared with 19% in the general population.

10. Are complications other than multiple gestations associated with the use of gonadotropins?
   On rare occasions patients who receive gonadotropins develop ascites, multiple ovarian cysts, and shock. To prevent this condition, called ovarian hyperstimulation syndrome, close monitoring is required in all patients.

11. Describe the most commonly performed assisted reproduction techniques.
   In vitro fertilization (IVF) intracytoplasmic sperm injection (ICSI), gamete intrafallopian transfer (GIFT), and intrauterine insemination are currently practiced assisted reproduction techniques. In IVF, ICSI, GIFT, and, frequently, intrauterine insemination, the mother undergoes ovulation induction with gonadotropins. The father's semen sample is collected and washed.
   IVF entails fertilization by incubation of the sperm and ova before implantation in the uterus. ICSI is a variation of IVF in which fertilization is achieved by injection of a single sperm into the cytoplasm of each harvested ovum. The procedure of GIFT consists of injection of the harvested eggs and sperm into the fallopian tube. During intrauterine insemination, sperm is injected into the uterus, usually after ovulation induction. Pregnancy rates of each of these techniques are reported to be about 20% per induced cycle. There have not been sufficiently large randomized, controlled studies to determine which technique is superior.

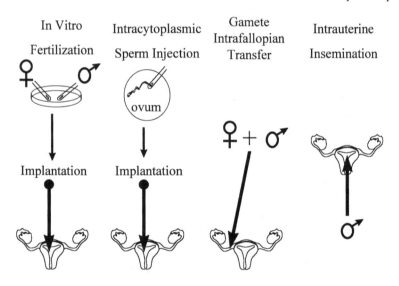

Assisted reproduction procedures.

12. How many semen samples are adequate to assess a man for fertility potential?
   Semen quality may vary widely on a day-to-day as well as a seasonal basis. Consequently, a minimum of two samples obtained within a 3-month period is required. If the results are disparate, additional samples should be collected.

13. How should a semen sample be obtained?
   Sexual abstinence for 48–72 hr but no longer than 7 days is necessary to ensure a representative volume of ejaculate without the complicating factor of necrospermia from autolysis. Masturbation is the preferred method for collection, but nonspermicidal condoms also

can be used to collect semen during intercourse. No matter how it is obtained, the entire sample must be submitted for analysis. Incomplete ejaculates should be discarded.

14. What may cause a transient reduction in semen quality?

Dramatic reductions in sperm concentration or motility may be observed during any febrile illness or during times of intense physiologic stress (e.g., strenuous physical exercise and high environmental temperatures). It may take as long as 3 months after resolution of the condition before semen parameters return to baseline.

15. What are the normal parameters for a semen analysis?

The World Health Organization offers the following criteria as representative of a normal ejaculate:

Criteria for Normal Semen Ejaculate

CRITERION	VALUE
Sperm concentration	$> 20 \times 10^6$ spermatozoa/ml
Total sperm in ejaculate	$> 40 \times 10^6$ spermatozoa/ejaculate
Motility	$> 50\%$ of sperm with forward progression
Morphology	$> 30\%$ with normal, oval forms
White blood cells	$< 1 \times 10^6$ WBC/mL

WBC = white blood cell.

16. Discuss the common causes of falsely low motility.

Asthenospermia or reduced sperm motility may result either from a primary disorder, such as Kartagener syndrome or the presence of immobilizing sperm antibodies, or from improper collection and handling of the specimen. An excessive delay in delivery of the sample to the laboratory or a delay in examination may result in a loss of sperm viability. The time between ejaculation and delivery must be as short as possible (<1 hr), and the sample must be analyzed within 30 minutes of liquefaction. Standard condoms are coated with spermicidal lubricants designed to immobilize sperm. Coitus interruptus is also unacceptable, because incomplete collections are common and the sample is frequently contaminated with vaginal secretions or bacteria that may impair motility. soaps or other lubricants may also be spermicidal and must be avoided. Lastly, care must be taken in the selection of the container. Because some plastics are spermicidal, a wide-mouthed sterile glass container is usually preferred.

17. What are the common causes of male infertility?

In an infertile but otherwise healthy man, the cause of infertility is usually not identified. Approximately one third of infertile men have a varicocele. A history of cryptorchidism, orchitis, or significant trauma is obtained in less than 15% of infertile men, and ductal obstruction occurs in less than 5%. Less common causes incude Klinefelter syndrome, Kallmann syndrome, or a history of chemotherapy or radiation therapy. Any systemic illness may temporarily reduce a man's fertility potential.

18. What are the reproductive consequences of a varicocele?

A varicocele is a palpable dilation or venous engorgement of the pampiniform plexus. It is the most frequent cause of potentially remediable infertility in men; however, not all men with varicoceles have primary infertility or any evidence of testicular dysfunction. The relationship between the presence of a varicocele and infertility is poorly understood. Recent studies have suggested that varicoceles may be implicated in secondary infertility. The clinical manifestations of a varicocele are reduced sperm number, diminished motility, and reduction in the percentage of normal oval spermatozoa. On occasion, a significant number of large, immature spermatozoa may be observed. This constellation of findings is sometimes called a "stress pattern" and usually portends a poorer prognosis for fertility. Men with varicoceles have other evidence of Sertoli cell impairment, including lower inhibin levels, higher basal FSH values, and an enhanced FSH response to GnRH.

19. How is azoospermia evaluated?

If the patient lacks evidence of Klinefelter syndrome, levels of seminal fluid fructose and serum FSH should be assessed. The finding of normal fructose levels verifies the presence of the seminal vesicles and excludes congenital absence of the vasa deferentia or the rare phenomenon of ejaculatory duct obstruction. If the FSH level is more than one and a half times the upper limit of normal, further evaluation is not warranted because of the high likelihood of severe, irreparable damage to seminiferous tubules. Otherwise, a vasogram to assess patency of the ejaculatory echanism and a testicular biopsy to evaluate spermatogensis are indicated.

20. How is male infertility treated?

Various regimens, including testosterone rebound, clomiphene, and bromocriptine, have been used to treat male infertility. Unfortunately, such empirical forms of therapy have not been demonstrated to be any more effective than nontreatment. As a result, the management of male infertility is frustrating for both physician and patient. The assisted reproductive technique of intracytoplasmic sperm injection shows great promise for the treatment of male infertility because only a single normal sperm is required to achieve fertilization. Two conditions, hypogonadotropic hypogonadism (Kallmann syndrome) and varicocele, merit special discussion, because treatment may enhance fertility potential in afflicted men. The use of pulsatile GnRH analogs or gonadotropins has been demonstrated to restore spermatogenesis in men with Kallmann syndrome. The effectiveness of varicocele repair by high ligation of the spermatic vein is more controversial, but most andrologists recommend the procedure because of its low morbidity and potential for great reward

21. What is the prognosis for conception in a couple seeking medical intervention?

Successful pregnancy varies with the reason for infertility. If anovulation is the cause, medical induction of ovulations results in an 80–90% chance of conception. If the female factor is not anovulation, a 30% chance of pregnancy is expected. Male factor infertility carries a poorer prognosis, but approximately 40% of men classified as infertile can ultimately father a child.

BIBLIOGRAPHY

1. Aksel S: Immunologic aspects of reproductive diseases. JAMA 268:2930–2934, 1992.
2. Dawood MY: In vitro fertilization, gamete intrafallopian transfer, and superovulation with intrauterine insemination: Efficacy and potential health hazards on babies delivered. Am J Obstet Gynecol 174:1208–1217, 1996.
3. Gilbaugh JH III, Lipshultz LI: Nonsurgical treatment of male infertility. Urol Clin North Am 21: 531–548, 1994.
4. Healy DL, Trounson AO, Andersen AN: Female infertility: Causes and treatment. Lancet 343: 1539–1544, 1994.
5. Howards SS: Treatment of male infertility. N Engl J Med 332:312–317, 1995.
6. Krysiewicz S: Infertility in women: Diagnostic evaluation with hysterosalpingography and other imaging techniques. AJR 159:253–261, 1992.
7. Nestler JE, Jakubowicz DJ, Evans WS, Pasquali R: Effects of metformin on spontaneous and clomiphene-induced ovulation in the polycystic ovary syndrome. N Engl J Med 338:1876–1880, 1998.
8. Schlegel PN, Girardi SK: In vitro fertilization for male factor infertility. J Clin Endocrinol Metab 82:709–716, 1997.
9. Silver SJ: Evaluation and treatment of male infertility. Clin Obstet Gynecol 43:854–888, 2000.
10. Skakkebaek NE, Giwercman A, de Kretser D: Pathogenesis and management of male infertility. Lancet 343:1473–1479, 1994.
11. Trantham P: The infertile couple. Am Fam Physician 54:1001–1010, 1996.

52. MENOPAUSE

William J. Georgitis, M.D., FACP

1. Define menopause.
Menopause represents the cessation of cyclic ovarian function. It encompasses approximately one third of a woman's life and spans the transition from the reproductive years to the final menstruation and then extends for the remainder of life. The final menstruation marks menopause for each woman. It can, by definition, be established only retrospectively.

2. When do ovulatory cycles decrease in frequency?
Ovulatory cycles usually decrease in frequency around age 38–42 years.

3. When does menopause usually occur?
The median age for the last menses is 51.4 years. The range for menopause is broad, but 90% of women cease menstruating by age 55.

4. What determines the timing of menopause?
Menses stop when the ovarian supply of oocytes is exhausted. The oocyte population peaks in utero with a subsequent loss of 80% of oocytes by birth. It is a curious fact that many more ovarian follicles vanish through atresia than by ovulation.

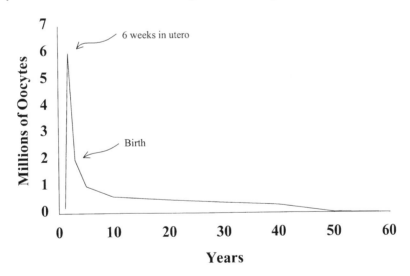

5. What is premature ovarian failure? What causes it?
Cessation of cyclic ovarian function before age 30 or 35 years is considered premature. It is attributed to either an inadequate complement of follicles from birth or accelerated attrition of follicles. Causes of premature ovarian failure include mumps oophoritis, irradiation, chemotherapy, autoimmune destruction, and genetic defects. The incidence of premature ovarian failure in women in the U.S. is about 0.3%, with approximately 146,000 cases projected for the year 2000.

6. Does the age of menopause vary with race, body size, age of menarche, geography, or socioeconomic conditions?

No. Evidence is currently sparse, but it is known that menopause occurs about 2 years earlier in cigarette smokers and that nulliparous women tend to experience an earlier menopause than multiparous women. More studies are being conducted to investigate these other potentially important factors.

7. Does the appearance of the ovaries change with menopause?

The menopausal ovary shrinks and its surface becomes wrinkled. A recent cross-sectional study employing transvaginal ultrasound in 58,673 women found the mean ovarian volume was 4.9 cm^3 in premenopausal women and 2.2 cm^3 in postmenopausal women. Cortical width diminishes, whereas interstitial and hilar cells become more prominent, giving the appearance of hyperplastic stroma.

8. What is the predominant circulating estrogen in menopause?

Estradiol is the most abundant serum estrogen during the reproductive years. In menopause, the biologically weaker hormone, estrone, becomes the principal estrogen. Estrone is predominantly derived from adipose tissue conversion of the adrenal androgen, androstenedione.

9. What is a hot flash? Or should it be called a flush?

These terms refer to menopausal spells lasting seconds to minutes or rarely as long as an hour. Symptoms include a sudden reddening of the skin accompanied by a warm sensation. In some women, this is followed by profuse sweating. Body surface temperature rises while core temperature falls; this is mediated by hypothalamic-directed, vasomotor dilation of surface blood vessels. The physiology of the flush or flash is complex and involves changes in catecholamines, prostaglandins, endorphins, and other neuropeptides.

Both expressions, flash and flush, appear in the medical literature. Each is appropriately descriptive. Flush aptly emphasizes vasodilation, whereas flash signifies the abrupt onset and brief duration. Many menopausal women also describe prodromal auras.

10. Hot flushes are accompanied by surges in luteinizing hormone. Does excess LH cause the spells?

No. The LH surge is an epiphenomenon. Hypophysectomized women lacking LH pulsatility still may experience menopausal hot flushes. Furthermore, women with gonadal dysgenesis have highly elevated levels of gonadotropins but fail to manifest hot flushes until after estrogen treatment and subsequent withdrawal. The hypothalamus appears to require priming with estrogens first before later demonstrating a response to estrogen deficiency with episodic vasomotor events.

11. Do all women develop menopausal vasomotor hot flushes? Do they last indefinitely?

About 85% of women experience vasomotor symptoms. The rate of change in estrogen levels seems to partly explain their severity. Women with abrupt declines in estrogen levels following ovariectomy are often bothered the most. Left untreated, hot flushes tend to diminish after 2–5 years.

12. Do any menopausal symptoms have an uncertain relation to estrogen?

Yes. A partial list of symptoms includes fatigue, nervousness, headaches, insomnia, depression, irritability, joint pain, muscle pain, dizziness, palpitations, and formication. Formication is a paresthesia resembling the sensation of ants crawling over the skin.

13. What important physiologic changes accompany menopause?

Hot flushes, urogenital atrophy, loss of bone calcium, increased rates of coronary heart disease, and alterations in serum lipids, including rises in LDL cholesterol and triglycerides with declines in HDL cholesterol, occur during menopause.

14. What is the principal cause of death in postmenopausal women?

Cardiovascular disease. One in two women will die of heart disease or stroke, whereas only one in twenty-five will die of breast cancer.

15. Does male menopause exist?

Not really. Although hypogonadal men may suffer spells and accelerated loss of bone mineral similar to hypogonadal women, such symptoms do not represent a physiologically programmed event. A man complaining of hot flushes should prompt testing to confirm hypogonadism first followed by an investigation for the cause.

16. Historical records indicate the age of menarche has decreased over the centuries, perhaps as a result of improved nutrition and general health. Is this also true for the timing of menopause?

No. While the average age for first menstruation may have become lower as a result of improved nutrition and general health, a downward shift in the average age of menopause has not been recorded. Perhaps ongoing studies will confirm such changes in the future.

17. How does one establish a diagnosis of menopause?

In a woman older than 45 years with secondary amenorrhea of 12 months' duration, historical evidence alone suggests a diagnosis of menopause. Pelvic examination may or may not help confirm the impression by showing signs of vaginal atrophy.

Laboratory tests alone are not reliable for diagnosis. Toward the end of a woman's fertile years, serum levels of follicle-stimulating hormone (FSH) gradually rise. Anovulatory periods occur and may be accompanied by menorrhagia. Once amenorrhea is well established, gonadotropins may become tonically elevated. FSH rises 10–20-fold, while elevations in LH of 3-fold are more moderate. Levels of FSH above 40 IU/L are generally considered diagnostic of ovarian failure. However, hot flashes and gondatropin elevations may be prevented by obesity, and, on the other end of the spectrum, elevated gonadotropin levels alone may be misleading because LH and FSH can reach menopausal range values during the midcycle surge just prior to ovulation.

18. What regimens of menopausal hormone replacement are in common use?

Numerous regimens are currently used for replacement. They vary by route of administration, composition of a variety of estrogens and progestogens, and by timing of administration of the various components. Too many permutations exist to discuss except in generality and by example.

ERT refers to estrogen replacement alone and HRT to hormone replacement with some combination or sequence of estrogen along with a progestogen. Routes of administration include oral, topical, and vaginal. Schemes for delivering the hormones include sequential dosing of estrogen and progestogen to mimic the normal hormone level variations through the menstrual cycle, continuous combined administration of estrogen and progestogen, and long cycle therapy in which the progestogen is administered a few times each year rather than on a repeating monthly schedule.

It is very difficult to determine which replacement regimen will be acceptable for each patient because individual tolerance varies unpredictably. Breast tenderness and bleeding of endometrial origin are commonly reported by postmenopausal women commencing replacement with any of the regimens. Although bleeding and mastalgia lessen over time, long-term compliance remains poor, perhaps owing to coexisting fear of breast cancer and thrombotic complications. There is at present no ideal treatment for women seeking replacement free from endometrial bleeding.

For those who have no endometrium, continuous daily replacement with estrogen alone is appropriate. Conjugated equine estrogens in daily doses ranging from 0.625 to 1.25 mg are commonly prescribed. Combination therapy with estrogen plus progesterone is prescribed for women who have not had hysterectomies in order to prevent endometrial hyperplasia and neoplasia, both of which increase in incidence with dose and duration of exposure to estrogen unopposed by progestogen. An example of a cyclic combination regimen is conjugated estrogens, 0.625–1.25 mg daily on days 1–25 of each month, and medroxyprogesterone acetate, 5–10 mg daily on days 13 through 25. During the last 5 days of the month, neither hormone is administered; withdrawal bleeding is common with this type of sequential therapy. An alternative approach is to use a continuous combination of conjugated estrogens, 0.625–1.25 mg, and medroxyprogesterone acetate, 2.5–5.0 mg, every day of the month. Oral estradiol 1–2 mg/day can be substituted for conjugated estrogens in any of the above regimens. Topical therapy with estradiol patches, applied as a 0.05–0.1 mg/day patch every 3 days or every 7 days, can also be used in either a cyclic or a continuous fashion. Again, spotting may occur with any therapy, including intravaginal estrogen alone. Persistent bleeding, especially early in the cycle of sequential therapy, may necessitate an endometrial biopsy. Intravaginal ultrasound and reliance on the timing of bleeding to assess risk of endometrial disease have proved to be unreliable.

19. What about testosterone replacement?

This issue remains controversial. In eugonadal women, circulating testosterone is roughly half ovarian and half adrenal in origin. Serum testosterone declines 50% in premenopausal women following bilateral oophorectomy compared with an 80% decline in serum estradiol.

Improvements in sexual function and psychosocial well-being were reported with topical testosterone replacement (patches) in a placebo-controlled dose response study of middle-aged women with surgical primary hypogonadism. Hot flushes averaged less than two per week at entry and were not affected by testosterone treatment. Adverse effects on lipids, acne, hirsutism, liver function, glucose, insulin, and blood counts were not seen, but serious study-related events, not all attributable to testosterone, occurred in 1 out of 15 subjects in the trial and 1 out of 16 women withdrew from the study. The number needed to treat (NTT) for any specified benefit in this study could not be derived. The placebo response was substantial, and, like prior short-term studies with testosterone implants or injections delivering excessive replacement doses, the long-term risk-benefit ratio of androgen replacement could not be determined and still requires additional investigation.

20. What are the most common indications for menopausal hormone replacement therapy?

The most common indications are for relief of vasomotor symptoms or symptoms associated with urogenital atrophy. For relief of these problems, short-term treatment may be sufficient and a commitment to chronic or life-long use may not be necessary.

21. What are the benefits?

Vasomotor symptoms improve, dyspareunia is reduced, and the frequency of cystitis may be decreased. Deaths attributable to cardiovascular disease in women each year now exceed those for men. Recent surveys show cardiovascular disease is underdiagnosed and receives less aggressive treatment in women than in men. Women have less favorable outcomes than men following myocardial infarction and even have higher complication rates with coronary revascularization. Whether hormone replacement therapy decreases the risk of vascular disease events, however, remains contentious. Reductions in LDL and increases in HDL cholesterol levels with hormone replacement therapy have been demonstrated in some, but not all, studies. Since lipid intervention trials with cardiovascular endpoints show greater benefit for women than men and since HMG-CoA reductase inhibitor therapy is clearly superior to hormone replacement therapy in causing favorable lipids changes, lipid lowering medications should be used when LDL treatment goals are not met by hormone replacement therapy alone.

There is less controversy about the beneficial effects of hormone replacement on the skeleton, where prevention of bone loss and reductions in the relative risk of osteoporosis associated fractures are substantial and clinically relevant. The suggestion that estrogen may affect the incidence and natural history of senile dementia deserves further investigation to determine the relevance of those observations in that debilitating disease.

22. What are the potential detrimental effects?

Estrogen administration is associated with small increases in the risk of several serious complications, and these risks rise with longer duration of hormone use. Estrogen treatment without the addition of a progestin increases the risk of endometrial hyperplasia or carcinoma 4–8 fold. In a reexamination of 51 studies comprised of 150,000 cases and controls, breast cancer risk was found to be increased 1.35-fold for women who had used hormone replacement for 5 years or more. The risk of venous thromboembolic events also increases about 3-fold with estrogen replacement. Progesterone, which markedly decreases the risk of endometrial carcinoma, can cause fluid retention and may also lower HDL and raise LDL cholesterol levels.

Long-term compliance is low with estrogen replacement therapy; up to 70% of women refuse it initially or discontinue it on their own accord. Only 30% of women for whom estrogen therapy is prescribed continue it for more than 3 years. Uterine bleeding, breast pain, fear of breast cancer, and thromboembolism, as well as the patient's recognition that treatment alternatives exist for osteoporosis and dyslipidemia, contribute to the poor adherence to treatment.

23. What about weight gain with hormone replacement therapy?

Although it is a common perception that hormone replacement causes weight gain, evidence suggests instead that menopause itself is associated with weight gain, in part attributed to reductions in the resting metabolic rate. In hormone treatment trials, untreated controls often gain as much weight as the hormone-treated groups. Furthermore, the distribution of body fat differs in that untreated control subjects tend to develop more androgenous obesity with increases in their waist to hip ratios. This form of obesity carries associations with insulin resistance, dyslipidemia, and hypertension.

24. Insomnia is a troublesome symptom. Does hormone replacement alter sleep?

Evidence from objective sleep laboratory studies suggests that estrogen replacement improves sleep quality, decreases the time to onset of sleep, and increases rapid eye movement (REM) sleep.

25. What levels of estradiol and estrone are achieved with replacement?

Oral conjugated equine estrogens (0.625 mg), micronized estradiol (1.0 mg), and estrone sulfate (1.25 mg) deliver peak estradiol levels of 30–40 pg/ml and peak estrone levels of 150–250 pg/ml. Intravaginal estrogens yield levels about one fourth those achieved with oral regimens.

26. Can gonadotropin levels be used to monitor adequacy of replacement?

No. Unlike primary hypothyroidism, in which the serum TSH can be used to individualize requirements for thyroxine replacement, gonadotropin levels remain elevated despite sex steroid replacement in many postmenopausal women. This elevation may result from a deficiency in inhibin, a polypeptide hormone normally produced by ovarian granulosa cells to inhibit secretion of FSH. Menopausal hormone replacement therapy must be gauged by the response in symptoms and signs, not by gonadotropin levels.

27. What alternative therapies may be used for the menopausal woman with contraindications for estrogen replacement?

Clonidine may be tried at bedtime for the relief of hot flushes, but hypotensive side effects may limit its use. Medroxyprogesterone in a daily pill or as a depot injection every 3 months also may relieve hot flushes. Herbal preparations and dietary supplements are not regulated by the FDA and safety and efficacy data are lacking. Widely used alternatives to prescribed hormones for hot flushes include black cohosh and soy, which have benefits attributed to phytoestrogens and side effects that have prompted regulatory agencies of some countries to recommend use for no longer than 6 months.

28. What web sites might you recommend to patients who seek information about menopause?

Two places to start include acog.org and menopause.org, representing the American College of Obstetricians and Gynecologists and the North American Menopause Society, respectively.

BIBLIOGRAPHY

1. Amundsen, DW, Diers CJ: The age of menopause in medieval Europe. Hum Biol 45:605–612, 1973.
2. Daly E, Gray A, Barlow D, et al: Measuring the impact of menopausal symptoms on the quality of life. BMJ 307:836–840, 1993.
3. Doren M: Hormonal replacement regimens and bleeding. Maturitas 34: Suppl 1 S17–S23, 2000.
4. McKinlay SM, Brambilla DJ, Posner JG: The normal menopause transition. Maturitas 14: 103–115, 1992.
5. Pavlik EJ, DePriest PD, Gallion HH, et al: Ovarian volume related to age. Gynecol Oncol 77: 410–412, 2000.
6. Schiff I, Regesein Q, Tulchinsky D, Ryan KJ: Effect of estrogens on sleep and psychological state of hypogonadal women. JAMA 242:2405–2407, 1979.
7. Shifren JL, Braunstein GD, Simon JA, et al: Transdermal testosterone treatment in women with impaired sexual function after oophorectomy. N Engl J Med 343:682–688, 2000.
8. Stamm WE, Raz Raul: Factors contributing to susceptibility of postmenopausal women to recurrent urinary tract infections. Clin Infect Dis 28:723–725, 1999.
9. Walsh BW, Schiff I, Rosner B, et al: Effects of postmenopausal estrogen replacement on the concentrations and metabolism of plasma lipoproteins. N Engl J Med 323:1196–1204, 1990.
10. Wenger NK: Lipid management and control of other coronary risk factors in the postmenopausal woman. J Women's Health Gend Based Med 9:234-243, 2000.

53. USE AND ABUSE OF ANABOLIC-ANDROGENIC STEROIDS

Rodney J. Sparks, M.D., and Homer J. LeMar, Jr., M.D.

1. What are anabolic-androgenic steroids (AASs)?

AASs are a group of steroid hormones derived from chemical modification of testosterone. Their name is often shortened to anabolic steroids. The term *anabolic* refers to their ability to promote positive nitrogen balance and accretion of lean body mass. *Androgenic* refers to masculinization induced by these hormones. Although potency varies among different AASs, all possess both androgenic and anabolic properties.

2. What are some of the biologic effects of AASs?

Endogenous AASs have diverse effects. The most prominent are effects on male sexual differentiation and secondary sexual characteristics, including growth and development of the prostate, seminal vesicles, penis and scrotum, beard, pubic, chest, and axillary hair; thickening of the vocal cords' and enlargement of the larynx. AASs promote nitrogen retention, increase lean body mass, and alter fat distribution. They increase sebum production and acne. They also stimulate hepatic synthesis of clotting factors and renal synthesis of erythropoietin (EPO) with a secondary increase in hematocrit. They may play a role in the development and maintenance of bone mass in men and contribute to the lower HDL and higher LDL cholesterol levels in men compared with women.

3. How do AASs exert their effects?

AASs act by binding to a specific receptor known as the androgen receptor. Both androgenic and anabolic effects appear to be mediated through the same receptor. Androgen receptors are present in many tissues, including the reproductive organs, skeletal muscle, bone, kidney, and liver as well as the brain, cardiac muscle, skin, fat, hematopoietic tissue, larynx, and thymus. Testosterone may bind directly to the androgen receptor or be converted by 5-alpha-reductase to dihydrotestosterone, which binds to the receptor more tightly than does testosterone. Some testosterone is converted to estradiol by an enzyme in peripheral tissues called aromatase. Estradiol can then bind to the estrogen receptor.

4. Why and how is testosterone modified to make clinically useful AASs? What are the routes of administration?

When administered orally, testosterone is rapidly metabolized by the first-pass effect through the gut and liver. The first-pass effect prevents any significant rise in plasma testosterone levels with oral intake of unmodified testosterone. Intramuscular injection of unmodified testosterone is also not very useful because absorption is too rapid and duration of action is too short.

Alkylation of testosterone at the 17-alpha position confers resistance to hepatic metabolism and results in AASs that can be administered orally. Esterification of testosterone at the 17-B hydroxy position results in a hydrophobic molecule, which allows testosterone to be mixed with a fatty vehicle (sesame oil) and given by intramuscular injection. Absorption is delayed, and the duration of action is prolonged sufficiently for therapeutic use. Testosterone is now also available in patch and gel forms that are applied to the skin, allowing testosterone to be absorbed transdermally. Sublingual and sustained-release preparations are under investigation. The following table lists some AASs available in the United States.

Anabolic-Androgenic Steroids Available in the United States

ANABOLIC-ANDROGENIC STEROID	USE
Parenteral agents	
Testosterone cypionate	Male hypogonadism
Testosterone enanthate	Male hypogonadism; delayed puberty; metastatic breast cancer (skeletal) 1–5 yr after menopause
Testosterone propionate	Male hypogonadism; delayed puberty
Transdermal testosterone patches	Male hypogonadism; delayed puberty
Transdermal testosterone gel	Male hypogonadism; delayed puberty
Oral agents (17-alpha-methylated)	
Methyl testosterone	Male hypogonadism; combined with estrogen for menopausal vasomotor symptoms; metastatic breast cancer (skeletal) 1–5 yr after menopause; delayed puberty
Oxandrolone	Promotes weight gain after extensive surgery, trauma, chronic infections, prolonged corticosteroid therapy; bone pain in osteoporosis
Stanozolol	Hereditary angioedema
Danazol	Endometriosis; fibrocystic breast disease; hereditary angioedema
Fluoxymesterone	Male hypogonadism; delayed puberty; androgen-responsive breast cancer (recurrent) 1–5 yr after menopause

5. What are the indications for AAS therapy?

AASs are indicated for use in male hypogonadism, constitutional delay of growth and puberty, hereditary angioneurotic edema, endometriosis, and fibrocystic breast disease; they also can benefit patients with aplastic or hypoplastic anemias. AASs are available in low doses combined with estrogens for the treatment of postmenopausal vasomotor symptoms. An oral AAS, oxandrolone, has been approved for promoting weight gain in patients with extensive surgery, severe trauma, chronic infections, and prolonged therapy with corticosteroids. AASs also may be used in selected women with metastatic (skeletal) breast cancer. Androgens are useful in the anemia of end-stage renal disease but have been largely replaced by recombinant erythropoietin. Indications of specific agents are listed in the table in question 4.

6. Are there any other potential uses for AASs?

AASs may help elderly men by increasing body weight and muscle mass, preventing bone loss, and improving the hematocrit. They also may be useful as male contraceptives. Both areas are under investigation. AASs are potentially useful in many other disorders, including severe chronic obstructive pulmonary disease and other wasting syndromes, autoimmune disorders, other hematologic disorders, alcoholic hepatitis, Turner syndrome (by improving height), and osteoporosis.

7. Which of the indications in question 5 is the most common use of AASs?

Most likely none. The illegal use of AASs to enhance sports performance or physical appearance probably represents the single most common use. Abuse is widespread based on the belief that their anabolic properties will enhance the response to physical training, especially weight training.

8. How common is abuse of AASs?

The true prevalence of AAS abuse is not known. An estimated 2–3 million American athletes have used AASs. Fifty to 80% of body builders, weight lifters, and power lifters may use AASs. Use is probably highest among body builders and participants in sports favoring larger and/or stronger athletes, but it is not limited to these sports. Because AASs increase the hematocrit via enhanced erythropoietin production, even athletes participating in endurance-oriented sports may try them. Nonathletes have used AASs solely to improve appearance. Surveys have revealed a 5–11% prevalence of use among high school students. Most users are men, but women also use AASs. Androgen sales have increased 20–30% per year in the U.S., and illicit use is likely to account for a significant portion.

9. Do AASs truly help athletes? How?

Both athletes and coaches are likely to answer unequivocally, "Yes." AASs used in conjunction with adequate protein and carbohydrate intake and proper training in experienced athletes seem to induce greater and more rapid gains than training and diet alone. In the past, studies were unable to show consistent gains in size and strength from AAS use in eugonadal men, largely because of design flaws and failure to control for confounding variables. However, a recent study comparing supraphysiologic doses of testosterone enanthate with placebo in eugonadal men found clear increases in muscle size and strength, with or without weight-training exercise. This study proves that AASs enhance size and strength and may lead to improved performance in some sports. Proposed mechanisms for increased size and strength include the anabolic effects of increased nitrogen retention and protein synthesis, anti-catabolic effects of blocking cortisol at its receptor, and the psychologic effect of increased motivation.

10. What doses of AASs are used in attempts to enhance sports performance and appearance?

Doses used for illicit purposes are markedly higher (10-fold or more) than therapeutic doses. Furthermore, multiple agents are often used in so-called stacking regimens or arrays. The drugs are often taken in 6–12 week cycles with variable periods off the drugs, but some athletes may use them as long as 1 year or more. Regimens may be complex with escalating and tapering doses of multiple drugs, each entering the cycle at different times. Human chorionic gonadotropin may be used at the end of a cycle to stimulate gonadal function. Little is known about precise doses or stacking regimens, and they appear to vary widely. Some anecdotal information is available, and examples of doses are given in the table below in comparison with the usual therapeutic doses.

Comparison of Doses in Therapeutic Use vs. Abuse of Anabolic-Androgenic Steroids*

AAS	THERAPEUTIC DOSE	ABUSE
Testosterone cypionate	200 mg every 2 weeks	200–800 mg/week
Testosterone enanthate	200 mg every 2 weeks	200–800 mg/week
Oxandrolone	2.5 mg 2–4 times/day	2.5 up to 8 mg or more/day
Stanozolol	2 mg 3 times/day, then once daily on alternate days	8–12 mg/day

* The doses for abuse are estimates from anecdotal data and may vary considerably in individual users. Two to 5 or more AASs are often combined at these or higher doses, yielding even higher total doses.

11. How do athletes get AASs?

AASs may be smuggled into the U.S. from countries where they are easily purchased without prescription. Some physicians also may prescribe them, and some AASs may be obtained from veterinarians. A significant black market exists, in which some of the preparations are fraudulent and potentially dangerous.

12. What are the potential adverse effects of AAS use?

A wide range of side effects have occurred with AAS use and abuse. AASs may cause weight gain as a result of fluid retention and increased lean body mass. Reproductive effects in men include testicular atrophy, oligospermia or azoospermia, and priapism, especially in elderly men. These effects may occur with any AAS.

Adverse hepatic effects are seen predominantly with the 17-alkylated oral agents. Examples include cholestatic hepatitis, pelioses hepatis (hemorrhagic liver cysts), and both benign and malignant hepatic tumors.

Cardiovascular risks may be increased because of lipid profile changes induced by AASs. The most consistent observation has been a reduction of HDL cholesterol, which is also seen predominantly with the alkylated, orally administered AASs but has been reported with high doses of parenteral esters. Increases in platelet count and aggregation also may occur, and ventricular thrombosis and systemic embolism have been reported in the literature. Stroke and myocardial infarction have been reported in weight lifters using AASs. Behavioral changes also have been blamed on AAS abuse. Excessive aggressiveness ("roid rage"), psychotic symptoms, and dependence/withdrawal have been observed. Whether behavioral abnormalities are caused by or precede AAS use is debated. Behavioral changes have not been observed in all studies of AASs, even when supraphysiologic doses were used.

Other side effects include acne, gynecomastia from aromatization to estradiol, male pattern baldness, induction or exacerbation of sleep apnea, erythrocytosis, possible prostatic hypertrophy or carcinoma in elderly men, and thrombotic events with supraphysiologic doses. AASs also may change structural and biomechanical properties of tendons, resulting in increased risk of injury. Finally, needle sharing among users increases the risk of AIDS and hepatitis.

13. What about side effects in women and children?

All of the adverse effects mentioned above may occur in women and children. Women may experience oligomenorrhea or amenorrhea with inhibition of gonadotropin secretion. Such effects may reverse with cessation of AAS use. Virilizing effects, including hirsutism, clitoromegaly, and deepening of the voice, may not be reversible. Premature epiphyseal closure with a reduction in final adult height is an additional concern in adolescents using AASs.

14. Which AASs have the least potential to cause adverse effects?

All AASs can cause significant adverse effects. However, hepatic toxicity and lipid derangements are seen predominantly with the oral alkylated AASs. The parenteral esters, patches and gels are safer in these respects. An orally active ester, testosterone undecanoate, does not appear to have the liver toxicity of the alkylated AASs. It is not currently available in the United States.

15. What is being done to prevent AAS abuse?

1. Under Sections 351, 352, 353, and 355 of the Food, Drug, and Cosmetic Act. 21 USCA, these substances came under FDA regulation, requiring a prescription from a licensed physician. In 1988, legislation was added to provide for criminal prosecution. The Anabolic Steroids Control Act of 1990 made AAS schedule III controlled substances. Possession with an intent-to-sell constitutes a federal felony.

2. With regards to their use by athletes, routine and random drug screening has been implemented. As professional and serious amateur athletes spend vast amounts of energy, time, and resources in preparing for and competing in their sport, it is believed that the fear of being precluded from competition will serve as an effective deterrent.

16. Have testosterone precursors such as androstenedione been shown to raise serum testosterone levels?

These compounds are marketed and advertised to be metabolized to testosterone or other active metabolites. However, the current literature to substantiate these claims is sparse and the results are mixed.

BIBLIOGRAPHY

1. Bhasin S, Bremner WJ: Emerging issues in androgen replacement therapy. J Clin Endocrinol Metab 82:3–8, 1997.
2. Bhasin S, Storer TW, Berman N, et al: Testosterone replacement increases fat-free mass and muscle size in hypogonadal men. J Clin Endocrinol Metab 82:407–413, 1997.
3. Catlin DH: Anabolic steroids. In DeGroot LJ, et al (eds): Endocrinology, 3rd ed. Philadelphia, WB Saunders, 1995, pp 2362–2376.
4. Cooper CJ, Noakes TD, Dunne T, et al: A high prevalence of abnormal personality traits in chronic users of anabolic-androgenic steroids. Br J Sports Med 30:246–250, 1996.
5. Dickerman RD, McConathy WJ, Zachariah NY: Testosterone, sex-hormone binding globulin, lipoproteins, and vascular disease risk. J Cariovasc Risk 4(5-6):363–366, 1997.
6. DuRant RH, Escobedo LG, Heath GW: Anabolic-steroid use, strength training, and multiple drug use among adolescents in the United States. Pediatrics 96:23–28, 1995.
7. King DS, Sharp RL Brown GA, et al: Effect of oral androstenedione on serum testosterone and adaptations to resistance training in young men: A randomized controlled trial. JAMA 281(21): 2020–2028, 1999.
8. Kouri EM, Pope HG Jr, Oliva PS: Changes in lipoprotein-lipid levels in normal men following administration of increasing doses of testosterone cypionate. Clin J Sports Med 6:152–157, 1996.
9. Kouri EM, Lukas SE, Pope HG Jr, Olivas PS: Increased aggressive responding in male volunteers following the administration of gradually increasing doses of testosterone cypionate. Drug Alcohol Depend 40(1):73–79, 1995.
10. Leder BZ, Longcope C, Catlin DH, et al: Oral androstenedione administration and serum testosterone concentrations in young men. JAMA 283(6):779–782, 2000.
11. Mendenhall CL, Moritz TE, Roselle GA, et al: Protein energy malnutrition in severe alcoholic hepatitis: Diagnosis and response to treatment. The VA Cooperative Study Group. J Parenter Enter Nutr 19:258–265, 1995.
12. Nilsson KO, Albertsson-Wiklund K, Alm J, et al: Improved final height in girls with Turner's syndrome treated with growth hormone and oxandrolone. J Clin Endocrinol Metab 81:635–640, 1996.
13. Ozata M, Yildirimkaya M, Bulur M, et al: Effects of gonadotropin and testosterone treatments on lipoprotein (a), high density lipoprotein particles, and other lipoprotein levels in male hypogonadism. J Clin Endocrinol Metab 81:3372–3378, 1996.
14. Ravaglia G, Forti P, Maioli F, et al: Body composition, sex steroids, IGF-1, and bone mineral status in aging men. J Gerontol A Biol Sci Med Sci 55(9):m516–521, 2000.
15. Sambrook PN, Eisman JA: Osteoporosis prevention and treatment. Med J Aust 172(5):226–229, 2000.
16. Sands R, Studd J: Exogenous androgens in postmenopausal women. Am J Med 98:765–795, 1995.
17. Wallace MB, Lim J, Cutler A, Bucci L: Effects of dehydroepiandrosterone vs androstenedione supplementation in men. Med Sci Sports Exerc 31(12):1788–1792, 1999.
18. Wang C, Alexander G, Berman N, et al: Testosterone replacement therapy improves mood in hypogonadal men—a clinical research center study. J Clin Endocrinol Metab 81:3578–3583, 1996.
19. Zgliczynski S, Ossowski M, Slowinska-Srzednicka J, et al: Effect of testosterone replacement therapy on lipids and lipoproteins in hypogonadal and elderly men. Atherosclerosis 121:35–43, 1996.

VII. Miscellaneous

54. MULTIPLE ENDOCRINE NEOPLASIA

Arnold A. Asp, M.D.

1. What are the multiple endocrine neoplasia syndromes?

There are three well-characterized, inherited pluriglandular disorders in which several endocrine glands simultaneously undergo neoplastic transformation and become hyperfunctional. All of these disorders are genetically transmitted in an autosomal dominant fashion. Briefly, these disorders include:

MEN 1: Hyperplasia or neoplastic transformation of the parathyroids, pancreatic islets, and pituitary.

MEN 2A: Hyperplasia or neoplastic transformation of the thyroid parafollicular cells (medullary carcinoma of the thyroid), parathyroid glands, and adrenal medulla (pheochromocytoma).

MEN 2B: Hyperplasia or neoplastic transformation of the thyroid parafollicular cells (medullary carcinoma of the thyroid) and adrenal medulla (pheochromocytoma) with concomitant development of mucosal neuromas.

2. How can so many various endocrine organs be affected in these syndromes?

This question is a matter of controversy and ongoing research. The cells that comprise many endocrine organs are able to decarboxylate various amino acids and convert the molecules to amines or peptides that act as hormones or neurotransmitters. These cells have been classified as APUD cells (amine precursor uptake and decarboxylation) and are considered to be embryologically of neuroectodermal origin. APUD cells contain markers of their common neuroendocrine origin, including neuron-specific enolase and chromogranin A. Neoplastic transformation of APUD cells long after organogenesis is complete appears to be due to a germline mutation (loss of a tumor suppressor gene in MEN 1 or mutation of a protooncogene to an oncogene in MEN 2A and 2B) in a gene that is expressed only in neuroectodermal cells. When neuroectodermal cells later migrate to specific developing organs, the genetic mutation likewise is distributed to those organs. This may explain the eventual development of tumors in so many diverse tissues.

3. What is Wermer's syndrome?

This is the eponym for the MEN 1 syndrome. Wermer first recognized the association of parathyroid hyperplasia, multicentric pituitary tumors, and pancreatic islet cell tumors in several kindreds and described the syndrome in 1954. Wermer's syndrome is the most common form of MEN. It is characterized by a high degree of penetrance; expression increases with age. Prevalence of the disorder is estimated to vary between 2 and 20 per 100,000 population. Although neoplastic transformation occurs most commonly in the parathyroids, pituitary, and pancreas, hyperplastic adrenal cortical and nodular thyroid disorders have been described. Carcinoid tumors, especially involving the foregut (thymus, lung, stomach, and duodenum), are uncommon but also have been reported in the MEN 1 syndrome.

4. Is hyperparathyroidism in MEN 1 similar to sporadic primary hyperparathyroidism?

No. Hyperparathyroidism associated with MEN 1 results from hyperplasia of all four glands, whereas sporadic primary hyperparathyroidism usually is characterized by adenoma-

tous change in a single gland. Hyperparathyroidism is the most common and earliest manifestation of MEN 1, occurring in 80–95% of cases. It has been described in patients as young
as 17 years of age and will develop in nearly all patients with MEN 1 by the age of 40.

Hyperplasia of parathyroid glands affected by MEN 1 occurs as a result of expansion of
multiple cell clones, while sporadic parathyroid adenomas result from activation of a single
cell clone. Several groups have described a mitogenic factor (probably basic fibroblast
growth factor) in the sera of patients with MEN 1. This factor potentiates the hyperplastic
growth of parathyroid tissue. Complications of MEN 1 hyperparathyroidism are similar to
those of sporadic hyperparathyroidism; they include nephrolithiasis, osteoporosis, mental
status changes, and muscular weakness.

Therapy of both sporadic adenomas and MEN 1–associated hyperplastic glands
depends on surgical resection. In sporadic primary hyperparathyroidism, removal of the
solitary adenoma is curative in 95% of cases. In MEN 1–associated hyperplasia, at least 3½
hyperplastic glands must be resected to restore normocalcemia. Only 75% of patients are
normocalcemic postoperatively; 10–25% are rendered hypoparathyroid. Unfortunately, the
parathyroid remnants in the patient with MEN 1 have a great propensity to regenerate; 50%
of cases become hypercalcemic again within 10 years of surgery. This recurrence rate dic-
tates that surgery be delayed until complications of hypercalcemia are imminent or gastrin
levels are elevated, as discussed below.

5. What type of pancreatic tumors are found in MEN 1 syndrome?

Neoplastic transformation of the pancreatic islet cells is the second most common manifestation of MEN 1, occurring in approximately 66–80% of cases. Such tumors are usually
multicentric and are often capable of elaborating several peptides and biogenic amines.
They are, by convention, classified on the basis of the clinical syndrome produced by the
predominant secretory product. This group of tumors characteristically progresses from
hyperplasia to malignancy with metastases, making curative resection unlikely. Tumors of
the pancreas may arise from normal islet cells (eutopic) or cells that are not normal constituents of the adult pancreas (ectopic).

Gastrinomas are the most common pancreatic tumors in the MEN 1 syndrome (47–78%
of cases). They are ectopic tumors; G-cells are normally present in the fetal pancreas only.
Gastrinomas also may occur independently of MEN 1 (only 15–48% of all patients with a
gastrinoma are later found to have MEN 1). Gastrinomas associated with MEN 1 are multiple and often extra-pancreatic, occurring in the duodenal wall and retroperitoneal lymphatics. Excessive gastrin secretion by these tumors causes prolific production of gastric
acid with resultant duodenal and jejunal ulcers and diarrhea. Basal acid output exceeds 15
mmol/hr, and basal fasting serum gastrin levels usually exceed 300 pg/ml. Hypergastrinemia also may result from any condition that stimulates normal gastrin secretion (hypercalcemia) or that interferes with normal gastric acid production and feedback to the G-cells
(achlorhydria, gastric outlet obstruction, retained antrum with a Billroth II procedure, vagotomy, and the use of H_2 blockers and proton pump inhibitors). Hyperparathyroidism (see
question 4) can therefore falsely elevate serum gastrin levels. A secretin stimulation test may
aid in the differentiation of gastrinomas from other hypergastrinemic states; serum gastrin
levels in patients with gastrinomas increase by at least 200pg/ml.More information about gastrinomas is included in Chapter 56.

Insulinomas are the second most common pancreatic islet cell tumor in the MEN 1 syndrome (12–36% of islet cell tumors) and the most common eutopic type. Persistent or disordered insulin secretion causes severe hypoglycemia; inappropriately elevated concentrations of insulin, proinsulin, and C-peptide are present in the serum. Insulinomas associated
with MEN 1 syndrome are more frequently multicentric and malignant than are the sporadic
tumors. Approximately 1–5% of all patients with an insulinoma are eventually discovered

to have MEN 1. An excellent discussion of the diagnosis and therapy of insulinomas is found in Chapter 56.

Pancreatic tumors less frequently associated with MEN 1 include glucagonomas, somatostatinomas, and vasoactive intestinal polypeptide–secreting tumors (VIPomas). Associated syndromes and therapy are also described in Chapter 56.

6. How are the most common pancreatic tumors of MEN 1 treated?

Multicentric gastrinomas are rarely surgically cured (10–15% of cases). Fortunately, symptoms of hypergastrinemia can be pharmacologically controlled with H_2 blocker, proton-pump inhibitor, or octreotide administration. Metastases to the liver become increasingly common when gastrinomas exceed 3 cm in diameter, prompting most surgeons to reserve excision for tumors larger than 3 cm. Gastrinomas express surface receptors for somatostatin, potentiating the use of somatostatin-receptor scintigraphy in combination with annual MRI/CT surveillance to monitor tumor progression.

Insulinomas, unlike gastrinomas, produce devastating hypoglycemia, which is difficult to counteract medically. Without effective long-term pharmacotherapy, surgical resection of the tumor(s) is required in most patients. Fortunately, when the largest tumor is excised, many of the patient's symptoms are ameliorated. Localization is accomplished pre-operatively with endoscopic ultrasonography, MRI/CT, or by comparison of insulin levels in the right hepatic vein following selective infusion of the intrapancreatic arteries with calcium gluconate. Intraoperative ultrasonography may also assist precise localization at the time of surgery.

7. Which pituitary tumors are associated with MEN 1?

Pituitary tumors occur in 50–71% of cases of MEN 1. They may result either from neoplastic transformation of anterior pituitary cells with clonal expansion to a tumor or from excessive stimulation of the pituitary by ectopically produced hypothalamic releasing factors elaborated by carcinoids or pancreatic islet cells.

Prolactinomas are the most common pituitary tumors associated with MEN 1, constituting 60% of the total. The symptoms of hyperprolactinemia (galactorrhea and amenorrhea in women; impotence in men) are the third most common manifestation of MEN 1. The tumors are typically multicentric and large but respond to dopamine agonists such as bromocriptine. In earlier series, many pituitary tumors described as chromophobe adenomas were, in reality, prolactinomas that contained sparse poorly staining secretory granules. These tumors are also discussed in Chapter 21.

The second most commonly encountered pituitary tumor type is the growth hormone–producing tumor, which is reported in 10–25% of patients. Overproduction of growth hormone results in gigantism in children and acromegaly in adults. The tumors are often multicentric and may result from secretion of growth hormone–releasing hormone by pancreatic or carcinoid tumors. Diagnosis and therapy is described in Chapter 22.

Finally, corticotropin (ACTH)–producing tumors that cause Cushing's syndrome may be associated with MEN 1. Such tumors result from neoplastic transformation of the pituitary or elaboration of corticotropin-releasing hormone by pancreatic or carcinoid tumors. Diagnosis and therapy are described in Chapter 24.

8. What causes MEN 1?

The gene predisposing to the development of MEN 1 (MEN 1 susceptibility gene) is located on the long arm of chromosome 11 (11q13) and encodes a protein known as menin, which functions as a tumor suppressor. The proband inherits an allele predisposing to MEN 1 from the affected parent, whereas a normal allele is passed down from the unaffected parent. The gene for this tumor suppressor is unusually susceptible to mutation. When a somatic mutation later inactivates the normal allele, suppressor function is lost, permitting hyperplasia of the gland to occur.

9. How should a kindred be screened after the proband is identified?

Carriers of the genetic defect must first be identified, the extent of their organ involvement determined, and their family screened for additional carriers of the susceptibility gene. As mentioned above, mutations in the gene coding for the tumor suppressor, menin, are apparent in patients with MEN 1 and may be used to identify carriers of the disorder in the near future. Because mutational analysis using polymerase chain reaction techniques is currently restricted to research laboratories, periodic measurement of associated hormones is the next best alternative to detect disease within affected kindreds. Manifestations of MEN 1 syndrome rarely occur before the age of 15; therefore, individuals at risk should not undergo endocrine screening before that time. Nearly all individuals at risk develop the disorder by the age of 40 years; screening may be unnecessary in members older than 50 who are proved to be disease-free.

Because hyperparathyroidism is temporally the first manifestation of MEN 1 syndrome, serum calcium concentrations constitute the best screening test to identify asymptomatic carriers. Biochemical evidence of hyperparathyroidism in a member of a MEN 1 kindred establishes a presumptive carrier state. Evaluation then should focus on delineation of pancreatic and pituitary involvement. Serum levels of gastrin disclose the presence of a gastrinoma, whereas levels of prolactin most often reveal the presence of pituitary disease (especially in women). The latter two tests are cost-effective only in established disease and should not be used for preliminary screening of the kindred (unless symptoms of hypergastrinemia or prolactinoma are present). The frequency of screening has not been prospectively studied, but recommended intervals range from 2–5 years.

10. What is Sipple's syndrome?

This is the eponym for MEN 2A. In 1961, Sipple recognized and described a patient who expired with an intracerebral aneurysm and was found at autopsy to have medullary carcinoma of the thyroid (MCT), pheochromocytomas, and hyperparathyroidism. This disorder is inherited in an autosomal dominant fashion and exhibits a high degree of penetrance and variable expressivity. It is less common than MEN-1 syndrome.

11. Is the form of medullary carcinoma of the thyroid (MCT) associated with MEN 2A similar to the sporadic form of MCT?

No. MCT results from malignant transformation of the parafollicular cells (or C cells) that normally elaborate calcitonin and are scattered throughout the gland. MCT comprises 2–10% of all thyroid malignancies. The sporadic form of MCT, as described in Chapter 38, is more common (75% of all MCT), occurs in a solitary form (< 20% multicentric), and metastasizes to local lymphatics, liver, bone, and lung early in the course of disease (metastasis may occur with primary tumors less than 1 cm in diameter). Sporadic MCT occurs more commonly in an older population (peak age: 40–60 years) and is usually located in the upper two thirds of the gland.

MCT associated with MEN 2A, on the other hand, is multicentric (90% at the time of diagnosis), occurs at a younger age (as young as 2 years of age), but generally has a better prognosis than the sporadic form. MCT occurs in nearly 95% of all cases of MEN 2A and is usually the first tumor to appear. Calcitonin or other peptides elaborated by the tumor may cause a secretory diarrhea that is present in 4–7% of patients at the time of diagnosis, but develops in 25–30% during the course of the disease. Parafollicular cells in patients with MEN 2A characteristically progress through a state of C-cell hyperplasia to nodular hyperplasia to malignant degeneration over a variable period. It is imperative that patients at risk be diagnosed while still in the C-cell hyperplasia stage; total thyroidectomy will preclude malignant degeneration and metastases. Detection of C-cell hyperplasia is facilitated by the pentagastrin stimulation test. MCT also expresses peptides and hormones not commonly elaborated by parafollicular cells, including somatostatin, thyrotropin-releasing hormone, vasoactive intestinal peptide, proopiomelanocortin, carcinoembryonic antigen, and neurotensin.

12. If MCT is the most common neoplasm associated with MEN 2A, what is the second most common neoplasm?

Pheochromocytomas occur in 50–70% of cases of MEN 2A and are bilateral in up to 84% of patients. Compared with the sporadic form, pheochromocytomas associated with MEN 2A secrete greater amounts of epinephrine. Hypertension is therefore less common, and urinary excretion of catecholamines may become supranormal later in the course of the disease. Surgical resection is indicated, but controversy surrounds the need for prophylactic resection of contralateral uninvolved adrenals, 50% of which develop pheochromocytomas within 10 years of the original surgery. The diagnosis and management of pheochromocytomas are discussed in Chapter 29.

13. Is hyperparathyroidism associated with MEN 2A similar to that found in MEN 1?

Yes, but it is encountered much less commonly, involving only 40% of cases. No mitogenic factor (as in MEN 1) has been described in the sera of these patients.

14. What is the genetic basis for the MEN 2A syndrome?

MEN 2A is caused by an activating mutation of the *RET* protooncogene located on chromosome 10q11.2. The gene codes for a receptor tyrosine kinase that phosphorylates and activates enzymes critical to cellular development. The ligand that normally activates the tyrosine kinase is glial cell–derived neurotropic factor (GDNF). When GDNF binds, two receptors bond together (homodimerization) and phosphorylation of enzymes occurs downstream.

Mutation of the *RET* protooncogene to an oncogene results in constitutive activation of the enzyme, causing unregulated phosphorylation of other critical enzymes. Inheritance of one *RET* oncogene from one affected parent is sufficient to cause MEN 2A syndrome in offspring. Five distinct mutations involving exons 10 and 11 have been described in 98% of 203 kindreds with the disorder.

15. How should a kindred be screened after the proband with MEN 2A is identified?

As explained in question 9, screening initially entails the differentiation of gene carriers from uninvolved family members and the subsequent delineation of organ involvement in the affected members. But unlike MEN 1, direct DNA sequencing of the *RET* oncogene causing MEN 2A is clinically available. With appropriate repeat analysis of positive and negative test results, the assay offers near 100% accuracy in identification of affected individuals. Genetic analysis of the kindred should be performed to identify the specific *RET* oncogene mutation; characterization of the familial oncogene precludes the need for repetitive biochemical screening of non-carriers in subsequent generations.

Because C-cell hyperplasia has been described in gene carriers as young as 2 years of age, total thyroidectomy is suggested in affected individuals before the age of 5. An alternative to pre-emptive thyroidectomy is to perform annual pentagastrin stimulation tests and withhold surgery until a positive result is obtained. Because MEN 2A–associated pheochromocytoma may produce large amounts of epinephrine that do not cause hypertension, annual timed urine collections for catecholamines should be obtained in all gene carriers. Serum levels of calcium should be assessed every 2 years. Once the presence of the syndrome is established, screening for adrenal and parathyroid involvement should continue through life.

16. What comprises the MEN 2B syndrome?

MEN 2B syndrome is the association of MCT and pheochromocytoma with multiple mucosal neuromas in an affected individual or kindred. Hyperparathyroidism is not associated with MEN 2B. This syndrome is less common than the MEN 2A and is more commonly sporadic than familial, but if inherited, it is transmitted in an autosomal dominant fashion.

The occurrence of multiple mucosal neuromas on the distal tongue, lips, and along the gastrointestinal tract should always raise the possibility of MEN 2B. Other manifestations of MEN 2B include marfanoid habitus (without ectopia lentis or aortic aneurysms), hypertrophic corneal nerves, and slipped femoral epiphysis.

The MCT associated with this syndrome is more aggressive than other forms; metastatic lesions have been described in infancy. Because of the propensity toward early metastasis, many advocate that children with the syndrome should undergo total thyroidectomy as soon as surgery can be tolerated. Pheochromocytomas occur in nearly one half of all patients and follow a clinical course similar to those in the MEN 2A syndrome. Overall mortality in MEN 2B is more severe; the average age of death for patients with MEN 2A is 60 years, whereas in patients with MEN 2B the average age of death is 30 years.

Screening of family members with pentagastrin stimulation for MCT should begin at birth and continue through life if thyroidectomy is deferred. Screening for pheochromocytoma should begin at 5 years and continue for life.

17. What is the cause of MEN 2B?

Over 95% of the kindreds with MEN 2B have been found to carry a mutation of the *RET* protooncogene at codon 918 (exon 16). This oncogene codes for a methionine-to-threonine substitution, resulting in activation of the innermost tyrosine kinase moiety of the same receptor associated with MEN 2A.

18. Have the clinical presentations and prognoses of the MEN syndromes changed since the time of their original descriptions?

Yes. When the MEN syndromes were initially described, most patients presented with involvement of all of the aforementioned organ systems because diagnostic capabilities were limited. In the present, early diagnosis of the proband and aggressive screening of the kindred may permit detection of hyperplasia and prompt prophylactic surgery or medical therapy that limits morbidity and mortality.

BIBLIOGRAPHY

1. Benson L, Ljunghall S, Akerstrom G, Oberg K: Hyperparathyroidism presenting as the first lesion in multiple endocrine neoplasia type 1. Am J Med 82:731–737, 1987.
2. Brandi ML, Auerbach GD, Fitzpatrick LA, et al: Parathyroid mitogenic activity in plasma from patients with familial multiple endocrine neoplasia type 1. N Engl J Med 314:1287–1293, 1986.
3. Cadiot G, Laurent-Piug P, Thuille B, et al: Is the multiple endocrine neoplasia type 1 gene a suppressor for fundic argyrophil tumors in Zollinger-Ellison syndrome? Gastroenterology 105:579–582, 1993.
4. Chandrasekharappa SCV, Guru SC, Manickam P, et al: Positional cloning of the gene for multiple endocrine neoplasia type 1. Science 276:404–407, 1997.
5. Doris-Keller H, Dou S, Chi D, et al: Mutations in the RET proto-oncogene are associated with MEN 2A and FMTC. Hum Mol Genet 2:851–856, 1993.
6. Eng C: The RET proto-oncogene in multiple endocrine neoplasia type 2 and Hirschsprung's disease. N Engl J Med 335:943–951, 1996.
7. Eng C, Clayton D, Schuffenecker I, et al: The relationship between specific RET proto-oncogene mutations and disease phenotype in multiple endocrine neoplasia type 2. JAMA 276:1575–1579, 1996.
8. Gagel RF: Multiple endocrine neoplasia. In Wilson JD, Foster DW (eds): Williams' Textbook of Endocrinology, 9th ed. Philadelphia, W.B. Saunders, 1998, pp 1637–1649.
9. Gicquel C, Bertherat J, Le Bouc Y, et al: The pathogenesis of adrenocortical incidentalomas and genetic syndromes associated with adrenocortical neoplasms. Endocrinol Metab Clin North Am 29:1–13, 2000.
10. Grauer A, Raue F, Gagel RF: Changing concepts in the management of hereditary and sporadic medullary thyroid carcinoma. Endocrinol Metab Clin North Am 19:613–635, 1990.

11. Herman V, Draznin NZ, Gonsky R, Melmed S: Molecular screening of pituitary adenomas for gene mutations and rearrangements. J Clin Endocrinol Metab 77:50–55, 1993.
12. Marx SJ, Vinik AI, Santen RJ, et al: Multiple endocrine neoplasia type 1: Assessment of laboratory tests to screen for the gene in a large kindred. Medicine 65:2226–2241, 1986.
13. Marx SJ, moderator: Multiple endocrine neoplasia type 1: Clinical and genetic topics. Ann Intern Med 129:484-494, 1998.
14. Phay JE, Moley JF, Lairmore TL. Multiple endocrine neoplasias. Semin Surg Oncol 18:324–332, 2000.
15. Saad MF, Ordenez NG, Rashid RK, et al: Medullary carcinoma of the thyroid. Medicine 63:319–342, 1984.
16. Santoro M, Carlomagno F, Romano A, et al: Activation of RET as a dominant transforming gene by germline mutations of MEN 2A and MEN 2B. Science 267:381–383, 1995.
17. Veldius JD, Norton JA, Wells SA, et al: Surgical versus medical management of multiple endocrine neoplasia (MEN) Type 1. J Clin Endocrinol Metab 82:357–364, 1997.

55. AUTOIMMUNE POLYGLANDULAR SYNDROMES

Arnold A. *Asp,* M.D.

1. Define the autoimmune polyglandular syndromes. How many clinical forms are there?

The autoimmune polyglandular syndromes (APSs) are disorders in which two or more endocrine glands are simultaneously hypo- or hyperfunctional as the result of autoimmune dysfunction. It is theorized that a defect in the T-suppressor cell subset inadvertently permits activation of the cellular and humoral arms of the immune system. The nature of this dysfunction is unknown. The two widely recognized clinical forms are appropriately designated APS type 1 and APS type 2. The common clinical link between the syndromes is adrenal insufficiency.

2. Is evidence of nonendocrine autoimmune dysfunction associated with APSs?

Yes. Connective tissue diseases and hematologic and gastrointestinal autoimmune disorders are commonly associated with the APSs.

3. What constitutes APS type 1?

APS type 1 is a pediatric disorder manifested by the presence of a combination of two of the following three disorders: hypoparathyroidism, adrenal insufficiency, and chronic mucocutaneous candidiasis. Usually hypoparathyroidism and candidiasis present by the age of 5 years. Adrenal insufficiency occurs by the age of 12 years, and all manifestations are present by the age of 15 years. Some affected individuals develop only one manifestation. Other endocrine conditions may also occur; the largest series of patients have noted the following endocrine manifestations:

Hypoparathyroidism	89%	Thyroid disease	12%
Adrenal insufficiency	60%	Diabetes mellitus, type 1	1–4%
Gonadal failure	45%		

4. Are nonendocrine manifestations associated with APS type 1?

Yes. Chronic mucocutaneous candidiasis occurs in 75% of patients, celiac disease in 25%, alopecia in 20%, pernicious anemia in 16%, and chronic autoimmune hepatitis in 9%. Dystrophy of the dental enamel, vitiligo, keratography, and hypoplasia of the teeth and nails also may occur, prompting the alternative designation for APS type1: autoimmune polyendocrinopathy–candidiasis–ectodermal dystrophy (APECED).

5. What is the etiology of APS type 1?

The etiology is largely unknown. The clustering of disease among equal numbers of boys and girls within a single sibship (not multiple generations) raises the possibility of autosomal recessive inheritance. There appears to be no HLA association. The cause of the candidiasis is not known, although delayed hypersensitivity is defective in affected patients. Antibodies to adrenal enzymes (21-hydroxylase, an enzyme in the biosynthetic pathway for aldosterone and cortisol) and to poorly characterized parathyroid antigens have been described by some groups.

6. What therapy can be offered?

Annual screening of levels of serum calcium, cosyntropin-stimulated cortisol, and liver-associated enzymes is performed in affected sibships until the age of 15 years. Adrenal insufficiency and hypoparathyroidism are treated with glucocorticoids and oral calcium supplementation, respectively. Mucocutaneous candidiasis is treated with fluconazole. Use of prophylactic immunosuppressives, such as cyclosporine, is not recommended.

7. What disorders are associated with APS type 2?

APS type 2 occurs in adulthood and consists of autoimmune adrenal insufficiency with autoimmune thyroid disease and/or diabetes mellitus, type 1. The age of onset tends to be between 20 and 30 years; one half of the cases are sporadic and one half are familial. Endocrine organ involvement is as follows:

Adrenal insufficiency	100%	Diabetes mellitus, type 1	50%
Autoimmune thyroid disease	70%	Gonadal failure	5–50%

Adrenal insufficiency is the presenting disorder in one-half of cases, whereas adrenal insufficiency with diabetes mellitus or thyroid disease is present at the time of diagnosis in 20% of cases. In the remaining 30%, adrenal insufficiency occurs after other endocrine dysfunction. Between 69–90% of patients have circulating antibodies to 21-hydroxylase.

Thyroid disorders associated with APS type 2 include Graves' disease (50%) and Hashimoto's disease or atrophic thyroiditis (50%). As expected, thyroid-stimulating immunoglobulins (TSI) are present in cases of hyperthyroidism, whereas antibodies to thyroid peroxidase or thyroglobulin are present in cases of hypothyroidism.

Cytoplasmic islet cell antibodies (ICA) are present in individuals with APS type 2 and diabetes mellitus; however, the significance of these antibodies is questionable. APS type 2 patients who have ICA but not diabetes may have no compromise of beta-cell function and subsequently develop diabetes at a rate of 2% per year, whereas ICA-positive first-degree relatives of non-APS, type 1 diabetic individuals develop diabetes at a rate of 8% per year.

Gonadal failure is more common in women than in men and is associated with antibodies to gonadal tissue. Very rarely geriatric hypoparathyroidism may be encountered in elderly patients with APS type 2.

8. Are nonendocrine abnormalities described in APS type 2?

Yes. In about 5% of cases, other autoimmune disorders are found, including vitiligo, pernicious anemia, alopecia, myasthenia gravis, celiac disease, Sjögren's syndrome, and rheumatoid arthritis.

9. How should kindreds with suspected APS type 2 be screened?

Because APS type 2 appears in multiple generations and because 20 years may lapse between the development of various endocrine organ failures, affected patients should be screened by assessing levels of serum glucose, thyrotropin (TSH), and vitamin B_{12} every 3–5 years. Symptoms of adrenal insufficiency should be investigated by assessing levels of cosyntropin-stimulated cortisol. First-degree relatives of the proband should be educated about the syndrome and advised to undergo screening every 3–5 years. Antibodies to thyroid peroxidase or thyroglobulin are so common in the general population as to preclude their use as a screening test.

10. What is the etiology of APS type 2?

The genetic basis of APS type 2 is uncertain, although it appears to be associated with an HLA-DR3 phenotype that may be permissive for the development of autoimmunity. Organ-specific antibodies may cause organ dysfunction—for example, TSI may cause

Graves' disease and antiacetylcholine receptor antibodies may cause myasthenia gravis—or, like antithyroglobulin antibodies, they may be epiphenomena of disease. The only consistent abnormality noted in affected patients is decreased function of T-suppressor cells.

11. What is POEMS syndrome?

POEMS syndrome is a disorder of unknown etiology, unrelated to either APS type 1or type 2, that appears to have an immunologic basis. The acronym highlights the cardinal features of the syndrome: polyneuropathy, organomegaly, endocrinopathy, monoclonal component, and skin changes. All of the symptoms are considered to be secondary to a plasma cell dyscrasia (MGUS; plasmacytoma; osteosclerotic, osteolytic or mixed myeloma) that produces the monoclonal gammopathy.

12. What is an eponym associated with POEMS?

Another name for the disorder is Crow-Fukase syndrome.

13. How does the disorder usually present?

The majority of patients are Asian males 45–55 years of age, but any ethnic group of either gender is susceptible. The most common presentation is that of a distal, symmetric peripheral sensorimotor neuropathy. There is usually loss of pin-prick and vibratory sense, and decreased deep tendon reflexes predominantly in the lower extremities. The neuropathy is slowly progressive. Electromyelograms and nerve biopsies are most consistent with both demyelination and axonal degeneration. Autonomic neuropathy has not been observed. Papilledema is present in 40–80% of cases. Nerve damage may result from myelin cross-reactivity with monoclonal IgA or IgG M proteins produced by plasmacytomas in sclerotic bone lesions, but evidence of intraneural immunoglobulin deposition has not been found in all series.

14. How does the organomegaly manifest?

Hepatomegaly (uncommon in multiple myeloma) and/or splenomegaly is noted in approximately two thirds of POEMS cases. The hepatomegaly may be associated with fibrosis and liver dysfunction.

15. Which endocrine systems are involved?

Diabetes mellitus, type 2, is commonly encountered in either gender (28-48%), as is primary hypothyroidism (45–59%) or, rarely, adrenal insufficiency. Both males and females manifest elevated serum estrogen levels, which may promote hyperprolactinemia with galactorrhea and amenorrhea or impotence. Antibodies to the thyroid or adrenal glands have not been consistently detected.

16. What skin changes have been encountered?

Skin changes include sclerosis, hypertrichosis, hyperpigmentation, and hyperhidrosis.

17. How is POEMS treated?

Treatment of POEMS is based on elimination of plasmacytomas with radiation or chemotherapy, which, if successful, results in amelioration of the polyneuropathy and reduction in organomegaly. Endocrine deficiencies are treated with replacement hormones.

BIBLIOGRAPHY

1. Ahonen P, Myllarniemi S, Sipila I, Perheentupa J: Clinical variation of autoimmune poly-endocrinopathy–candidiasis–ectodermal dystrophy (APECED) in a series of 68 patients. N Engl J Med 322:1829–1836, 1990.

2. Betterle C, Grehhio NA, Volpato M. Autoimmune polyglandular syndrome type 1. J Clin Endocrinol Metab 83: 1049-1055, 1998.
3. Eisenbarth GS, Verge CF: The immunoendocrinopathy syndromes. In Wilson JD, Foster DW (eds): Williams' Textbook of Endocrinology, 9th ed. Philadelphia, W.B. Saunders, 1998, pp 1651–1662.
4. Kutteh WH: Immunology of multiple endocrinopathies associated with premature ovarian failure. Endocrinologist 6:462–466, 1996.
5. Leshin M: Polyglandular autoimmune syndromes. Am J Med Sci 290:77–88, 1985.
6. Neufeld M, Maclaren NK, Blizzard RM: Two types of autoimmune Addison's disease associated with different polyglandular autoimmune (PGA) syndromes. Medicine 60:355–362, 1981.
7. Soubrier M, Dubost JJ, Sauvezie B: POEMS syndrome: a study of 25 cases and a review of the literature. Am J Med 97: 543-553, 1994.
8. Soubrier M, Sauron C, Souweine B, et al: Growth factors and proinflammatory cytokines in the renal involvement of POEMS syndrome. Am J Kid Dis 34:633-638, 1999.

56. PANCREATIC ENDOCRINE TUMORS

Michael T. McDermott, M.D.

1. What are the pancreatic endocrine tumors?

These tumors arise from the islet cells of the pancreas and are generally named for the hormones they secrete. They include tumors that secrete insulin (insulinomas), gastrin (gastrinomas), vasoactive intestinal polypeptide (VIPomas), glucagon (glucagonomas), somatostatin (somatostatinomas), corticotropin–releasing factor (CRFomas), ACTH (ACTHomas), growth hormone–releasing factor (GRFomas) and pancreatic polypeptide (PPomas).

Gastrinoma
60-80%

Insulinoma
20-40%

VIPoma
<1%

Glucagonoma
<1%

Somatostatinoma
<1%

Pancreatic islet cell tumors.

2. Are pancreatic endocrine tumors usually benign or malignant?

Insulinomas are usually benign (80–90%), whereas the other pancreatic endocrine tumors are frequently malignant (50–80%).

3. Are pancreatic endocrine tumors associated with other endocrine disorders?

Up to 10% of pancreatic endocrine tumors occur as part of the multiple endocrine neoplasia type 1 (MEN I) syndrome. This inherited disorder consists of pituitary tumors, pancreatic endocrine tumors and hyperparathyroidism. Hyperparathyroidism usually occurs before pituitary or pancreatic tumors appear. The condition is caused by an inherited mutation in the Menin gene.

4. What are insulinomas?

Insulinomas are discreet insulin-producing tumors within the pancreas. They belong to a larger group of hyperinsulinemic pancreatic beta cell disorders that include insulinomas, islet cell hyperplasia, and nesidioblastosis (neo-proliferation of beta cells along the pancreatic ducts).

5. What is Whipple's triad?

Whipple's triad is the following combination:
1. Hypoglycemia
2. Symptoms during hypoglycemia
3. Relief of symptoms with correction of hypoglycemia

6. What glucose levels are considered to be hypoglycemia?

The exact criteria for hypoglycemia continue to be disputed. However, glucose levels of < 50 mg/dl in men and < 40 mg/dl in women are commonly considered to be hypoglycemia.

7. What are the symptoms of hypoglycemia?

Hypoglycemic symptoms are generally classified according to the their type and their timing in relation to meals. Symptoms such as confusion, slurred speech, blurred vision, seizures, and coma result from inadequate delivery of glucose to the brain (neuroglycopenia). Symptoms such as tremors, sweating, palpitations and nausea likely result from a counterregulatory discharge of catecholamines (adrenergic). When symptoms occur within 5 hours of the previous meal, they are considered to be "postprandial," whereas if they occur more than 5 hours after a meal, they are considered to be "fasting." Insulinomas most commonly cause fasting neuroglycopenic symptoms, although fasting and postprandial adrenergic symptoms may also occur.

8. How is the diagnosis of an insulinoma made?

The diagnosis of insulinoma requires documentation of the presence of both Whipple's triad and endogenous hyperinsulinemia. Although some patients present to the provider during a hypoglycemic episode, more commonly the physician must attempt to provoke hypoglycemia when this diagnosis is suspected. The test procedure of choice is a prolonged fast (up to 48 hours) with blood sampling for serum glucose, insulin, and C-peptide levels every 6–12 hours and during any symptoms that occur.

The criteria for hyperinsulinemia in a hypoglycemic patient are a serum insulin level > 6 μU/ml or an insulin:glucose ratio of $\geq$ 0.33 (although these values are disputed). Measurement of serum C-peptide is also necessary in order to document that the hyperinsulinemia is endogenous. C-peptide comes from the cleavage of proinsulin into insulin and C-peptide molecules in the pancreatic islet cells before insulin is secreted; because it is co-secreted in equimolar amounts with insulin, serum C-peptide measurements can be used to assess endogenous pancreatic insulin secretion. A serum C-peptide level of > 0.2 nmol/L strongly suggests that the hyperinsulinemia is due to an insulinoma. Elevated serum proinsulin levels are also indicative of a probable insulinoma.

The differential diagnosis of hyperinsulinemic hypoglycemia includes insulinomas, surreptitious insulin administration, and sulfonylurea use. The following table illustrates how testing can be used to distinguish these three entities.

Test	Insulinoma	Surreptitious Insulin Use	Sulfonylurea Use
Insulin	↑	↑	↑
C-Peptide	↑	↓	↑
Proinsulin	↑	↓	nl
Sulfonylurea screen	neg	neg	pos

9. How can an insulinoma be localized?

A CT scan or MRI is usually the first localization procedure, although the reported sensitivity of these techniques has varied anywhere from 15-90% in recent studies. Endoscopic ultrasound of the pancreas has higher sensitivity (56-93%) and can detect tumors as small as 2-3 mm in size. Intra-arterial pancreatic calcium infusions with measurement of insulin changes in the right hepatic vein yields similar or superior results but is clearly a more invasive technique. Intraoperative ultrasound is also highly accurate and is particularly useful for finding small tumors that could not be localized preoperatively. Octreotide scintigraphy (octreoscan) has proved to be of little value in localizing insulinomas.

10. What is the treatment for an insulinoma?

Surgery is the treatment of choice. When surgery is not desired, or when tumors are unresectable, medical therapy consists of multiple (usually 6 or more) small meals per day and the use of medications that inhibit insulin secretion. The most effective drug for this purpose is oral diazoxide; other medications that may be useful include propranolol, calcium channel blockers, thiazide diuretics, and phenytoin. Octreotide is rarely beneficial. Chemotherapy using streptozotocin with doxorubicin or with 5-fluorouracil reduces symptoms and improves survival in patients with malignant insulinomas.

11. What are the clinical manifestations of gastrinomas?

Gastrinomas secrete excessive gastrin, which stimulates prolific secretion of gastric acid. Patients develop severe peptic ulcer disease, often associated with secretory diarrhea. This disorder is also known as the Zollinger-Ellison syndrome.

12. Do gastrinomas always arise from pancreatic islet cells?

No. Gastrinomas may arise from the pancreatic islets but also may occur in the duodenum and stomach.

13. How is the diagnosis of gastrinoma made?

The diagnosis is made by demonstrating the presence of high gastric acidity (pH < 3.0) in association with a fasting serum gastrin level > 1000 pg/ml or a moderately elevated gastrin that increases by more than 200 pg/ml within 15 minutes after the intravenous administration of secretin.

14. What is the best way to localize a gastrinoma?

Localization of the tumor may be pursued with various techniques including CT scan, MRI, endoscopic ultrasonography, octreotide scanning, transhepatic portal venous sampling, and selective arterial secretin infusions with right hepatic vein gastrin measurements.

15. What is the treatment for gastrinoma?

Most benign and some malignant gastrinomas can be cured by surgery. Otherwise, attention should be directed toward reduction of gastric acid overproduction. Proton pump inhibitors (omeprazole, lanzoprazole) are the drugs of choice for this purpose. Octreotide (Sandostatin; 50–500 μg bid–tid SQ) or long acting octreotide (Sandostatin LAR; 10–30 mg q month, intragluteal) is also a highly effective agent for this condition. High dose H2 blockers may also be useful but are rarely adequate by themselves. Refractory patients may require total gastrectomy and vagotomy for symptom relief.

Since most gastrinomas are malignant, chemotherapy is often necessary. The most effective chemotherapy combinations include the following: streptozotocin, 5-fluorouracil and leucovorin; lomustine and 5-fluorouracil; etoposide, doxorubicin, and 5-fluorouracil; cisplatin, dacarbazine and alpha interferon. Finally, tumor embolization in conjunction with direct intra-arterial infusions of chemotherapy agents has shown additional promise as a palliative procedure.

16. What are the characteristics of glucagonomas?

Glucagon antagonizes the effects of insulin in the liver by stimulating glycogenolysis and gluconeogenesis. Glucagonomas, which secrete excessive glucagon, cause diabetes mellitus, weight loss, anemia and a characteristic skin rash, necrolytic migratory erythema. Affected patients also have a thromboembolic diathesis. The diagnosis depends on finding an elevated level of serum glucagon (> 500 pg/ml). Techniques similar to those used for gastrinomas are useful for localizing these tumors.

17. How are glucagonomas treated?

Treatment options include surgery for localized disease, octreotide to reduce glucagon secretion, and chemotherapy regimens similar to those used for gastrinomas. Chronic anticoagulation to reduce the risk of thromboembolic events should also be considered. Finally, zinc supplements and intermittent amino acid infusions may help to reduce the skin rash and to improve the patient's overall sense of well-being.

18. What are the characteristics of somatostatinomas?

Among its multiple systemic effects, somatostatin inhibits secretion of insulin and pancreatic enzymes, production of gastric acid, and gallbladder contraction. Somatostatinomas secrete excess somatostatin, causing diabetes mellitus, weight loss, steatorrhea, hypochlorhydria, and cholelithiasis. The diagnosis is made by finding an elevated level of serum somatostatin.

19. What is the treatment for somatostatinoma?

Surgery is the treatment of choice. When surgery is not possible, somatostatin secretion and tumor size may be reduced by the same chemotherapy regimens used for other pancreatic endocrine tumors.

20. What are the characteristics of vasoactive intestinal polypeptide–secreting tumors (VIPomas)?

VIPomas cause watery diarrhea, hypokalemia, and achlorhydria (WDHA syndrome, pancreatic cholera). This is also known as the Verner-Morrison syndrome. The diagnosis is made by finding an elevated level of serum VIP.

21. How are VIPomas treated?

Surgery is the treatment of choice. Octreotide effectively reduces diarrhea in most patients. Radiation therapy and chemotherapy also may effectively reduce diarrhea and tumor size.

22. Briefly discuss the remaining pancreatic endocrine tumors.

The remaining pancreatic endocrine tumors are very rare. CRFomas and ACTHomas lead to the development of Cushing's syndrome and GRFomas cause acromegaly. PPomas are initially asymptomatic but may eventually enlarge to produce mass effects without a recognizable hormone hypersecretion syndrome. Localization procedures and treatments are similar to those described above for other pancreatic endocrine tumors.

BIBLIOGRAPHY

1. Arnold R, Simon B, Wied M: Treatment of neuroendocrine GEP tumors with somatostatin analogues. Review. Digestion 62 Suppl S1:84–91, 2000.
2. Boukhman MP, Karam JM, Shaver J, et al: Localization of insulinomas. Arch Surg 134:818–22; discussion 822–823, 1999.
3. Doppman JL, Chang R, Fraker DL, et al: Localization of insulinomas to regions of the pancreas by intra-arterial stimulation with calcium. Ann Intern Med 123:269–273, 1995.
4. Hirshberg B, Livi A, Bartlett DL, et al: Forty-eight hour fast: The diagnostic test for insulinoma. J Clin Endocrinol Metab 85: 3222–3226, 2000.
5. Jaffe BM: Current issues in the management of Zollinger-Ellison syndrome. Surgery 111: 241–243, 1992.
6. Jensen RT: Pancreatic endocrine tumors: Recent advances. Ann Oncol 10 Suppl 4:160–170, 1999.
7. Krejs GJ, Orci L, Conlon M, et al: Somatostatinoma syndrome: Biochemical, morphologic and clinical features. N Engl J Med 301:283–292, 1979.
8. Leichter SB: Clinical and metabolic aspects of glucagonoma. Medicine 59:100–113, 1980.

9. Moertel CG, Johnson CM, McKusick MA, et al: The management of patients with advanced carcinoid tumors and islet cell carcinomas. Ann Intern Med 120:302–309, 1994.

10. Moertel CG, Lefkopoulo M, Lipsitz S, et al: Streptozocin-doxorubicin, streptozocin-fluorouracil, or chlorozotocin in the treatment of advanced islet-cell carcinoma. N Engl J Med 326:519–523, 1992.

11. Perry RR, Vinik AI: Diagnosis and management of functioning islet cell tumors. J Clin Endocrinol Metab 80:2273–2278, 1995.

12. Ricke J, Klose K: Imaging procedures in neuroendocrine tumors. Digestion 62 Suppl S1:39–44, 2000.

13. Service FJ, McMahon MM, O'Brien PC, Ballard DJ: Functioning insulinomas—incidence, recurrence, and long-term survival of patients: A 60-year study. Mayo Clin Proc 66:711–719, 1991.

14. Service FJ: Classification of hypoglycemic disorders. Endocrinol Metab Clin North Am 28:501–517, 1999.

15. Tomassetti P, Migliori M, Corinaldesi R, Gullo L: Treatment of gastroenteropancreatic neuroendocrine tumours with octreotide LAR. Ailment Pharmacol Ther 14:557–560, 2000.

16. Warner RRP: Gut neuroendocrine tumors. In Bardin CW (ed): Current Therapy in Endocrinology and Metabolism, 6th ed. New York, Mosby, 1997, p. 606–614.

17. Wermers RA, Fatourechi V, Kvols LK: Clinical spectrum of hyperglucagonemia associated with malignant neuroendocrine tumors. Mayo Clin Proc 71:1030–1038, 1996.

57. CARCINOID SYNDROME

Michael T. McDermott, M.D.

1. What are carcinoid tumors?

Carcinoid tumors are neoplasms that arise from enterochromaffin or Kulchitsky cells.

2. How are carcinoid tumors classified anatomically?

Carcinoid tumors are classified as originating in the foregut (bronchus, stomach, duodenum, bile ducts, pancreas), midgut (jejunum, ileum, appendix, ascending colon), or hindgut (transverse colon, descending and sigmoid colon, rectum). They also occasionally occur in the ovaries, testes, prostate, kidney, breast, thymus, or skin.

3. What is the carcinoid syndrome?

The carcinoid syndrome is a humorally mediated disorder that consists of cutaneous flushing (90%), diarrhea (75%), bronchospasm (20%), endocardial fibrosis (33%), right-heart valvular lesions, and occasionally pleural, peritoneal, or retroperitoneal fibrosis.

4. What are the biochemical mediators of the carcinoid syndrome?

Carcinoid tumors produce a variety of humoral mediators, including serotonin, bradykinin, tachykinins, histamine, prostaglandins, neurotensin, motilin, and substance P. Diarrhea and fibrous tissue formation may be caused by serotonin, whereas flushing and wheezing are likely due to kinins, histamine, or prostaglandins.

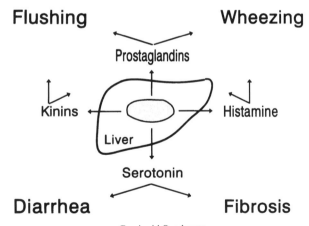

Carcinoid Syndrome

5. Why does pellagra sometimes accompany the carcinoid syndrome?

Pellagra is due to niacin deficiency that results when the tumor diverts tryptophan from synthesis of niacin to synthesis of serotonin.

6. Why do intestinal carcinoid tumors so infrequently cause carcinoid syndrome?

For the carcinoid syndrome to occur, humoral mediators must reach the systemic circulation. Mediators secreted by intestinal carcinoids enter the portal circulation but are almost totally metabolized in the liver and never reach the systemic circulation. Thus carcinoid syndrome does not usually occur with these tumors unless there are hepatic metastases that impair metabolism of the mediators or that secrete mediators directly into the hepatic vein. Extraintestinal carcinoids, however, may cause carcinoid syndrome in the absence of metastases because they secrete mediators into venous systems that do not first pass through the liver.

7. Do carcinoid tumors cause any other humoral syndromes?

Yes. Carcinoids, particularly bronchial and pancreatic carcinoids, may secrete corticotropin-releasing factor (CRF) or corticotropin (ACTH), which cause Cushing's syndrome, or growth hormone–releasing factor (GRF), which causes acromegaly.

8. How is the diagnosis of carcinoid syndrome made?

The diagnosis depends on the demonstration of increased serum concentrations of serotonin, neurotensin, or substance P or increased urinary excretion of 5-hydroxyindoleacetic acid (5-HIAA), a breakdown product of serotonin. Serum levels of chromogranin A are often elevated in these patients also.

9. What is the treatment for carcinoid syndrome?

Surgery may occasionally be curative when the carcinoid syndrome results from an extraintestinal carcinoid tumor that has not metastasized. Most patients with the carcinoid syndrome, however, have extensive metastases at the time of diagnosis. The goal of therapy, therefore, is usually not to cure but to provide palliation and to prolong survival. Medications to control symptoms (flushing, diarrhea, bronchospasm) and chemotherapy to reduce the tumor burden are the most effective general management strategies.

10. How does one control the symptoms of carcinoid syndrome?

The most troublesome symptoms patients with carcinoid syndrome experience are intense flushing and frequent diarrhea. Octreotide, a somatostatin analogue, is highly effective in controlling most carcinoid symptoms. The following tables list the various medications or combinations that may be tried for symptom relief.

Medications to Control Carcinoid Flushing

Octreotide (Sandostatin)	100–150 μg BID-TID, SQ
Octreotide, long acting (Sandostatin LAR)	20–30 mg q month, intragluteal
Phentolamine (Regitine)	25–50 mg q day–TID
Phenoxybenzamine (Dibenzyline)	30 mg q day
Cyproheptadine (Periactin)	2–4 mg TID–QID
Methysergide (Sansert)	2 mg TID
Prochlorperazine (Compazine)	5–10 mg q 4–6 h
Chlorpromazine (Thorazine)	10–25 mg q 4–6 h
Clonidine (Catapres)	.1–.2 mg BID
Methyldopa (Aldomet)	250 mg TID
Cimetidine (Tagamet), plus	300 mg QID
Diphenhydramine (Benadryl)	50 mg QID
Glucocorticoids	

Medications to Control Carcinoid Diarrhea

Standard anti-diarrheal measures	
Octreotide (Sandostatin)	100–150 μg BID–TID, SQ
Octreotide, long acting (Sandostatin LAR)	20-30 mg q month, intragluteal
Clonidine (Catapres)	.1–.2 mg BID
Cyproheptadine (Periactin)	2–4 mg TID–QID
Methysergide (Sansert)	2 mg TID
Ondansetron (Zofran)	8 mg TID

11. What chemotherapy regimens are most effective in carcinoid tumors?

Although not generally curative, chemotherapy may reduce the total tumor burden sufficiently to reduce carcinoid symptoms. The following chemotherapy regimens have thus far shown the greatest efficacy in these patients: streptozotocin, 5-fluorouracil and leucovorin; lomustine and 5-fluorouracil; etoposide, doxorubicin, and 5-fluorouracil; cisplatin, dacarbazine, and alpha interferon. Another promising approach for hepatic tumor debulking has been hepatic artery embolization along with direct intra-arterial chemotherapy infusions.

12. What is a carcinoid crisis?

A carcinoid crisis is an acute episode of severe flushing, bronchospasm, and hypotension. These episodes are most commonly provoked by the administration of adrenergic agents, such as epinephrine and sympathomimetic amines, or monoamine oxidase (MAO) inhibitors in patients with underlying carcinoid tumors. Patients need not have previously experienced symptoms of the carcinoid syndrome to have a carcinoid crisis.

13. How can a carcinoid crisis be prevented?

Patients with known carcinoid syndrome should not be given epinephrine, sympathomimetic amines, or MAO inhibitors. When these patients require a surgical procedure, they should be pretreated with octreotide (Sandostatin) 100 μg subcutaneously 30–60 minutes prior to the operation. Anesthesiologists should be specifically notified that the patient has carcinoid syndrome.

Patients who have known carcinoid tumors but who have not exhibited features of carcinoid syndrome can be tested for their potential to develop a carcinoid crisis. This is most commonly done with an epinephrine provocation test. In this test, patients receive progressive intravenous boluses of epinephrine every 5 minutes, starting with a dose of 1 μg and increasing, if necessary, to 10 μg, while monitoring heart rate and blood pressure every 60 seconds. A positive response consists of flushing or a blood pressure drop of 20 mm Hg systolic or 10 mm Hg diastolic 45–120 minutes after an injection. All patients undergoing this test must have indwelling intravenous catheters and be monitored carefully throughout the test; intravenous phentolamine (Regitine) 5 mg and methoxamine (Vasoxyl) 3 mg preparations must also be available to reverse a crisis should it occur.

14. How should a carcinoid crisis be treated?

An effective treatment for an acute carcinoid crisis is the administration of intravenous octreotide and hydrocortisone. If this does not successfully abort the episode, other options include methotrimeprazine (an anti-serotonin agent), methoxamine (a direct vasoconstrictor), phentolamine (an alpha adrenergic blocker), ondansetron (a serotonin receptor antagonist), and glucagon. It is critical to avoid the use of adrenergic and sympathomimetic agents in patients with suspected carcinoid crisis as these drugs can significantly worsen the condition. Effective medication dose regimens for this condition are listed below.

Medication	Dose Regimen
Octreotide (Sandostatin)	50 μg IV over 1 min., then 50 μg IV over 15 min
Hydrocortisone (Solu-Cortef)	100 mg IV over 15 min
Methotrimeprazine (Levoprome)	2.5–5.0 mg slow IV push
Methoxamine (Vasoxyl)	3-5 mg slow IV push, followed by an infusion
Phentolamine (Regitine)	5 mg slow IV push
Ondansetron (Zofran)	20 mg IV over 15 min
Glucagon	.5–1.5 mg slow IV push

BIBLIOGRAPHY

1. Fehmann HC, Wulbrand U, Arnold R: Review. Treatment of endocrine gastroenteropancreatic tumors with somatostatin analogues. Recent Results Cancer Res 153:15–22, 2000.
2. Feldman JM: The carcinoid syndrome. Endocrinologist 3:129–135, 1993.
3. Galanis E, Kvols LK, Rubin J: Carcinoid syndrome. J Clin Oncol 16:796–798, 1998.
4. Janmohamed S, Bloom SR: Review. Carcinoid tumours. Postgrad Med J 73:207–214, 1997.
5. Kulke MH, Mayer RJ: Review. Carcinoid tumors. N Engl J Med 340:858–868, 1999.
6. Lamberts SWJ, van der Lely A-J, de Herder WW, Hofland LJ: Octreotide. N Engl J Med 334: 246–254, 1996.
7. Metcalfe DD: Differential diagnosis of the patient with unexplained flushing/anaphylaxis. Allergy Asthma Proc 21:21–24, 2000.
8. Moertel CG, Johnson CM, McKusick MA, et al: The management of patients with advanced carcinoid tumors and islet cell carcinomas. Ann Intern Med 120:302–309, 1994.
9. Oberg K: Carcinoid tumors: Current concepts in diagnosis and treatment. Oncologist 3:339–345, 1998.
10. O'Toole D, Ducreaux M, Bommelaer G, et al: Treatment of carcinoid syndrome: A prospective crossover evaluation of lanreotide versus octreotide in terms of efficacy, patient acceptability, and tolerance. Cancer 88:770–776, 2000.
11. Soga J, Yakuwa Y, Osaka M: Carcinoid syndrome: A statistical evaluation of 748 reported cases. J Exp Clin Cancer Res 18:133–141, 1999.
12. Warner RRP: Gut neuroendocrine tumors. In Bardin CW (ed): Current Therapy in Endocrinology and Metabolism, 6th ed. New York, Mosby, 1997, pp. 606–614.

58. CUTANEOUS MANIFESTATIONS OF DIABETES MELLITUS AND THYROID DISEASE

James E. Fitzpatrick, M.D.

1. How often do patients with diabetes mellitus demonstrate an associated skin disorder?

Most published studies report that 30–50% of patients with diabetes mellitus ultimately develop a skin disorder attributable to their primary disease. However, if one includes subtle findings such as nail changes, vascular changes, and alteration of the cutaneous connective tissue, the incidence approaches 100%. Skin disorders most often present in patients with known diabetes mellitus, but cutaneous manifestations also may be an early sign of undiagnosed diabetes.

2. Are any skin disorders pathognomonic of diabetes mellitus?

Yes. Bullous diabeticorum (bullous eruption of diabetes, diabetic bullae) is specific for diabetes mellitus, but it is uncommon. Bullous diabeticorum most often occurs in patients with severe diabetes, particularly those with associated peripheral neuropathy. In general, all other reported skin findings may be found to some extent in normal individuals without diabetes. However, some cutaneous conditions (e.g., necrobiosis lipoidica diabeticorum) demonstrate strong associations with diabetes.

3. What are the skin disorders most likely to be encountered in diabetics?

The most common skin disorders are finger pebbles, nail bed telangiectasia, red face, skin tags (acrochordons), diabetic dermopathy, yellow skin, yellow nails, and pedal petechial purpura. Less-common cutaneous disorders that are closely associated with diabetes mellitus include necrobiosis lipoidica diabeticorum, bullous eruption of diabetes, acanthosis nigricans, and scleredema adultorum.

Common Cutaneous Findings in Diabetes Mellitus

CUTANEOUS FINDING	INCIDENCE IN CONTROLS (%)	INCIDENCE IN DIABETICS (%)
Finger pebbles	21	75
Nail bed telangiectasia	12	65
Rubeosis (red face)	18	59
Skin tags	3	55
Diabetic dermopathy	Uncommon	54
Yellow skin	24	51
Yellow nails	Uncommon	50
Erythrasma	Uncommon	47
Diabetic thick skin	Uncommon	30

4. Define finger pebbles.

Finger pebbles are multiple, grouped minute papules that tend to affect the extensor surfaces of the fingers, particularly near the knuckles. They are asymptomatic and may be extremely subtle in appearance. Histologically, finger pebbles are caused by increased collagen in the dermal papillae. The pathogenesis is not understood.

5. What is acanthosis nigricans?

Acanthosis nigricans is a skin condition due to papillomatous (wartlike) hyperplasia of the skin. It is associated with various conditions, including diabetes mellitus, obesity, acromegaly, Cushing's syndrome, certain medications, and underlying malignancies. The acanthosis nigricans that occurs in patients with insulin-dependent diabetes has been associated with insulin resistance by three different mechanisms: type A (receptor defect), type B (antireceptor antibodies), and type C (postreceptor defect). It is proposed that in insulin-resistant states, there is hyperinsulinemia which competes for the insulin-like growth factor receptors on keratinocytes, and thus stimulates epidermal growth. In the case of hypercortisolism (Cushing's syndrome), the associated insulin resistance is similarly believed to induce epidermal growth.

6. Describe what acanthosis nigricans looks like.

It is most noticeable in axillary, inframammary, and neck creases, where it appears as

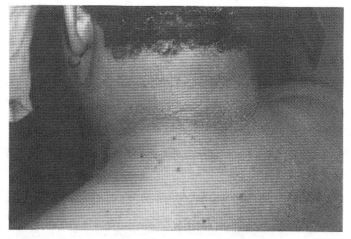

Acanthosis nigricans. Characteristic velvety hyperpigmentation of flexural areas.

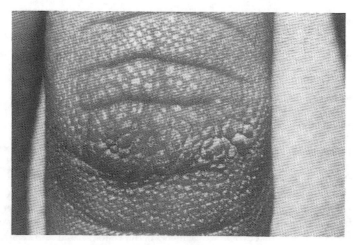

Acanthosis nigricans. Typical lesions over the knuckles demonstrating the papillomatous nature of this cutaneous finding.

hyperpigmented velvety skin that has the appearance of being "dirty." The tops of knuckles may also demonstrate small papules that resemble finger pebbles, except they are more pronounced.

7. What is diabetic dermopathy? What is the pathogenesis?

Diabetic dermopathy (shin spots or pretibial pigmented patches) is a common affliction of diabetics that initially presents as erythematous to brown to brownish-red macules that typically measure 0.5–1.5 cm with variable scale on the pretibial surface. They heal with varying degrees of atrophy and hyperpigmentation over 1–2 yr. The lesions are typically asymptomatic but are occasionally pruritic or are associated with a burning sensation. Patients with diabetic dermopathy are more likely to have retinopathy, nephropathy, and neuropathy.

The pathogenesis is unknown, and similar lesions are less commonly seen in nondiabetics. Skin biopsies from the lesions demonstrate diabetic microangiopathy characterized by a proliferation of endothelial cells and thickening of the basement membranes of arterioles, capillaries, and venules. It is not clear whether the lesions are attributable entirely to vascular changes or whether other secondary factors, such as trauma or venous stasis, are required. Although many physicians attribute these lesions to trauma, this is not supported by an unusual study in which patients with diabetes mellitus did not develop lesions after being struck on the pretibial surface with a hard rubber hammer! There is no known effective treatment.

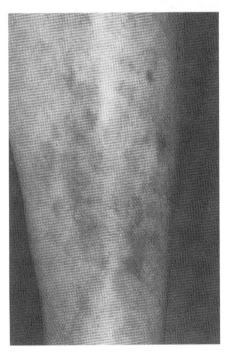

Diabetic dermopathy. Characteristic brown macules of pretibial areas..

8. Define necrobiosis lipoidica diabeticorum.

Necrobiosis lipoidica diabeticorum is a disease that most commonly occurs on the pretibial areas, although it may occur at other sites. Early lesions present as nondiagnostic erythematous papules or plaques that evolve into annular lesions characterized by a yellowish color, dilated blood vessels, and central epidermal atrophy. Developed lesions are characteristic and usually can be diagnosed by clinical appearance. Less commonly, ulcers may develop.

Biopsies demonstrate palisaded granulomas that surround large zones of necrotic and sclerotic collagen. Additional findings include dilated vascular spaces, plasma cells, and increased neutral fat. Biopsies of developed lesions are usually diagnostic, although some cases may be difficult to separate from granuloma anulare. The pathogenesis is not known, but proposed causes include an immune complex vasculitis and a platelet aggregation defect.

9. What is the relationship of necrobiosis lipoidica diabeticorum to diabetes mellitus?

In a major study of patients with necrobiosis lipoidica diabeticorum, 62% had diabetes. Approximately one half of the nondiabetic patients had abnormal glucose tolerance tests, and almost one half of the nondiabetics gave a family history of diabetes. However, necrobiosis lipoidica diabeticorum is present in only 0.3% of patients with diabetes. Some dermatologists prefer the term *necrobiosis lipoidica* for patients who have the disorder without associated diabetes. Because of the strong association between these conditions, patients who present with necrobiosis lipoidica should be screened for diabetes; patients who test negative should be re-evaluated periodically.

10. Describe how necrobiosis lipoidica diabeticorum should be treated.

Necrobiosis lipoidica occasionally may resolve without treatment. It does not seem to respond to treatment of diabetes in new cases or to tighter control of established diabetes. Early lesions may respond to treatment with potent topical or intralesional corticosteroids. More severe cases may respond to oral treatment with either acetylsalicylic acid and dipyridamole or pentoxifylline, although many cases show no response. Severe cases with recalcitrant ulcers may require surgical grafting.

11. Are skin infections more common in diabetics than in control populations?

Yes. But skin infections are probably not as common as most medical personnel believe. Studies show that an increased incidence of skin infections strongly correlates with elevated levels of mean plasma glucose.

12. What are the most common bacterial skin infections associated with diabetes mellitus?

The most common serious skin infections associated with diabetes mellitus are diabetic foot and amputation ulcers. One autopsy study revealed that 2.4% of all diabetics had infectious skin ulcerations of the extremities compared with 0.5% of a control population. Staphylococcal skin infections, including furunculosis and staphylococcal wound infections, are usually described in textbooks as more common and more serious in diabetics than in the nondiabetic population. Although it is universally accepted that staphylococcal infections are more serious and difficult to manage in diabetics, no well-controlled studies prove that the incidence is higher in diabetics. This controversial issue remains to be resolved. Erythrasma, a benign superficial bacterial infection caused by *Corynebacterium minutissimum*, was present in 47% of adult diabetics in one study. Clinically it presents as tan to reddish-brown macular lesions with slight scale in intertriginous areas, usually of the groin; however, the axilla and toe web spaces also may be affected. Because the organisms produce porphyrins, the diagnosis can be made by demonstrating a spectacular coral red fluorescence with a Wood's lamp.

13. What are the most common fungal skin infections associated with diabetes mellitus?

The most common mucocutaneous fungal infection associated with diabetes is candidiasis, usually caused by *Candida albicans*. Women are particularly prone to get vulvovaginitis. One study demonstrated that two-thirds of all diabetics have positive cultures for *Candida albicans*. In women with signs and symptoms of vulvitis, the incidence of positive cultures approaches 99%. Similarly, positive cultures are extremely common in diabetic men and women who complain of anal pruritus. Other mucocutaneous forms of candidiasis include thrush, perleche (angular cheilitis), intertrigo, erosio interdigitalis blastomycetica

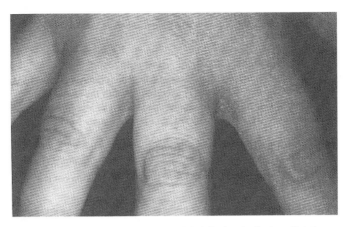

Erosio interdigitalis blastomycetica chronica. *Candida* infection in the interdigital spaces in a diabetic patient. A very long name for a very small infection!

chronica (see figure above), paronychia (infection of the soft tissue around the nail plate), and onychomycosis (infection of the nail). The mechanism appears to be due to increased levels of glucose that serve as a substrate for *Candida* species to proliferate. Patients with recurrent cutaneous candidiasis of any form should be screened for diabetes. Diabetics in ketoacidosis are particularly prone to develop mucormycosis (zygomycosis) caused by various zygomycetes, including *Mucor, Mortierella, Rhizopus,* and *Absidia* species. Fortunately, such fulminant and often fatal infections are rare. Although early studies had suggested that dermatophyte infections were more common in diabetics than in controls, more recent epidemiologic data do not support this association.

14. Why are diabetics in ketoacidosis especially prone to mucormycosis?

These fungi are thermotolerant, prefer an acid pH, grow rapidly in the presence of high levels of glucose, and are one of the few fungi that utilize ketones as a growth substrate. Thus, diabetics in ketoacidosis provide an ideal environment for the proliferation of these fungi.

15. Are any skin complications associated with the treatment of diabetes mellitus?

Yes. Adverse reactions to injected insulin are relatively common. The reported incidence varies from 10–56%, depending on the study. In general these complications may be divided into three categories: reactions due to faulty injections (e.g., intradermal injection), idiosyncratic reactions, and allergic reactions. Several types of allergic reactions have been described, including localized and generalized urticaria, Arthus reactions, and localized delayed hypersensitivity. Oral hypoglycemic agents occasionally may produce adverse cutaneous reactions, including photosensitivity, urticaria, erythema multiforme, and erythema nodosum. Chlorpropamide in particular may produce a flushing reaction when consumed with alcohol.

16. What is scleredema adultorum?

Scleredema adultorum is a woody induration that most commonly presents on the posterior neck, upper back, and shoulders. Less commonly it may be more extensive and involve the face, abdomen, and extremities. It is most commonly associated with insulin-dependent diabetes and less commonly associated with monoclonal gammopathies and following streptococcal infections. Biopsies demonstrate increased dermal collagen and hyaluronic acid (dermal mucin). The pathogenesis is not understood. When associated with insulin-dependent diabetes, scleredema adultorum is chronic and recalcitrant to therapy.

17. Discuss the most important cutaneous manifestations of the hypothyroid state.

Generalized myxedema is the most characteristic cutaneous sign of hypothyroidism. Other skin findings include xerosis (dry skin), follicular hyperkeratosis, diffuse hair loss (especially the outer one third of the eyebrows), dry brittle nails, yellowish discoloration of the skin, and thyroid acropachy. These skin changes are all reversible with appropriate thyroid replacement.

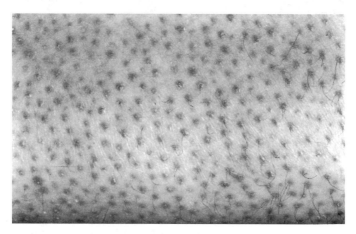

Marked follicular hyperkeratosis and hair loss in a hypothyroid patient. These changes quickly disappeared with thyroid replacement therapy.

18. Why do hypothyroid patients often have yellow skin?

The yellow color is due to the accumulation of carotene (carotenoderma) in the top layer of the epidermis (stratum corneum). Carotene is excreted by both the sweat glands and sebaceous glands and tends to concentrate on the palms, soles, and face. The increased levels of carotene are probably secondary to impaired hepatic conversion of beta-carotene to vitamin A.

19. Describe the clinical findings in generalized myxedema.

Generalized myxedema is characterized by pale, waxy, edematous skin that does not

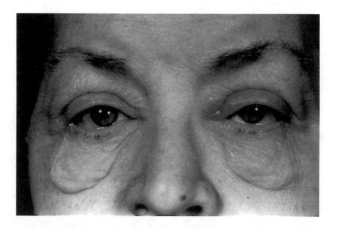

Marked pale, waxy skin of the upper eyelids associated with extensive pendulous edematous skin below the lower eyelids. These changes quickly disappeared with thyroid replacement therapy.

demonstrate pitting. These changes are most noticeable in the periorbital area but may also be observed in the distal extremities, lips, and tongue.

20. What is the pathogenesis of generalized myxedema?

The skin demonstrates an increased accumulation of dermal acid mucopolysaccharides, of which hyaluronic acid (ground substance) is the most important. Studies also have demonstrated that an increased transcapillary escape of serum albumin into the dermis adds to the edematous appearance. Neither of these changes are permanent; both are reversible with replacement therapy.

21. What is the difference between generalized myxedema and pretibial myxedema?

Generalized myxedema is associated only with the hypothyroid state, whereas pretibial myxedema is characteristically associated with Graves' disease. Patients with pretibial myxedema may be hypothyroid, hyperthyroid, or euthyroid when the skin disorder appears. The pathogenesis has not been proven, but it has been demonstrated that serum from patients with pretibial myxedema will stimulate the production of acid mucopolysaccharides by fibroblasts. Fibroblasts from the pretibial area appear to be more sensitive to stimulation than fibroblasts from other areas; this would account for the tendency for these lesions to occur in pretibial areas. The nature of this circulating factor is unknown, but antithyroid immunoglobulins that bind to fibroblasts may be the culprit. It has also been postulated that activated T cells can induce pretibial fibroblast proliferation and the production of acid mucopolysaccharides.

22. Describe the clinical manifestations of pretibial myxedema.

Pretibial myxedema occurs in about 3–5% of patients with Graves' disease. The major-ity of patients have associated exophthalmos. Thyroid acropachy is also present in 1% of patients with Graves' disease (see figure, below left). Clinically pretibial myxedema is char-acterized by edematous, indurated plaques over the pretibial areas, although other sites of the body also may be involved. The plaques are usually sharply demarcated, but diffuse

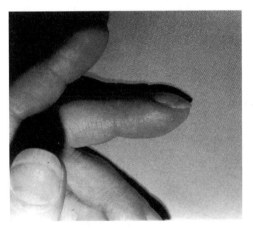

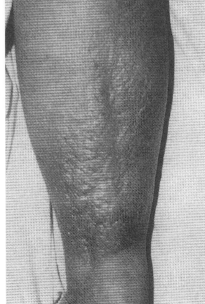

Left, Patient with Graves' disease and thyroid acropachy demonstrating swelling of soft tissues and increased curvature of the nail plate.

Right, **Pretibial myxedema.** Indurated plaques of pretibial area. This case demonstrated a brownish-red color, but lesions may be skin-colored.

variants are also reported. The overlying skin surface is usually normal, although it may be studded with smaller papules. The color varies from skin-colored to brownish-red (see figure, below right). Overlying hypertrichosis may be present on rare occasions. Histologically, pretibial myxedema demonstrates massive accumulation of dermal hyaluronic acid.

23. How is pretibial myxedema treated?

Studies comparing different treatment modalities have not been performed. Because the condition is not harmful to patients, treatment is not always indicated. Many cases respond to potent topical corticosteroids under occlusion or intralesional corticosteroids. More extensive cases may be treated with oral systemic corticosteroids. Treatment of the thyroid disease does not affect the cutaneous findings.

24. Discuss the skin manifestations of hyperthyroidism.

Studies have shown that as many as 97% of all patients with hyperthyroidism develop skin manifestations. Common cutaneous findings include cutaneous erythema, evanescent flushing, excoriations, smooth skin, hyperpigmentation, moist skin (due to increased sweating), pretibial myxedema, pruritus (itching), and warm skin. Nails are often brittle and may separate from the underlying bed (onycholysis). The hair also may be thinner than normal.

BIBLIOGRAPHY

1. Bodman M, Friedman S, Clifford LB: Bullous diabeticorum. A report of two cases with review of the literature. J Am Podiatr Med Assoc 81:561–563, 1991.
2. Freinkel RK, Freinkel N: Hair growth and alopecia in hypothyroidism. Arch Dermatol 106:349–352, 1972.
3. Goette DK: Thyroid acropachy. Arch Dermatol 116:205–206, 1980.
4. Hollister DS, Brodell RT: Finger "pebbles." A dermatologic sign of diabetes mellitus. Postgrad Med 107:209–210, 2000.
5. Huntley AC: The cutaneous manifestations of diabetes mellitus. J Am Acad Dermatol 7:427–455, 1982.
6. Lang PG Jr, Sisson JC, Lynch PJ: Intralesional triamcinolone therapy for pretibial myxedema. Arch Dermatol 110:197–202, 1975.
7. Lipsky BA, Berendt AR: Principles and practice of antibiotic therapy of diabetic foot infections. Diabetes Metab Res Rev 16(Suppl 1):S42–S46, 2000.
8. Montes LF, Dobson H, Dodge BG, Knowles WR: Erythrasma and diabetes mellitus. Arch Dermatol 99:674–680, 1969.
9. Muller SA, Winkelmann RK: Necrobiosis lipoidica diabeticorm: A clinical and pathological investigation of 171 cases. Arch Dermatol 93:272–281, 1966.
10. Mullin GE, Eastern JS: Cutaneous consequences of accelerated thyroid function. Cutis 37:109–112, 1986.
11. Quimby SR, Muller SA, Schroeter AL, et al.: Necrobiosis lipoidica diabeticorum: Platelet survival and response to platelet inhibitors. Cutis 43:231–236, 1989.
12. Parving HH, Hansen JM, Nielsen SL, et al: Mechanism of edema formation in myxedema: Increased protein extravasation and relatively slow lymphatic drainage. N Engl J Med 301:460–465, 1979.
13. Plourde PV, Marks JG, Hammond JM: Acanthosis nigricans and insulin resistance. J Am Acad Dermatol 10:887–891, 1984
14. Rapoport B, Alsabeh R, Aftergood D, McLachlan SM: Elephantiasic pretibial myxdema: insight into and a hypothesis regarding the pathogenesis of the extrathyroidal manifestations of Graves's disease. Thyroid 10:685–692, 2000.
15. Shemer A, Bergman R, Linn S, et al.: Diabetic dermopathy and internal complications in diabetes mellitus. Int J Dermatol 37:113–115, 1998.
16. Sibbald RG, Landolt SJ, Toth D: Skin and diabetes. Endocrinol Metab Clin North Am 25:463–472, 1996.

59. INHERITED HORMONE RESISTANCE SYNDROMES

Michael T. McDermott, M.D.

1. Name some of the well-characterized genetic hormone resistance syndromes.

There are well-described syndromes caused by inherited resistance to insulin, thyroid hormone, parathyroid hormone (PTH), vitamin D, androgens, cortisol, vasopressin, growth hormone, and estrogen.

2. What are the causes of inherited insulin resistance?

Inherited insulin resistance may result from a variety of abnormalities. Prereceptor disorders include genetic mutations that produce abnormal insulin molecules or that result in inability to cleave proinsulin into insulin and c-peptide, resulting in high circulating serum proinsulin levels. Receptor disorders result from a multitude of inactivating genetic mutations that affect the insulin receptor. Postreceptor disorders include loss-of-function mutations involving insulin-receptor substrate 1 (IRS-1), glucose transporters, intracellular signaling proteins, and the enzymes involved in intracellular glucose metabolism.

3. What are the manifestations of insulin resistance?

Insulin resistance is characterized by normal or elevated levels of plasma glucose in the presence of moderate-to-extreme elevations of the serum insulin concentration. Patients may be asymptomatic or may have symptoms of hyperglycemia. Obesity, acanthosis nigricans, and excessive secretion of androgens are often seen in patients with insulin resistance.

4. What role does insulin resistance play in the development of atherosclerosis?

Mild-to-moderate insulin resistance is commonly associated with hypertension, elevated serum triglycerides, low serum HDL cholesterol, and small, dense LDL particles. Referred to as syndrome X, this combination of coronary artery disease risk factors appears to be particularly atherogenic.

5. What causes the thyroid hormone resistance syndromes?

Generalized resistance to thyroid hormone (GRTH) results from genetic mutations of the thyroid hormone receptor that alter the T_3-binding region, causing reduced T_3-binding affinity. Resistance to thyroid hormone feedback at the pituitary level results in hypersecretion of TSH, which in turn stimulates excessive production of T_4 and T_3 by the thyroid gland. Symptomatic thyrotoxicosis does not occur, however, because peripheral tissues are also resistant to thyroid hormone effects.

6. What are the clinical manifestations of thyroid hormone resistance?

Patients with GRTH are clinically euthyroid or hypothyroid but have elevated serum levels of total and free T_4 and T_3 and inappropriately normal or elevated serum TSH levels. Hyperactivity–attention deficit disorder, low IQ, hearing impairment, and heart disease are sometimes associated.

7. What causes the parathyroid hormone resistance syndromes?

PTH receptors are normal but postreceptor signaling is defective, most often because of inactivating genetic mutations affecting the Gs alpha protein that normally couples the PTH receptor to the cyclic adenosine monophosphate (cAMP) response cascade. Some cases are due to abnormalities at other sites in the signal pathways. Lack of PTH effect causes hypocalcemia and hyperphosphatemia despite an increased serum level of PTH. This disorder is also termed pseudohypoparathyroidism.

8. What are the clinical manifestations of parathyroid hormone resistance?

Affected patients often have short stature, short fourth and fifth metacarpals, mental retardation, and calcification of the basal ganglia. Biochemically, the serum calcium is low, phosphorus is high, and PTH is moderately to greatly elevated.

9. What causes the vitamin D resistance syndromes?

The two major disorders are congenital 1-alpha-hydroxylase deficiency (C1HD) and congenital resistance to 1,25-dihydroxyvitamin D (CRVD). C1HD is caused by genetic mutations that inactivate 1-alpha-hydroxylase, the enzyme that converts 25-hydroxyvitamin D to 1,25-dihydroxyvitamin D. CRVD is due to inactivating mutations involving vitamin D receptors. A third condition, congenital hypophosphatemic rickets, was initially termed "vitamin D–resistant rickets," but the predominant defect is now known to be renal phosphate wasting.

10. What are the manifestations of vitamin D resistance?

Vitamin D resistance causes short stature, rickets, and muscle weakness; patients with CRVD also may have alopecia. Biochemically, both disorders exhibit hypocalcemia, hypophosphatemia, and elevated levels of serum PTH. However, serum levels of 1,25-dihydroxyvitamin D are low in C1HD and normal or elevated in CRVD. In contrast, patients with congenital hypophosphatemic rickets have normal serum calcium concentrations but very low serum phosphate levels associated with increased urinary phosphate excretion.

11. What causes the androgen resistance syndromes?

There are two main categories of androgen resistance syndromes. Genetic mutations producing abnormal androgen receptors may cause partial or complete androgen resistance in all tissues; complete androgen resistance is termed testicular feminization. In contrast, deficiency of 5-alpha-reductase, the enzyme that converts testosterone to dihydrotestosterone (DHT), causes androgen resistance only in DHT-dependent tissues, such as the external genitalia.

12. What are the clinical manifestations of androgen resistance?

The androgen resistance syndromes have thus far been recognized only in individuals who are genetic males. Depending on their severity, androgen receptor abnormalities can produce a spectrum of disorders ranging from simple oligospermia to ambiguous genitalia to a phenotypic female (genetic male) who fails to develop menses (testicular feminization). Hormone testing reveals normal or elevated male-range levels of testosterone and elevated serum luteinizing hormone (LH) levels. Deficiency of 5-alpha-reductase in genetic males produces phenotypically female or ambiguous genitalia, which then undergo partial masculinization at puberty when secretion of testosterone greatly increases.

13. What causes the cortisol resistance syndromes?

Cortisol resistance syndromes are due to inactivating genetic mutations involving cortisol receptors. Lack of normal cortisol receptors in the central nervous system results in ineffective suppression of ACTH by circulating cortisol. The resultant hypersecretion of ACTH stimulates increased adrenal production of cortisol, aldosterone, and androgens. Because of defective function of cortisol receptors, however, the body responds only to the excess of aldosterone and androgens and does not exhibit clinical features of hypercortisolism.

14. What are the clinical manifestations of cortisol resistance?
Men with cortisol resistance develop mainly hypertension, whereas affected women tend to exhibit hypertension, hirsutism and virilization. Serum levels of cortisol, aldosterone, and testosterone are all elevated, and ACTH is inappropriately normal or high.

15. What causes congenital resistance to vasopressin?
Congenital resistance to vasopressin has been found to be due to genetic mutations producing abnormal renal vasopressin receptors; some patients, however, may have abnormalities in the Gs alpha protein that couples the receptors to cAMP activation. In either case, the result is an inability of the renal collecting ducts to conserve water in response to vasopressin. The condition also has been termed congenital nephrogenic diabetes insipidus.

16. What are the clinical manifestations of vasopressin resistance?
Affected patients develop polyuria soon after birth. The increased urinary output does not respond to water deprivation or to the administration of vasopressin. When testing is available, levels of vasopressin are elevated. If fluid intake is not adequate, severe volume depletion may result.

17. What causes the growth hormone resistance syndromes?
The best studied disorder, Laron dwarfism, is due to inactivating genetic mutations involving the growth hormone receptor. The result is an inability of growth hormone to stimulate hepatic production of insulin-like growth factor–1 (IGF-1), which is the major factor that stimulates peripheral growth.

18. What are the clinical manifestations of growth hormone resistance?
Affected patients have moderate-to-severe growth retardation. Serum levels of growth hormone are elevated, but IGF-1 levels are low.

19. What causes estrogen resistance?
Estrogen resistance results from an inactivating genetic mutation of the estrogen receptor.

20. What are the clinical manifestations of estrogen resistance?
Estrogen resistance has thus far been described only in a genetic male. This patient presented with osteoporosis, unfused epiphyses, acanthosis nigricans, glucose intolerance, and hyperinsulinemia and was subsequently found to have premature coronary artery disease. His serum testosterone level was normal, but his serum levels of estradiol, estrone, FSH, and LH were all elevated as a result of impaired function of the estrogen receptor.

BIBLIOGRAPHY
1. Amselem S, Duquesnoy P, Attree O, et al: Laron dwarfism and mutations of the growth hormone–receptor gene. N Engl J Med 321:989–995, 1989.
2. Amselem S, Sobrier M-L, Duquesnoy P, et al: Recurrent nonsense mutations in the growth hormone receptor from patients with Laron dwarfism. J Clin Invest 87:1098–1102, 1991.
3. Breslau NA: Pseudohypoparathyroidism: Current concepts. Am J Med Sci 298(2):130–140, 1989.
4. Farfel Z, Brickman AS, Kaslow HR, et al: Defect of receptor-cyclase coupling protein in pseudohypoparathyroidism. N Engl J Med 303:237–242, 1980.
5. Flier JS: Lilly lecture: Syndromes of insulin resistance; from patient to gene and back again. Diabetes 41:1207–1219, 1992.
6. Griffin JE: Androgen resistance—the clinical and molecular spectrum. N Engl J Med 325: 611–618, 1992.
7. Holtzman EJ, Harris HW Jr, Kolakowski LF Jr, et al: Brief report: A molecular defect in the vasopressin V2-receptor gene causing nephrogenic diabetes insipidus. N Engl J Med 238:1534–1537, 1993.

8. Javier EC, Reardon GE, Malchoff CD: Glucocorticoid resistance and its clinical presentations. Endocrinologist 1:141–148, 1991.

9. Kristjansson K, Rut AR, Hewison M, et al: Two mutations in the hormone binding domain of the vitamin D receptor cause tissue resistance to 1,25 dihydroxyvitamin D_3. J Clin Invest 92:12–16, 1993.

10. Malchoff DM, Brufsky A, Reardon G, et al: A mutation of the glucocorticoid receptor in primary cortisol resistance. J Clin Invest 91:1918–1925, 1993.

11. McDermott MT, Ridgway EC: Thyroid hormone resistance syndromes. Am J Med 94:424–432, 1993.

12. McPhaul MJ, Marcelli M, Zoppi S, et al: Genetic basis of endocrine disease 4: The spectrum of mutations in the androgen receptor gene that causes androgen resistance. J Clin Endocrinol Metab 76:17–23, 1993.

13. Merendino JJ Jr, Spiegel AM, Crawford JD, et al: Brief report: A mutation in the vasopressin V2-receptor gene in a kindred with X-linked nephrogenic diabetes insipidus. N Engl J Med 238:1538–1543, 1993.

14. Moller DE, Flier JS: Insulin resistance—mechanisms, syndromes, and implications. N Engl J Med 325:938–948, 1991.

15. Smith EP, Boyd J, Frank GR, et al: Estrogen resistance caused by a mutation in the estrogen-receptor gene in a man. N Engl J Med 331:1056–1061, 1994.

16. Sudhir K, Chou TM, Chatterjee K, et al: Premature coronary artery disease associated with a disruptive mutation in the estrogen receptor gene in a man. Circulation 96:3774–3777, 1997.

17. Taylor SI: Lilly lecture: Molecular mechanisms of insulin resistance; lessons from patients with mutations in the insulin-receptor gene. Diabetes 41:1473–1490, 1992.

18. Yagi H, Oxono K, Miyake N, et al: A new point mutation in the deoxyribonucleic acid–binding domain of the vitamin D–receptor in a kindred with hereditary 1,25-dihydroxyvitamin D-resistant rickets. J Clin Endocrinol Metab 76:509–512, 1993.

60. AGING AND ENDOCRINOLOGY

Robert S Schwartz, M.D., and Wendy M Kohrt, Ph.D.

AGE-RELATED CHANGES IN BODY COMPOSITION

1. Describe the body weight changes that occur with aging.

Aging is associated with several important changes in body composition that might be related to changes in endocrine status and that can have important endocrine/metabolic consequences. In cross-sectional studies, body weight increases until about age 55 yr and then there is a significant drop off. This finding is probably due to a "die off" effect in the heaviest patients during middle age. Prospective studies suggest that there may be a decline in weight that occurs after age 65–70 yr. Unlike what is seen in studies in younger populations, this reduction in body weight appears to be associated with an increase in mortality, morbidity and disability. The untoward effects of weight loss in older individuals do not appear to be explained simply by unintentional weight loss due to illness or disease, as similar effects have been noted in individuals who espouse intentional weight loss. The explanation for this is not clear but may be due to the fact that any sustained weight loss may, in fact, be unintentional, as intentional weight loss is always quite difficult to maintain. Weight loss in the face of illness or disease that may raise cytokine levels may predispose to the loss of the preponderance of weight as lean body mass (muscle mass) and thus worsen the age-related sarcopenia and lead to a state of cachexia. Small clinical studies (unpublished) of intentional weight loss in *carefully screened* healthy older men have noted a distribution of weight loss that is similar to that seen in younger individuals on moderate caloric restriction.

2. What are the changes in lean body mass and muscle mass that occur with aging?

A loss of lean body mass, mostly skeletal muscle mass, also occurs with aging. This has been termed "sarcopenia" and has been blamed for much (but not all) of the age-related decline in muscle strength and power. In cross-sectional studies, a loss of 20–30% of lean mass has been detected between ages 30 and 80 yr. This would suggest an even larger loss of muscle mass. The decline in strength is even greater, with longitudinal studies finding up to a 60% loss from age 30 to 80. The loss of strength is greatest at the older ages; a 25% decline has been detected between 70 and 75 yr. Power (work per unit time) may decline at double the rate of strength, 3% per year from ages 65–84. These changes in lean mass, muscle mass, strength and power have complex but important functional consequences for older individuals.

3. Discuss the changes in adiposity and fat distribution that occur with aging.

The changes in adiposity and fat distribution with age have important effects on metabolism. While lean mass is declining with age, fat mass increases (at least until age 65 yr). Furthermore, the central and intra-abdominal depots of fat increase preferentially. This increase in central adiposity begins following puberty in males but primarily after menopause in females. This increment in visceral adiposity (along with the decline in physical activity) plays an important role in the age-associated decrement in insulin sensitivity and probably the high incidence and prevalence of type 2 diabetes mellitus and insulin resistance syndrome that occurs with age.

4. Does the menopause trigger an increase in abdominal obesity in women?

Cross-sectional comparisons of women across the age spectrum suggest that waist size increases more rapidly in women aged 50 yr and older than in younger women. Similarly, comparisons of young and older women, utilizing soft-tissue scanning techniques (i.e., computed tomography, magnetic resonance imaging), suggest that intra-abdominal fat depots do not increase markedly until after the menopause. These findings were corroborated by a 6-yr prospective study of age-matched women who either remained premenopausal over the period of study or underwent the menopausal transition. Body fat content increased only in the latter group (+2.5 kg), and this was accompanied by an increase in the waist-to-hip circumference ratio, indicating a preferential deposition of fat in the abdominal region.

The results of the Postmenopausal Estrogen/Progestin Intervention trial provided evidence that estrogens modulate fat metabolism. Postmenopausal women were randomized to receive estrogens alone, estrogens and medroxyprogesterone acetate, or placebo treatment for 3 yr. The hormone-treated groups gained less weight and had less of an increase in waist size than the placebo-treated group. The group treated with unopposed estrogens tended to have the smallest gains in body weight and waist girth. It has not yet been determined whether estrogens specifically prevent or attenuate intra-abdominal fat accumulation.

5. What are the changes in bone mass and density that occur with aging?

Prospective data indicate that peak bone mass occurs during the late teenage years in women and about a decade later in men. Because of the intimate structural and functional link between muscle and bone, the occurrence of peak bone mass likely corresponds with peak skeletal muscle development. It is generally thought that bone mass is maintained, or decreases slowly (<0.2% per year), at least through age 40 yr in women and age 50 in men. Intuitively, the decline in physical activity during middle age might be expected to induce an even faster rate of bone loss. However, the increase in body weight that typically also occurs during middle age probably counters this to a large extent, by increasing mechanical loading forces acting on the skeleton during weight-bearing activity. There is inarguably an accelerated decline in bone mineral density around the time of menopause in women. What remains somewhat controversial is whether the menopause-induced increase in resorption diminishes after a few years or persists into old age. In this regard, observational studies of women aged 65 yr and older indicate that the rate of bone loss continues to increase with age, particularly in the hip region. This is corroborated by observations that serum markers of bone turnover increase at the menopause and remain elevated into old age. In elderly women and men, the decrease in bone mineral at the hip appears to be accelerated (~1% per year) relative to the changes at the spine. However, vertebral compression fractures and the development of extravertebral osteophytes lead to an increase in bone mineral density, but this does not reflect increased vertebral strength. The utility of spine bone mineral density for the diagnosis of osteoporosis is therefore compromised.

6. Can weight-bearing exercise prevent the menopause-related loss of bone mineral in women?

It is unlikely that even vigorous weight-bearing exercise can effectively counteract the deleterious effects of estrogen deficiency on bone mineral density. Older female athletes not on hormone replacement therapy have decreased bone mineral density relative to premenopausal athletes. Moreover, young female athletes with menstrual dysfunction can have bone mineral density levels in the osteopenic (1–2.5 SD below the average peak bone mineral density) and even osteoporotic range (>2.5 SD below the average peak bone mineral density), despite their participation in sports that involve high levels of mechanical loading (e.g., gymnastics, distance running). Although the direct effects of estrogens on bone metabolism are well known, there is growing evidence that estrogens, and possibly androgens, also specifically modulate the responses of bone cells to mechanical stress. In animal models, the effects of mechanical stress in the presence of estrogens (in females) or androgens (in males) on the bone proliferative response have been found to be synergistic (i.e., more than additive). There is also evidence for additive or synergistic effects of exercise and estrogens on bone mineral density in postmenopausal women.

AGE-RELATED CHANGES IN THE GROWTH HORMONE/INSULIN-LIKE GROWTH FACTOR-I AXIS

7. Describe the changes in the growth hormone/insulin-like growth factor-I axis with aging.

Aging is associated with a significant decline in the growth hormone (GH) area under the curve as well as number of GH peaks and peak amplitude. These changes in GH secretion are associated with a steady decline in insulin-like growth factor-I (IGF-I) after age 30 yr. By age 65, a majority of individuals have an IGF-I concentration that is near or below the lower limit of normal for young healthy individuals. This decline in the GH/IGF-I axis appears to occur above the level of the pituitary since chronic treatment with growth hormone–releasing hormone (GHRH) and/or other growth hormone secretagogues (GHS) can mitigate much of this decline. The cause of the fall-off in this axis is not entirely clear but could be explained by age-related changes in GHRH, somatostatin or ghrelin tone. This last peptide has recently been discovered and appears to be the natural ligand for the GHS receptor.

8. Might the decline in the GH/IGF-I axis be related to age-related changes in body composition and function?

Many of the body compositional changes that occur with aging seem consistent with what might be expected in a GH/IGF-I –deficient state. The strongest evidence for this potential association comes from studies of GH-deficient adults. These patients have many of the same physiological abnormalities seen in older individuals, including: 1) reduced lean body and muscle mass; 2) reduced strength and aerobic capacity; 3) excess overall adiposity, and central and intra-abdominal fat; 4) high incidence of insulin resistance syndrome; 5) reduced bone mass and density; 6) reduced or absent slow-wave sleep; and 7) high incidence of mood disturbance (depression). More importantly, most of these abnormalities reverse with GH *replacement* in these patients. Recently there have been several clinical trials of either GH or GHRH *supplementation* in older individuals with low IGF-I concentrations. These have consistently demonstrated the ability to increase IGF-I concentrations and lean body/muscle mass and reduce both total and central/intraabdominal adiposity. However, changes in strength, function, and bone density have been difficult to demonstrate.

It is possible that some of the most potentially important effects of supplementing the GH/IGF-I axis will be on the brain. The elderly as a group often experience lack of sleep and feeling tired during the day. This may be due to the almost total loss of slow-wave sleep (stages 3 and 4). Of interest, the periods of slow wave sleep in younger individuals coincide exactly with the nighttime peaks of GH secretion. Indeed, there are animal and some human data that suggest that GHRH supplementation may be able to restart pulsatile GH secretion and also stimulate slow-wave sleep. There is also a recent abstract that suggests that chronic GHRH supplementation may improve cognitive function, specifically psychomotor and perceptual processing speed, as well as fluid memory.

The adverse effects profile for GH administration (but not GHRH) has been substantial, with development of carpal tunnel syndrome, gynecomastia, and edema and worsening of glucose tolerance, insulin sensitivity and osteoarthritis. An increase in the risk for certain cancers (breast, prostate) has been postulated but thus far has not been detected. While it is possible that the most correct doses of GH, GHRH, or GHS for supplementation have not been defined yet, it would appear reasonable that significant improvements in strength and function may require not only hormone supplementation but also the appropriate stimulus, such as exercise. Nevertheless, considerable interest in supplementation of this axis continues to exist, especially for the treatment or prevention of frailty and recovery from hip fracture.

AGE-RELATED CHANGES IN ANDROGEN CONCENTRATIONS IN MEN

9. What are the changes in testosterone concentration with aging?

Like IGF-I, testosterone concentration appears to decline steadily after age 30 in men. However, because of coincident increases in sex hormone binding globulin, the decline in total testosterone concentration is difficult to detect in many studies. When either free or "bio-available" testosterone is measured, the decline with age is more apparent. Estimates of "hypogonadism" in older men run from 30-70%.

10. Might the decline in the testosterone concentration be related to age-related changes in body composition and function?

Similar to what is discussed above, there is a close relationship between many of the physiological findings in young hypogonadal men and those found in older men. Furthermore, reversibility has been noted with testosterone replacement in hypogonadal young men and in patients with acquired hypogonadism associated with human immunodeficiency infection. To date, there have been only a few studies that have investigated the effects of testosterone supplementation in older men. The largest published study found improvements in muscle and fat mass but no significant effects on bone mineral density or strength. Unpublished studies suggest that small but detectable changes in strength do occur with testosterone supplementation in older men.

Recently, there has been considerable interest in the effect of testosterone supplementation on bone density in older men. While large clinical trials are still in the planning stages, there is evidence of potential efficacy. However, recent work suggests that much, if not all, of the effect may be due to concomitant elevations of estrogen levels through aromatization. Similarly, it is possible that some of the recently noted cognitive effects of testosterone may be due to estrogen effects on the brain.

The dose of testosterone required for supplementation has not been adequately defined and may vary depending on whether an exercise stimulus is included in the study. The potential side effect profile of testosterone supplementation includes erythrocytosis, prostate enlargement, stimulation of prostate cancer growth, elevation of liver enzymes, edema, acne, and worsening of obstructive sleep apnea.

AGE-RELATED CHANGES IN DEHYDROEPIANDROSTERONE

11. What are the changes in dehydroepiandrosterone concentration with aging?

Dehydroepiandrosterone (DHEA) and its sulfate (DHEAS), collectively referred to as DHEA/S, are the most abundant steroid hormones in humans; approximately 95% are secreted from the adrenal glands. DHEAS is one of the best biological markers of human aging. Peak serum DHEAS levels are reached early in the third decade and then decline steadily: By age 60–70 yr, circulating levels are only about 20% of peak levels. The decrease in DHEAS with aging does not represent a general decline in adrenal function, as similar changes in other adrenal hormones do not occur.

12. What are the biological effects of DHEA/S?

Despite the abundance of DHEA/S and its distinctive age-related changes, little is known regarding the biological effects of DHEA/S in humans. Because it can be converted to testosterone and aromatized to estrogens, the decline in DHEA/S with aging may contribute to physiological changes that occur as a result of or that are augmented by sex hormone deficiency (e.g., the loss of bone and muscle mass). DHEA administration has potent antiobesity, antidiabetogenic, and antiatherogenic effects in rodents. However, it is not clear that these findings are relevant to humans, because physiologic DHEA/S levels in rodents are negligible. In humans, studies of DHEA *supplementation* in young adults have typically involved pharmacologic doses (1,600 mg/day). An early study indicated that DHEA use at this dose by young, healthy men for 1 month resulted in a large increase in lean mass and a large decrease in fat mass. However, a subsequent similar study of obese young men by the same investigators found no such effects. Several other studies of short-term DHEA supplementation in young and middle-age individuals had negative outcomes. More recently, studies of DHEA *replacement* in older adults with low DHEA/S levels suggest that DHEA can increase lean mass and bone mineral density and decrease fat mass. Other reports suggest that DHEA replacement in the elderly has beneficial effects on immune and cognitive function. The replacement dose for women and men 60 yr and older is ~50 mg/day. Most of the studies in older adults have involved small numbers of subjects, and not all have been randomized, placebo-controlled trials. Larger clinical trials of DHEA replacement in humans are currently in progress.

The mechanisms for the observed changes in body composition and other outcomes in response to DHEA replacement are not clear. The reported increases in serum IGF-1 and testosterone that occur in both women and men in response to DHEA could have anabolic effects on lean mass and bone mineral density. Serum levels of estrogens do not appear to increase markedly in response to DHEA, but a shift toward more estradiol and less estrone and a decrease in sex hormone binding globulin could result in increased biological activity of estrogens.

BIBLIOGRAPHY

1. Bassey EJ, Fiatarone MA, O'Neill, et al.: Leg extensor power and functional performance in very old men and women. Clin Sci 82:321–327, 1992.
2. Bhasin S, Bagatel CJ, Bremner WJ, et al.: Issues in testosterone replacement in older men. J Clin Endocrinol Metab 83:3435–3447, 1998.
3. Cheng M., Zaman G, Rawlinson SC, et al.: Enhancement by sex hormones of the osteoregulatory effects of mechanical loading and prostaglandins in explants of rat ulnae. J Bone Miner Res 12:1424–1430, 1997.
4. Ensrud KE, Palermo L, Black DM, et al.: Hip and calcaneal bone loss increase with advancing age: longitudinal results from the study of osteoporotic fractures. J Bone Miner Res 10:1778–1787, 1995.
5. Espeland MA, Stefanick ML, Kritz-Silverstein D, et al.: Effect of postmenopausal hormone therapy on body weight and waist and hip girths. J Clin Endocrinol Metab 82:1549–1556, 1997.
6. Kohrt WM: Abdominal obesity and associated cardiovascular comorbidities in the elderly. Coronary Artery Disease 9:489–494, 1998.
7. Kohrt WM, Ehsani AA., Birge SJ: HRT preserves increases in bone mineral density and reductions in body fat after a supervised exercise program. J Appl Physiol 84:1506–1512, 1998.
8. Labrie FA, Belanger A, Van LT, et al.: DHEA and the intracrine formation of androgens and estrogens in peripheral target tissues: its role during aging. Steroids 63:322–328, 1998.
9. Lamberts SWJ, van den Beld AW, van der Lely A-J: The endocrinology of aging. Science 278:419–424, 1997.
10. Merriam GR, Buchner DM, Prinz PN, et al.: Potential applications of GH secretagogs in the evaluation and treatment of the age-related decline in growth hormone secretion. Endocrine 7:49–52, 1997.
11. Rosen CJ, Strom BL: Effect of testosterone treatment on body composition and muscle strength in men over 65 years of age. J Clin Endocrinol Metab 84:2653, 1999.

12. Schwartz RS: Trophic factor supplementation: Effect on the age-associated changes in body composition. J Gerontol A Biol Sci Med Sci 50:151–156, 1995.
13. Snyder PJ, Peachey H, Hannoush P, et al.: Effect of testosterone treatment on body composition and muscle strength in men over 65 years of age. J Clin Endocrinol Metab 84:2647–2653, 1999.
14. Villareal DT, Holloszy JO, Kohrt WM: Effects of DHEA replacement on bone mineral density and body composition in elderly women and men. Clin Endocrinol 53:561–568, 2000.
15. Wallace JI, SchwartzRS" Involuntary weight loss in elderly outpatients: recognition, etiologies, and treatment. Clin Geriatr Med 13:717–735, 1997.

61. ENDOCRINE SURGERY

Christopher D. Raeburn, M.D., and Robert C. McIntyre, Jr., M.D.

THYROID

Nodules and Cancer

1. Can operative management of thyroid nodules be based solely on fine needle aspiration (FNA)?

No. FNA of thyroid nodules is a powerful means of assisting in preoperative surgical decision-making. The sensitivity, specificity and accuracy of FNA for thyroid cancer are approximately 90%, 95%, and 95%, respectively. A lesion found to be benign by FNA can be safely followed. Patients with an FNA result of "suspicious" for papillary cancer should undergo surgery with an intraoperative frozen section; if frozen section confirms papillary cancer, a definitive procedure is done. Patients with obvious FNA findings of cancer can undergo a definitive cancer operation. Because of the high specificity of FNA for papillary cancer, no further testing is needed; a standard cancer operation can be performed without intraoperative frozen section. An FNA result of follicular neoplasm requires at least a lobectomy. A frozen section may reveal a follicular variant of papillary cancer, allowing a definitive procedure; however, it cannot distinguish between benign and malignant follicular tumors. The diagnosis of follicular cancer requires the finding of capsular, vascular, or lymphatic invasion on permanent section. If the final pathology is consistent with follicular carcinoma, then completion thyroidectomy may be done if indicated.

2. Describe the appropriate therapy when FNA of a lateral neck mass reveals "normal thyroid follicular cells."

This finding, sometimes erroneously referred to as "lateral aberrant thyroid," most likely represents metastatic, well-differentiated papillary thyroid carcinoma in a cervical lymph node. Appropriate therapy includes near total or total thyroidectomy with a modified neck dissection.

3. What is the appropriate extent of thyroidectomy for differentiated thyroid carcinoma?

Well-differentiated thyroid cancer (papillary and follicular) can be separated into low-, intermediate-, and high-risk groups by considering certain patient and tumor factors. Patient factors such as age and gender and tumor factors including size, local invasion and distant metastases all influence outcome. For those patients who stratify into a high-risk category (males, age > 45, size > 4 cm, local invasion or distant metastases), near-total (leaving less than 1 g of visible thyroid tissue) or total thyroidectomy should be performed. Minimal or occult papillary thyroid cancers (size < 1 cm, no local invasion, and no distant metastases) do well with total lobectomy and isthmusectomy. Minimally invasive follicular carcinoma (fewer than three areas of capsular) microinvasion also has a good outcome with lobectomy alone. For intermediate risk patients, total or near-total thyroidectomy lowers local recurrence rates with minimal additional morbidity. This approach allows improved postoperative cancer surveillance by increasing the sensitivity of radioiodine scans and thyroglobulin levels. More aggressive variants of well-differentiated carcinoma (Hurthle cell and islet cell) should be treated by near-total or total thyroidectomy.

4. Discuss the appropriate surgical management for medullary thyroid carcinoma.

Total thyroidectomy is the only treatment for medullary thyroid carcinoma, as this tumor is not sensitive to radioiodine or thyroid stimulatory hormone suppression. Due to this tumor's propensity for spreading to regional lymph nodes early in the course of disease, appropriate surgical management includes routine central neck dissection, with the addition of modified radical (lateral) neck dissection for clinically positive nodes. Some surgeons advocate routine bilateral modified neck dissection because of the high incidence of lateral nodal metastases (approximately 75% ipsilateral and 50% contralateral to the thyroid tumor). This therapeutic approach, when implemented early in the course of medullary thyroid carcinoma, results in normalization of calcitonin levels in up to 25% of patients.

5. Is there a role for surgery in anaplastic carcinoma of the thyroid?

Unfortunately, anaplastic carcinoma of the thyroid is one of the most aggressive solid tumors known, with greater than 50% of patients having distant metastases at the time of diagnosis resulting in a dismal outcome regardless of therapeutic strategy. Surgery is rarely curative and in most cases should be restricted to a diagnostic or palliative role. Attempts at curative total thyroidectomy with postoperative chemotherapy may be indicated for patients without evidence of distant disease and a tumor felt to be entirely contained within the thyroid gland. Palliative surgical debulking and tracheostomy should be reserved for symptoms of dysphagia or airway compromise, respectively, as they do not prolong survival. Care should be taken to distinguish anaplastic carcinoma from medullary carcinoma or lymphoma, which have considerably better prognoses and require different therapeutic approaches.

6. What is the role of surgery for primary lymphoma of the thyroid?

Primary lymphoma of the thyroid is a relatively uncommon occurrence, representing less than 1% of all thyroid malignancies. Lymphoma of the thyroid often develops in patients with a history of Hashimoto's thyroiditis. The development of a rapidly enlarging thyroid mass often accompanied by compressive symptoms is a common presentation of this tumor. The majority of primary thyroid lymphomas are of the large B-cell type and typically are very sensitive to both chemotherapy (cyclophosphamide, doxorubicin, vincristine, and prednisone) and radiation. Thus, combined modality therapy is the standard treatment, with surgery being relegated to a purely diagnostic role. FNA or core biopsy is often adequate for diagnosis, but incisional biopsy is sometimes necessary; when it is performed, a fresh specimen should be sent directly to the pathologist so that immunohistochemical analysis can be performed as needed.

7. What are a central and modified neck dissections?

A central neck dissection removes all the perithyroidal and tracheoesophageal groove nodes from the thyroid notch superiorly down to the thoracic inlet. Laterally, the dissection extends from carotid to carotid artery. The lateral spread of disease usually involves high, middle, and low jugular lymph nodes (levels II–IV) and occasionally lateral (level V) nodes. A modified neck dissection, sometimes referred to as a functional dissection, spares the internal jugular vein, sternocleidomastoid muscle and spinal accessory nerve, because sacrificing these structures does not improve outcome.

8. When should formal node dissection be performed versus "berry picking"?

For well-differentiated thyroid cancers, formal node dissection is indicated in all patients with clinically positive nodes. "Berry picking" (removing only the obviously abnormal nodes) is associated with increased local recurrence compared with formal node dissection and disrupts surgical planes, making subsequent dissection much more difficult. Microfoci of cancer in regional lymph nodes are found in 80% of differentiated thyroid cancers. The presence of these clinically occult lymph node metastases does not worsen prognosis in younger patients but may affect outcome in older patients. Therefore, prophylactic node dissection for younger patients without clinically positive nodes does not impact survival; however, some surgeons do advocate ipsilateral nodal dissections for older patients.

9. When is surgery indicated for recurrent thyroid cancer?

The appropriate treatment of recurrent thyroid cancer depends on whether the cancer takes up radioiodine and whether it is a macroscopic (clinically detected) or microscopic (scintigraphically detected) recurrence. Although the recurrence rate for differentiated thyroid cancer is low, about 50% of patients whose cancer recurs will ultimately die of the disease, making early detection and treatment paramount to successful outcome. Scintigraphically detected recurrences that are not clinically evident are best treated by radioiodine ablation, while clinically evident recurrences should be surgically resected followed by radioiodine ablation. Medullary thyroid cancer and Hurthle cell cancers do not typically concentrate radioiodine; therefore, surgical resection of any residual thyroid tissue and meticulous nodal dissection when indicated may be the only chance for cure. Inoperable recurrences may be amenable to external radiation therapy.

10. How many times should a thyroid cyst be aspirated if it reaccumulates fluid? Should the cyst fluid be sent for cytology?

Thyroid cysts are fairly common and most often benign. The initial diagnostic and therapeutic procedure is aspiration. The complete disappearance of a palpable lesion is adequate therapy for thyroid cysts; however, about 50% will reaccumulate fluid. If the cyst recurs after repeat aspiration, it should be considered for surgical excision. Fluid cytology results are typically nonspecific; however, it may be prudent to perform cytology on cysts that reaccumulate fluid. If the nodule does not completely disappear after aspiration, it may be a complex cyst, which is associated with higher malignant potential. Therefore, FNA of the solid component should be performed

Hyperthyroidism

11. List the indications for thyroidectomy in hyperthyroidism.

In the United States, thyroidectomy is not commonly performed for hyperthyroidism unless secondary to a single hyperfunctioning adenoma or because of a goiter containing a suspicious nodule. Despite the excellent success, low recurrence rate, safety and more rapid return to a euthyroid state, fewer than 10% of patients with hyperthyroidism undergo thyroidectomy. Possible indications for thyroidectomy for hyperthyroidism are listed below:

- Failure of antithyroid medications
- Large goiter and low iodine uptake
- Compression symptoms such as dysphagia, stridor or hoarseness
- Nodules suspicious for cancer
- Patient is a child
- Patient is pregnant and difficult to treat medically
- Patient is a young female who wants to become pregnant in the near future
- Patient is noncompliant
- There are cosmetic concerns
- Severe Graves' ophthalmopathy

12. How should patients with hyperthyroidism be prepared for surgery?

It is important to render patients euthyroid prior to surgery for hyperthyroidism to avoid perioperative thyroid storm. Antithyroid medications administered for 4 weeks prior to surgery are usually adequate. Some surgeons also prefer using Lugol's solution (potassium iodine) for 3–5 days prior to surgery to decrease the vascularity of the goiter and reduce the risk of bleeding. Patients who are very symptomatic may benefit from preoperative beta-blockade. For more rapid induction of a euthyroid state, patients may also be given dexamethasone, which can return T4 and T3 to within the normal range in < 7 days.

13. What is the extent of thyroidectomy for hyperthyroidism?

The controversy over the appropriate extent of thyroidectomy for hyperthyroidism resides in the desire to render the patient euthyroid without inducing hypothyroidism while balancing the risk of recurrence. Many surgeons prefer to perform near-total thyroidectomy, which successfully cures hyperthyroidism in nearly 100% of patients; however, it does so with the drawback of uniform hypothyroidism. Patients willing to accept the risk of recurrent hyperthyroidism may undergo subtotal thyroidectomy, which leaves approximately 4–8 g of visible thyroid tissue with an adequate blood supply. A recent meta-analysis revealed subtotal thyroidectomy to result in an euthyroid state (no need for postoperative thyroid replacement therapy) in approximately 60% of patients, but it has a 5–10% incidence of persistent or recurrent hyperthyroidism.

Miscellaneous

14. What are the complications of thyroidectomy?

Thyroidectomy is a safe procedure with a mean length of hospitalization in large series of < 1.5 days. The incidence of specific complications after thyroidectomy are listed below.

- Hemorrhage 1%
- Recurrent laryngeal nerve injury, 1%
- Superior laryngeal nerve injury, 1%
- Hypoparathyroidism, 1–3%
- Mortality, 0.3%

15. What's the appropriate therapy for an intrathoracic goiter?

Intrathoracic goiters are typically cervical goiters with mediastinal extension, although primary intrathoracic goiters do occur secondary to abnormal descent of the thyroid during development. The incidence of carcinoma residing in intrathoracic goiters is reported as high as 17%; moreover, approximately 40% of patients present with compressive symptoms resulting from impingement on the airway, esophagus, vascular structures or nerves. Radioiodine ablation is not typically recommended because of the risk of transient enlargement of the goiter during initiation of therapy, potentially resulting in life threatening airway compromise. Thus, the presence of an intrathoracic goiter is generally accepted as an indication for thyroidectomy. Since the arterial supply of intrathoracic goiters originates in the neck, the vast majority of these tumors can be resected through a cervical approach. Extension into the posterior mediastinum, malignancy or compression of the vena cava may necessitate a combined cervical and sternotomy approach, although this is required in < 5% of cases.

16. When should thyroglossal duct cysts be removed? Describe the operation.

During the embryologic development of the thyroid, a diverticulum forms from the foramen cecum at the base of the tongue and descends as the thyroglossal duct to the future anatomical position of the thyroid overlying the anterolateral surface of the upper tracheal rings. The thyroglossal duct normally disappears during further development but in rare cases will persist as a patent duct or as a thyroglossal duct cyst. Patients may complain of infection, pain or compressive symptoms or may have cosmetic concerns. Because of the risk of infection, most surgeons feel that all thyroglossal duct cysts should be removed; this requires excision of the entire cyst and cyst tract from the origin at the foramen cecum down to the cyst itself. Since the tract nearly always passes through the hyoid bone, the center of the hyoid should be resected to lower the risk of recurrence; this causes no disability and requires no repair.

PARATHYROID

Hyperparathyroidism

17. Discuss the indications for parathyroidectomy.

When carefully questioned, approximately 95% of patients with primary hyperparathyroidism report at least one symptom referable to the disease and 95% report symptomatic improvement postoperatively. The indication for parathyroidectomy in symptomatic hyperparathyroidism is clear; however, there is controversy about asymptomatic patients. In 1990, the National Institutes of Health (NIH) Consensus Development Conference Panel recommended surgery for asymptomatic hyperparathyroidism in patients with complicating coexistent illnesses, for younger patients (< 50 yr), and for those in whom consistent long-term follow-up could not be ensured. Surveillance might be justified in patients whose calcium levels are only mildly elevated (< 1 mg/dL above normal) and whose renal and bone status are normal. On the other hand, the high success and low morbidity of parathyroidectomy when performed by experienced surgeons supports a more liberal approach to operation. Parathyroidectomy, even when performed for asymptomatic hyperparathyroidism, results in improved bone mineral density and reduced cardiovascular risk. Moreover, studies have shown that the expense of surgery equals that of medical follow-up for hyperparathyroidism at 5–6 yr, again tipping the scales in favor of early parathyroidectomy.

18. When should preoperative parathyroid localization studies be performed?

The NIH consensus statement concluded that preoperative localization studies are neither necessary nor cost-effective when an experienced surgeon plans the initial operation for primary hyperparathyroidism in patients without a prior history of neck surgery. Patients with a prior history of neck surgery and certainly all patients with persistent or recurrent hyperparathyroidism should undergo preoperative localization studies prior to planned re-exploration. The best localization study available is the ^{99m}technetium sestamibi scan, although ultrasound, computed tomography (CT) scan, magnetic resonance imaging (MRI), and arteriography with or without venous sampling may all be useful in certain situations. Another indication for preoperative localization is to enable minimally invasive parathyroidectomy (directed unilateral, radioguided or endoscopic).

19. Describe when intraoperative intact parathyroid hormone (iPTH) assay should be utilized.

A rapid assay for iPTH allows intraoperative assessment of the functional success of the operation. This test is performed by drawing a sample of blood before the operation and 5–10 min after the suspected abnormal gland(s) has/have been removed. The test typically takes 10–15 min to run, and a reduction of the iPTH to 50% of the preoperative level and into the normal range predicts successful removal of all abnormal glands and the surgery is terminated. iPTH is most useful in patients with hyperplasia and those undergoing reoperation and during minimally invasive parathyroidectomy.

20. What is the expected success of surgery for primary hyperparathyroidism?

Parathyroidectomy is highly successful for primary hyperparathyroidism, correcting hypercalcemia in more than 95% of patients when performed by an experienced surgeon. Nearly all patients experience improvement in the general symptoms of hyperparathyroidism. Bone density increases in the vast majority of patients. The complications of kidney stones, gout and peptic ulcer disease typically all improve. Improvement in longevity is also seen, presumably through a decrease in cardiovascular morbidity and mortality.

21. Describe the appropriate management of a "missing" parathyroid.

Despite meticulous operative technique during conventional parathyoidectomy (identification of all four glands), the surgeon will occasionally encounter a "missing gland." A systematic search of the most common ectopic locations is required for successful outcome in these patients. When three normal glands have been identified and the fourth gland is not in a normal position, the most likely ectopic location depends on whether it is a missing upper or lower gland. The lower parathyroid glands descend during development from the 3rd branchial pouch and are more likely to descend too far rather than too little. Therefore, a search for a missing lower gland should proceed from the thyroid inferiorly to the thyrothymic ligament, the thymus and the mediastinum outside the thymus; if not located inferiorly, a search for an undescended lower gland should ensue. The upper glands descend from the 4th branchial pouch. A search for a missing upper gland should first proceed posterior to the thyroid and inferiorly along the tracheoesophageal groove, followed by the posterior-superior mediastinum and finally an intrathyroidal position. When four normal glands have been identified without an obvious adenoma or when an iPTH has failed to decrease, a search for a supernumerary gland should ensue. The position of supernumerary glands is less predictable; thus, all of the above locations may need to be examined.

22. When should autotransplantation of parathyroid tissue be performed?

A single adenoma is by far the most common cause of primary hyperparathyroidism; however, 10–15% of patients have hyperplasia. Patients with sporadic hyperplasia, a multiple endocrine neoplasia (MEN) syndrome or secondary and tertiary hyperparathyroidism must undergo either subtotal (removal of three and a half glands, static pelvic traction [SPTx]) or total parathyroidectomy with autotransplantation of parathyroid tissue (TPTX+AT). The success of either approach depends on finding all four glands. Autotransplantation is performed by placing 10–15 grafts of 1-mm pieces of parathyroid into two or three separate pockets formed in either the sternocleidomastoid muscle or a forearm muscle and marked with a nonabsorbable suture for easy identification. These two techniques have similar outcomes with respect to persistent or recurrent hypercalcemia and hypocalcemia (both 10-15%). The advantage of TPTx+AT is that persistent or recurrent hypercalcemia can be treated by partially or completely removing the grafts under local anesthesia, while the same complication occurring after SPTx requires repeat neck operation with higher morbidity. One prospective randomized trial demonstrated a clear benefit of TPTX+AT for secondary hyperparathyroidism in renal failure patients in that it resulted in a more rapid return of normal calcium homeostasis and relief of symptoms.

23. Define minimally invasive parathyroidectomy.

The combination of accurate preoperative localization studies and intraoperative iPTH assay have fostered the development of minimally invasive approaches to parathyroidectomy as an alternative to conventional parathyroidectomy (identifying all four glands). Minimally invasive parathyoidectomy is a viable option for patients found to have a single adenoma on preoperative imaging (up to 95% of patients). A directed unilateral approach utilizes preoperative imaging to limit the dissection to one side. If one normal gland and one adenomatous gland are identified, the adenoma is removed and the surgery is terminated. Many surgeons also utilize an intraoperative iPTH assay to exclude the possibility of a double adenoma. Minimally invasive radioguided parathyroidectomy is a second alternative to conventional parathyroidectomy and involves performing a technetium sestamibi scan the morning of the surgery and utilizing the images from the scan as well as an intraoperative gamma probe to localize the abnormal gland. A directed incision is then performed and the gland is removed. A third option is endoscopic parathyroidectomy, but this technique is only performed in a few centers. All of these minimally invasive approaches appear to be as safe and effective as conventional parathyroidectomy but may be more time- and cost-efficient as they limit the amount of dissection required and can be done without hospitalization.

24. List the complications of parathyroidectomy and their prevalence.
  * Persistent or recurrent hyperparathyroidism, 2–12%
  * Transient hypocalcemia, 25%
  * Permanent hypoparathyroidism in 2–5%
  * Permanent regional lymph node injury in < 1%; temporary in 3%
  * Mortality in < 0.5%

25. Discuss the options available for patients with persistent or recurrent hyperparathyroidism.
  Persistent hyperparathyroidism is defined as failure of calcium and PTH levels to normalize or remain normal in the initial 6 months after operation, whereas recurrent hyperparathyroidism is defined by recurrence of hypercalcemia after 6 months. The approach to patients with persistent or recurrent hyperparathyroidism requires confirmation of the diagnosis, estimation of disease severity, careful review of the operative and pathology reports and preoperative localization. Causes of failure include missed adenoma in a normal location, ectopic glands, inadequate resection in multiglandular disease and supernumerary glands. Preoperative localization is usually achieved by sestamibi scan. Repeat cervical exploration is successful in normalizing PTH levels in about 85% of patients and may be aided by intraoperative ultrasound and iPTH assay. Mediastinal parathyroid tissue is most often removed via the transcervical approach, but thoracoscopy or median sternotomy may be required 1–2% of the time. Angiographic ablation of mediastinal parathyroid tissue using high doses of ionic contrast may be successful in selected patients with high surgical risk.

Parathyroid Cancer

26. How does one recognize and manage parathyroid cancer?
  Parathyroid cancer is the rarest of all endocrine tumors, with a reported incidence of < 1% in patients with primary hyperparathyroidism. Patients may present with a palpable mass and typically have symptomatic hypercalcemia that is often severe (>14 mg/dL) and of rapid onset. Successful outcome requires early recognition and appropriate treatment. The diagnosis is rarely confirmed preoperatively and is often not obvious at the initial operation. Local invasion and pathologic nodes should be assumed to represent cancer. Any suspicious parathyroid lesions should be carefully removed without disrupting the parathyroid capsule, since this may result in tumor spillage and local recurrence. If a parathyroid gland is obviously abnormal and infiltrating other tissues, those tissues should be resected en bloc with the tumor whenever possible; this should include the ipsilateral thyroid lobe when necessary. The histopathalogic diagnosis of this cancer is also difficult; thus, intraoperative frozen section is rarely useful other than to confirm parathyroid tissue. Lymph nodes are rarely involved; however, any obviously enlarged nodes should be resected in an appropriate neck dissection. Prophylactic neck dissections have shown no benefit. The prognosis of parathyroid cancer varies depending on whether metastases are present at the time of initial surgery. Those without metastases tend to do well in the long term; a large study of metastatic parathyroid cancer including 40 patients revealed a 50% survival at 5 yrs.

ISLET CELL TUMORS

27. How should pancreatic islet cell tumors be imaged?

Due to the small size of most islet cell tumors, preoperative localization is often difficult, and the extent of preoperative imaging needed is controversial. Ultrasound, CT, MRI and angiography all have reported sensitivities around 60%. Octreotide scans are very sensitive (85%), especially for metastases, in locating most islet cell tumors, with the exception of insulinomas (50% sensitivity), which are the most common type. Provocative arterial stimulation (secretin for gastrinomas and calcium for insulinomas) and venous sampling have higher sensitivities, but their invasiveness and ability to only regionalize a tumor make them less desirable. Recent reports have shown endoscopic ultrasound to be the most sensitive preoperative test for localizing pancreatic islet cell tumors, although it is invasive and highly operator dependent. Due to the above difficulties, many surgeons feel that exhaustive efforts to localize these tumors preoperatively are unwarranted. They prefer to obtain a preoperative ultrasound or CT scan to identify obviously invasive or metastatic tumors and then rely on intraoperative palpation (90% sensitivity) with intraoperative ultrasound (sensitivity approaches 100%) to localize the tumor. All patients undergoing re-exploration for islet cell tumors should undergo preoperative localization studies.

28. What is the appropriate surgical approach for sporadically occurring islet cell tumors?

Insulinomas account for approximately 90% of nonfamilial islet cell tumors. The small size of these tumors and the rarity of malignancy allow simple enucleation or distal pancreatectomy in the vast majority of cases. Rarely, formal pancreaticoduodenectomy is required, most typically for malignant cases. Laparoscopy for enucleation or distal pancreatectomy is used selectively in some centers. The surgical approach to gastrinomas is more complex, as these tumors are more frequently malignant and occur outside the pancreas in up to 50% of cases. Tumors occurring distal to the pancreatic neck should be removed by formal pancreatic resection because of the high incidence of malignancy. Tumors in the pancreatic head can often be enucleated, reserving formal pancreaticoduodenectomy for more invasive tumors or those in close proximity to the pancreatic duct. When palpation with or without intraoperative ultrasound has failed to localize the tumor within the pancreas, careful evaluation of the duodenum by palpation, endoscopic transillumination or duodenotomy when necessary often identifies the tumor within the duodenal wall. Small submucosal lesions can be enucleated, but a full-thickness resection of the duodenal wall may be necessary. The propensity for these tumors to metastasize to lymph nodes necessitates a regional lymph node dissection of the celiac and porta hepatis basins in all patients. Other sporadically occurring islet cell tumors are typically large, and 50% are malignant, requiring an individualized surgical approach in these rare cases.

29. Should islet cell tumors occurring in patients with MEN type I be approached differently than those occurring sporadically?

Yes. Approximately 70% of patients with MEN type I develop pancreatic islet cell tumors, with gastrinoma being the most common tumor. Due to the multifocal nature and diffuse islet cell dysplasia seen in these patients, aggressive surgery rarely results in biochemical cure. The morbidity and mortality of aggressive surgical resection combined with low cure rate and the availability of effective palliative treatment options for symptomatic patients sway many clinicians to treat these patients medically unless there is suspicion of malignancy. Other surgeons take a more aggressive approach, citing the incidence of malignancy. Further, the larger tumors seen on preoperative imaging often account for symptoms, and therefore surgical extirpation of these tumors may be beneficial. Formal resection of the distal pancreas accompanied by enucleation of tumors in the pancreatic head is necessary.

30. Is there a role for surgery for liver metastases from islet cell tumors?

Yes. Patients who undergo resection of isolated liver metastases from islet cell tumors have prolonged survival (73% versus 29% 5-yr survival) compared with patients with similar tumor burdens not undergoing hepatic resection. Patients with unresectable liver metastases or those with prohibitive surgical risks may benefit from either cryosurgical or radiofrequency thermal ablation. These techniques have resulted in a 5-year survival rate of 25% when used for colorectal liver metastases and would likely result in survival rates similar to those for resection when used specifically for islet cell metastases.

ADRENAL

31. What are the available imaging studies for evaluating adrenal pathology?

The appropriate imaging study for adrenal lesions depends somewhat on the diagnosis. Aldosteronomas are typically ≤ 2 cm in diameter, and therefore the sensitivity of CT scans is only 85%. When CT scanning fails to demonstrate an adenoma, iodomethylnorcholesterol scans and adrenal venous sampling are often useful to differentiate small adenomas from bilateral hyperplasia. For cortisol-producing adenomas, CT scans are very accurate. Most pheochromocytomas are of considerable size by the time they are diagnosed, so CT scans are very accurate. MRI is essentially equivalent to CT for adrenal tumors; however, it may be superior in recurrent or metastatic disease and for pheochromocytomas. Meta-iodobenzylguanidine scans are best utilized for recurrent or nonadrenal pheochromocytomas.

32. Should all incidentally discovered adrenal masses be resected?

An adrenal incidentaloma is found in 0.3–5% of all abdominal CT scans. The two main criteria for deciding to remove a lesion are functionality and size. Work-up should include a thorough history and physical, with the minimum laboratory studies to include a serum sodium and potassium as well as 24-hr urine free cortisol, metanephrines and vanillylmandelic acid. Approximately 5% of incidentally discovered adrenal masses are ultimately found to be functional; in these cases, adrenalectomy is indicated. For nonfunctional tumors, no currently available imaging study is specific enough to distinguish benign versus malignant lesions; however, lesions > 6 cm have a much higher risk of being malignant. Consequently, nonfunctional lesions > 5 cm on the initial CT scan should be removed. If < 5 cm, the tumor should be followed with repeat CT scans and resected if there is any evidence of growth.

33. Describe the surgical techniques available for adrenalectomy.

There are many different surgical approaches to the adrenal glands. Conventional open adrenalectomy can be performed through an anterior (transperitoneal), an anterlolateral (extraperitoneal), or a posterior (retroperitoneal) approach. Rarely, a combined thoracoabdominal approach is required for extremely large or malignant lesions. Advances in laparoscopic surgical techniques have been applied to adrenalectomy over the past 8 yr; currently, most endocrine surgeons would agree that laparoscopic adrenalectomy is the procedure of choice for benign adrenal tumors, with open adrenalectomy reserved for malignant tumors. Laparoscopic adrenalectomy has been associated with decreased hospital stay, postoperative pain, blood loss, shorter recovery and overall increased patient satisfaction compared with the open techniques. Just as with open adrenalectomy, there are several different laparoscopic approaches being utilized. The most common technique is via an anterolateral approach, which provides excellent exposure but does not allow removal of both glands without repositioning the patient. An anterior approach provides access to both adrenal glands, but exposure is more difficult. A posterior endoscopic approach avoids entering the peritoneal cavity altogether; however, this approach provides a limited working space and may hinder removal of larger lesions.

34. What is the long-term success of adrenalectomy for functional tumors?

Adrenalectomy for aldosteronomas is at least 95% successful in normalizing the aldosterone level and correcting hypokalemia, but the long-term resolution of hypertension is variable. For younger patients with relatively recent onset hypertension, adrenalectomy usually results in normotension. In older patients with severe, long-standing hypertension, adrenalectomy may not normalize the blood pressure, but often results in easier control of hypertension with fewer or lower dose medications. Unilateral adrenalectomy is 95% effective in treating cortisol producing adenomas; bilateral adrenalectomy in patients failing hypophysectomy for adrenocorticotropic hormone–dependent Cushing's syndrome is slightly less effective, with approximately 25% of patients having persistent symptoms, hypertension or diabetes. These patients must also deal with hormone replacement. Adrenalectomy for nonfamilial benign pheochromocytomas is curative in most cases; however, a 5–10% late recurrence rate has been reported, and therefore these patients should undergo lifelong observation.

35. Describe the appropriate management of adrenal malignancies.

Adrenocortical carcinoma is a rare and aggressive cancer that is frequently metastatic by the time of diagnosis. Approximately 60% of adrenocortical carcinomas are functioning tumors. The overall 5-yr survival rate for this disease is around 25%, and the only chance for cure is surgery, which should be offered to all patients without metastases and of a reasonable surgical risk. Surgery should also be considered for young patients with an isolated, easily resectable metastasis. Approximately 10% of pheochromocytomas are malignant and the 5-yr survival is approximately 40% with surgical resection offering the only chance for cure. The adrenal glands are a relatively common site for metastases from other malignancies, but surgical resection is restricted to patients with isolated lesions.

CARCINOID

36. How are carcinoid tumors localized?

Carcinoid tumors develop from enterochromaffin tissue and can be divided into those arising in the foregut, midgut or hindgut. The most common locations of carcinoid tumors are the small intestine (35%), appendix (35%), rectum (15%) and bronchial system (10%). Bronchial carcinoids may present with hemoptysis or carcinoid syndrome, while tumors developing in the small intestine are typically diagnosed incidentally or after carcinoid syndrome develops secondary to metastases. Hindgut carcinoids do not usually produce active hormones and are typically found incidentally during endoscopy performed for other reasons. Once a patient is diagnosed with carcinoid syndrome, the tumor must then be localized; this may be difficult because of the small size of most carcinoid tumors. Tumors arise in the small bowel and appendix in nearly 70% of patients, and therefore a small bowel contrast study or abdominal CT scan is often the initial study performed. If these tests fail to localize the tumor, a chest x-ray and/or chest CT scan should be obtained to exclude a bronchial carcinoid. Metaiodobenzylguanidine or octreotide scintigraphy is sometimes able to localize tumors not found by conventional methods.

37. What is the appropriate surgical management for carcinoid tumors?

Bronchial carcinoids tend to spread locoregionally and therefore should be resected by formal lobectomy when possible. Gastric and small intestinal carcinoids without metastases should be excised by segmental resection and lymph node dissection. Appendiceal carcinoids are typically incidentally discovered and occur most commonly at the appendiceal tip. Distal lesions < 2 cm are adequately treated by appendectomy. The presence of a carcinoid near the appendiceal base, size > 2 cm or grossly involved lymph nodes requires formal right hemicolectomy. Rectal carcinoids often present with bleeding or are incidentally found on endoscopy. Extensive surgery for rectal carcinoids offers no survival advantage over local excision.

38. Is there a role for surgery in carcinoid syndrome?

The development of somatostatin analogues has allowed successful control of symptoms in most patients with carcinoid syndrome and diffuse hepatic metastases. Systemic chemotherapy and hepatic artery embolization have not been very effective in palliating these patients; however, selective hepatic artery chemoembolization has been successful in decreasing tumor burden and alleviating symptoms in up to 80% of patients. Patients who do not respond to medical palliation may benefit from aggressive tumor debulking by resecting the primary tumor and as many of the liver metastases as feasible. As with liver metastases from islet cell tumors, cryosurgical or radiofrequency thermal ablation may be useful for unresectable lesions in patients not responding to medical palliation.

BIBLIOGRAPHY

1. Barry MK, van Heerden JA, Farley DR, et al: Can adrenal incidentalomas be safely observed. World J Surg 22:599–604, 1998.
2. Chen H, Hardacre JM, Uzar A, et al: Isolated liver metastases from neuroendocrine tumors: does resection prolong survival? J Am Coll Surg 187:88–92, 1998.
3. Chen H, Zeiger MA, Clark DP, et al: Papillary carcinoma of the thyroid: Can operative management be based solely on fine-needle aspiration? J Am Coll Surg 184:605–610, 1997.
4. Clark OH, Duh QY: Textbook of Endocrine Surgery. Philadelphia, W.B. Saunders, 1997.
5. Crucitti F, Bellantone R, Ferrante A, Boscherini M, Crucitti P: The Italian Registry for Adrenal Cortical Carcinoma: analysis of a multiinstitutional series of 129 patients. The ACC Italian Registry Study Group. Surgery 119:161–170, 1996.
6. Doppman JL, Chang R, Fraker DL, et al: Localization of insulinomas to regions of the pancreas by intra-arterial stimulation with calcium. Ann Intern Med 123:269–273, 1995.
7. Fleming JB, Lee JE, Bouvet M, et al: Surgical strategy for the treatment of medullary thyroid carcinoma. Ann Surg 230:697–707, 1999.
8. Gagner M: Laparoscopic Adrenalectomy: Lessons learned from 100 consecutive procedures. Ann Surg 226:238–247, 1997.
9. Goldstein RE, O'Neill JA Jr, Holcomb GW 3rd, et al: Clinical experience over 48 years with pheochromocytoma. Ann Surg 229:755–764, 1999.
10. Hay ID, Grant CS, Bergstralh EJ, et al: Unilateral total lobectomy: Is it sufficient surgical treatment for patients with AMES low-risk papillary thyroid carcinoma? Surgery 124:958–964, 1998.
11. Jensen RT: Carcinoid and pancreatic endocrine tumors: recent advances in molecular pathogenesis, localization, and treatment. Curr Opin Oncol 12:368–377. 2000.
12. McIntyre RC Jr, Kumpe DA, Liechty RD: Reexploration and angiographic ablation for hyperparathyroidism. Arch Surg 129:499–503, 1994.
13. NIH Conference: Diagnosis and management of asymptomatic primary hyperparathyroidism: consensus development conference statement. Ann Intern Med 114:593–597, 1991.
14. Norton JA, Fraker DL, Alexander HR, et al: Surgery to cure the Zollinger-Ellison syndrome. N Engl J Med 341:635–644, 1999.
15. Patwardhan NA, Moront M, Rao S, et al: Surgery still has a role in Graves' hyperthyroidism. Surgery 114:1108–1112, 1993.
16. Rothmund M, Wagner PK, Schark C: Subtotal parathyroidectomy versus total parathyroidectomy and autotransplantation in secondary hyperparathyroidism: A randomized trial. World J Surg 15:745–50, 1991.
17. Udelsman R, Donovan PI, Sokoll LJ: One hundred consecutive minimally invasive parathyroid explorations. Ann Surg 232:331–339, 2000.
18. Wiedenmann B, Jensen RT, Mignon M, et al: Preoperative diagnosis and surgical management of neuroendocrine gastroenteropancreatic tumors: General recommendations by a consensus workshop. World J. Surg 22:309–318, 1998.
19. Wynne AG, van Heerden J, Carney JA, Fitzpatrick LA: Parathyroid carcinoma: Clinical and pathologic features in 43 patients. Medicine 71:197–205, 1992.

62. ENDOCRINOLOGY IN THE MANAGED CARE ENVIRONMENT

Elliot G. Levy, M.D.

1. What is "managed care"?

The American College of Physicians/American Society of Internal Medicine has defined "managed care" as "a system of health-care delivery provided by contracted providers in which the entities responsible for financing the cost of health care exert influence on the clinical decision-making of those who provide the health care in an attempt to provide health care that is cost effective, accessible, and of acceptable quality."

2. Is there only one type of "managed care"?

Managed care is actually a spectrum of health care delivery systems ranging from managed indemnity insurance through preferred provider organizations (PPOs), point of service plans (POSs), and various types of health maintenance organizations (HMOs). Collectively, these organizations are called "managed care organizations" (MCOs). To a greater or lesser extent, all managed care systems attempt to shift financial risk in one way or another to the providers of care.

3. Who actually provides the care in a managed care environment?

In most cases, the initial contact that a patient has is with a health care provider, conveniently called a "primary care provider" (PCP). This person is usually a physician such as a family medicine or family practice or general practice physician, but often can be a physician who has specialized in internal medicine or an internist with a subspecialty (such as endocrinology) who enjoys practicing primary care in addition to his or her subspecialty or does not have enough subspecialty work to fill his or her schedule. The PCP can also be a physician extender, such as a nurse practitioner or a physician assistant.

Some MCOs will utilize physicians in large clinic type settings in an effort to control costs. In other situations, PCPs will function out of their usual private practice offices, in a sense, mixing their private (or non-MCO) patients with their HMO or PPO patients. Regardless of the type of training, the PCP is usually the physician who makes initial contact with the patient. There has been a movement over the past few years to allow pediatricians to become PCPs for children and for obstetrics and gynecology specialists to become PCPs for women of child-bearing years who often have no need to see other types of physicians. It is only under the recommendation of a PCP that a patient is allowed to see a subspecialist, such as an endocrinologist. Usually, an endocrinologist is not allowed to function as both a PCP and as a subspecialist within a given HMO. In these situations, when a fully trained endocrinologist is serving as a PCP, he or she cannot even perform specialty type procedures and must refer them out to another endocrinologist.

Once an MCO has established itself in a community, it begins to develop a "panel" of all the providers it needs. This includes the PCPs, the medical subspecialists, the surgeons and surgical subspecialists, the pediatricians, ob-gyn specialists, and the dermatologists. Simultaneously, the MCO contracts with hospitals (strategically located around the community it wants to "penetrate"), nursing homes, home health agencies, physical therapy centers, dialysis centers, outpatient diagnostic centers, clinical (commercial) laboratories, and, sometimes, even things such as outpatient diabetes education centers or dietitians. All these providers are then published yearly in a directory that goes by a variety of names, such as preferred provider list, which is distributed to all participants of the MCO. This directory is sometimes called the "list." It is used by patients to determine which PCP is available for them to use (although in some HMOs the new patients are immediately assigned to a PCP of the HMO's choice). It is used by a PCP to know which subspecialists, which diagnostic center, and which laboratory to use. It is also used by the MCO itself as a marketing tool, trying to solicit business for itself by proudly showing which subspecialists are providers for this organization. It is, therefore, necessary to be on "the list" to ever be referred patients from this HMO, but just because you, as a subspecialist, are on the list, does not mean that you will ever be referred patients. There is another situation called "point of service option" that, in some cases, will allow a patient to see any specialist, although the reimbursement schedule is different, and, often the out of pocket expenses (the "co-payment")") are much larger. This POS option differs greatly among those insurance companies that offer them.

The health care for the MCO is then provided by this entire group of health care providers, all of whom are under contracts with the HMO to provide the care in the manner and for the price that is negotiated. Thus the MCO has managed to do what the health care system was never able to do by itself—organize all the health care into one unit. When one looks at this system from afar, it is not so different than any other business unit that has to negotiate with vendors to provide things that it cannot do on its own. Think of a business unit as the cruise ship industry, which negotiates with its own employees, as well as entertainers, doctors, food suppliers, fuel suppliers, ports, and travel agents to provide for its customers (its passengers) a total package for their enjoyment. So have the MCOs attempted to organize the United States health care system. It is clearly a private, non–government-regulated, for-profit (in most cases) system whose primary goal is to earn a profit for its shareholders, while attempting to contain costs for the entire health care system. Not-for-profit MCOs are not necessarily any more efficient in providing the care to its members, and often have the same fiscal problems as for-profit MCOs.

4. What is the difference between a PPO and an HMO?

PPO is a plan, as originally conceived 10–20 years ago, that contracts with independent providers at a discounted fee for service. When the PPO systems first started, their representatives would approach a PCP or a specialist and offer a discounted fee schedule to a physician in exchange for the potential of being specifically referred a group of patients who otherwise would not be able to see that physician. There developed the concept of "panels" (i.e., the "lists" discussed above) in which a list of accepted providers would be given to patients covered by the plan, who must agree to use only the physicians on such a panel in order for their care to be covered by the plan. This concept has been modified many times (see below). HMO was originally defined as a prepaid organization that provided comprehensive health care services to voluntarily enrolled members in return for a prepaid fixed amount of money. Nowadays, an HMO can be a health plan that places some providers at risk for medical expenses or a health plan that uses PCPs as gatekeepers.

5. Are there any other types of MCO plans?

As there has been pressure placed on employers of businesses that employ large numbers of employees who were not happy with the original types of plans, and as many employers were not happy with the costs involved with the yearly premiums of certain plans, many other different insurance options were created. Virtually every insurance company has its own types of plans that can vary from state to state or even from city to city within one state. Far from excluding every one of these options, such blended policies include PPO with an assigned PCP and full coverage for specialty referral within the network of contracted providers, but partial payment for use of specialists outside the network. Plans can have different deductibles for office visits, for hospitalizations, for brand name versus generic medications. HMOs may include ones in which an entire clinic provides all the health care and referrals must be made internally. Other HMOs might contract with certain physicians within a community to be PCPs and other physicians to be the specialists. Referrals may be scrutinized very carefully and the PCP indirectly penalized by withholding bonuses or even reprimanded when they refer too many patients to specialists. Other HMOs may offer a plan in which a patient can be seen by the subspecialist of his or her choice, but with a larger copayment, such as 50% of usual and customary fees or a fixed amount. These so-called point of service (POS) options are becoming more popular, but are not standardized between insurance companies. There are many more such plans as insurance companies are trying to provide options to employers that meet the needs of the employees but keep the cost down to the employer. In many MCOs, a physician must provide care for both HMO and PPO patients, although some times with different fee schedules. Some MCOs allow physicians to participate in one or the other.

6. How does an endocrinologist join an HMO?

As many options are there for a physician to practice, such are the options for joining MCOs. In some cases, an endocrinologist is employed by a faculty group practice of a large medical center or a very large group practice in which all members of this group are participants in the specific plan. That doctor would most likely become a provider as soon as his or her credentials are approved by the MCO. In some areas of the country, there is a shortage of endocrinologists, and when one relocates into that area of the country or even city, that doctor will be approached by many MCOs to participate immediately. For the most part, if an endocrinologist decides to practice solo or joins a group practice in an area where there are already established panels of endocrinologists and the MCO is satisfied with the doctors already on the panel, joining the HMO can be very difficult, take a lot of time, and, in some cases, may not ever be possible. That is one reason why trying to open up a solo office for general endocrinology in an area of great HMO penetration may be extremely difficult and frustrating, especially when a large percent of the residents of a community are covered by some form of MCO. Sometimes, however, the MCO is under pressure to increase the number of endocrinologists, especially in certain geographic areas, and it welcomes the applications of new doctors. Other times there are specific requests from patients or employers to include in their panels certain groups of doctors who were never participants. This could be an opportunity to participate in a MCO. In general, the process of application, review of application, and final approval for participation can be quite long, maybe even more than 6 months. During this time, a physician cannot see patients for the MCO.

7. How does an HMO patient get to your office?

Once a PCP determines that he or she does not have the experience or expertise to treat a certain endocrine problem, the patient is referred to your office. Sometimes the patient has his or her referral made by their HMO or "their center," as it is often called. The patient must have in hand a "referral form," either in the form of an authorization form or a special slip of paper giving you the specific authority to evaluate and treat this patient. It is important that the patient has that paper in hand or that his or her center sends the referral, or you will not be compensated for that consultation visit. It is essential that each subsequent visit is also authorized in the same manner or payment will be withheld. It can be frustrating when a patient arrives for follow-up at the physician's office without the authorization form. Naturally the doctor wants to see that patient and has the time blocked out in his or her schedule to see that patient, but the HMO will definitely refuse to back issue a referral form, and, most likely, the doctor will never receive compensation for that visit.

8. What can you expect to be able to do for that patient at the time of the initial consultation or at subsequent follow-up visits?

In general, you will be allowed to perform a history and physical exam of the patient and order simple diagnostic tests without any hassle. Blood tests should be allowed, although the samples usually have to be sent to the laboratory that the MCO has contracted with (see below). Other tests you request have to be approved in writing by the HMO center or by the main HMO office, depending upon the individual company's policy. Simple procedures such as thyroid scans, ultrasound studies, radioactive iodine treatment, and even fine-needle aspiration biopsies can take hours to days to get approval. Some HMOs require their PCPs to schedule all tests, which can be a problem since you may not know when or where the study is scheduled so as to know when to have the patient return to discuss the results. The more expensive a test is (such as an MRI), the more difficult it is to arrange.

9. Can you use your own physician office laboratory (POL) for HMO patients?

Although many endocrinologists have their own laboratories, accredited to perform certain endocrine tests, you usually cannot utilize them to perform tests for HMO patients. Often the HMO has arranged special fees with commercial labs to perform these tests. This can create some logistical problems in your office if you do work for several different HMOs, all of which use different commercial labs. Your laboratory technicians must keep straight which specimens go where. In addition, some HMOs require that the patient have all blood tests drawn at the office of the PCP. That is especially a problem because sometimes you will never know if your patient ever went to the PCP's office to have the blood drawn, and the test results may not be returned to you until the patient returns for a follow-up visit, and you have to call the PCP's office to have the results given to you over the phone or faxed to you.

Another potentially serious problem with a contracted lab has to do with pathology. One particular procedure often performed by endocrinologists is the fine-needle aspiration biopsy (FNA) of a thyroid nodule. Most endocrinologists trust the interpretations by one particular laboratory, often at a university setting. The MCO may not have a contract with that lab and may require you to use a totally different lab for FNA cytology interpretation. Sometimes the pathologists at that lab may not be used to interpreting thyroid FNAs, and the results you receive may not be as accurate. That last particular problem is being addressed at present by the American Thyroid Association and the College of American Pathologists.

10. What happens if your patient changes jobs and receives health insurance from a company that you are not providing services for or if the patient's employer switches insurance because the price of the original one was too high?

Obviously, this is a very frustrating problem for both patient and physician. The concept of long-term loyalty has been changed. There is occasionally the possibility of a point of service option being available in the new plan, but often the patient gets tired of paying the extra co-payment. Sometimes, a physician will give the patient a discount to see the patient. Other times a patient will feel so strongly about the opinion of his or her doctor for so many years that he or she will pay out of pocket to see that doctor, especially if the patient only has to be seen once or twice per year.

There are movements in Congress to try to allow the continuation of the patient-physician relationship. Until such time, the physician has to understand that losing patients in this way may be unavoidable. He or she should always welcome the patient back to his or her practice when the insurance situation changes.

11. Are there any special problems regarding submission of claims, and prompt, reliable reimbursement?

Some HMOs have been accused rightly or wrongly of frequent improper handling of claims They have been accused of holding claims for extraordinarily long periods of time before payment. They have been accused of finding mistakes in claims, losing claims, or never receiving claims, despite the fact that most physicians submit claims electronically and these claims are scrutinized by the software to make sure that they are properly completed. Other HMOs have been accused of "downcoding" claims. This refers to a process of stating that a level of service submitted by a physician is too high, despite the fact that the doctor has adequate documentation in his or her records to indicate proper services were submitted. This means that no matter what fee schedule is agreed upon between physician and MCO, the MCO can set its own fees by lowering the level of care, usually without an acceptable process. All of these matters are currently being investigated by a committee of the American Association of Clinical Endocrinologists (AACE).

12. Is it advisable to continue seeing patients for MCOs if such problems exist?
This becomes a personal and financial decision that a physician or a physicians' group practice has to make. Some doctors work for a company on a strict salary basis. Seeing all patients is just part of what he or she has to do. Other physicians are in solo practice or in small groups. These doctors need to be aware of all the problems so that the decision to begin or continue seeing patients is done for the right economic reasons. Many doctors react out of fear and anger, the worst emotions to invoke when an economic decision has to be made. Doctors need to be involved in all aspects of the MCO relationship, from contract negotiation to ongoing monitoring of day-to-day problems in seeing patients for the particular MCO to being aware of the reimbursement problems discussed above. The practice needs to monitor collections, to be on top of claims, to resubmit claims that were rejected, claims that were down-coded, and claims that were held for a long time without payment. The doctor needs to be involved to make sure that the collection of claims is not forgotten, and that all claims are actively pursued, especially when there is third party payment (i.e., from an insurance company) involved. The doctor or his staff must have a policy in force to ensure that referrals are obtained, claims submitted on time, and proper payments are received.

In addition, doctors in small groups must make sure that the MCO in question is contributing a significant amount to the gross revenue of the practice to be worth the "hassle" involved in seeing their patients. As a particular doctor gets busier and busier, it might be more worthwhile to substitute seeing patients from a particular HMO that has a low reimbursement schedule for patients from other HMOs with higher schedules. Perhaps the doctor could see only patients covered by higher paying PPOs or choose not to be involved in MCOs at all, if there are enough patients to fill his or her schedule. For those new in practice, it might be worthwhile to see more and more patients, despite the problems associated with seeing them.

The decision to join MCO panels or to resign from a particular panel should not be an emotional one, such as fear that if you do not accept a contract with what you consider an inadequate reimbursement schedule, another endocrinologist will do so. In addition, do not make a decision in anger, when a company denies payment or down-codes a series of claims without good reason. Work out the economics associated with leaving rather than resign out of anger. In fact, first try to work it out with the MCO, then look at all the above issues, and then decide whether resignation is the proper thing to do for economic reasons, not emotional ones.

13. Does the physician have to be a good business person to survive in today's managed care environment?
Unfortunately, yes. Most physicians go to medical school to learn how to become a good doctor. They work hard during their residency and fellowship to learn as much inter-

nal medicine and then endocrinology as they can. Most likely, there is nothing taught to them about practice management, contract negotiation skills, and cost-effective medical care. In addition, the old traditional role of a physician as a healer of the sick without concern for compensation because doctors "always made a good living" is no longer applicable. It is becoming too expensive to run an office without being aware of the costs of every aspect of the practice, the revenue stream, and the "bottom line." Some doctors sell their practices in order to not have to deal with these problems, only to find out that working for a physician management company or a hospital that acquires practices or very large groups creates an entirely different set of problems that they never expected.

In order to be successful financially in practice, the doctor today has to have a totally different attitude than one generation ago. The doctor has to view practice as a business, with the providing of health care only one part of the practice. It takes time, effort, experiential learning, and even mistakes to be successful.

Doctors have high intellectual abilities. They need to apply these abilities into learning the business aspects of their practices. Combining a career in clinical endocrinology with a successful income stream is certainly possible and should be the goal of all practicing endocrinologists today.

BIBLIOGRAPHY

1. Levy EG: On entering private practice: A personal perspective. A guide for the young endocrinologist about to embark on a career in private practice. Endocrinologist 9:119, 1999.

63. ENDOCRINE CASE STUDIES

Michael T. McDermott, M.D.

1. A 34-year-old woman has new-onset hypertension. Her serum potassium level is 2.7 mmol/L. Initial hormone screening shows a plasma aldosterone of 55 ng/dl (nl, 1–16) and a plasma renin of 0.1 ng/ml/hr (nl, 0.15–2.33). Subsequent testing reveals the following: plasma aldosterone after a saline infusion = 54 ng/dl (nl, 1–8), 4-hour upright plasma aldosterone = 32 ng/dl (nl, 4–31), 4-hour upright plasma renin = 0.1 ng/ml/hr (nl, 1.31–3.95), and serum 18-hydroxycorticosterone = 108 ng/dl (normal < 30). What is the probable diagnosis?

This patient has hypertension and hypokalemia, which should alert the provider to the possibility of primary aldosteronism (Conn's syndrome). The initial plasma aldosterone level is elevated, the renin is suppressed, and the aldosterone to renin ratio is greater than 20, strongly suggesting that primary aldosteronism is present. This diagnosis is confirmed by demonstrating that the high plasma aldosterone cannot be suppressed by volume expansion with saline. Once the diagnosis of primary aldosteronism is made, one must determine if it is caused by an aldosterone-producing adenoma or bilateral adrenal hyperplasia. The very low basal serum potassium, the significant drop in plasma aldosterone during the 4-hour posture test, and the elevated level of 18-hydroxycorticosterone are most consistent with an adrenal adenoma. The next step would be an abdominal CT scan to localize the tumor. The treatment for an aldosterone-producing adrenal adenoma is surgical removal. Spironolactone should be given to control blood pressure and to normalize the serum potassium preoperatively. (Chapter 28)

2. A 32-year-old female business executive develops amenorrhea. She has not recently lost weight but states that her job is very stressful. Evaluation reveals the following laboratory results: serum estradiol = 14 pg/ml (nl, 23–145), LH = 1.2 mIU/ml (nl, 2–15), FSH = 1.5 mIU/ml (nl, 2–20), prolactin = 6.2 ng/ml (nl, 2–25), TSH = 1.2 μU/ml (nl, 0.5–5.0), and a serum pregnancy test is negative. An MRI scan of her pituitary gland is normal. What is the probable diagnosis?

The patient has secondary amenorrhea with low levels of estradiol and gonadotropins. This clinical picture is most consistent with hypothalamic amenorrhea, which sometimes occurs in women who exercise excessively or who have stressful jobs. The disorder results from reduced frequency of gonadotropin-releasing hormone (GnRH) pulses in the hypothalamus. Treatment consists of stress management and, if menses don't resume, estrogen replacement therapy. (Chapter 48)

3. A nulliparous 48-year-old woman presents with symptoms of thyrotoxicosis. She has a modest, nontender goiter and no exophthalmos. The following results are found on thyroid evaluation: free T_4 = 3.5 ng/dl (nl, 0.7–2.7), TSH < 0.1 μU/ml, 24-hour radioactive iodine uptake (RAIU) = 1% (nl, 20–35%), thyroglobulin = 35 ng/ml (nl, 2–20), and sedimentation rate = 10 mm/hr. What is the likely diagnosis?

The patient has clinical and biochemical thyrotoxicosis but the RAIU is low. The differential diagnosis includes subacute thyroiditis, silent thyroiditis, postpartum thyroiditis, factitious thyrotoxicosis, and iodine-induced thyrotoxicosis. The elevated level of serum thyroglobulin suggests thyroiditis. She has never been pregnant. The nontender gland and normal sedimentation rate are therefore most consistent with silent thyroiditis. A transient

(1–3 months) thyrotoxic phase followed by a transient (1–3 months) hypothyroid phase are expected before the condition resolves; 20% of patients, however, remain hypothyroid. If symptomatic, the thyrotoxic phase is best treated with beta blockers and the hypothyroid phase can be managed, if necessary, with levothyroxine. (Chapter 36)

4. A 38-year-old man has coronary artery disease, xanthomas of the Achilles tendons, and the following serum lipid profile: cholesterol = 482 mg/dl, triglycerides = 152 mg/dl, HDL cholesterol = 42 mg/dl, and LDL cholesterol = 410 mg/dl. What is the probable diagnosis?

Significant elevations of total cholesterol and LDL cholesterol, normal triglycerides, tendon xanthomas, and premature coronary artery disease are most consistent with the diagnosis of heterozygous familial hypercholesterolemia. This disorder is due to deficient or abnormal LDL receptors. Aggressive lipid lowering with combinations of statins and bile acid resins and/or niacin and, in some cases, plasmapheresis is indicated. (Chapter 8)

5. A 28-year-old man presents because of infertility. He is found to have small, firm testes and gynecomastia. Lab testing shows the following abnormalities: testosterone = 2.6 ng/ml (nl, 3.0–10.0), LH = 88 mIU/ml (nl, 2–12), and FSH = 95 mIU/ml (nl, 2–12). What is the likely diagnosis?

The patient has hypergonadotropic hypogonadism with small firm testes and gynecomastia, which is most consistent with a diagnosis of Klinefelter's syndrome. Such patients usually have a 47 XXY karyotype. Androgen replacement therapy is the treatment of choice. (Chapter 45)

6. A 38-year-old nurse presents in a stuporous state; the blood glucose level is 14 mg/dl. Additional blood is drawn, and the patient is quickly resuscitated with intravenous glucose. Further testing on the saved serum reveals the following: serum insulin = 45 mU/ml (normal < 22), C-peptide = 4.2 ng/ml (nl, 0.5–2.0), and proinsulin = 0.6 ng/ml (nl, 0–0.2). A sulfonylurea screen is negative. What is the probable diagnosis?

The patient has hyperinsulinemic hypoglycemia. The differential diagnosis includes insulinoma, surreptitious insulin injection and oral sulfonylurea ingestion. The elevated serum C-peptide and proinsulin levels are most consistent with an insulinoma. After an appropriate localizing procedure, surgical removal is the treatment of choice. (Chapter 56)

7. A 28-year-old woman with type 1 diabetes mellitus develops amenorrhea. Further testing reveals the following serum hormone values: estradiol = 15 pg/ml (nl, 23–145), LH = 78 mIU/ml (nl, 2–15), FSH = 92 mIU/ml (nl, 2–20), prolactin = 12 ng/ml (nl, 2–25), TSH = 1.1 μU/ml and a pregnancy test is negative. What is the most likely diagnosis?

The patient has secondary amenorrhea with low levels of estradiol and elevated gonadotropins. The differential diagnosis includes premature ovarian failure and the resistant ovary syndrome. In a patient with another autoimmune disease (type 1 diabetes mellitus), the most likely diagnosis is premature ovarian failure. Hormone replacement therapy is the treatment of choice. (Chapter 48)

8. A 34-year-old woman presents with galactorrhea, amenorrhea, headaches, fatigue, and weight gain. Laboratory evaluation reveals the following: prolactin = 58 ng/ml (nl, 2–25), free T$_4$ = 0.2 ng/dl (nl, 4.5–12) and TSH > 60 μU/ml (nl, 0.5–5.0). She has an enlarged pituitary gland on MRI scan. What is the probable diagnosis?

The patient has moderately increased serum prolactin levels, pituitary enlargement, and severe primary hypothyroidism. Her entire clinical picture is most likely explained solely by the hypothyroidism, which is well known to cause secondary hypersecretion of prolactin and pituitary enlargement due to thyrotroph hyperplasia. All abnormalities should resolve after adequate thyroid hormone replacement is established. (Chapters 35 and 21)

9. A 6-year-old girl develops breast enlargement, pubic hair, and monthly vaginal bleeding. Laboratory tests produce the following results: estradiol = 40 pg/ml (nl, 23–145), LH = 12 mIU/ml (nl, 2–15), FSH = 14 mIU/ml (nl, 2–20), prolactin = 8 ng/ml (nl, 2–25), TSH = 1.9 µU/ml (nl, 0.5–5.0), and a normal pituitary MRI scan. What is the probable diagnosis?

The patient has gonadotropin-dependent true precocious puberty. The etiology includes pituitary and hypothalamic tumors, but most cases in girls are idiopathic. The normal pituitary MRI points to a diagnosis of idiopathic precocious puberty. A long-acting GnRH analogue should successfully arrest her premature development and allow her to enter puberty at a later, more appropriate time. (Chapter 44)

10. A 19-year-old man presents with excessive thirst and urination. Laboratory evaluation shows the following: serum glucose = 88 mg/dl, serum sodium = 146 mmol/L, serum osmolality = 298 mOsm/kg, and urine volume = 8800 ml/24 hr. A water deprivation test is performed and shows a baseline urine osmolality of 90 mOsm/kg with no response to water deprivation and an increase in urine osmolality to 180 mOsm/kg after the administration of vasopressin. What is the likely diagnosis?

The patient has polyuria and polydipsia with maximally dilute urine. The differential diagnosis includes central diabetes insipidus, nephrogenic diabetes insipidus, and primary polydipsia. The lack of response to water deprivation and the more than 50% increase in urine osmolality after administration of vasopressin are most consistent with central diabetes insipidus. This may be caused by inflammatory or mass lesions in the hypothalamus, but is often idiopathic. An MRI of the pituitary–hypothalamic region should be performed. The treatment of choice is desmopressin (DDAVP) nasal spray. (Chapter 25)

11. A 25-year-old woman presents with a cushingoid appearance. The results of hormone testing are as follows: 24-hour urine cortisol = 218 mg (nl, 20–90), morning serum cortisol = 28 µg/dl (nl, 5–25), and morning plasma ACTH = 65 pg/ml (nl, 10–80). After an 8-mg oral bedtime dose of dexamethasone, the morning serum cortisol = 3 µg/dl. What is the probable diagnosis?

Cushingoid features and elevated urinary excretion of cortisol confirm the diagnosis of Cushing's syndrome. The etiology is usually an ACTH-secreting pituitary adenoma (65–80%), ectopic production of ACTH (10–15%), or a cortisol-producing adrenal adenoma (10–15%). The normal plasma level of ACTH, which is inappropriate for the elevated serum cortisol level, and suppression of serum cortisol with high-dose dexamethasone are most consistent with a pituitary adenoma (Cushing's disease). This should be confirmed with an MRI of the pituitary gland and/or inferior petrosal sinus sampling. Transsphenoidal surgical removal is the treatment of choice. (Chapter 24)

12. An 8-year-old boy with known adrenal insufficiency complains of paresthesias of the lips, hands and feet and intermittent muscle cramps. He has a positive Chvostek sign and a positive Trousseau sign on examination. Results of blood testing are as follows: calcium = 6.2 mg/dl (nl, 8.5–10.2), phosphorous = 5.8 mg/dl (nl, 2.5–4.5), intact PTH = 6 pg/ml (nl, 10–65), and 25-hydroxyvitamin D = 42 ng/ml (nl, 16–74). What is the most likely diagnosis?

Hypocalcemia, hyperphosphatemia, and a low serum PTH level are diagnostic of primary hypoparathyroidism. This disorder, which is autoimmune in nature, may occur in association with adrenal insufficiency as part of the polyendocrine failure type I syndrome. The treatment of this condition is calcium supplementation along with calcitriol (Rocaltrol) administration. Calcitriol is necessary because the lack of PTH makes these patients unable to convert 25-hydroxyvitamin D into 1,25-dihydroxyvitamin D in the kidneys and the latter vitamin D metabolite is necessary for normal intestinal calcium absorption. (Chapters 17 and 55)

13. A 52-year-old man has a personal and family history of early coronary artery disease, minimal alcohol consumption and no xanthomas on examination. He has the following results on serum testing: cholesterol = 328 mg/dl, triglycerides = 322 mg/dl, HDL = 35 mg/dl, LDL = 229 mg/dl, apoprotein B = 175 mg/dl (nl, 60–130), apoprotein E phenotype = E3/E3, TSH = 2.1 mg/ml (nl, 0.1–4.5), and glucose = 85 mg/dl. What is the probable diagnosis?

The patient has elevations of both serum cholesterol and triglycerides and no detected disorders that cause secondary dyslipidemia. The differential diagnosis of this profile includes familial combined hyperlipidemia and familial dysbetalipoproteinemia. The elevated level of apoprotein B and the normal apoprotein E phenotype are most consistent with familial combined hyperlipidemia. The top treatment priority is LDL reduction with a statin. Once LDL cholesterol is under the NCEP goal level, persistent triglyceride elevations should be addressed with the possible addition of a fibrate or niacin. (Chapter 8)

14. A 58-year-old man has recently developed diabetes mellitus, weight loss, and a skin rash that is most prominent on the buttocks; a dermatologist diagnoses this as necrolytic migratory erythema. What is the probable underlying diagnosis?

Diabetes mellitus, weight loss, and necrolytic migratory erythema are virtually diagnostic of a glucagon-secreting pancreatic endocrine tumor (glucagonoma). The diagnosis can be confirmed by finding an elevated serum level of glucagon. After appropriate localizing procedures, surgery is the treatment of choice, if possible. Chemotherapy should be considered for unresectable malignant tumors or tumor remnants. (Chapter 56)

15. A 39-year-old HIV-positive man with *Pneumocystis carinii* pneumonia has the following serum thyroid hormone values: T_4 = 4.0 μg/dl (nl, 4.5–12.0), T_3 = 22 ng/dl (nl, 90–200), T_3 resin uptake = 48% (nl, 35–45%) and TSH = 4.3 μU/ml (nl, 0.5–5.0). What is the most likely endocrine diagnosis?

A very low T_3, a mildly low T_4, an elevated T_3 resin uptake, and normal TSH are most consistent with the euthyroid sick syndrome. This is not a primary thyroid disorder but instead is a set of circulating thyroid hormone abnormalities that occur in the presence of non-thyroidal illnesses; it corrects when the underlying illness resolves. Treatment of the condition with thyroid hormone administration, though controversial, is not currently recommended. (Chapter 40)

16. An 18-year-old girl has not yet begun menstruating. She has a height of 56 inches, a small uterus, and no breast development. The results of hormone tests are as follows: estradiol = 8 pg/ml (nl, 23–145), LH = 105 mIU/ml (nl, 2–15), FSH = 120 mIU/ml (nl, 2–20), prolactin = 14 ng/ml (nl, 2–15), and TSH = 1.8 μU/ml (nl, 0.5–5.0). What is the probable diagnosis?

Primary amenorrhea, short stature, a low serum estradiol level, and elevated gonadotropins are most consistent with a diagnosis of Turner's syndrome. This disorder, which is characterized by ovarian dysgenesis, is associated with a 45 XO karyotype. These patients should be given hormone replacement therapy with estrogen and progesterone. Growth hormone therapy should also be considered, as it has been shown to improve longitudinal growth and final height. (Chapter 48)

17. A 29-year-old woman has asymptomatic hypercalcemia. Her mother and a sister also have hypercalcemia and have had failed neck explorations for presumed parathyroid tumors. Further testing reveals the following: serum calcium = 11.0 mg/dl (nl, 8.5–10.2), phosphorous = 3.0 mg/dl (nl, 2.4–4.5), intact PTH = 66 pg/ml (nl, 10–65), 25-hydroxyvitamin D = 42 ng/ml (nl, 16–74), and 24-hour urinary calcium excretion = 13 mg (nl, 100–300). What is the probable diagnosis?

Although the vast majority of patients with hypercalcemia and a mildly elevated serum PTH level have hyperparathyroidism, the presence of very low urinary excretion of calcium and a family history of hypercalcemia and unsuccessful parathyroidectomies points to a probable diagnosis of familial hypocalciuric hypercalcemia. The diagnosis is confirmed by finding a calcium/creatinine clearance ratio (urine calcium x serum creatinine/serum calcium x urine creatinine) of < .01. This autosomal dominant disorder results from a heterozygous inactivating mutation in the gene that encodes the calcium receptor. These mutant receptors, present in parathyroid cells and renal tubular cells, have a raised threshold for recognition of calcium. The result is a physiologic equilibrium in which hypercalcemia coexists with mild elevations of PTH and low urinary calcium excretion. The disorder does not cause any morbidity and does not require treatment. (Chapters 14 and 15)

18. A 62-year-old woman presents for evaluation of recent nephrolithiasis and low back pain. Her estimated calcium intake is 800 mg/day, and she takes no vitamins. Her physical examination is unremarkable. Spinal x-rays reveal osteopenia and a compression fracture at L2. Laboratory evaluation shows the following: serum calcium = 13.0 mg/dl (nl, 8.5–10.5), phosphorus = 2.3 mg/dl (nl, 2.5–4.5), albumin = 4.4 g/dl (nl, 3.2–5.5), intact PTH = 72 pg/ml (nl, 11–54), and 24-hour urine calcium = 312 mg (nl, 100–300). What is the most likely diagnosis?

Hypercalcemia, hypophosphatemia, and elevated serum PTH levels are characteristic of hyperparathyroidism. The only other cause of hypercalcemia associated with increased serum PTH levels is familial hypocalciuric hypercalcemia, which can be distinguished by the finding of very low urinary calcium excretion (calcium/creatinine clearance ratio < .01). Most non-familial cases of hyperparathyroidism are due to solitary parathyroid adenomas, whereas patients with familial hyperparathyroidism or one of the multiple endocrine neoplasia (MEN) syndromes more often have 4-gland hyperplasia. Indications for surgical treatment of hyperparathyroidism include serum calcium levels > 1 mg/dl above the upper limits of normal, urine calcium > 300 mg/24 hr, kidney stones, renal impairment, osteoporosis and symptoms related to hyperparathyroidism. Estrogens, bisphosphonates, or observation alone may be appropriate for some patients with mild, asymptomatic disease. (Chapter 15)

19. A 52-year old woman complains of a 1 year history of progressive fatigue, puffy eyes, dry skin and mild weight gain. She was treated with transsphenoidal surgery and radiation therapy for acromegaly 10 years ago. Physical examination shows normal visual fields, mild periorbital edema and dry skin. Lab testing reveals the following: growth hormone = 1.2 ng/ml (nl, < 2.0), IGF-1 = 258 μg/ml (nl, 182-780), TSH = 0.2 μU/ml (nl, 0.5-5.0) and free T4 = 0.6 ng/dl (nl, 0.7 -2.7). What is the most likely cause of this patient's symptoms?

This patient has central hypothyroidism due to pituitary damage from the combined effects of surgery and radiation treatment of her pituitary tumor 10 years earlier. Such a lengthy delay in the development of this condition is not uncommon. The diagnosis of central hypothyroidism is based on the presence of symptoms of thyroid hormone deficiency, a low serum free T_4 and a low or low-normal serum TSH. Treatment consists of levothyroxine replacement in doses sufficient to relieve symptoms and to maintain the serum free T_4 level in the mid-normal or upper-normal range. Because TSH secretion is impaired, the serum TSH level cannot be used to monitor this patient's response to therapy. (Chapter 35)

20. A 32-year-old woman presents with the recent onset of fatigue, palpitations, profuse sweating, and emotional lability. She gave birth to her second child 8 weeks ago. Her pulse is 100/min, and she has mild lid retraction, a fine hand tremor and a slightly enlarged, non-tender thyroid gland. Laboratory tests are as follows: TSH < .03 μU/ml (nl, 0.5–5.0), free T_4 = 3.8 ng/dl (nl, 0.7–2.7). Radioactive iodine uptake is < 1% at 4 and 24 hours. What is the probable diagnosis?

Hyperthyroidism occurring in the postpartum period is most often due to Graves' disease or postpartum thyroiditis. The radioactive iodine uptake (RAIU) will distinguish the two; the RAIU is generally very high in Graves' disease and very low in postpartum thyroiditis. This patient has postpartum thyroiditis. The condition is caused by lymphocytic inflammation with leakage of thyroid hormone from the inflamed gland. There is often a hyperthyroid phase (lasting 1–3 months) followed by a hypothyroid phase (lasting 1–3 months) and eventual return to euthyroidism, although approximately 20% remain permanently hypothyroid. Treatment consists of beta blockers, if needed, for symptom control in the hyperthyroid phase, and levothyroxine, if needed, for symptom control in the hypothyroid phase and for those who remain permanently hypothyroid. (Chapter 36)

21. A 70-year old man complains of a 1-year history of weakness, weight loss and hand tremors. He has been treated with amiodarone for nearly 3 years for a diagnosis of paroxysmal atrial flutter. Laboratory tests show the following: TSH < .01 μU/ml (nl, 0.5–5.0), and free T_4 = 3.35 ng/dl (nl, .7–2.7). Radioiodine uptake was 2.7% at 6 hours and 4.1% at 24 hours. Thyroid scan showed scant patchy tracer uptake. What is the likely diagnosis?

This man most likely has amiodarone-induced thyrotoxicosis (AIT). This condition occurs in up to 10% of patients using amiodarone, which has a very high iodine content. There are 2 pathophysiological subtypes. Type 1 AIT results from iodine overload and occurs mainly in patients with underlying goiters. Type 2 AIT results from iodine-induced thyroid follicular damage. The distinction between the two types is often difficult, although the presence of a pre-existing goiter is more common in type 1 and a high serum level of interleukin 6 (IL-6) suggests type 2 disease. Treatment of type 1 AIT consists of the administration of thionamides with or without potassium perchlorate, whereas type 2 AIT may respond to steroid therapy. Difficult cases may require plasmapheresis, dialysis, or thyroidectomy. (Chapter 34)

22. A 32-year-old man complains of impotence and retro-orbital headaches intermittently for the past year. He is adopted and does not know his natural family history. He has bitemporal visual field loss, but his examination is otherwise normal. Lab tests reveal the following: serum calcium = 11.8 mg/dl (nl, 8.5–10.5), phosphorus = 2.5 mg/dl (nl, 2.5–4.5), albumin = 4.8 g/dl (nl, 3.2 - 5.5), intact PTH = 58 pg/ml (nl, 11–54), prolactin = 2650 ng/ml (nl, 0–20). What is the likely diagnosis?

This patient most certainly has a prolactinoma, manifested by impotence, headaches, bitemporal hemianopsia, and a significantly elevated serum prolactin level. Hypercalcemia associated with an elevated serum PTH level indicates that he also has hyperparathyroidism. He most likely has the multiple endocrine neoplasia type 1 syndrome (MEN 1), which consists of hyperparathyroidism, pituitary tumors, and pancreatic endocrine tumors. MEN 1 results from an inherited mutation in the gene now referred to as the Menin gene. This patient should be screened for a gastrinoma and insulinoma by measuring serum gastrin, insulin, proinsulin, and glucose following an overnight fast. After appropriate pituitary imaging studies, he should be treated with a dopamine agonist and/or transsphenoidal surgery, and subsequently parathyroid surgery. (Chapter 54)

23. A 20-year-old man presents for failure to enter puberty. He has small, soft testes, no gynecomastia, normal visual fields, and decreased sense of smell. Laboratory evaluation is as follows: serum testosterone = 0.7 ng/ml (nl, 3.0–10.0), LH = 2.0 mIU/ml (nl, 2–12), FSH = 1.6 mIU/ml (nl, 2–12), prolactin = 7 ng/ml (nl, 2–20), TSH = 0.9 μU/ml (nl, 0.5-5.0). An MRI of the pituitary gland is normal. What is the probable diagnosis?

This picture is most consistent with idiopathic hypogonadotropic hypogonadism, also known as Kallmann's syndrome. This disorder is due to a deficiency of gonadotropin-releasing hormone (GnRH), resulting from failure of fetal migration of the GnRH-secreting neurons from the olfactory placode to the hypothalamus. Olfactory lobe maldevelopment causes the associated anosmia. Androgen therapy is indicated to promote appropriate masculinization. When desired, these patients can also become fertile by receiving treatment with GnRH or gonadotropin preparations. (Chapter 45)

24. A 32-year old woman complains of deep pain in both thighs. She was diagnosed as having type 1 diabetes mellitus at age 20. She currently has 3–4 bowel movements each day; she used to have more but noted that eliminating bread from her diet reduced her stool frequency. Her menses are normal. Physical examination is normal except for bowing of the legs. Skeletal x-rays reveal pelvic narrowing and a pseudofracture of the left femur. Bone densitometry reveals a T-score of –2.1 in the spine and –3.4 in the hip. Laboratory studies show the following: serum calcium = 7.2 mg/dl (nl, 8.5–10.5), phosphorous = 2.3 mg/dl (nl, 2.5–4.5), alkaline phosphatase = 312 U/L (nl, 25–125), PTH = 155 pg/ml (nl, 11–54), 25 hydroxyvitamin D = 7 ng/ml (nl, 16–74). Explain the clinical, radiographic, densitometry and biochemical findings in this patient and suggest a probable underlying diagnosis.

Deep thigh pain, pelvic narrowing, and pseudofractures are characteristic clinical features of osteomalacia. Densitometry testing reveals disproportionate loss of bone in the hip relative to the spine, a finding that always suggests PTH-mediated bone loss. Her biochemical profile of hypocalcemia, hypophosphatemia, elevated alkaline phosphatase, and significant secondary hyperparathyroidism suggests vitamin D deficiency; this is confirmed by the low serum 25-hydroxyvitamin D level. The history of increased stool frequency that decreased with elimination of bread from her diet suggests an underlying diagnosis of celiac disease (gluten-sensitive enteropathy). This condition is more common in patients with type 1 diabetes mellitus, another autoimmune disorder. The diagnosis of celiac disease can be confirmed by the measurement of anti-endomysial or anti-gliadin antibodies or by a small bowel biopsy. The treatment is elimination of gluten (wheat, rye, barley, and oats) from the diet and supplementation with calcium and vitamin D. (Chapter 12)

25. A 68-year-old man complains of a 10-year history of progressive pain in the shins, knees, and left arm. His right knee pain has become disabling. He also notes that his hearing has significantly deteriorated over the past 2 years. Physical examination reveals tenderness above the left elbow and enlarged, bowed shins. Skeletal x-rays show enlargement of the tibias with multiple focal lytic and sclerotic areas, and there is swelling along with reactive bone formation in the distal left humerus. Laboratory evaluation shows the following: serum calcium = 9.8 mg/dl (nl, 8.5–10.5) and alkaline phosphatase = 966 U/L (nl, 25–125). What is the probable diagnosis?

Bone pain and deformity, reduced hearing and markedly elevated serum alkaline phosphatase levels suggest a diagnosis of Paget's disease. Characteristic findings on skeletal radiographs confirm this diagnosis, which could also be made by finding intense focal radioisotope accumulation on bone scanning. The treatment options of choice are analgesics, intermittent high-dose oral bisphosphonates, and calcitonin, all of which may control but will not cure the disease. (Chapter 13)

26. A 42-year-old man presents for evaluation of a skin rash that recently developed over most of his body. He has type 2 diabetes mellitus and hypertension. He does not smoke but drinks 2–3 alcoholic beverages several nights each week. On physical examination, he has eruptive xanthomas (red papules with golden crowns) all over his body, most prominently on the buttocks, thighs, and forearms. His initial laboratory studies reveal the following: glucose = 310 mg/dl, HbA1C = 12.9%, cholesterol = 1082 mg/dl, and triglycerides = 8900 mg/dl. Discuss the cause and treatment of this lipid disorder.

This patient has severe hypertriglyceridemia. His LDL cholesterol cannot be determined with serum triglyceride levels this high. This condition is likely the result of combining an inherited triglyceride disorder (familial hypertriglyceridemia or familial combined hyperlipidemia) with a secondary cause of hypertriglyceridemia (uncontrolled diabetes mellitus, excess alcohol consumption). Because he is at a significant risk of developing acute pancreatitis, the top priority is to quickly lower his serum triglyceride level to less than 1000 mg/dl. The most effective measures to achieve this goal are a temporary very low fat (< 5%) diet, aggressive control of his blood glucose, and discontinuation of alcohol intake. Triglyceride levels should fall on this regimen by about 20% per day. A fibrate medication (gemfibrozil or fenofibrate) should be added at this point, and he should be switched to maintenance on an American Heart Association diet. Good diabetes control must be continued, and further alcohol intake should be discouraged. When the triglyceride level is below 400 mg/dl, serum LDL cholesterol should be evaluated and treated to a goal level of less than 100 mg/dl. (Chapter 8)

27. A 26-year-old woman requests to be tested for a type of thyroid cancer that has recently been found in her mother and two of five siblings. She notes that she has had intermittent headaches and palpitations for the past year. Her blood pressure is 164/102. She has a 1-cm left-sided thyroid nodule without associated lymphadenopathy. Laboratory testing shows the following results: serum calcium = 11.2 mg/dl (nl, 8.5–10.5) phosphorus = 2.4 mg/dl (nl, 2.5– 4.5), albumin = 4.5 g/dl (nl, 3.2–5.5), intact PTH = 55 pg/ml (nl, 11–54), calcitonin = 480 pg/ml (nl, 0–20) and 24 hour urine catecholamines = 1225 μg (nl, 0–200). Discuss her diagnosis and management.

This patient has a 1-cm thyroid nodule, an elevated serum calcitonin level, and a strong family history of thyroid cancer; she almost certainly has medullary thyroid cancer. Her hypertension, headaches, palpitations and elevated urinary excretion of catecholamines indicate the probable coexistence of a pheochromocytoma. She also has hyperparathyroidism manifested by hypercalcemia associated with an elevated serum PTH level. The combination of medullary thyroid carcinoma, pheochromocytoma and hyperparathyroidism is known as multiple endocrine neoplasia type 2A syndrome (MEN 2A). This autosomal dominant condition results from a germline-activating mutation in the Ret gene, which codes for the Ret receptor in tissues of neuroectodermal descent. Screening for MEN 2A in at-risk family members can be done by testing for the Ret/MCT oncogene. After appropriate adrenal imaging studies, alpha blocker administration, and blood pressure control, treatment of this patient would consist of surgical removal of the pheochromocytoma(s) followed by surgery to remove the abnormal thyroid and parathyroid glands. (Chapter 54)

28. A 19-year-old man has experienced fatigue, muscle weakness, and dizziness for the past 3 weeks. This morning, he fainted when he went outdoors to exercise. His blood pressure is 95/60, and his pulse is 110. His skin is cool, dry and tanned. His thyroid feels normal. Laboratory testing shows the following: hematocrit = 36%, glucose = 62 mg/dl, sodium = 120 meq/L, potassium = 6.7 meq/L, creatinine = 1.4 mg/dl, BUN = 36 mg/dl. What endocrine disorder should be considered and evaluated?

Hyponatremia with hyperkalemia should make one think immediately of adrenal insufficiency. This patient's fatigue, muscle weakness, hypotension, tanned skin, anemia, azotemia, and relatively low blood glucose are also very consistent with this diagnosis. The most common cause of this is autoimmune destruction of the adrenal glands (Addison's disease). The diagnosis can be confirmed by an ACTH stimulation test, which will show a low basal serum cortisol level that fails to increase after ACTH administration. In the setting of an adrenal crisis, one does not, however, have time to wait for the results of this test. In this case, the best approach would be to immediately draw blood for a serum cortisol measurement and then start treatment with intravenous fluids and dexamethasone 2 mg intravenously. ACTH can then be administered and cortisol measured again 30 minutes later (dexamethasone does not interfere with the cortisol assay). Afterwards, hydrocortisone 100 mg should be given intravenously every 6 hours along with continued fluid resuscitation. Infections must be actively sought and treated, if present. Once the patient is stable, he can be switched to therapy with oral hydrocortisone and Florinef for maintenance. In the near future, the diagnosis should be confirmed by repeat ACTH stimulation testing and/or measurement of anti-adrenal antibodies. (Chapter 31)

64. FAMOUS PEOPLE WITH ENDOCRINE DISORDERS

Kenneth J. Simcic, M.D. FACP

1. Despite his type 1 diabetes, this former National Hockey League star led the Philadelphia Flyers to back-to-back Stanley Cup championships in 1973–1974 and 1974–1975.

Bobby Clarke. Clarke's diabetes was diagnosed at age 13.

2. This female track star recovered from Graves' disease and went on to win the title of "Fastest Woman in the World" at the 1992 Summer Olympics in Barcelona.

Gail Devers. (Devers repeated as champion in the women's 100 meters at the 1996 Olympics in Atlanta.)

3. Actor Gary Coleman starred on the television series *Different Strokes*. His short stature was caused by what medical illness?

Kidney failure.

4. Composer Ludvig van Beethoven (1770–1827) began to lose his hearing before he reached the age of 30. What bone disorder may have been the cause of his hearing loss?

Paget's disease of bone.

5. Name the dwarf actor who gained fame for his role as Tattoo on the television series *Fantasy Island*.

Herve Villechaize (1943–1993).

6. Television and film actress Mary Tyler Moore has what endocrine disorder?

Type 1 diabetes.

7. What famous male singer has a skin disorder that is often associated with autoimmune gland diseases?

Michael Jackson (vitiligo).

8. George Bush and his wife Barbara were both diagnosed with Graves' disease during the Bush presidency (1989–1993). How did the president's Graves' disease present clinically?

Atrial fibrillation.

9. In addition to hyperthyroidism, what other complication of Graves' disease did Mrs. Bush experience?

Ophthalmopathy. She was treated with glucocorticoids and orbital radiation therapy.

10. Name the University of Oklahoma linebacker who was banned from the 1987 Orange Bowl after testing positive for anabolic steroids.

Brian Bosworth.

11. At the 1988 Summer Olympics in Seoul, what Canadian sprinter was stripped of his gold medal after testing positive for anabolic steroids?

Ben Johnson.

12. What late actor, who appeared in the film *Young Frankenstein*, had obvious Graves' ophthalmopathy?

Marty Feldman (1933–1982).

13. Ancient Egyptian sculptures and paintings suggest that Tutankhamun (1357–1339 B.C.) and other pharaohs had what endocrine disorder?

Gynecomastia.

14. Elected to Baseball's Hall of Fame in 1987, this late pitcher was undefeated in three World Series with the Oakland Athletics. He had type 2 diabetes. Who was he?

Jim "Catfish" Hunter (1946–1999).

15. What male ice-skater overcame growth failure related to a childhood illness to win the gold medal at the 1984 Winter Olympics in Sarajevo?

Scott Hamilton. As a child, Hamilton suffered from Shwachman syndrome, a rare disorder of the pancreas. (Hamilton was diagnosed with testicular cancer in 1997.)

16. Despite a diagnosis of diabetes at age 26 years, which National Football League (NFL) quarterback played for 10 seasons with the Minnesota Vikings and appeared in the Pro Bowl in 1988?

Wade Wilson.

17. In 1999, Tipper Gore, the wife of former Vice President Al Gore, had surgery for what endocrine condition?

Thyroid nodule (benign).

18. Name the late professional wrestler (and actor) who was well known for his acromegalic features.

Andre the Giant (1947–1993).

19. Charles Sherwood Stratton (1838–1883) reached an adult height of only 3 feet, 4 inches. What was his circus name?

General Tom Thumb.

20. Comedian and talk-show host Jay Leno has facial features suggestive of what benign endocrine disorder?

Benign prognathism.

21. Name some other famous people with apparent benign prognathism.

Pittsburgh Steelers' coach Bill Cowher
Green Bay Packers' quarterback Brett Favre
San Francisco 49ers' linebacker Ken Norton, Jr.
Hockey player Mark Messier
Rock singer Bruce Springsteen
Cartoon characters Fred Flintstone and Beavis.

22. Professional golfer Ben Crenshaw has been treated for what endocrine disorder?

Graves' disease.

23. Chris Dudley plays professional basketball for the New York Knicks. At age 16, he was diagnosed with what endocrine disorder?

Type 1 diabetes.

24. Kerri Strug, the heroine of the 1996 Women's Olympic Gymnastics Team, had an endocrine disorder shared by many young elite female athletes. What is it?

Delayed puberty. Strug was 18 years old when she competed in the 1996 Summer Olympics in Atlanta.

25. Ron Santo won six Golden Glove Awards and played in nine All Star games while playing third base for the Chicago Cubs. He was diagnosed with type 1 diabetes at what age?

Eighteen years, just after signing his first contract to play major league baseball.

26. Name the 3-foot, 7-inch, 65-pound dwarf who batted one time for the St. Louis Browns on August 19, 1951.

Eddie Gaedel. He was walked by Detroit Tigers' pitcher Bob Cain.

27. Gheorghe Muresan of the Washington Bullets is the tallest player in the history of the National Basketball Association (7 feet, 7 inches). What treatments has he received for his acromegaly and gigantism?

Transsphenoidal pituitary surgery, pituitary radiation, and somatostatin injections. (*Note:* Shaquille O'Neal is 7 feet, 1 inch tall.)

28. What is Muresan's shoe size?

Nineteen.

29. What was Muresan's height at age 14?

Six feet, 9 inches.

30. Nicole Johnson was 24 years old when she was crowned Miss America 1999. At age 19, she was diagnosed with what endocrine disorder?

Type 1 diabetes.

31. Did Nicole Johnson wear her insulin pump for the entire 1999 Miss America Pageant competition?

No. She removed it for the swimsuit competition.

32. Baseball legend Jackie Robinson (1919–1972) and jazz legend Ella Fitzgerald (1917–1996) shared the same endocrine disorder. What was it?

Diabetes.

33. Jackie Robinson's diabetes was diagnosed at what age?

Age 38, just 1 year after his retirement from baseball.

34. Willie Shoemaker is only 4 feet, 11 inches tall, but he is considered one of the most successful members of his profession. What is his profession?

Racehorse jockey.

35. The biblical giant Goliath was killed by a stone hurled from the sling of David. What visual disorder may have contributed to his demise?

Bitemporal hemianopia caused by a growth hormone–secreting pituitary tumor.

36. What medical disorder may account for the short stature of the fictional character Tiny Tim from Charles Dickens' *A Christmas Carol?*

Distal renal tubular acidosis—type I.

37. Naim Suleymanoglu of Turkey is only 4 feet, 11 inches tall and weighs only 141 lbs. At the 1995 Summer Olympics, he won a weightlifting gold medal with a lift of 413 lbs in the clean-and-jerk event. Because of his strength and short stature, he is also known by what other name?
Pocket Hercules.

38. Comedian/actor Joe Piscopo has been treated for what type of thyroid cancer?
Medullary thyroid cancer.

39. Track star Carl Lewis competed in 5 consecutive Olympics. He is one of only 2 athletes who have won 9 gold medals in an Olympic career. With what endocrine disorder was he diagnosed at age 35?
Primary hypothyroidism (secondary to Hashimoto's thyroiditis).

40. Name the American swimmer who was diagnosed with type 1 diabetes 18 months before he won 2 gold medals at the 2000 Olympics in Sydney, Australia.
Gary Hall, Jr.

41. Carla Overbeck, women's soccer star and captain of the United States 1996 gold medal Olympic team, was diagnosed with what endocrine disorder at age 32?
Graves' disease.

BIBLIOGRAPHY

1. Dawson LY: Skating at the cutting edge: Bobby Clarke. Diabetes Forecast March:16–19, 1994.
2. Kubba AK, Young M: Ludwig van Beethoven: A medical biography. Lancet 347:167–170, 1996.
3. Lewis DW: What was wrong with Tiny Tim? Am J Dis Child 146:1403–1407, 1992.
4. Mandernach M: Short hitter, long memory. Sports Illustrated September 2:5, 1996.
5. Mansfield S: Kerri's struggles. USA Weekend February 21–23, pp 4–5, 1997.
6. Montville L: Giant. Sports Illustrated October 2:50–56, 1995.
7. Naiken VS: Did Beethoven have Paget's disease of bone? Ann Intern Med 74:995–999, 1971.
8. Paulshock BZ: Tutankhamun and his brothers: Familial gynecomastia in the eighteenth dynasty. JAMA 244:160–164, 1980.
9. Sprecher S: David and Goliath. Radiology 176:288, 1990.
10. Mazur ML. Here She Is Miss America. Diabetes Forecast. July:49-51, 1999.
11. Drimmer F: Very Special People. New York, Carol Publishing Group, 1991.

65. INTERESTING ENDOCRINE FACTS AND FIGURES

Michael T. McDermott, M.D.

1. Who is the tallest man on record?

The man with the greatest medically documented height was Robert Wadlow of Alton, Illinois. He was 7 feet, 1¾ inches at age 13 years and 8 feet, 11.1 inches when he died in 1940, at the age of 22 years. He weighted 439 lbs. His condition was the result of a growth hormone-secreting pituitary tumor that developed before closure of the skeletal epiphyseal plates (gigantism).

2. Name the tallest woman on record.

Zeng Jinlian of Hunan Province, China, is the tallest woman on record. She was 7 feet, 1½ inches tall at age 13 years and reached 8 feet, 1¾ inches just before her death at age 17 in 1982. She also had a growth hormone–secreting tumor that developed during childhood.

3. How tall was the shortest man on record?

Calvin Phillips of Bridgewater, Massachusetts was 26½ inches tall and weighed 12 pounds at the age of 19 years. He died at age 22 in 1812. He had progeria, which is characterized by dwarfism and premature senility.

4. Who is the shortest woman on record?

The shortest adult woman on record was Pauline Musters of The Netherlands. She was 23.2 inches tall and weighed 9 pounds shortly before her death at age 19 years in 1895. Because of her relatively normal proportions, she is believed to have had a pituitary growth hormone deficiency, although growth hormone measurements were clearly not available in 1895.

5. Who had the most variable adult stature?

Adam Rainer of Austria was a 3-foot, 10.45-inch dwarf at the age of 21 years but rapidly grew into a 7-foot, 1¾-inch giant at age 32 years in 1931.

6. What is the tallest tribe in Africa?

The Watusi (or Tutsi) tribe of Sudan, Rwanda, Burundi, and Central African Republic are the tallest in the world. The men average 6 feet, 5 inches, and the women average 5 feet, 10 inches. Their tall stature is believed to be a genetic adaptation.

7. What is the shortest tribe?

The Mbuti pygmies of Zaire and Central African Republic have the lowest mean height. The men average 4 feet, 6 inches, and the women 4 feet, 5 inches. Their short stature is thought to result from genetic resistance to growth hormone, possibly owing to deficient growth hormone receptors.

8. Who was the heaviest man on record?

Jon Brower Minnoch of Bainbridge Island, Washington, was 6 feet, 1 inch tall and weighed approximately 1400 pounds when he was admitted to the hospital at age 37 years in congestive heart failure. He remained in the hospital for 2 years on a 1,200-calorie diet and was discharged at 476 lbs. He weighed 798 lbs when he died at age 42 years in 1983. His wife weighed 110 lbs.

9. How much did the heaviest woman on record weigh?

The heaviest woman on record was Mrs. Percy Pearl Washington of Milwaukee, Wisconsin, who was 6 feet tall and weighed 880 pounds. She died in 1972.

10. What is the largest recorded waist size?

Walter Hudson of New York, who stood 5 feet, 10 inches, had a peak weight of 1197 pounds and a waist size of 119 inches.

11. Who are the heaviest twins on record?

Billy and Benny McCrary of Hendersonville, North Carolina weighed 743 pounds and 723 pounds, respectively. Both had 84-inch waists. One brother died in a motorcycle accident, but the other is alive at the time of this printing.

12. What is the greatest known number of children born to one woman in a lifetime?

A peasant woman from Shuya, east of Moscow, Russia, gave birth to 69 children from 1725 to 1765. She had 27 pregnancies, producing 16 pairs of twins, 7 sets of triplets, and 4 sets of quadruplets. Sixty-seven of the children survived infancy.

13. Who is the oldest known woman to give birth?

In 1956, Ruth Alice Kistlen of California gave birth to a daughter at the age of 57 years, 129 days. She is the oldest medically verified mother to have become pregnant and delivered a child without a medically assisted reproductive method. Newer technologies have allowed this record to be eclipsed. In 1996, a 63-year-old woman gave birth to a healthy baby following implantation of an ovum from a younger woman.

14. What is the highest reported number of multiple births for a single gestation?

Ten births (decaplets) were reported in Brazil (1946), China (1936), and Spain (1924). Nine births (nonuplets) were recorded in Australia (1971), Philadelphia (1972), and Bangladesh (1977).

15. What is the largest tumor ever reported?

In 1905, a 329-pound ovarian cyst was removed from a woman in Texas.

16. What is the longest hair ever recorded?

In 1780, a 52-year-old peasant woman from Poland was recorded to have hair 12 feet long. Because hair grows at approximately ½ inch per month, this would have required at least 24 years of continuous growth. Most hairs fall out and are replaced before they are 3 feet long.

17. Who has the largest chest and arm muscles on record?

Isaac "Dr. Size" Nesser of Greensburg, Pennsylvania, has a 68.06-inch chest and 26⅛-inch biceps. He is 5 feet, 10 inches tall and weighs 351 pounds.

18. Did King David of Israel have an endocrine disorder?

"When King David was old and advanced in years, though they spread covers over him, he could not keep warm. His servants therefore said to him, 'Let a young virgin be sought to attend you, lord king, and to nurse you. If she sleeps with your royal majesty, you will be kept warm.'. . . The maiden, who was very beautiful, nursed the king and cared for him, but the king did not have relations with her" (I Kings 1:1–4). Some speculate King David was afflicted with hypothyroidism.

19. What endocrine disorder might Goliath of Gath have had?

Goliath of Gath, who was killed by a stone from David's sling (I Samuel 17:1–51), probably stood about 6 feet, 10 inches. His tall stature may have resulted from a growth hormone-secreting pituitary tumor. Others add that the ease with which David's stone became embedded in Goliath's skull may have been due to hyperparathyroidism and his bizarre behavior may have resulted from hypoglycemia due to an insulinoma. He may thus be the earliest known case of MEN 1 syndrome.

20. What endocrine disorder did President John F. Kennedy have?

Kennedy had primary adrenal insufficiency—Addison's disease. He was sustained throughout the later years of his life and his presidency by therapy with oral glucocorticoids.

BIBLIOGRAPHY

1. McFarlan D (ed): The Guiness Book of World Records. New York, Bantam Books, 1991.
2. Baumann G, Shaw MN, Merimee TJ: Low levels of high affinity growth hormone–binding protein in African Pygmies. N Engl J Med 320:1705–1709, 1989.
3. The New American Bible. Catholic Publishers, Inc., 1971.

INDEX

Page numbers in **boldface type** indicate complete chapters.